Geriatric Psychopharmacology

Medical Psychiatry

Series Editor

William A. Frosch, M.D.
Cornell University Medical College
New York, New York

1. Handbook of Depression and Anxiety: A Biological Approach, *edited by Johan A. den Boer and J. M. Ad Sitsen*
2. Anticonvulsants in Mood Disorders, *edited by Russell T. Joffe and Joseph R. Calabrese*
3. Serotonin in Antipsychotic Treatment: Mechanisms and Clinical Practice, *edited by John M. Kane, H.-J. Möller, and Frans Awouters*
4. Handbook of Functional Gastrointestinal Disorders, *edited by Kevin W. Olden*
5. Clinical Management of Anxiety, *edited by Johan A. den Boer*
6. Obsessive-Compulsive Disorders: Diagnosis • Etiology • Treatment, *edited by Eric Hollander and Dan J. Stein*
7. Bipolar Disorder: Biological Models and Their Clinical Application, *edited by L. Trevor Young and Russell T. Joffe*
8. Dual Diagnosis and Treatment: Substance Abuse and Comorbid Medical and Psychiatric Disorders, *edited by Henry R. Kranzler and Bruce J. Rounsaville*
9. Geriatric Psychopharmacology, *edited by J. Craig Nelson*

ADDITIONAL VOLUMES IN PREPARATION

Geriatric Psychopharmacology

edited by

J. Craig Nelson
Yale University School of Medicine, and
Yale-New Haven Hospital
New Haven, Connecticut

MARCEL DEKKER, INC. NEW YORK • BASEL • HONG KONG

ISBN: 0-8247-9851-1

The publisher offers discounts on this book when ordered in bulk quantities. For more information, write to Special Sales/Professional Marketing at the address below.

This book is printed on acid-free paper.

MARCEL DEKKER, INC.
270 Madison Avenue, New York, New York 10016
http://www.dekker.com

Current printing (last digit):
10 9 8 7 6 5 4 3 2 1

PRINTED IN THE UNITED STATES OF AMERICA

Series Introduction

Recent decades have seen a dramatic shift in the world's demographics: there has been a striking increase in both the number and percentage of the old and the very old. Current projections suggest that in the year 2030 nearly 20% of the population of the United States will be over 65. In addition, the older we are, the older we are likely to become. In 1994, life expectancy at 65 was for an additional 17.4 years, at 75 an additional 11.0 years, and at 85 an additional 6.1 years. Improved nutrition; a variety of public health measures, such as wide availability of soap and clean water, elimination of smallpox, immunization against a variety of diseases; and medical advances, such as the development and availability of antibiotics and antihypertensive drugs, have all played a role in increasing human longevity. In the developed, industrialized West, the young old—65 to 80—are generally healthy and active and have sustainable or better incomes. However, as we age and become the very old—over 80—we are likely to be exposed to increasing numbers of phase-related stresses: a series of losses and their accompanying bereavements, a slowly or rapidly failing brain and body, and creeping financial impoverishment.

Despite, as well as because of, the advances of medicine, the chances of serious illnesses increase with age. The fields of gerontology, geriatric medicine, and geriatric psychiatry have been created in response to increased need. The old are different, as children are different, in their physiological and psychological responses. Their coping skills differ, their metabolic functions are altered, the presentation of illness and responses to treatments are not the same as those of the nonelderly. It is essential that physicians and psychiatrists improve their knowledge of these differences and alter their practices accordingly.

This new text will help all of us achieve these goals. It brings together a pantheon of modern geriatric psychiatrists, who tell us what they have learned and, also important, point out the gaps in current knowledge. We can all hope that future editions will provide further information to help us as we enter the population of the aged.

William A. Frosch

Preface

Treatment of psychiatric disorders in the elderly puts the clinician to the test. During the past decade, the number of pharmacological agents available for treatment of the major psychiatric disorders has increased substantially. For some disorders, such as dementia, new treatments have been developed and marketed. Evidence that these treatments are effective encourages their use. At the same time, the treatment of elderly patients presents a challenge for the clinician. The presence of comorbid medical illness, concurrent use of other medications, and pharmacokinetic and pharmacodynamic changes with aging compicate treatment. The clinician may conclude it is easier to make the patient worse than better!

In geriatric psychopharmacology, a sophisticated understanding of the medications employed, and how they are affected by the complicating factors referred to above, is crucial for enhancing outcome and avoiding adverse consequences. The psychiatrist, as the psychopharmacology expert on the mental health team, will be expected to have a sophisticated knowledge of psychopharmacology in the elderly. All mental health professionals will be expected to be informed about pharmacological treatments. Medical physicians, in the current health care market, will be expected to treat a larger number of depressed and anxious older patients. For these reasons, acquisition of knowledge by clinicians working in the field is most important.

The development of empirically based treatment in geriatric psychiatry has been hampered by the frequent exclusion of elderly patients from clinical research. Although this may be understandable, it nevertheless limits the growth of knowledge about treatment of older patients. If age alone is not reason for exclusion, medical illness may be. Yet medical illness is the norm rather than the exception in elderly patients and is another factor that limits the study of this group. As a result of these considerations, geriatric psychopharmacology has been relatively more dependent on "clinical lore" than most other areas of psychopharmacology. This increases the chance that mistaken beliefs are passed along.

This book has been organized around empirically based areas of knowledge. Rather than starting with a comprehensive list of topics in geriatric psychiatry, the chapters were selected on the basis of their importance and the extent to which there was a body of supporting clinical research. The contributors are research clinicians who are experts in their area. Some of the contributors may not be recognized as "geriatric psychiatrists," but they are recognized for their expertise in an area that clearly relates to geriatric psychiatry. Each of the contributors was asked to emphasize the empirical basis of what we know, and to challenge myths about practice.

The varying chapter lengths are intentional. In some cases a topic was important to include, but supporting research was limited. In some areas—for example, the treatment of psychosis in Parkinson's disease—although the patients may be few in number, the problem has important implications for our understanding of the neuropharmacology of psychotic disorders. The interface of psychiatry and medicine is becoming increasingly important, and research on the interaction of psychiatric disorders and medical illness is accelerating. Because of the importance of this information, several chapters on depression in different medical disorders have been included.

The book begins with three chapters that provide information basic to all the following chapters. These chapters on neurochemistry in aging, pharmacokinetics in the elderly, and drug interactions provide a foundation for the subsequent chapters, that focus on specific disorders.

The development of this book was a collaborative effort. Many of the contributors not only wrote their chapter, but made suggestions about other areas to cover and who should write about them. Their suggestions greatly enhanced the quality of the final product and I am very grateful to this outstanding group of contributors.

Researchers and academics will find this text helpful. The chapters provide authoritative reviews of clinical research in several areas. Ultimately, the book will be judged by its value to clinicians. The authors, after reviewing the state of the knowledge in their area, were asked to put the information in a clinical context at the end of their chapter. How would a clinician use this information? What drug do you start with? In this manner, we intend to provide an empirically based and clinically relevant description of the state of the art in geriatric psychopharmacology.

J. Craig Nelson

Contents

Series Introduction *William A. Frosch* *iii*
Preface *v*
Contributors *xi*

I. GENERAL PRINCIPLES

1. Neurochemistry of Aging 1
Kaj Blennow and C. G. Gottfries

2. Pharmacokinetics of Psychotropic Drugs 27
David J. Greenblatt, Lisa L. von Moltke, and Richard I. Shader

3. Drug Interactions 43
Bruce G. Pollock

II. DEPRESSION

4. Treatment of Major Depression in the Elderly 61
J. Craig Nelson

5. Treatment of Psychotic Depression 99
Barnett S. Meyers

6. Treatment of Major Depressions During Bereavement 115
Selby Jacobs and Sidney Zisook

7. Maintenance Therapies for Late-Life Recurrent Major Depression: Research and Review Circa 1996 127
Charles F. Reynolds III, Ellen Frank, James M. Perel, Sati Mazumdar, and David J. Kupfer

III. TREATMENT OF DEPRESSION WITH ASSOCIATED CONDITIONS

8. Depression and Cardiac Disease 143
Steven P. Roose

9. Treatment of Poststroke Psychiatric Disorders 161
Robert G. Robinson, Susan K. Schultz, and Sergio Paradiso

10. Depression and Cancer 187
Herbert Ward and Dwight L. Evans

11. Depression and Parkinson's Disease 199
Norman Sussman

12. The Assessment and Treatment of Depressed-Demented Patients 223
George S. Alexopoulos

13. Use of Stimulants in Depressed Patients with Medical Illness 245
George B. Murray and Edwin Cassem

IV. BIPOLAR DISORDER

14. Use of Lithium in Bipolar Disorder 259
Robert C. Young

15. Lithium Toxicity in the Elderly 273
James W. Jefferson

16. Anticonvulsants in Bipolar Elderly 285
Charles L. Bowden

V. LATE-LIFE PSYCHOSIS

17. Treatment of Psychosis in Late Life 301
John H. Eastham, Jonathan P. Lacro, James B. Lohr, and Dilip V. Jeste

18. Treatment of Psychosis in Parkinson's Disease 327
Jonathan M. Meyer and George M. Simpson

VI. ANXIETY DISORDERS

19. Sedative-Hypnotics in the Elderly Population 347
Philip G. Janicak and Frank J. Ayd, Jr.

20. The Treatment of Generalized Anxiety Disorder, Panic Disorder, and Obsessive–Compulsive Disorder in the Elderly 367
Malcolm Lader and Raymond Ancill

VII. DEMENTIA

21. Use of Cognitive Enhancers in Dementing Disorders 381
Steven C. Samuels and Kenneth L. Davis

22. Neuroleptics for Behavioral Complications of Dementia 405
D. P. Devanand

23. Nonneuroleptic Treatment of Complications of Dementia: Applying Clinical Research to Practice 427
Pierre N. Tariot and Lon S. Schneider

Index *455*

Contributors

George S. Alexopoulos, M.D. Department of Psychiatry, Cornell University Medical College, White Plains, New York

Raymond Ancill, M.A., M.B., F.R.C.P.(C) Department of Psychiatry, St. Vincent's Hospital, Vancouver, British Columbia, Canada

Frank J. Ayd, Jr., M.D. Editor, International Drug Therapy Newsletter, Baltimore, Maryland

Kaj Blennow, M.D., Ph.D. Department of Psychiatry and Neurochemistry, Institute of Clinical Neuroscience, University of Göteborg, and the Swedish Medical Research Council, Mölndal, Sweden

Charles L. Bowden, M.D. Department of Psychiatry, The University of Texas Health Science Center at San Antonio, San Antonio, Texas

Edwin Cassem, M.D. Department of Psychiatry, Massachusetts General Hospital, and Harvard Medical School, Boston, Massachusetts

Kenneth L. Davis, M.D. Department of Psychiatry, Mount Sinai School of Medicine, and Mount Sinai Medical Center, New York, New York

D. P. Devanand, M.D. New York State Psychiatric Institute, and College of Physicians and Surgeons, Columbia University, New York, New York

John H. Eastham, Pharm.D. Department of Psychiatry, University of California, San Diego, La Jolla, and Psychiatry Services, San Diego Veterans Affairs Medical Center, San Diego, California

Dwight L. Evans, M.D. Department of Psychiatry, College of Medicine, University of Florida, Gainesville, Florida

Ellen Frank, Ph.D. Western Psychiatric Institute and Clinic, University of Pittsburgh Medical Center, Pittsburgh, Pennsylvania

C. G. Gottfries, M.D., Ph.D. Department of Psychiatry and Neurochemistry, Institute of Clinical Neuroscience, University of Göteborg, Mölndal, Sweden

David J. Greenblatt, M.D. Department of Pharmacology and Experimental Therapeutics, Tufts University School of Medicine, and New England Medical Center, Boston, Massachusetts

Selby Jacobs, M.D. Department of Psychiatry, Yale University School of Medicine, New Haven, Connecticut

Philip G. Janicak, M.D. Department of Psychiatry, The University of Illinois at Chicago, Chicago, Illinois

James W. Jefferson, M.D. Dean Foundation for Health, Research and Education, Middleton, Wisconsin

Dilip V. Jeste, M.D. Department of Psychiatry, University of California, San Diego, La Jolla, and Psychiatry Services, San Diego Veterans Affairs Medical Center, San Diego, California

David J. Kupfer, M.D. Department of Psychiatry, Western Psychiatric Institute and Clinic, University of Pittsburgh Medical Center, Pittsburgh, Pennsylvania

Jonathan P. Lacro, Pharm.D. Department of Psychiatry, University of California, San Diego, La Jolla, and Psychiatry Services, San Diego Veterans Affairs Medical Center, San Diego, California

Malcolm Lader, O.B.E., D.Sc., Ph.D., M.D., F.R.C.Psych. Department of Psychiatry, Institute of Psychiatry, University of London, London, England

James B. Lohr, M.D. Department of Psychiatry, University of California, San Diego, La Jolla, and Psychiatry Services, San Diego Veterans Affairs Medical Center, San Diego, California

Sati Mazumdar, Ph.D. Graduate School of Public Health, University of Pittsburgh, Pittsburgh, Pennsylvania

Jonathan M. Meyer, M.D. Department of Psychiatry and the Behavioral Sciences, Los Angeles County–USC Medical Center, University of Southern California, Los Angeles, California

Barnett S. Meyers, M.D. Department of Psychiatry, Cornell University Medical College, and Westchester Division, The New York Hospital–Cornell Medical Center, White Plains, New York

George B. Murray, M.D. Department of Psychiatry, Massachusetts General Hospital, and Harvard Medical School, Boston, Massachusetts

J. Craig Nelson, M.D. Department of Psychiatry, Yale University School of Medicine, and Yale-New Haven Hospital, New Haven, Connecticut

Sergio Paradiso, M.D., Ph.D. Department of Psychiatry, College of Medicine, University of Iowa, Iowa City, Iowa

James M. Perel, Ph.D. School of Medicine, Departments of Psychiatry and Pharmacology, University of Pittsburgh, and Western Psychiatric Institute and Clinic, University of Pittsburgh Medical Center, Pittsburgh, Pennsyvania

Bruce G. Pollock, M.D., Ph.D., F.R.C.P.(C) Department of Psychiatry, Western Psychiatric Institute and Clinic, University of Pittsburgh Medical Center, Pittsburgh, Pennsylvania

Charles F. Reynolds III, M.D. Department of Psychiatry and Pharmacology, Geriatric Psychopharmacology Program, Western Psychiatric Institute and Clinic, University of Pittsburgh Medical Center, Pittsburgh, Pennsylvania

Robert G. Robinson, M.D. Department of Psychiatry, College of Medicine, University of Iowa, Iowa City, Iowa

Stephen P. Roose, M.D. Department of Psychiatry, College of Physicians and Surgeons, Columbia University, New York, New York

Steven C. Samuels, M.D. Department of Psychiatry, Mount Sinai School of Medicine, and Mount Sinai Medical Center, New York, New York

Lon S. Schneider, M.D. Departments of Psychiatry and the Behavioral Sciences, and Department of Neurology, and the Leonard Davis School of Gerontology, School of Medicine, University of Southern California, Los Angeles, California

Susan K. Schultz, M.D. Department of Psychiatry, College of Medicine, University of Iowa, Iowa City, Iowa

Richard I. Shader, M.D. Department of Pharmacology and Experimental Therapeutics, Tufts University School of Medicine, and New England Medical Center, Boston, Massachusetts

George M. Simpson, M.D. Department of Psychiatry and the Behavioral Sciences, Los Angeles County–USC Medical Center, University of Southern California, Los Angeles, California

Norman Sussman, M.D. Department of Psychiatry, School of Medicine, New York University, and Psychopharmacology Research and Consultation Service, Bellevue Hospital Center, New York, New York

Pierre N. Tariot, M.D. Departments of Psychiatry, Medicine, and Neurology, University of Rochester School of Medicine, and Department of Psychiatry, Monroe Community Hospital, Rochester, New York

Lisa L. von Moltke, M.D. Department of Pharmacology and Experimental Therapeutics, Tufts University School of Medicine, and New England Medical Center, Boston, Massachusetts

Herbert Ward, M.D. Department of Psychiatry, College of Medicine, University of Florida, Gainesville, Florida

Robert C. Young, M.D. Department of Psychiatry, Westchester Division, The New York Hospital– Cornell Medical Center, White Plains, New York

Sidney Zisook, M.D. Department of Psychiatry, University of California, San Diego, La Jolla, California

1

Neurochemistry of Aging

Kaj Blennow
University of Göteborg, and the Swedish Medical Research Council, Mölndal, Sweden

C. G. Gottfries
University of Göteborg, Mölndal, Sweden

I. INTRODUCTION

Human beings have the longest senium of all species, if "senium" is defined as the time elapsing between the end of the reproductive period and death. The reason why human beings have such a long senium is a subject of speculation. The length of the senium has no obvious significance for the survival of the species. This "extra" survival time must depend on factors that, per se, are not intended to prolong survival. One possibility may be that our large reserve capacities, which are of use for survival, also provide higher resistance to involution processes.

Theoretically one can separate normal aging, adaptive processes, and age-related diseases. Changes develop slowly in normal aging, which is a process assumed to occur at a subcellular level without immediate signs or symptoms. Ultimately, however, when the reserve capacities of the brain decline, and the compensatory mechanisms are exhausted, symptoms and behavioral disturbances appear. Diseases usually have a more rapid progress.

Data from several sources indicate that the involution of the human brain proceeds at increased speed from the sixth or seventh decade of life (1–3). Whether this involution is a genetically determined process, the result of a less effective genetic program, or the result of environmental factors is still unknown. Aging may come about because there is a limit to the number of divisions that the non-neuron cells can accomplish. The genome may show increasing instability in time, with decreasing protection and repair activity.

Aging may also be the result of random errors in the protein synthesis, with abnormal metabolites that increasingly disturb the chain of cellular functions. A combination of these factors may well be assumed. An involution phase is part of the genetic program, but this part may be switched on earlier than normal due to adverse influences from environmental factors. The influence of the genome on the aging process has been investigated from different viewpoints, and new lines of investigation suggest that some genes of aging (gerontogenes) are responsible for the apoptosis phenomenon or programmed cell death that has been demonstrated in several types of cells. Apoptosis is the process whereby cells die in a controlled manner, apparently following an intrinsic program. This process can be triggered in a variety of cell types by different mechanisms. It can be assumed that apoptosis also takes place in neuron cell death in neurodegenerative disorders such as Alzheimer's disease and Parkinson's disease (4).

II. COMPENSATORY MECHANISMS

It is clear that there is an involution of the human brain, especially after the sixth decade of life. However, the brain is an organ with great reserve capacities, which explains why cognitive and emotional functions may be maintained well into old age and signs and symptoms of mental insufficiency may be absent or unnoticed until the eighth or ninth decade of life.

What reserves and mechanisms does the brain have, which compensate for the loss caused by the involution process? First, the original number of neurons in the brain is very large. In several nuclei, function is maintained even when the number of neurons has been reduced by 50% or more. Second, neurons are capable of increasing their metabolism if necessary. This means that neurons can produce more neurotransmitters and thereby compensate for the loss of other neurons (2). Third, the individual nerve terminal is able to increase in size and take over the function of lost neighboring terminals. Last, receptors, the target for the neurotransmitters, can increase their sensitivity and thus continue to respond adequately, although the number of released neurotransmitters is reduced (5). When all these compensatory mechanisms are exhausted, symptoms of insufficiency appear (e.g., depression, confusion, impaired motor performance, cognitive impairment, and changes in personality).

Dementia is a term used for disorders in which cognitive impairment is so severe that the individual can no longer cope with the activities of daily living without support. It can be assumed that, if the individual lives long enough, the brain changes included in the concept of "normal aging" will cause such severe cognitive impairment that the individual fulfills the criteria for dementia. Although the involution is intensified in the sixth decade of life, it takes at least another two decades for the involution process to bring the individual's state down to the level of dementia (Fig. 1). Involution of the brain is a slow and silent process that manifests itself as a mild decline in mental functions. Exposure to stress, however, may lower the individual's thresholds for depressive disorders, confusion, and anxiety states.

There is no common name for disorders in which the capacity of an individual's brain is reduced but not enough to justify a diagnosis of dementia. The suggested name "dysmentia" (6) seems appropriate in contrast to names such as "benign senescent forgetfulness" and "age-associated memory impairment" (Fig. 1).

III. THE BIOLOGICAL AGING OF THE BRAIN

Based on studies of postmortem human brain material, morphological and neurochemical changes in the human brain have been described in individuals who had not suffered from neurological, psychiatric, or aging disorders prior to death. Their brains have been compared to brains of patients who had suffered from pathological aging or neurodegenerative disorders. Data have

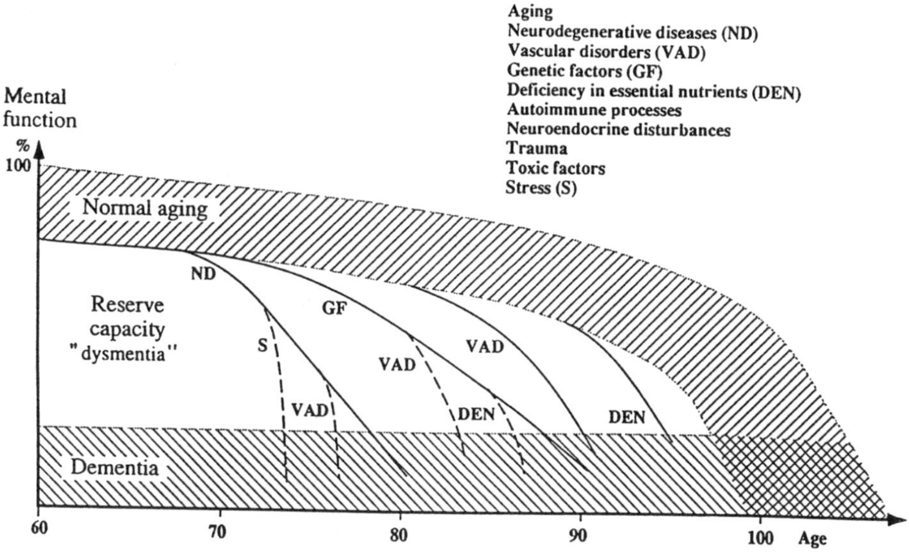

FIGURE 1 Factors influencing the decline of mental functioning. Accelerating factors are suggested. Dementia is an end stage and syndromes between normal aging and dementia are named dysmentia.

accumulated that describe morphological and neurochemical changes both in normal and in pathological aging. In the living individual, cerebrospinal fluid (CSF) samples have been investigated and neuroendocrine disturbances that can be related to aging have been recorded. Morphological and neurochemical changes in normal and pathological aging are discussed below.

A. Morphological Changes in the Normal Aging Brain

Age-related morphological changes in the brain can be listed as follows: decrease in brain volume; decrease in brain weight; decrease in volume of neurons; reduction in number of neurons; changes in glial cells; loss of dendrites and synapses; lipofuscin pigmentation; senile plaques; neurofibrillary tangles; granulovacuolar degeneration; congophil angiopathy; and white matter lesions.

It has long been known that there are structural changes in normal aging (7). A widening of the ventricles occurs in advanced age and the volume of the brain declines to around 80% of its original volume (8). At the time of birth, the brain weighs around 350 g. It reaches its maximum weight at the age of 20. The brain weight depends on environmental factors. The average brain weight has increased during the last century, most likely because of the increasingly improved nutritional status. In a recent investigation (9), 151 subjects were studied. The estimated brain weight at 20 years of age was 1.422 kg ± 47 g for females and 1.633 kg ± 27 g for males. The brain weight began to diminish at the age of 20, and the estimated value at the age of 100 was 1.155 kg ± 25 g for females and 1.244 kg ± 25 g for males, which means that the decrease was 20% for female brains and 24% for male brains.

The volume and number of neurons also change with age, but regional differences exist. Fairly dramatic reductions in the number of nerve cells were often reported earlier. There may have been overestimations, as changes in the volume of neurons were not taken into account. Some studies have shown that the reduction is principally in the volume and only to a lesser extent in the number of neurons (10). Studies have also shown that there is a loss of dendritic processes and spines at older ages. A simultaneous compensatory growth of dendrites, especially an elongation, also occurs. Age-related brain tissue changes differ in various brain areas. They are most pronounced in the neocortical areas, hippocampus, amygdala, cerebellum, locus coeruleus, dorsal nucleus of the vagus nerve, and substantia nigra.

The production of glial cells in neuronal aging was also investigated recently. In the aging brain there are glial precursors and astrocytes at various stages of maturation (11). Astrocytes are being acknowledged as major production sites for a variety of cytokines serving the maintenance of neurons, renewal of glial cells, and control of responses to lesions. There is abundant evidence that these neurotropins influence astroblast differentiation and proliferation. To elucidate pathogenetic factors in degenerative disorders such as Alzheimer's disease (AD), Parkinson's disease (PD), and amyotropic lateral sclerosis (ALS) (12) it is also essential to understand the mechanism that underlies the regulation of growth factors.

Senile plaques (SPs) are round to ovoid lesions with a diameter of 15–200 μm, located within the neuropil and consisting of a central core of amyloid fibers surrounded by numerous dystrophic, degenerating neurites, and reactive astrocytes and microglia (13). Although SPs are regarded as characteristics of AD, they are also found in increasing numbers in normal aging. They are rarely found in individuals under 40 years of age but are found in 60–75% of those aged 80 or more (14,15). In advanced age, there is relatively large overlap in SP counts between nondemented individuals and AD patients (16–20).

Cerebral amyloid angiopathy (CAA), or "congophil angiopathy," is located in the leptomeningeal (=pia and arachnoid) and intracortical arterioles and capillaries, and is characterized by an acellular, amyloid thickening of the walls of the blood vessels (21). The prevalence of CAA in nondemented individuals increases with age (21).

Amyloid deposition in SPs and CAA consists of a specific protein termed β-amyloid protein (Aβ) (22). Aβ is a 39–42 amino acid cleavage product from a set of much larger precursors, collectively referred to as amyloid precursor protein (APP), encoded by a single gene on chromosome 21 (23).

Deposits of Aβ in the form of diffuse plaques occur in the brain without evidence of dementia or neuronal damage as an inevitable consequence of aging. Diffuse plaques are found in about 45% of 70–80-year-olds, 80% of 80–90-year-olds, and 100% of centenarians (24,25).

It is known that the deposits in the core of SPs and in CAA contain different truncated forms of Aβ, with predominantly 42 amino acids in SP cores (26) and 39–40 amino acids in CAA (27), suggesting that different proteases may be involved in the production of Aβ.

The physiological function of APP is incompletely known. APP undergoes fast axonal transport to the synaptic region where it interacts with extracellular matrix (28), suggesting that APP may be important for neuronal plasticity. The secretory form of APP is identical to protease nexin-II (29), suggesting a role in growth regulation or neurite outgrowth (30,31). Several lines of evidence also suggest a role for APP in the tissue damage repair process (32,33). Thus a disturbance of the normal function or metabolism of APP may be important in the pathogenesis of Aβ deposition.

Neurofibrillary tangles (NFTs) are intracytoplasmatic changes, manifest as bundles of paired helical filaments (PHFs) (13). The prevalence of NFTs in nondemented individuals increases with age, particularly after the age of 65

(17). NFTs are very rare before the age of 40, but present in all individuals over 90 (14,15). As with SPs, there is a relatively large overlap in NFT counts between nondemented individuals and AD patients at older ages (16–20).

The principal component of paired helical filaments (PHFs), which make up the characteristic NFTs, neuropil threads and senile plaque neurites, is probably a hyperphosphorylated form of tau protein (PHFtau) (34). PHFtau is also called A68 (35), Alzheimer's disease–associated proteins (ADAP) (36), and tau 64/69 (37).

Granulovacuolar degeneration (GVD) consists of vacuoles (about 5-μm diameter), each containing a granule, in the pyramidal cells of the hippocampus (13). In nondemented individuals GVD is rare before the age of 65, but after that age its prevalence increases, and by the ninth decade GVD is a common finding, present in about 75% of all individuals (8).

Studies in the late 1970s and early 1980s—after the introduction of high-resolution CT—showed that white matter lesions (WMLs) are common in aged individuals. WMLs found on CT are characterized by patchy or diffuse, bilateral, symmetric, hypodense areas in the periventricular white matter. The neuropathological finding is demyelination in the periventricular white matter, accompanied by hyaline arteriolosclerosis in the penetrating arteries (38). Neurochemically, WMLs in AD are characterized by a reduced amount of myelin lipids (phospholipid, cholesterol, sulfatide, and cerebroside), with the normal proportion preserved between them (39).

WMLs are associated with aging; that is, they are more common in old age (40,41). In nondemented aged people the prevalence of WMLs established by CT varies between 2% and 19% (40).

Lipofuscin pigments, neurofibrillary tangles, senile plaques, and granulovacuolar degeneration are found in the aging brain, but these pathological changes occur to a much greater extent in patients with dementia. Changes in terms of β-amyloid deposition are found in healthy elderly individuals, but these β-amyloid-containing plaques are mostly "diffuse plaques" with morphological distinctions from the neuritic plaques (25,42).

B. Neurochemical Changes in the Normal Aging Brain

Neurotransmitter release is a key event in neurotransmission. Several neurotransmitters are known [e.g., acetylcholine (ACh); dopamine (DA); noradrenaline (NA); 5-hydroxytryptamine or serotonin (5-HT); γ-butyric acid (GABA); glycine; glutamate; and neuropeptides]. Neurotransmitters react with the respective receptors in postsynaptic membranes and in turn activate other neurons and transmit the neuronal signals to the target tissue. More than one neurotransmitter may be released from one and the same nerve ending.

Most studies on aging have focused on the synthesis and release of the neurotransmitters themselves, the concentrations of metabolites, and the enzyme activity involved in neurotransmitter metabolism. In Figure 2 some of the changes in neurotransmitter metabolism in normal aging are summarized. As shown in the figure, choline acetyltransferase (CAT) activity declines with age, but acetylcholinesterase (AChE) remains unchanged. With regard to changes in receptors, an increase in the numbers of muscarinic and nicotinic receptors in the thalamus and a decrease in the cortex have been recorded,

		Cortex	Hippocampus	Nucleus caudatus	Thalamus
ACh	CAT	↓	↓	↓	
	AChE	→	→	→	
	M-rec	↓	↓	→	↑
	N-rec	↓	↑		↑
5-HT	5-HT	↓	→	↓	→
	5-HIAA	→	→	→	→
NA	NA	↓	↓	→	→
	α-rec	→	→		
	ß-rec	→			
DA	DA	→	↓	↓	↓
	HVA	↑	→	↓	
	D1-rec			↑	
	D2-rec			↓	
MAO	MAO-B	↑	↑	↑	↑
GABA	GAD	↓		→	↓
	GABA-rec	↑			

FIGURE 2 Changes in the human brain neurotransmitter systems in aging. Arrows pointing downward or upward indicate significant age-sensitive changes. Abbreviations: ACh = acetylcholine; CAT = choline acetyltransferase; AChE = acetylcholinesterase; M = muscarinic; N = nicotinic; -rec = receptors; 5-HT = 5-hydroxytryptamine or serotonin; 5-HIAA = 5-hydroxyindoleacetic acid; NA = noradrenaline; DA = dopamine; HVA = homovanillic acid; MAO-B = monoamine oxidase B; GAD = glutamic acid decarboxylase; GABA-rec = γ-aminobutyric acid receptors.

while a decrease in muscarinic receptors and an increase in nicotinic receptors have been recorded in the hippocampus (for review, see Ref. 43).

Reduced concentrations of DA in discrete brain areas and an age-correlated loss of DA uptake sites have been reported (1,44). Data about the end metabolite homovanillic acid (HVA) vary and so do those about DA receptor changes with aging.

Serotonin metabolism is also sensitive to aging. Reduced concentrations of serotonin in discrete brain areas have been recorded (for review, see Ref. 45). The end metabolite of serotonin metabolism, 5-hydroxyindoleacetic acid (5-HIAA), does not seem to be reduced with age. This may indicate that, although the number of 5-HT neurons is reduced, as reflected in the reduced serotonin concentration, the loss of neurons is compensated for by an increased turnover rate of the remaining neurons. This is possibly attributable to the compensatory mechanism of the neurons (2). The notion of a decline in serotonin metabolism with age is further supported by reduced activity of tryptophan hydroxylase and carboxylase, the enzymes that synthesize serotonin. 5-HT receptors are still not mapped out with regard to age-related changes.

The concentrations of NA also decline with age in some discrete brain areas, but these changes are less impressive and the end metabolite, 3-methoxy-4-hydroxyphenylglycol (HMPG) has not been reported to be reduced with age.

Human brain monoamine oxidase (MAO) activity can be divided into two forms: MAO-A, which is mainly responsible for the oxidative deamination of 5-HT, NA, and partially DA, and MAO-B, which catalyzes the oxidative deamination of several exogenous amines, as well as part of DA. MAO-B activity in the human brain increases with age (46), but MAO-A activity remains unchanged. MAO-B is localized to glial cells and an increase in MAO-B is assumed to represent gliosis. Whether increased MAO-B activity is of biological importance is uncertain.

A loss of dopaminergic and noradrenergic neurons in the substantia nigra and locus coeruleus has also been demonstrated in relation to age (47).

Neuropeptidergic systems have been sparsely examined in relation to aging. Most of these studies, mainly confined to measurements of tissue levels, report few changes (48), but there are some data that suggest age-associated changes (49–51).

Not only cell metabolism may change with aging but also more substantial elements of the brain tissue. In 118 subjects, aged 20–100 years, Svennerholm and coworkers (9) investigated the composition of membrane lipids from the frontal and temporal cortex and the white matter. From 20 years of age the total solids, phospholipids, and cholesterol from the frontal and temporal cortex diminished linearly. In the frontal and temporal white matter, however, the total solids, phospholipids, cholesterol, cerebroside, and sulfatide showed a curvilinear diminution with a somewhat faster decline above the age of 60. Ganglioside concentration, which is a measure of axonal/dendritic outgrowth, showed no diminution before 70 years of age; only after the age of 80 did the changes become pronounced.

C. Pharmacological Implications of Neurochemical Changes in the Aging Brain

The neurochemical changes in the aging brain reduce the reserve capacities and make the balance between neurotransmitter systems more delicate. This leads to increased sensitivity to neuropsychopharmacological drugs. Sensitivity to drugs with anticholinergic effects is well known in elderly people. Several drugs with anticholinergic effects (e.g., anti-Parkinsonian drugs, tricyclic antidepressants, and neuroleptics) may precipitate attacks of delirium in the elderly if used carelessly. This sensitivity to neuroleptics is due to already reduced activity in the DA systems, and these drugs further block DA receptors. Even small doses may elicit extrapyramidal symptoms and dyskinesia. Drugs with more selective effects, for instance, selective serotonin reuptake inhibitors (SSRI), are preferable in elderly people. With the increased MAO-B activity in elderly people, MAO inhibitors such as selegeline may seem attractive, but we do not think that the increase in MAO-B activity is of such magnitude that it has biological importance. Yet, as has been shown in several studies, treatment with selegeline may be successful in, for instance, Parkinson's disease.

D. Discussion of Age-Related Changes in the Human Brain

It seems rational to divide the elderly into two groups, younger elderly and older elderly, with a dividing line around the age of 80. The younger elderly are a rapidly growing group of retired people who are physically and mentally vigorous. They are relatively healthy, relatively well off, well educated, and active, and they are therefore an important group in society. It can be assumed that changes of involution occur in this group, but that the brain's reserve capacities are so great that no symptoms or signs of deficiency appear. It is only when these individuals are exposed to stress that symptoms may manifest themselves. In the older elderly, however, the compensatory mechanisms of the brain are more exhausted and symptoms of insufficiency therefore appear. Motor functioning disturbances, impaired cognition, and emotional disturbances, especially in the form of depressed mood, are some of the more important disorders seen in the elderly.

Neuroendocrine function also changes with age. As shown by Swaab and coworkers (49), there is increased activity of neuropeptides in the hypothalamus of elderly people. According to findings by Raadsheer (52), the activity of hypothalamic corticotropin-releasing hormone (CRH) neurons is increased in aging, Alzheimer's disease, and depression. These findings indicate that CRH neurons change their activity at older ages and also express arginine vasopressin. This is in agreement with the finding of increased hypothalamic–pituitary–adrenal (HPA) axis activity in elderly people. It is not known whether the increased HPA axis activity is due to reduced inhibitory control over the hypothalamus from the neurotransmitter systems or to disturbed feedback from other systems that regulate the hypothalamus.

IV. NEUROCHEMISTRY OF PATHOLOGICAL AGING

In this section, only neurochemical changes in dementia disorders are discussed. The concept of dementia is not well defined. It is a syndrome in which the decline in memory and thinking is sufficient to impair functioning of the daily living. Deterioration of emotional functions and impairment of motor performance may also be included in the symptomatology. For a reliable diagnosis to be established, the syndrome should be present in clear consciousness. The two main groups of dementias are idiopathic and vascular dementias. Idiopathic dementia includes frontal lobe dementia, Alzheimer's disease, and some more uncommon disorders: Huntington's chorea, Parkinsonism with dementia, and ALS with dementia. The most common idiopathic dementia is Alzheimer dementia, which is divided into two subgroups: early-onset pure Alzheimer's disease (AD) and senile dementia of the Alzheimer type (SDAT). Vascular dementia (VAD) is also divided into subgroups, which include multi-infarct dementia, dementia due to small vessel disturbances, and disorders associated with hypoxia.

A. Alzheimer-Type Dementia

Although senile plaques (SPs) accompany normal aging, these changes are found in greater abundance in AD. There are two schools of thought regarding whether SPs are primary phenomena (i.e., the direct cause of the symptoms), or whether they are secondary to the neuronal and synaptic degeneration. Many researchers believe that amyloid deposition and SPs are the "central event" (53), or play the "central role" (54) in the etiology and pathogenesis of AD, while other researchers challenge the amyloid hypothesis (55,56).

According to the amyloid cascade hypothesis, deposition of Aβ is the central event in the pathogenesis of AD, which is regarded as an amyloid storage disease of the brain (53,54). Amyloid deposition is thought to start a cascade of events that finally results in the dementia that brings the patient to the physician. The essential premise in the amyloid cascade hypothesis is that Aβ, or aggregates thereof, are neurotoxic, as has been suggested in experimental studies using cell cultures or animal systems.

Other researchers agree that Aβ deposition and SPs accompany AD, but claim that more research is needed to settle the question of whether Aβ deposition is the factor that causes the neuronal dysfunction and dementia, or whether it is a pathological by-product of the disease without direct pathogenetic importance. Deposition of Aβ in the brain at levels greater than would be expected at the patient's age is a nonspecific phenomenon, which is found in AD and other conditions such as in the periphery of cerebral infarcts (57), around arteriovenous malformations (58), in non-Down's syndrome mentally retarded individuals (59), after acute severe cerebral trauma (60), and after chronic repeated cerebral trauma (i.e., in dementia pugilistica) (61).

Thus there is evidence both supporting and not supporting the etiological importance of Aβ deposition. We believe that the real test of the amyloid cascade hypothesis will not occur until drugs that prevent amyloid deposition in animal models can be tested in living patients. Then we will find out whether AD can be arrested or cured by such prevention.

Like SPs, neurofibrillary tangles accompany normal aging, but are found in much greater abundance in AD. Their disease specificity is low; besides being present in AD, they inevitably accompany aging, and are also found in a wide range of disorders (62). This lack of disease specificity suggests that PHFtau and NFTs are nonspecific indices of brain damage.

The concentration of PHFtau is increased in cortical AD brain homogenates (35,36,63–65), whereas the concentration of normal tau protein is reduced (64,65), suggesting hyperphosphorylation of normal tau protein rather than an increased synthesis.

Although our knowledge of both APP/Aβ and tau protein/PHFtau has increased greatly, the relationship between deposition of amyloid (and the development of SPs) and hyperphosphorylation of tau protein (and the development of paired helical filaments and NFTs) is unknown.

The processes related to neurotransmitter release are proposed to be mediated by membrane-bound proteins. These can be divided into two major groups: synaptic vesicle membrane proteins and presynaptic membrane proteins.

The principal component in intraneuronal communication is the synapse, a specialized junctional complex between axons and dendrites emerging from various neurons. The presynaptic component contains synaptic vesicles, in which neurotransmitters are stored. As a first step of synaptic transmission, the synaptic vesicles fuse with the presynaptic plasma membrane. Then the neurotransmitters are released into the synaptic gap, and finally they bind to specific postsynaptic receptors.

Evidence of a marked synaptic loss in several cortical regions in AD has been established using various methods, including electron microscopy (66), immunohistochemistry, and quantitative immunoblotting with the synaptic vesicle proteins synapsin I, synaptophysin, and synaptotagmin (67–70).

The major part of the synaptic pathology in AD is localized in the neuropil, without relation to SPs or NFTs (71,72). Moreover, the degree of synapse pathology correlates well with clinical measures of the dementia, whereas SPs and NFTs show no correlation at all or only a weak correlation (68,72). Therefore, it has been suggested that the central event in the pathogenesis of AD is synaptic degeneration and loss, whereas SPs and NFTs are secondary nonspecific indices of brain damage.

Apolipoprotein E (ApoE) is a protein that is a constituent of several plasma lipoproteins and is essential in the transport and metabolism of lipids, by mediating the uptake of lipoproteins by interaction with specific receptors (73). It is known that the ApoE gene shows polymorphism with three different alleles (Apoε2, ε3, and ε4), which give rise to three isoforms (ApoE2, E3, and E4) that only differ on two amino acids (74). ApoE3 is the most common isoform, present in 77–78% of the general population, while ApoE2 is found in 7–8%, and ApoE4 in 14–16%.

Recent data indicate that ApoE is involved in the pathogenesis of AD. In 1991, antibodies to ApoE were found to label SPs and congophil angiopathy (75). In 1993, several papers reported an increased frequency of the E4 allele in both familial and sporadic AD (76–79). Since then, numerous papers have confirmed these findings.

The leading hypothesis about the pathogenetic mechanism of ApoE in AD is an involvement in Aβ deposition. ApoE immunoreactivity is found in the SPs and in CAA (75). In vitro studies have also found EpoE4 to have greater affinity to Aβ than EpoE3 has (80). In vitro experiments have further shown that incubation of Aβ with ApoE gives rise to Aβ/ApoE complexes that precipitate to amyloidlike fibrils (81,82). It has therefore been suggested that ApoE may act as a "pathological chaperone" that binds to normally soluble Aβ, making it insoluble and thus sequestered in the senile plaques and cerebral blood vessels, and/or preventing it from proteolysis (83). In brain tissue from AD patients, however, immunoreactivity to ApoE is markedly more limited than immunoreactivity to Aβ (84), and is preferentially found in the core of classical SPs (consisting of fibrillar Aβ) (84). These findings do not support the notion that ApoE is involved at the early stages of fibrillar amyloid formation. Moreover, the binding between ApoE and Aβ is unspecific, since ApoE has been found to bind to amyloid in virtually any amyloid-associated disease (83), suggesting that ApoE might merely be absorbed by various kinds of already existing hydrophobic amyloid fibrils.

ApoE immunoreactivity is also found in NFTs (75). It has been shown that ApoE3 but not ApoE4 binds to tau protein. This finding has led to the hypothesis that, by binding to tau protein, ApoE3 slows down the degree of phosphorylation and self-assembly into PHFs (85).

ApoE has also been implicated in the regulation of the mobilization and transport of lipids during neuronal repair and reactive synapsogenesis after injury (73,86,87). In short, after experimental lesions in animals, astrocytes engulf the presynaptic terminals and their axons, which are then stored within the astrocytes where the accumulation of cholesterol induces a synthesis of ApoE (88). The lipids form ApoE lipoprotein particles, which may then be directed to specific target sites within the CNS (87), resulting in uptake of ApoE lipid complexes by specific receptor-mediated endocytosis in the neuronal growth cones (89). After uptake of ApoE lipoprotein particles/LDL receptor complexes, cholesterol is released within the neurons, and can be transported to the terminals for synapse formation (87).

This ApoE repair process may also be isoform-dependent. In cultures of dorsal root ganglion neurons, ApoE3 increased and ApoE4 decreased neurite outgrowth in the presence of β-VLDL, which suggests that the isoforms may be specific to either the LDL or the LRP receptor (90). It has been suggested that ApoE4 might interfere with the normal compensatory synaptogenesis through the ApoE/LDL receptor system (87). In this model ApoE4 carriers may have impaired reactive synaptogenesis to compensate for the age-related nerve cell loss (87).

In a study by Svennerholm and Gottfries (91) membrane components were studied in AD, SDAT, and controls. Gangliosides, phospholipids, cholesterol, cerebroside, and sulfatide were determined in the frontal gray matter, the temporal gray matter, the caudate nucleus, the hippocampus, and the frontal white matter. In all areas the concentrations of gangliosides were significantly lower in the AD group than in the SDAT group and age-matched controls. Phospholipids were also significantly reduced in all gray matter areas in AD compared with the SDAT group. Membrane lipids in the white matter showed an opposite turn. Significantly reduced concentrations were recorded for phospholipids, cholesterol, cerebroside, and sulfatide in the SDAT group. The data indicate biochemical differences in the two major forms of Alzheimer-type dementia. In AD the loss of gangliosides indicates a reduction in neuronal processing, whereas loss of myelin lipids is the major characteristic of the SDAT form. Evidently the two dementia forms do not have the same pathogenesis.

Several investigations have focused on neurotransmitter disturbances in the gray matter in patients with AD/SDAT (for review, see Ref. 92). As is evident from Figure 3, most of the neurotransmitters are disturbed in AD/SDAT. The reductions in concentrations and enzyme system activity are greater than

		Cortex cerebri					Subcortical areas				
		Front.	Temp.	Cinguli	Hippoc.	Unspec.	Hypothal.	Caudat.	Putam.	Thalam.	Hippoc.
ACh	CAT	↓	↓			↓	↓	↓			↓
	AChE	↓			↓	↓					↓
5-HT	5-HT	↓	↓			↓	↓	↓			↓
	5-HIAA	↓	↓			↓	↓				↓
	Imipramine binding	↓	↓	↓					↓		
NA	NA	↓	↓			↓	↓	↓	↓		↓
	HMPG					↓		↑			↓
	DBH	↓	↓								↓
	TH					↓					
DA	DA				↓		↓	↓	↓	↓	
	HVA	↓	↓	↑				↓	↓		
	GBR 12935 binding								↓		
MAO	MAO-A					↑		↑		↑	
	MAO-B	↑	↑	↑	↑			↑	↑	↑	
GABA	GABA		↓			↓					
	GABA-T	↓	↓					↓			
Neuro-peptides	Somatostatin		↓				↑				↓
	Vasopressin					↓	↑	↓			↓
	CRF					↓		↑			
	Substance P					↓		↑			↓
	Neuropeptide Y					↓	↑				↓
	Galanin	↑				↑	↑	↑			
	VIP					↓					

FIGURE 3 Changes in human brain neurotransmitter systems in dementia of the Alzheimer type (AD/SDAT). Arrows pointing downward or upward indicate significant changes. Abbreviations: ACh = acetylcholine; CAT = choline acetyltransferase; AChE = acetylcholinesterase; 5-HT = 5-hydroxytryptamine or serotonin; 5-HIAA = 5-hydroxyindoleacetic acid; NA = noradrenaline; HMPG = 3-methoxy-4-hydroxyphenylglycol; DBH = dopamine-β-hydroxylase; DA = dopamine; HVA = homovanillic acid; DDC = dopamine decarboxylase; TH = tyrosine hydroxylase; MAO = monoamine oxidase; GABA = γ-aminobutyric acid; GAD = glutamic acid decarboxylase; GABA-T = γ-aminobutyrate aminotransferase; CRF = corticotropin-releasing factor; Subst. = substance; VIP = vasoactive intestinal peptide.

those seen in normal aging, and usually AD-afflicted brains are more severely damaged than brains of patients with SDAT. Several findings indicate severe disturbances of the acetylcholine (ACh) system. One of the first reports actually dates back to 1964, when Pope and associates (93) demonstrated a loss of AChE activity in biopsy brain tissue. Several other studies later reported reduced activity of AChE. Reports of reduced activity in choline acetyltransferase (CAT) followed, and there is also evidence that, in AD/SDAT, the number of cell bodies is reduced in the nucleus basalis of Meynert (94). According to Nordberg and Winblad (43), there is also an increased number of muscarinic receptors and a decreased number of nicotinic receptors in Alzheimer-afflicted brains. The disturbed function in the cholinergic system has been given great importance for AD/SDAT, as CAT activity in neocortical areas is also related to dementia scores (95). There is also evidence from animal studies that the ACh systems are important for memory and learning and that cholinergic drugs are important for memory and cognitive functions in humans.

It is evident that neurotransmitter systems other than ACh are disturbed in AD/SDAT. A dementia-related reduction in homovanillic acid (HVA) in the caudate nucleus of patients with AD/SDAT was known from postmortem investigations already in 1969 (96). The catecholamines dopamine and noradrenaline were later shown to be reduced in discrete brain areas, but their end metabolites, HVA and HMPG, are not reduced. In fact, one study found a significant increase in HMPG in the caudate nucleus (97). With regard to serotonin activity in Alzheimer-afflicted brains, it is evident that it is relatively severely damaged. Serotonin, as well as its end metabolite 5-HIAA, has been found to be significantly reduced in several brain areas investigated (for review, see Ref. 98).

Glutamate is an excitatory transmitter probably to some degree involved in most CNS functions. It activates AMPA, NMDA and metabotropic receptors. In animal experiments the concentration of extracellular glutamate has been shown to rise rapidly upon the initiation of ischemia or trauma. It is also well known that overactivity of glutamate causes an excitotoxic effect, presumably by enabling CA influx to the cell. It has been suggested that neurodegeneration of the substantia nigra in Parkinson's disease may be due to an excitotoxic effect of glutamate. There is also a glutamatergic hypothesis of AD. Association pathways in the cortex are disrupted in AD and results in loss of NMDA receptor (for review, see Ref. 99).

In a study by Adolfsson and associates (100) MAO activity in brains of patients with AD/SDAT was compared with that of age-matched controls. A significant selective increase in MAO-B activity was found in two of four regions investigated (hippocampus and cortex gyrus cinguli). MAO-B was also drastically increased in the white matter (71%). One simple explanation of the

MAO-B increase would be that degenerative processes that occur as a result of, for instance, aging or AD/SDAT, induce the growth of extra neuronal cells (e.g., glia) containing about the same amount of MAO-A activity but being relatively richer in MAO-B activity than the original tissue. MAO-B activity can then be considered a marker for gliosis. It is of interest that AD/SDAT patients also have increased MAO activity (the MAO-B form) in platelets when these patients are compared with controls. However, as Regland and associates (101) have shown, increased MAO activity in platelets seems to be a phenomenon different from increased MAO activity in brain tissue. Due to vitamin B_{12} deficiency, immature platelets are produced that contain high MAO activity. Enzyme activity is normalized when vitamin B_{12} and folic acid are supplemented.

The concentrations of several neuropeptides have been measured in postmortem human brain studies in patients with AD/SDAT. In a critical review (102), it was reported that somatostatin, vasopressin, corticotropin-releasing hormone, substance P, and neuropeptide Y are significantly reduced in cortical and subcortical brain areas in patients with AD/SDAT. The neuropeptide galanin is increased. It is of interest that changes in the hypothalamus are different from those in cortical areas and subcortical nuclei. Thus, according to some investigators, somatostatin, vasopressin, and neuropeptide Y are significantly increased in the hypothalamus together with galanin. The increased concentrations of some neuropeptides in the hypothalamus may possibly be the consequence of lost inhibitory control over the hypothalamus due to failing feedback of stress systems. In contrast to other neuropeptides, galanin seems to be increased in the demented brain, an unusual finding which, together with clinical data, suggests a role for this peptide in the impairment of learning and memory that is characteristic of dementia disorders. Galanin is present throughout the human brain and is abundant in the basal forebrain region. It is expressed in the cholinergic projection neurons from the nucleus basalis of Meynert to the hippocampus and it is a powerful inhibitor of hippocampal ACh release.

B. Pharmacological Implications of Neurochemical Changes in Alzheimer's Disease

The neurochemical changes that occur in the Alzheimer-afflicted brain have been the theoretical basis for formulating pharmacological treatment strategies. So far there is only symptomatic pharmacological treatment, as the etiology of the disorder is unknown. In treatment trials, efforts have been made to counteract failing neurotransmitter systems by substitution. Most well known are the efforts to activate the cholinergic system. To some extent, they have been successful. Tetrahydroaminoacridine (THA, Cognex) is now registered in several countries for treatment of AD/SDAT. This drug inhibits the breakdown of ACh in the synaptic cleft. The success is modest, however; only about one-third of the patients benefit from the treatment. It can be assumed that for a favorable outcome there must be a certain number of active cholinergic neurons to maintain the synthesis of ACh. This assumption is supported by the clinical observation that patients with mild dementia react more favorably to "cholinergic drugs" than those with moderate or severe dementia. One way to test "the cholinergic hypothesis" is to use a receptor agonist. Tests with muscarinic receptor agonists have been performed but have not been very promising so far.

It is known that the serotonergic system has importance for normal functions such as mood level, appetite, temperature, rhythms around the clock, and sexual activity. It is also known that this system has pathogenetic importance for mood disturbances, anxiety, suicidal behavior, and aggressiveness. In one study, the SSRI citalopram was used in the treatment of Alzheimer's disease. Improvement was seen not only in the mood level but also in anxiety, fear–panic, restlessness, and emotional bluntness, but cognitive impairment was unchanged (103). Other studies have found citalopram to be beneficial in the treatment of poststroke depression and poststroke pathological crying (104,105). There is, indeed, a great need for further studies of SSRI preparations in degenerative neuropsychiatric disorders.

As the dopaminergic system is disturbed and Parkinsonlike symptoms appear in AD, it is of interest to test L-dopa treatment. Some studies have been performed, with a marginal effect. It must be kept in mind, however, that the symptoms in Parkinson's disease may be attributable to an imbalance between the cholinergic and dopaminergic systems due to deficient dopaminergic activity. In AD, it is primarily the cholinergic system that is deficient and only to a lesser extent the dopaminergic system. The simple principle for treatment of Parkinson's disease is therefore not applicable to Alzheimer's disease.

It is of interest to study drugs with effects on the glutamatergic system, which is assumed to be deficient both in vascular dementia and AD (99). The activation of NMDA receptors is problematic, however, since excessive activation may cause excitotoxicity and degeneration of the neurons. A group of drugs, to which amantadine and memantine belong, are blockers of NMDA channels, and they are tested in degenerative brain disorders (99).

C. Vascular Dementia (VAD)

VAD is cognitive impairment caused by changes in the blood circulation of the brain. Neurochemical investigations of noninfarcted brain tissue from patients with VAD show general changes (for review, see Ref. 106). Serotonin metabolism is reduced, and so is CAT activity. MAO-B is significantly increased in the white matter. It is obvious that, in brains with large-vessel or small-vessel pathology and in which chronic hypoxia can be assumed, a disturbance of the glutamatergic system may be present. It is well known from animal experiments that hypoxia and ischemic attacks elicit an excitotoxic effect due to increased release of glutamate.

A severe decrease in myelin components indicates white matter disturbances of such a degree that they must be of pathogenetic importance. The levels of some neuropeptides in the hypothalamus are increased and the pattern of the increased concentrations is similar to that found in AD/SDAT. This postmortem finding is in agreement with clinical findings of high hypothalamic-pituitary-adrenal (HPA) axis activity in patients with VAD. Around 70% of these patients have a pathological dexamethasone suppression test, indicating overactivity in the HPA axis. In AD/SDAT there is also increased activity in the HPA axis, but less pronounced than in VAD.

REFERENCES

1. Carlsson A, Winblad B. Influence of age and time interval between death and autopsy on dopamine and 3-methoxytyramine levels in human basal ganglia. J Neural Transm 1976; 38:271–276.
2. Carlsson A. Neurotransmitters in old age and dementia. In: Heffner H, Moschel G, Sartorius N, eds. Mental Health in the Elderly: a Review of the Present State of Research. Berlin: Springer, 1986:154–161.
3. Gottfries CG. Nosological aspects of differentia typology of dementia of Alzheimer type. In: Bergener M, Ermini M, Stähelin HB, eds. Dimensions in Aging. London: Academic Press, 1986:207–217.
4. Bredesen DE. Neural apoptosis. Ann Neurol 1995; 38:839–851.
5. Wesemann W, Arnold N, Rodden A, Weiner N. In: Riederer P, Usdin E, eds. Transmitter Biochemistry of Human Brain Tissue. London: MacMillan, 1981:55–69.
6. Chiu E. What's in a name—dementia or dysmentia? (Editorial) Intern J Geriatr Psychiatry 1994; 9:1–4.
7. Arnold G. The brain in aging. In: Hume Adams J, Corsellis JAN, Duchen LW, eds. Greenfield's Neuropathology. 5th ed. London: Edward Arnold, 1992:1290–1317.
8. Tomlinson BE, Corsellis JAN. Ageing and the dementias. In: Hume Adams J, Corsellis JAN, Duchen LW, eds. Greenfield's Neuropathology. London: Edward Arnold, 1984:951–1025.
9. Svennerholm L, Broström K. Jungbjer B, Olsson L. Membrane lipids of adult human brain: lipid composition in frontal and temporal lobe in subjects of age 20 to 100 years. J Neurochem 1994; 63:1802–1011.
10. Terry RD, Peck A, DeTeresa R, Schechter R, Horoupian BS. Neocortical cell counts in normal human adult aging. Ann Neurol 1987; 21:530–539.

11. Leek KS, Vernadakis A. Comparative biochemical, morphological, and immunocytochemical studies between C-6 glial cells of early and late passages and advanced passages of glial cells derived from aged mouse cerebral hemispheres. Clia 1992; 6:245–257.
12. Otto D, Unsicker K. FGF-2 in the MTPT model of Parkinson's disease: effects on astroglial cells. Glia 1994; 11:47–56.
13. Brun A. An overview of light and electron microscopic changes. In: Reisberg B, ed. Alzheimer's Disease. New York: The Free Press, 1983:48–56.
14. Tomlinson BE. Morphological changes and dementia in old age. In: Lynn Smith W, ed. Aging and Dementia. New York: Spectrum Publications, 1977:25–56.
15. Matsuyama H. Incidence of neurofibrillary change, senile plaques, and granulovacuolar degeneration in aged individuals. In: Reisberg B, ed. Alzheimer's Disease. New York: The Free Press, 1983:149–154.
16. Rotschild D. Pathologic changes in senile psychoses and their psychobiologic significance. Am J Psychiatry 1937; 97:757–788.
17. Dayan AD. Quantitative histological studies on the aged human brain, II. Senile plaques and neurofibrillary tangles in senile dementia. Acta Neuropath (Berlin) 1970; 16:95–102.
18. Sourander P, Sjögren H. The concept of Alzheimer's disease and its clinical implications. In: Wolstenholme GEW, O'Connors M, eds. Alzheimer's Disease. Ciba Foundation Symposium. London: Churchill, 1970:11–36.
19. Constantinides J. Is Alzheimer's disease a major form of senile dementia? Clinical, anatomical and genetic data. In: Katzman R, Terry RD, Bick KL, eds. Alzheimer's Disease: Senile Dementia and Related Disorders (Aging Vol. 7). New York: Raven Press, 1978:15–25.
20. Hansen LA, DeTeresa R, Davies P, Terry RD. Neocortical morphometry, lesion counts, and choline acetyltransferase levels in the age spectrum of Alzheimer's disease. Neurology 1988; 38:48–54.
21. Vinters HV. Cerebral amyloid angiopathy: a critical review. Stroke 1987; 18:311–324.
22. Glenner GG, Wong CW. Alzheimer's disease: initial report of purification and characterization of a novel cerebrovascular amyloid protein. Biochem Biophys Res Commun 1984; 120:885–890.
23. Kang J, Lemaire HG, Unterbeck A, Salbaum JM, Masters CL, Grzeschik KH, Multhaup G, Beyreuther K, Müller-Hill B. The precursor of Alzheimer's disease amyloid A4 protein resembles a cell-surface receptor. Nature 1987; 325:733–736.
24. Davies L, Wolska B, Hilbich C, Multhaup G, Martins R, Simms G, Beyreuther K, Masters CL. A4 amyloid protein deposition and the diagnosis of Alzheimer's disease: prevalence in aged brains determined by immunocytochemistry compared with conventional neuropathologic techniques. Neurology 1988; 38:1688–1693.
25. Delaere P, Fayep G, Duyckaerts C, Hauw JL. β-A4 deposits are constant in the brain of the oldest old: an immunocytochemical study of 20 French centenarians. Neurobiol Aging 1993; 14:191–194.
26. Rohrer AE, Lowenson JD, Carke S, Woods AS, Cotter RJ, Gowing E, Ball MJ. Beta-amyloid-(1-42) is a major component of cerebrovascular amyloid deposits:

implications for the pathology of Alzheimer disease. Proc Natl acad Sci USA 1993; 90:10836–10840.
27. Joachim CL, Duffy LK, Morris JH, Selkoe DJ. Protein chemical and immunocytochemical studies of minogovascular β-amyloid protein in Alzheimer's disease and normal aging. Brain Res 1988; 474:100–111.
28. Klier FG, Cole G, Stallcup W, Schubert D. Amyloid β-protein precursor is associated with extracellular matrix. Brain Res 1990; 515:336–342.
29. van Nostrand WE, Wagner SL, Suzuki M, Choi BH, Farrow JS, Geddes JW, Cotman CW, Cunningham DD. Protease nexin-II, a potent antichymotrypsin, shows identity to amyloid β-protein precursor. Nature 1989; 341:546–549.
30. Saitoh T, Sundsmo M, Roch JM, Kumura N, Cole G, Schubert D, Oltersdorf T, Schenk DB. Secreted form of amyloid β protein precursor is involved in the growth regulation of fibroblasts. Cell 1989; 58:615–622.
31. Whitson JS, Glabe CG, Shintani E, Abcar A, Cotman CW. β-amyloid protein promotes neuritic branching in hippocampal cultures. Neurosci Lett 1990; 110:319–324.
32. Beyreuther K, Masters CL. Amyloid precursor protein (APP) and βA4 amyloid in the etiology of Alzheimer's disease: precursor-product relationships in the derangement of neuronal function. Brain Pathol 1991; 1:241–251.
33. Mattson MP, Barger SW, Cheng B, Lieberburg I, Smith-Swintosky VL, Rydel RE. Beta-amyloid precursor protein metabolites and loss of neuronal Ca^{2+} homeostasis in Alzheimer's disease. Trends Neurosci 1993; 16:409–414.
34. Grundke-Iqbal I, Iqbal K, Tung YC, Quinian M, Wisniewski HM, Binder LI. Abnormal phosphorylation of the microtubule-associated protein τ (tau) in Alzheimer cytoskeletal pathology. Proc Natl Acad Sci 1986; 83:4913–4917.
35. Wolozin B, Davies P. Alzheimer-related neuronal protein A68: specificity and distribution. Ann Neurol 1987; 22:521–526.
36. Bissette G, Smith WH, Dole KC, Crain B, Ghanbari H, Miller B, Nemeroff CB. Alterations in Alzheimer's disease-associated protein in Alzheimer's disease frontal and temporal cortex. Arch Gen Psychiatry 1991; 48:1009–1012.
37. Delacourte A, Flament S, Dibe EM, Hublau P, Sablonnière B, Hémon B, Shérrer V, Défossez A. Pathological proteins tau 64 and 69 are specifically expressed in the somatodendritic domain of the degenerating cortical neurons during Alzheimer's disease. Acta Neuropathol 1990; 80:111–117.
38. Brun A, Englund E. A white matter disorder in dementia of the Alzheimer type: a pathoanatomical study. Ann Neurol 1986; 19:253–262.
39. Gottfries CG, Karlsson I, Svennerholm L. Senile dementia—a "white matter" disease? In: Gottfries CG, ed. Normal Aging, Alzheimer's Disease and Senile Dementia. Brussels: Edition de l'Université, 1985:111–118.
40. Steingart A, Hachinski VC, Lau C, Fox AJ, Diaz F, Cape, Lee D, Inzitari D, Merskey H. Cognitive and neurological findings in subjects with diffuse white matter lucencies on computed tomographic scan (leuko-araiosis). Arch Neurol 1987; 44:32–35.
41. de Leon MJ, George AE, Kluger A, Franssen E, Ferris SH, Wolf AP. PET-dexyglucose, CT, and neuropathology of age-related whtie matter pathology in normals and Alzheimer's disease patients. Psychiatry Res 1989; 29:359–360.

42. Crystal HA, Dickson DW, Sliwinski MJ, Lipton RB, Grober E, Mark-Nelson H, Antis P. Pathological markers associated with normal aging and dementia in the elderly. Ann Neurol 1993; 34:566–573.
43. Nordberg A, Winblad B. Brain nicotinic and muscarinic receptors in normal aging and dementia. In: Fischer A, Hanin H, Lacman D, eds. Alzheimer's and Parkinson's Disease. New York: Plenum Press, 1986:95–108.
44. Allard P, Marcusson JO. Age-correlated loss of dopamine uptake sites labeled with [3H]GBR-12935 in human putamen. Neurobiol Aging 1989; 10:661–664.
45. Gottfries CG. Disturbance of the 5-hydroxytryptamine metabolism in brains from patients with Alzheimer's dementia. J Neural Transm 1990 (Suppl 30): 33–43.
46. Gottfries CG, Oreland L, Wiberg Å, Winblad B. Lowered monoamine oxidase activity in brains from alcoholic suicides. J Neurochem 1975; 25:667–673.
47. Palmer AM, DeKosky AT. Monoamine neurons in aging and Alzheimer's disease. J Neural Transm (Gen Section) 1993; 91:135–159.
48. Leake A, Ferrier IN. Alterations in neuropeptides in aging and disease. Drug Aging 1993; 3:408–427.
49. Swaab DF, Tiers E, Partiman TS. The suprachiasmatic nucleus of the human brain in the relation to sex, age and senile dementia. Brain Res 1985; 342:37–44.
50. Wallin A, Carlsson A, Ekman R, Gottfries CG, Karlsson I, Svennerholm L, Widerlöv E. Hypothalamic monoamines and neuropeptides in dementia. Eur J Neuropsychopharmacol 1991; 1:165–168.
51. Decker MW. The effects of aging on hippocampal and cortical projections of the forebrain cholinergic system. Brain Res Rev 1987; 12:423–438.
52. Raadsheer FC. Increased activity of hypothalamic corticotrophin-releasing hormone neurons in aging, Alzheimer's disease and depression: a study on human postmortem material. Ph.D. dissertation, University of Amsterdam, 1994.
53. Hardy J, Allsop D. Amyloid deposition as the central event in the aetiology of Alzheimer's disease. Trends Pharmacol Sci 1991; 12:383–388.
54. Joachim CL, Selkoe DJ. The seminal role of β-amyloid in the pathogenesis of Alzheimer's disease. Alz Dis Assoc Disord 1992; 6:7–34.
55. Regland B, Gottfries CG. The role of amyloid β-protein in Alzheimer's disease. Lancet 1992; 340:467–469.
56. Hoyer S. Sporadic dementia of Alzheimer's disease: role of amyloid in the etiology is challenged. J Neural Transm (P-D Section) 1993; 6:159–165.
57. Nukina N, Kanazawa I, Mannen T, Uchida Y. Accumulation of amyloid precursor protein and β-protein immunoreactivities in axons injured by cerebral infarct. Gerontology 1992; 38(Suppl 1):10–14.
58. Hart MN, Merz P, Bennet-Gray J, Menezes AH, Goeken JA, Schelper RL, Wisniewski HM. β-amyloid protein of Alzheimer's disease is found in cerebral and spinal cord vascular malformations. Am J Pathol 1988; 132:167–172.
59. Popovitch ER, Wisniewski HM, Barcikowska M, Silverman W, Bancher C, Sersen E, Wen GY. Alzheimer neuropathology in non-Down's syndrome mentally retarded adults. Acta Neuropathol 1990; 80:362–367.
60. Roberts GW, Gentleman SM, Lynch A, Graham DI. Beta A4 amyloid protein deposition after head trauma. Lancet 1991; 2:1422–1423.

61. Roberts GW, Allsop D, Bruton C. The occult aftermath of boxing. J Neurol Neurosurg Psychiatry 1990; 53:373–378.
62. Wisniewski K, George AJ, Moretz RC, Wisniewski HM. Alzheimer neurofibrillary tangles in diseases other than senile and presenile dementia. Ann Neurol 1979; 5: 288–294.
63. Harrington CR, Mukaetova-Ladinska EB, Hills R, Edwards PC, de Garcini EM, Novak M, Wischik CM. Measurement of distinct immunochemical presentations of tau protein in Alzheimer's disease. Proc Natl Acad Sci USA 1991; 88:5842–5846.
64. Bramblett GT, Trojanowski JQ, Lee VMY. Regions with abundant neurofibrillary pathology in human brain exhibit a selective reduction in levels of binding-component τ and accumulation of abnormal τ-isoforms (A68 proteins). Lab Invest 1992; 66:212–222.
65. Mukaetova-Ladinska EB, Harrington CR, Hills R, O'Sullivan A, Roth M, Wischik CM. Regional distribution of paired helical filaments and normal tau proteins in aging and in Alzheimer's disease with and without temporal lobe involvement. Dementia 1992; 3:61–69.
66. DeKosky ST, Scheff SW. Synapse loss in frontal cortex biopsies in Alzheimer's disease: correlation with disease severity. Ann Neurol 1990; 27:457–464.
67. Hamos JE, DeGennaro LJ, Drachman DA. Synaptic loss in Alzheimer's disease and other dementias. Neurology 1989; 39:355–361.
68. Terry RD, Masliah E, Salmon DP, Butters N, DeTeresa R, Hill R, Hansen LA, Katzman R. Physical basis of cognitive alterations in Alzheimer's disease: synapse loss is the major correlate of cognitive impairment. Ann Neurol 1991; 30:572–580.
69. Lassman H, Weiler R, Fischer P, Bancher C, Jellinger K, Floor E, Danielczyk W, Seitelberger F, Winkler H. Synaptic pathology in Alzheimer's disease: immunological data for markers of synaptic and large dense-core vesicles. Neuroscience 1992; 46:1–8.
70. Davidsson P, Jahn R, Bergquist J, Ekman R, Blennow K. Synaptotagmin, a synaptic vesicle protein, is present in human cerebrospinal fluid: a new biochemical marker for synaptic pathology in Alzheimer's disease? Mol Chem Neuropathol 1996; 27:195–210.
71. Masliah E, Hansen L, Albright T, Mallory M, Terry RD. Immunoelectron microscopic study of synaptic pathology in Alzheimer's disease. Acta Neuropathol 1991; 81:428–433.
72. Blennow K, Bogdanovic N, Alafuzoff I, Ekman R, Davidsson P. Synaptic pathology in Alzheimer's disease: relation to severity of dementia, but not to senile plaques, neurofibrillary tangles, or the ApoE4 allele. J Neural Transm (P-D Section) 1996; 103:603–618.
73. Mahley RW. Apolipoprotein E: cholesterol transport protein with expanding role in cell biology. Science 1988; 240:622–630.
74. Zannis VI, Breslow JL, Utermann G, Mahley RW, Weisgraber KH, Havel RJ, Goldstein JL, Brown MS, Schonfeld G, Hazzard WR, Blum C. Proposed nomenclature of apoE isoproteins, apoE genotypes, and phenotypes. J Lipid Res 1982; 23:911–914.
75. Namba Y, Tomonaga M, Kawasaki H, Otomo E, Ikeda K. Apolipoprotein E immunoreactivity in cerebral amyloid deposits and neurofibrillary tangles in Alz-

heimer's disease and kuru plaque amyloid in Creutzfeldt-Jakob disease. Brain Res 1991; 541:163–166.
76. Corder EH, Saunders AM, Strittmatter WJ, Schmechel DE, Gaskell PC, Small GW, Roses AD, Haines JL, Pericak-Vance MA. Gene dose of apilipoprotein E type 4 allele and the risk of Alzheimer's disease in late onset families. Science 1993; 261:921–923.
77. Poirier J, Davignon J, Bouthillier D, Kogan S, Bertrand P, Gauthier S. Apolipoprotein E polymorphism and Alzheimer's disease. Lancet 1993; 342:697–699.
78. Saunders AM, Strittmatter WJ, Schmechel D, St George-Hyslop PH, Pericak-Vance MA, Joo SH, Rosi BL, Gusella JF, Crapper-MacLachlan DR, Alberts MJ, Hulette C, Crain B, Goldgaber D, Roses AD. Association of apolipoprotein E allele ε4 with late-onset familial and sporadic Alzheimer's disease. Neurology 1993; 43:1467–1472.
79. Strittmatter WJ, Saunders AM, Schmechel D, Pericak-Vance M, Enghild J, Salvesen GS, Roses AD. Apolipoprotein E: high-avidity binding to β-amyloid and increased frequency of type 4 allele in late-onset familial Alzheimer's disease. Proc Natl Acad Sci USA 1993; 90:1977–1981.
80. Strittmatter WJ, Weisgraber KH, Huang DY, Dong LM, Salvesen GS, Pericak-Vance M, Schmechel D, Saunders AM, Goldgaber D, Roses AD. Binding of human apolipoprotein E to synthetic amyloid β peptide: isoform-specific effects and implications for late-onset Alzheimer's disease. Proc Natl Acad Sci USA 1993; 90:8098–8102.
81. Ma J, Yee A, Brewer Jr HB, Das S, Potter H. Amyloid-associated proteins α1-antichymotrypsin and apolipoprotein E promote assembly of Alzheimer β-protein into filaments. Nature 1994; 372:92–94.
82. Sanan DA, Weisgraber KH, Russel SJ, Mahley RW, Huang D, Saunders A, Schmechel D, Wisniewski T, Frangione B, Roses AD, Strittmatter WJ. Apolipoprotein E associates with β amyloid peptide of Alzheimer's disease to form novel monofibrils. J Clin Invest 1994; 94:860–869.
83. Wisniewski T, Frangione B. Apolipoprotein E: a pathological chaperone protein in patients with cerebral and systemic amyloid. Neurosci Lett 1992; 135:235–238.
84. Kida E, Golabek AA, Wisniewski T, Wisniewski KE. Regional differences in apolipoprotein E immunoreactivity in diffuse plaques in Alzheimer's disease. Neurosci Lett 1994; 167:73–76.
85. Strittmatter WJ, Weisgraber KH, Goedert M, Saunders AM, Huang D, Corder EH, Dong LM, Jakes R, Alberts MJ, Gilbert JR, Han SH, Hulette C, Einstein G, Schmechel D, Pericak-Vance MA, Roses AD. Hypothesis: microtubule instability and paired helical filaments formation in the Alzheimer's disease brain are related to apolipoprotein E genotype. Exp Neurol 1994; 125:163–171.
86. Snipes GJ, McGuire CB, Norden JJ, Freeman JA. Nerve injury stimulates the secretion of apolipoprotein E by nonneuronal cells. Proc Natl Acad Sci USA 1986; 83:1130–1134.
87. Poirier J. Apolipoprotein E in animal model of CNS injury and in Alzheimer's disease. TINS 1994; 17:525–530.
88. Poirier J, Hess M, May PC, Pasinetti G, Finch CE. Astroglial gene expression in the hippocampus following partial deafferentiation in the rat and in Alzheimer's

disease. In: Nagatsu T, ed. Basic, Clinical, and Therapeutic Aspects of Alzheimer's and Parkinson's diseases. New York: Plenum Press, 1990:191–194.
89. Ignatius MJ, Shooter EM, Pitas RE, Mahley RW. Lipoprotein uptake by neuronal growth cones in vitro. Science 19878; 236:959–962.
90. Nathan BP, Bellosta S, Sanan DA, Weisgraber KH, Mahley RW, Pitas RE. Differential effects of apolipoproteins E3 and E4 on neuronal growth in vitro. Science 1994; 264:850–852.
91. Svennerholm L, Gottfries CG. Membrane lipids selectively diminished in Alzheimer brains suggest synapse loss as primary event in early onset form (Type I) and demyelination in late onset form (Type II). J Neurochemistry 1994; 62:1039–1047.
92. Francis PT, Cross AJ, Bowen DM. Neurotransmitters and neuropeptides. In: Terry RD, Katzman R, Bick KL, eds. Alzheimer Disease. New York: Raven Press, 1994: 247–262.
93. Pope A, Hess HH, Lewis E. Studies on microchemical pathology of human cerebral cortex. In: Cohen MM, Snider RS, eds. Morphological and Biochemical Correlates of Neural Activity. New York: Harper, 1964:98–111.
94. Whitehouse PJ, Price DL, Struble RG, Clark AW, Coyle JT, deLong MR. Alzheimer's disease and senile dementia: loss of neurons in the basal forebrain. Science 1982; 215:1237–1239.
95. Perry EK, Tomlinson BE, Blessed Y, Bergmann K, Gibson PH, Perry RH. Correlation of cholinergic abnormalities with senile plaques and mental test scores in senile dementia. Br Med J 1978; 2:1457–1459.
96. Gottfries CG, Gottfries I, Roos BE. The investigation of homovanillic acid in the human brain and its correlation to senile dementia. Br J Psychiatry 1969; 115: 563–574.
97. Gottfries CG, Adolfsson R, Aquilonius SM, Carlsson A, Eckernäs SÅ, Nordberg A, Oreland L, Svennerholm L, Wiberg Å, Winblad B. Biochemical changes in dementia disorders of Alzheimer type (AD/SDAT). Neurobiol Aging 1983; 261–271.
98. Gottfries CG. Alzheimer's disease: a critical review. Compr Gerontol C 1988; 2:47–62.
99. Danysz W, Parsons C, Bresink I, Quack G. Glutamate in CNS disorders. Drug News Perspect 1995; 8:261–277.
100. Adolfsson R, Gottfries CG, Oreland L, Wiberg Å, Winblad B. Increased activity of brain and platelet monoamine oxidase in dementia of Alzheimer type. Life Sci 1980; 27:1029–1034.
101. Regland B, Gottfries CG, Oreland L. Vitamin B12-induced reduction of platelet monoamine oxidase activity in patients with dementia and pernicious anaemia. Eur Arch Psychiatry Clin Neurosci 1991; 240:288–291.
102. Gottfries CG, Frederiksen SO, Heilig M. Neuropeptides and Alzheimer's disease. Eur Neuropsychopharmacol 1995; 5:491–500.
103. Nyth AL, Gottfries CG. The clinical efficacy of citalopram in treatment of emotional disturbances in dementia disorders. A Nordic multicentre study. Br J Psychiatry 1990; 157:894–901.

104. Andersen G, Vestergaard K, Riis JO. Citalopram for post-stroke pathological crying. Lancet 1993; 342:837–839.
105. Andersen G, Vestergaard K, Lauritzen L. Effective treatment of post-stroke depression with the selective serotonin reuptake inhibitor citalopram. Stroke 1994; 25:1099–1104.
106. Gottfries CG, Blennow K, Karlsson I, Wallin A. The neurochemistry of vascular dementia. Dementia 1994; 5:163–167.

2
Pharmacokinetics of Psychotropic Drugs

David J. Greenblatt, Lisa L. von Moltke, and Richard I. Shader
Tufts University School of Medicine, and New England Medical Center, Boston, Massachusetts

The appropriate use of psychotropic drugs in the elderly assumes major importance in clinical medicine because emotional and psychiatric disorders are disproportionately prevalent in geriatric populations when compared to younger age groups (1–3). Older persons may respond uniquely to psychopharmacological treatment due to alterations in disease characteristics in aging, or because of age-related changes in drug sensitivity at the neuroreceptor site mediating drug action. Response to pharmacological treatment may also change in the elderly because of age-related alterations in pharmacokinetics.

Drug absorption, distribution, elimination, and clearance in elderly populations have been extensively studied during the past three decades (4–13). This chapter focuses on the principles of pharmacokinetics, alterations of drug disposition in the elderly, and implications for clinical psychopharmacology in the elderly.

I. PRINCIPLES OF PHARMACOKINETICS

A. Clearance

Clearance is an entity having units of volume divided by time (i.e., ml/min or l/h), that refers to the total amount of blood, serum, or plasma from which a substance is completely removed per unit time (14–18). Clearance may also be viewed as the rate of drug removal per unit of plasma concentration. Physicians and other health care professionals usually first encounter the principle of clearance in the context of renal function, in which creatinine clearance is used as an indicator of renal function. Assuming that creatinine, an endogenous substance, is completely cleared by the kidney, renal clearance of creatinine can be used to reflect glomerular filtration rate.

The same concept of clearance also applies to the removal of drugs and other foreign substances. Clearance is the single most reliable index of the capacity of a given patient to remove a given drug. For most clinically relevant drugs, hepatic biotransformation, renal excretion, or a combination of the two are the major mechanisms of clearance. For renally cleared drugs, a significant fraction of the administered drug is excreted unchanged in the urine. For drugs metabolized by the liver, biotransformation products may be recovered in the urine, but this does not mean that the parent drug undergoes renal clearance (Fig. 1).

Among psychotropic drugs, lithium is eliminated primarily by renal clearance (19,20), as are the hydroxylated metabolites of the cyclic antidepressants (21,22). Hepatic biotransformation accounts for clearance of essentially all other psychotropic drugs. Renal clearance of drugs excreted intact by the kidney is predictably related to age, since renal function on the average declines with increasing age (23,24). An age-related decline in clearance of lithium can therefore be anticipated. On the other hand, hepatic biotransformation of drugs is mediated by a number of enzyme systems whose activities are not predictably influenced by age (Fig. 2).

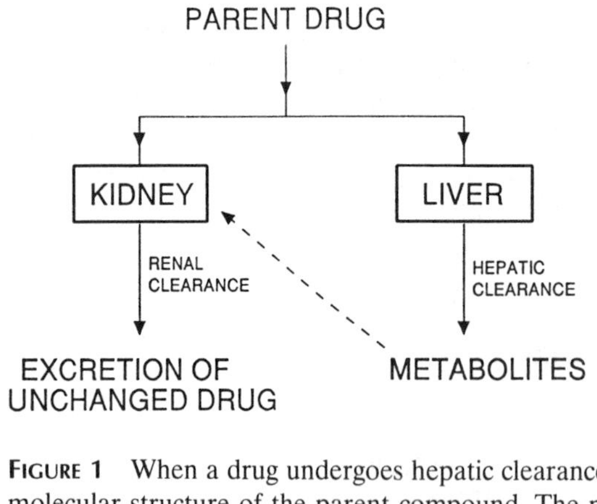

FIGURE 1 When a drug undergoes hepatic clearance, liver enzyme systems alter the molecular structure of the parent compound. The metabolites produced by hepatic biotransformation often appear in the systemic circulation and are excreted by the kidney (dashed line), but this does not imply renal clearance of the parent drug. When the parent drug undergoes renal clearance, a significant fraction of the dose is recovered in the urine in unchanged form.

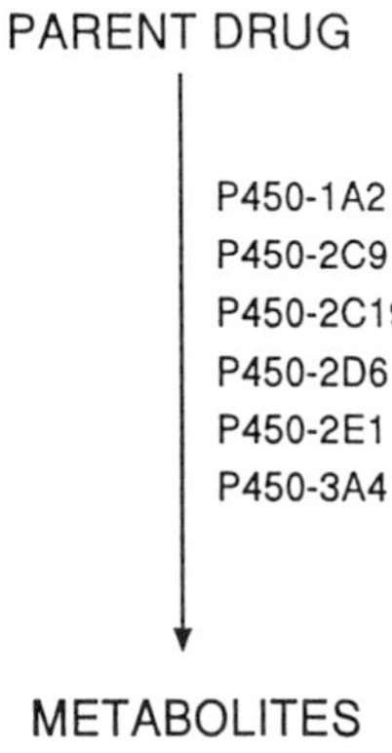

FIGURE 2 Cytochrome P450 enzymes most commonly involved in oxidative metabolism of drugs in humans.

Hepatic blood flow is the upper limit of clearance for drugs that are metabolized exclusively by the liver, since clearance cannot exceed the rate of drug delivery to the clearing organ. Hepatic blood flow in healthy individuals usually falls between 1500 and 1800 ml/min, although there is considerable individual variation, and no routinely available clinical test can be used for quantitation. Some studies suggest a decline in hepatic blood flow with age, but this is not clearly established.

The relation between drug clearance and hepatic blood flow has important clinical implications (15–18,25). Benzodiazepine derivatives (with the exception of triazolam and midazolam) and trazodone have low values of hepatic clearance (less than 20% of hepatic blood flow). First-pass metabolism or presystemic extraction of these drugs after oral dosage is relatively small, and absolute bioavailability after oral dosage usually exceeds 80%. For these low-clearance drugs, a reduction in hepatic clearance due to old age or a drug interaction will prolong elimination half-life, but have little effect on the peak plasma concentration after oral dosage. In contrast, most of the cyclic antidepressants, the selective serotonin reuptake inhibitor (SSRI) antidepressants, the "mixed" mechanism antidepressants nefazodone and venlafaxine, the benzodiazepine derivatives triazolam and midazolam, and antipsychotic agents have values of hepatic clearance greater than 40–50% of hepatic blood flow after oral administration. These drugs undergo substantial presystemic extraction, leaving a relatively small fraction that reaches the systemic circulation (Fig. 3). A reduction in hepatic clearance of such drugs may lead to a prolongation of half-life as well as an increase in the peak plasma concentration after oral dosage.

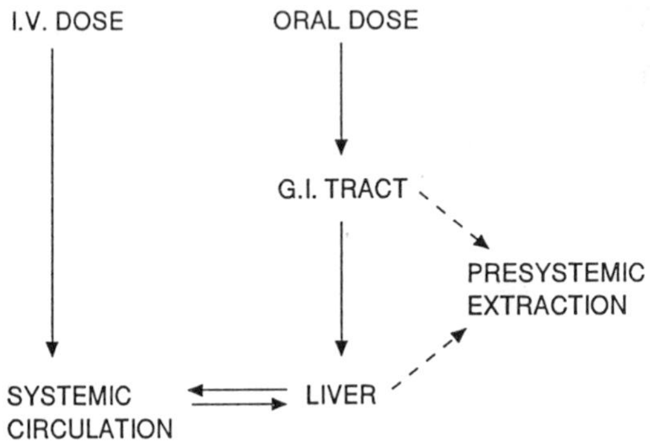

FIGURE 3 When a drug is given intravenously, the entire dose reaches the systemic circulation. However, after oral administration, a fraction of the dose may be metabolized by the gastrointestinal tract mucosa, by the liver during the "first pass," or both, prior to reaching the systemic circulation. This is collectively termed "presystemic extraction."

The predicted hepatic extraction ratio (ER) of a drug metabolized exclusively by the liver can be calculated as the ratio of clearance after intravenous dosage divided by hepatic blood flow. The maximum oral bioavailability administered dose (F) is calculated as:

$$F \leq 1 - \text{ER} \tag{1}$$

Thus, the greater a drug's intravenous clearance relative to hepatic blood flow, the lower is the maximum oral bioavailability. Significant amounts of human cytochrome P450-3A isoforms are present in gastrointestinal tract mucosa as well as liver (26). The gastrointestinal P450-3A component may contribute importantly to presystemic extraction of some psychotropic drugs (such as triazolam, midazolam, and nefazodone) that are biotransformed mainly by P450-3A isoforms (27). Since this component of clearance is largely bypassed after intravenous dosage, oral bioavailability of such drugs may be considerably below the maximum predicted by the extraction ratio using Eq. (1).

Clearance is the principal physiological determinant of steady-state plasma concentration (C_{ss}) during chronic administration. If a drug is given long enough for the steady-state to be reached, C_{ss} can be calculated as:

$$C_{ss} = \frac{\text{Dosing rate}}{\text{Clearance}} \tag{2}$$

Dosing rate is the "input" variable: the rate at which the drug is given to the patient. C_{ss} will theoretically increase in proportion to dosing rate in any given patient as long as clearance is constant. This assumes that *actual* dosing rate is equal to the *intended* dosing rate, and does not consider the possible influence of patient compliance. The denominator of this equation is clearance, which represents the capacity of that particular patient to eliminate the particular drug.

Clearance, which appears in the denominator, cannot be directly measured or predicted without actually giving that particular patient a test dose of the drug in question. If drug clearance declines with old age, C_{ss} will increase unless dosing rate is adjusted correspondingly (Fig. 4). Increases in C_{ss} may be associated with a greater likelihood of drug toxicity. For this reason, clearance is almost always a major focus of studies of altered drug disposition in the elderly.

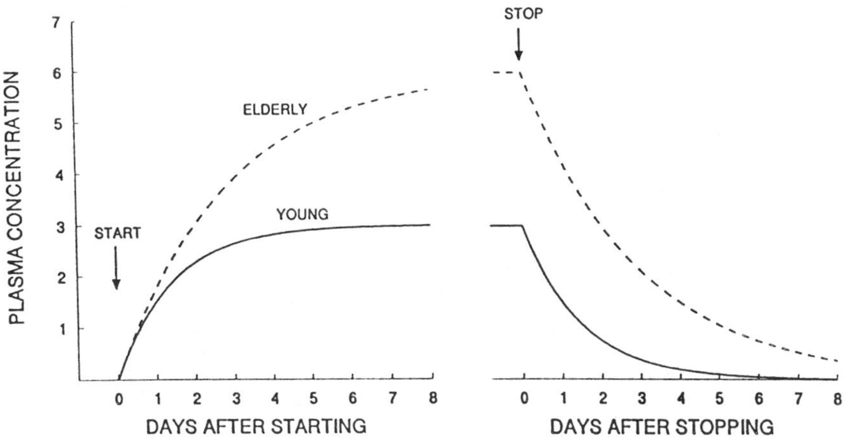

FIGURE 4 Effect of reduced clearance in old age on the rate and extent of drug accumulation during chronic dosage, and on the rate of elimination when treatment is stopped. In the young subject (solid line) it is assumed that $t_{1/2} = 1.0$ days. After initiation of a constant dosage regimen at time = 0 (arrow, left graph), the steady-state plasma concentration is 3.0 units, and approximately 4 days ($4 \times t_{1/2}$) are required for steady-state to be more than 90% attained. Assume the same volume of distribution and dosing rate, but a 50% lower value of clearance in an elderly subject. This results in an increased steady-state plasma concentration (6.0 units) as well as a longer time necessary to attain steady state (dashed line), since $t_{1/2}$ is prolonged to 2 days based on Eq. (4). When treatment is stopped (arrow, right graph), the time necessary for plasma concentrations to decline is similarly prolonged in the elderly subject.

B. Distribution

Drug distribution is determined by physicochemical properties: the drug's relative solubility in lipid as opposed to water (lipophilicity), its affinity for various body tissues, the blood flow to each of these tissues, and the drug's binding to plasma protein. Drug distribution is unrelated to and independent of clearance. For psychotropic drugs, only a small fraction of the total amount present in the body interacts with the specific neuroreceptor recognition site in the brain. Uptake of drug by peripheral sites, at which the drug is not pharmacologically active, will influence the amount that is available to specific binding sites in the brain.

The amount of adipose tissue relative to total body weight generally will increase as a person ages, while the fraction of lean body mass correspondingly decreases (28–31). This shift is not necessarily accompanied by a change in total body weight. The same pattern of age-related change will occur in both men and women, but, at any age, women have a higher fraction of body weight consisting of adipose tissue than do men. Since age and gender both influence body habitus (29), gender is a potential confounding factor in pharmacokinetic studies of the elderly.

Drug distribution can be quantitated using the pharmacokinetic concept of volume of distribution (V_d). This hypothetical quantity has units of volume (liters) and is defined as follows:

$$V_d = \frac{\text{Amount of drug in the body}}{\text{Concentration in reference compartment}} \tag{3}$$

The "reference compartment" usually refers to blood, serum, or plasma, and V_d therefore represents the amount of drug in the body divided by the blood or plasma concentration. Most psychotropic agents are lipophilic and have large values of V_d, indicating that the plasma concentration is small relative to the amount of drug in the body. For cyclic antidepressants, for example, the pharmacokinetic V_d may be ten or more times the size of the body, whereas hydrophilic drugs such as lithium will have values of V_d smaller than body size, indicating that a larger fraction of what is present in the body is found in blood, serum, or plasma. It must be emphasized that the pharmacokinetic V_d does not refer to the actual volume of any specific anatomical entity.

Pharmacokinetic V_d for many drugs will change with increasing age because of age-related changes in body habitus (7,29). V_d for lipophilic drugs generally is larger in elderly as compared to young subjects of the same gender, even when total body weight does not differ between groups. Conversely, V_d of hydrophilic drugs may be reduced in the elderly relative to young controls.

V_d and its potential changes with aging are of importance because elimination half-life depends on both V_d and clearance (see below). Furthermore, the duration of action of many lipophilic psychotropic drugs after single doses is dependent more on distribution than on elimination or clearance. The duration of action of some psychotropic drugs may theoretically change in the elderly as a consequence of a change in distribution, but this possibility has not been validated in controlled studies.

C. Elimination

Elimination half-life is used to quantitate the rate of drug disappearance in the postdistributive phase after a single dose, or after termination of multiple-dose treatment. The same half-life applies to the rate of attainment of steady state after initiation of multiple-dose therapy (without a loading dose), or the rate of attainment of a new steady-state condition if the maintenance dose is increased or decreased (Fig. 4). Elimination half-life is potentially misleading as a pharmacokinetic variable, because it is a dependent quantity related to V_d and clearance as follows:

$$\text{Elimination half-life} = \frac{0.693 \cdot V_d}{\text{Clearance}} \tag{4}$$

The intuitively logical inverse relationship of elimination half-life and clearance is valid only in situations when V_d is relatively constant, an assumption that may be incorrect when pharmacokinetic properties are being evaluated in relation to age. Since V_d or clearance, or both, may be affected by aging, elimination half-life cannot be a valid single index of the capacity for drug removal. The relationship of half-life to V_d is most evident in pharmacokinetic studies of lipophilic drugs in obese individuals, in which elimination half-life greatly increases in obese persons only because of their increased V_d rather than a difference in clearance (32–34).

D. Absorption

Structural and functional changes in the aging gastrointestinal tract are well recognized (35–39). Gastrointestinal cytochrome P450-3A isoforms may potentially change in content or activity with increasing age, although this has not been verified. Such observations have led to speculation that absorption of orally administered medications may be reduced and/or delayed in the elderly. However, systematic studies of drug absorption in old age fail to confirm this presumption. The rate and extent of absorption of several orally administered psychotropic medications are not importantly changed in elderly subjects when compared to young controls (Table 1).

TABLE 1 Psychotropic Drugs for Which the Rate and Extent of Absorption After Oral Dosage Is Uninfluenced by Age

Chlordiazepoxide
Diazepam
Lorazepam
Midazolam
Trazodone
Flumazenil

E. Protein Binding

Many psychotropic drugs are extensively bound to plasma protein. For some drugs, such as diazepam, the extent of binding is very high, with an unbound fraction of only 1–2% of the total concentration in plasma. Albumin and α_1-acid glycoprotein (AAG) are the two plasma proteins usually responsible for drug binding (40–45).

Drug binding to plasma protein may be reduced in old age, particularly for drugs bound to plasma albumin. Since albumin concentrations tend to decline with age (46), the extent of drug binding may also be reduced, leaving higher unbound fractions in plasma. Age-related changes in plasma binding of drugs bound to AAG are not clearly established (47).

It is often incorrectly assumed that reduced plasma binding of psychotropic drugs in the elderly produces increased amounts of unbound drug available for pharmacological action, and therefore a greater intensity of drug action. A drug's free fraction (FF) in plasma can be calculated as the free (unbound) concentration divided by total (free plus bound) concentration. This equation is arithmetically correct but biologically wrong (40). The biologically correct form of the equation is:

$$\text{Total concentration} = \frac{\text{Free concentration}}{\text{Free fraction}} \tag{5}$$

The independent variables are on the right side of the equation. FF is a physicochemical variable determined by the concentration of binding protein, the drug concentration, and the drug's affinity for the binding protein. Free concentration, in the numerator, is completely independent of FF, and depends on the dosing rate and the liver's capacity to remove the free drug, assuming that only the unbound drug is available for clearance. The dependent variable, on the left side of the equation, is total concentration. In a clinical situation with constant dosing rate and constant free clearance, free concentration is therefore constant. If plasma protein binding decreases (FF increases), total concentrations will fall. Thus a change in FF alone will influence total drug concentration, but by itself has no effect on either free concentration or the drug's pharmacological activity. Since most drug assays measure total rather than free concentration, interpretation of total concentrations may be influenced by changes in FF (40,48). In studies of clinical situations (such as old age) in which drug binding to plasma protein may be altered, FF must be measured to assure correct interpretation of pharmacokinetic data based on total (free plus bound) plasma concentrations.

II. PSYCHOTROPIC DRUG DISPOSITION IN OLD AGE

A. The Available Data Base

The pharmacokinetics of psychotropic drugs in elderly humans have been reviewed in prior publications. The data base is convincing in the case of benzodiazepine derivatives and buspirone (6,8). Reasonable data are also available for a number of cyclic antidepressants (49–52) and for trazodone (34), nefazodone (53,54), and venlafaxine (55). Some data are available for the SSRI antidepressants, although the information has been slow to reach the peer-reviewed medical literature. Data on the neuroleptic agents are sparse, largely due to ethical considerations in studies of normal volunteers, and difficulties with analytical methodology.

Most benzodiazepines are metabolized by microsomal oxidation, with cytochrome P450-3A4 identified as a major responsible cytochrome (Table 2). Most studies indicate impairment of clearance of these drugs in old age, particularly among men. For benzodiazepines metabolized by glucuronide conjugation, the data indicate that age has only a small effect on clearance. A similar conclusion can be drawn for nitrazepam, which is biotransformed by nitroreduction. Since clonazepam is metabolized by the same pathway, it can be expected that age would not greatly influence its clearance. However, this has not been studied, and it is reported that P450-3A isoforms may be involved in clonazepam metabolism.

Among cyclic antidepressants, clearance of imipramine (also mediated in part by P450-3A4) appears to be impaired in old age. Some data suggest that amitriptyline clearance may also be reduced in the elderly, but this is not consistently reported. Clearance of trazodone, nefazodone, and sertraline appears to be impaired in old age, particularly among men (34,53–56). For several other antidepressants, studies of age effects on clearance either are conflicting or are affected by methodological drawbacks that make definitive interpretation difficult (51).

TABLE 2 Psychotropic Drugs Whose Hepatic Clearance Is Impaired in Healthy Elderly Subjects

Alprazolam[a]
Adinazolam[a]
Bromazepam
Chlordiazepoxide
Clobazam
Desalkylflurazepam
Desmethyldiazepam
Diazepam[a]
Imipramine[a]
Loprazolam
Midazolam[a]
Nefazodone[a]
Sertraline
Trazodone
Triazolam[a]

[a]Established as probable substrates for cytochrome P450-3A isoforms.

Nortripytline, desipramine, venlafaxine, and several neuroleptics are primarily cleared by the 2D6 pathway. Although there are some conflicting data, there is a growing body of evidence to suggest that clearance of drugs metabolized by 2D6 is either not affected or minimally affected by age. Abernethy et al. (49) examined the pharmacokinetics of desipramine in normal volunteers. They found age had a minimal effect on the clearance of orally administered desipramine. Population studies of desipramine, including a sample of patients over 75 years of age (57), indicate no effect of age on the plasma concentration achieved (57–60). Although two studies of steady-state nortriptyline concentrations found blood levels increased with age (61,62), four others found no relationship between age and nortriptyline levels (63–66). In addition, in the oldest sample reported (67), Katz et al. found that the mean dose necessary to reach a level of 100 ng/ml, in patients 80 years and older, was 80 mg/day, a dose similar to that needed in younger patients. Finally, studies of dextromethorphan, a substrate of 2D6, suggest no significant differences in the clearance of this agent in older subjects (68). Although questions remain, these findings contradict the view that clearance necessarily declines with age. Rather, there appear to be differences between drugs and differences between their metabolic pathways with respect to how they are affected by age. This has important clinical implications. For some drugs, dose reduction may

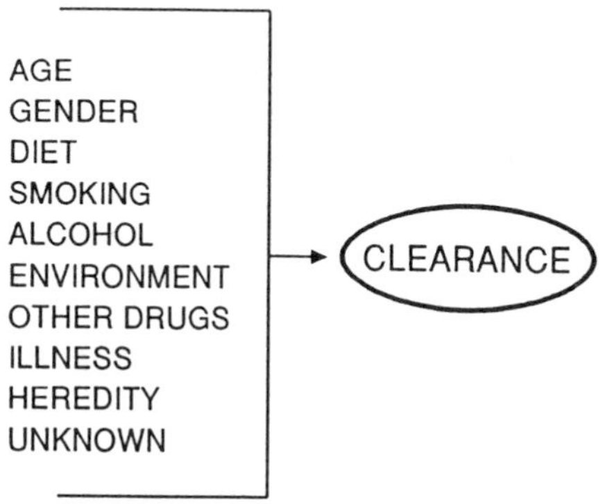

FIGURE 5 Factors that may contribute to individual variation in clearance of drugs.

be necessary in the elderly. For others, usual doses will be required to reach plasma concentrations similar to those in younger patients.

B. Issues of Research Design in Drug Development

Many psychotropic drugs marketed prior to the mid-1970s were released for clinical use with essentially no data available on pharmacokinetics and pharmacodynamics in geriatric populations which, in fact, might comprise one of the groups at highest risk for the target disorder. As an example, the benzodiazepine derivative diazepam became available for general clinical use in the early 1960s, but data on pharmacokinetics in the elderly were first published in the mid-1970s (6,8). With the evolution of industrial and regulatory approaches to drug development, pharmacogeriatric studies have now become a standard aspect of the development process. However, a consensus on how the topic should be studied unfortunately has not emerged along with the understanding of how important the topic is. A typically designed study might include a single-dose or multiple-dose protocol (or both) in groups of young male, young female, elderly male, and elderly female populations. Resources, time, and patience are usually stretched to the limit with sample sizes of 12 per cell. Even when adequate statistical power can be demonstrated, a negative study (i.e., no significant effect of age on clearance) may not lead to a confident assertion that clearance of the compound is uninfluenced by age in the general population. The literature contains a disquieting number of inconsistencies, even among similarly designed studies of the same drug. It is possible that studies aimed at evaluating "age" as the principal source of variance are actually overlooking other more important sources of variance (Fig. 5). Until such phenomena are more completely understood, outcomes of small-sample pharmacogeriatric studies should be generalized only with reservation.

ACKNOWLEDGMENTS

The authors are grateful for the collaboration and assistance of Jerold S. Harmatz. Supported by Grants MH-34223, DA-05258, MH-19924, MH-01237, and RR-00054 from the Department of Health and Human Services.

REFERENCES

1. Blazer D. Depression in the elderly. N Engl J Med 1989; 320:164–166.
2. Regier DA, Boyd JH, Burke JD, Rae DS, Myers JK, Kramer M, Robins LN, George LK, Karno M, Locke BZ. One-month prevalence of mental disorders in the United States. Arch Gen Psychiatry 1988; 45:977–986.
3. Uhlenhuth EH, Balter MB, Mellinger GD, Cisin IH, Clinthorne J. Symptom checklist syndromes in the general population: correlations with psychotherapeutic drug use. Arch Gen Psychiatry 1983; 40:1167–1173.
4. Durnas C, Loi C-M, Cusack BJ. Hepatic drug metabolism and aging. Clin Pharmacokinet 1990; 19:359–389.
5. Greenblatt DJ, Abernethy DR, Shader RI. Pharmacokinetic aspects of drug therapy in the elderly. Ther Drug Monit 1986; 8:249–255.
6. Greenblatt DJ, Harmatz JS, Shader RI. Clinical pharmacokinetics of anxiolytics and hypnotics in the elderly: therapeutic considerations. Clin Pharmacokinet 1991; 21:165–177, 262–273.
7. Greenblatt DJ, Sellers EM, Shader RI. Drug disposition in old age. N Engl J Med 1982; 306:1081–1088.
8. Greenblatt DJ, Shader RI, Harmatz JS. Implications of altered drug disposition in the elderly: studies of benzodiazepines. J Clin Pharmacol 1989; 29:866–872.
9. Loi C-M, Vestal RE. Drug metabolism in the elderly. Pharmacol Ther 1988; 36: 131–149.
10. Montamat SC, Cusack BJ, Vestal RE. Management of drug therapy in the elderly. N Engl J Med 1989; 321:303–309.
11. Schmucker DL. Aging and drug disposition: an update. Pharmacol Rev 1985; 37: 133–148.
12. Thompson TL, Moran MG, Nies AS. Psychotropic drug use in the elderly. N Engl J Med 1983; 308:134–138, 194–199.
13. Tumer N, Scarpace PJ, Lowenthal DT. Geriartric pharmacology: basic and clinical considerations. Annu Rev Pharmacol Toxicol 1992; 32:271–302.
14. Greenblatt DJ. Pharmacokinetic principles in clinical practice (Clinical Therapeutic Conference). J Clin Pharmacol 1992; 32:118–123.
15. Greenblatt DJ. Presystemic extraction: mechanisms and consequences. J Clin Pharmacol 1993; 33:650–656.

16. Greenblatt DJ, Koch-Weser J. Clinical pharmacokinetics. N Engl J Med 1975; 293:702–705, 964–970.
17. Wilkinson GR. Clearance approaches in pharmacology. Pharmacol Rev 1987; 39: 1–47.
18. Wilkinson GR, Shand DG. A physiological approach to hepatic drug clearance. Clin Pharmacol Ther 1975; 18:377–390.
19. Hardy BG, Shulman KI, MacKenzie SE, Kutcher SP, Silverberg JD. Pharmacokinetics of lithium in the elderly. J Clin Psychopharmacol 1987; 7:153–158.
20. Hewick DS, Newbury P, Hopwood S, Naylor G, Moody J. Age as a factor affecting lithium therapy. Br J Clin Pharmacol 1977; 4:201–205.
21. Nordin C, Bertilsson L. Active hydroxymetabolites of antidepressants: emphasis on E-10-hydroxy-nortriptyline. Clin Pharmacokinet 1995; 28:26–40.
22. Young RC. Hydroxylated metabolites of antidepressants. Psychopharmacol Bull 1991; 27:521–532.
23. Lindeman RD. Changes in renal function with aging: implications for treatment. Drugs Aging 1992; 2:423–431.
24. Nicoll SR, Sainsbury R, Bailey RR, King A, Frampton C, Elliot JR, Turner JG. Assessment of creatinine clearance in healthy subjects over 65 hears of age. Nephron 1991; 59:621–625.
25. Greenblatt DJ, von Moltke LL, Shader RI. The importance of presystemic extraction in clinical psychopharmacology. J Clin Psychopharmacol 1996; 16:417–419.
26. Watkins PB. Drug metabolism by cytochromes P450 in the liver and small bowel. Gastrointest Clin North Am 1992; 21:511–526.
27. Paine MF, Shen DD, Kunze KL, Perkins JD, Marsh CL, McVicar JP, Barr DM, Gillies BS, Thummel KE. First-pass metabolism of midazolam by the human intestine. Clin Pharmacol Ther 1996; 60:14–24.
28. Barlett HL, Puhl SM, Hodgson JL, Buskirk ER. Fat-free mass in relation to stature: ratios of fat-free mass to height in children, adults, and elderly subjects. Am J Clin Nutr 1991; 53:1112–1116.
29. Greenblatt DJ, Divoll M, Abernethy DR, Shader RI. Physiologic changes in old age: relation to altered drug disposition. J Am Geriatr Soc 1982; 30(Nov. suppl): s6–s10.
30. Schwartz RS, Shuman WP, Bradbury VL, Cain KC, Fellingham GW, Beard JC, Kahn SE, Stratton JR, Cerqueira MD, Abrass IB. Body fat distribution in healthy young and older men. J Gerontol 1990; 45:M181–185.
31. Shimokata H, Tobin JD, Muller DC, Elahi D, Coon PJ, Andres R. Studies in the distribution of body fat: I. Effects of age, sex, and obesity. J Gerontol 1989; 44: M66–73.
32. Abernethy DR, Greenblatt DJ. Pharmacokinetics of drugs in obesity. Clin Pharmacokinet 1982; 7:108–124.
33. Abernethy DR, Greenblatt DJ. Drug disposition in obese humans: an update. Clin Pharmacokinet 1986; 11:199–213.
34. Greenblatt DJ, Friedman H, Burstein ES, Scavone JM, Blyden GT, et al. Trazodone kinetics: effect of age, gender, and obesity. Clin Pharmacol Ther 1987; 42: 193–200.
35. Evans MA, Triggs EJ, Cheung M, Broe GA, Creasy H. Gastric empyting rate in the elderly: implications for drug therapy. J Am Geriatr Soc 1981; 29:201–205.

36. Geokas MC, Haverback BJ. The aging gastrointestinal tract. Am J Surg 1969; 117: 881–892.
37. Holt PR, Balint JA. Effects of aging on intestinal lipid absorption. Am J Physiol 1993; 264:G1–G6.
38. Horowitz M, Maddern GJ, Chatterton BE, Collins PJ, Harding PE, Shearman DJC. Changes in gastric emptying rates with age. Clin Sci 1984; 67:213–218.
39. Moore JG, Tweedy C, Christian PE, Datz FL. Effect of age on gastric emptying of liquid-solid meals in man. Dig Dis Sci 1983; 28:340–344.
40. Greenblatt DJ, Sellers EM, Koch-Weser J. Importance of protein binding for the interpretation of serum or plasma drug concentrations. J Clin Pharmacol 1982; 22: 259–263.
41. Koch-Weser J, Sellers EM. Binding of drugs to serum albumin. N Engl J Med 1976; 294:311–316, 526–531.
42. Rothschild MA, Oratz M, Schreiber SS. Serum albumin. Hepatology 1988; 8:385–401.
43. Salive ME,Cornoni-Huntley J, Phillips CL, Guralnik JM, Cohen HJ, Ostfeld AM, Wallace RB. Serum albumin in older persons: relationship with age and health status. J Clin Epidemiol 1992; 45:213–221.
44. du Souich P, Verges J, Erill S. Plasma protein binding and pharmacological response. Clin Pharmacokinet 1993; 24:435–440.
45. Wood M. Plasma drug binding: implications for anesthesiologists. Anesth Analg 1986; 65:786–804.
46. Greenblatt DJ. Reduced serum albumin concentration in the elderly: a report from the Boston Collaborative Drug Surveillance Program. J Am Geriatr Soc 1979; 27:20–22.
47. Abernethy DR, Kerzner L. Age effects on alpha-1-acid glycoprotein concentration and imipramine plasma protein binding. J Am Geriatr Soc 1984; 32: 705–708.
48. Friedman H, Greenblatt DJ. Rational therapeutic drug monitoring. J Am Med Assoc 1986; 256:2227–2233.
49. Abernethy DR, Greenblatt DJ, Shader RI. Imipramine and desipramine disposition in the elderly. J Pharmacol Exp Ther 1985; 232:183–188.
50. Benetello P, Furlanut M, Zara G, Baraldo M. Imipramine pharmacokinetics in depressed geriatric patients. Int J Clin Pharmacol Res 1990; 10:191–195.
51. von Moltke LL, Greenblatt DJ, Shader RI. Clinical pharmacokinetics of antidepressants in the elderly: therapeutic implications. Clin Pharmacokinet 1993; 24: 141–160.
52. Furlanut M, Benetello P. The pharmacokinetics of tricyclic antidepressant drugs in the elderly. Pharmacol Res 1990; 22:15–25.
53. Barbhaiya RH, Shukla UA, Greene DS. Single-dose pharmacokinetics of nefazodone in healthy young and elderly subjects and in subjects with renal or hepatic impairment. Eur J Clin Pharmacol 1995; 49:221–228.
54. Barbhaiya RH, Buch AB, Greene DS. A study of the effect of age and gender on the pharmacokinetics of nefazodone after single and multiple doses. J Clin Psychopharmacol 1996; 16:19–25.

55. Klamerus KJ, Parker VD, Rudolph RL, Derivan AT, Chiang ST. Effects of age and gender on venlafaxine and O-desmethylvenlafaxine pharmacokinetics. Pharmacother 1996; 16:915–923.
56. Ronfeld RA, Tremaine LM, Wilner KD. Pharmacokinetics of sertraline and its N-demethyl metabolite in elderly and young male and female volunteers. Clin Pharmacokinet 1997; 32(suppl 1):22–30.
57. Nelson JC, Mazure CM, Jatlow PI. Desipramine treatment of major depression in patients over 75 years of age. J Clin Psychopharmacol 1995; 15:99–105.
58. Nelson JC, Jatlow PI, Mazure CM. Desipramine plasma levels and response in elderly melancholics. J Clin Psychopharmacol 1985; 217–220.
59. Cutler NR, Zavadil AP, Eisdorfer C, Ross RJ, Potter WZ. Concentrations of desipramine in elderly women. Am J Psychiatry 1981; 138:1235–1237.
60. Amsterdam JD, Brunswick DJ, Potter L, Winokur A, Rickels K. Desipramine and 2-hydroxydesipramine plasma levels in endogenous depressed patients. Arch Gen Psychiatry 1985; 42:361–364.
61. Dawling S, Crome P, Heyer EJ, Lewis RR. Nortriptyline therapy in elderly patients: dosage prediction from plasma concentration at 24 hours after a single 50 mg dose. Br J Psychiatry 1981; 139:413–416.
62. Kragh-Sorensen P, Larsen NE. Factors influencing nortriptyline steady-state kinetics: plasma and saliva levels. Clin Pharmacol Ther 1980; 28:796–803.
63. Smith RC, Reed K, Leelavathi DE, et al. Pharmacokinetics and the effects of nortriptyline in geriatric depressed patients. Psychopharmacol Bull 1980; 16:54–57.
64. Ziegler VE, Biggs JT. Tricyclic plasma levels: effect of age, race, sex, and smoking. J Am Med Assoc 1977; 238:2167–2169.
65. Bertilsson L, Mellstrom B, Sjoqvist F. Pronounced inhibition of noradrenaline uptake by 10-hydroxy metabolites of nortriptyline. Life Sci 1979; 25:1285–1292.
66. Young RC, Alexopoulos GS, Shamoian CA, Manley MW, Dhar AK, Kutt H. Plasma 10-hydroxy-nortriptyline in elderly depressed patients. Clin Pharmacol Ther 1984; 35:540–544.
67. Katz IR, Simpson GM, Jethanandani V, Cooper T, Muhly C. Steady state pharmacokinetics of nortriptyline in the frail elderly. Neuropsychopharmacology 1989; 2:229–236.
68. Laurent-Kenesi MA, Jacqz-Aigrain E, LeJonc JL, Jaillon P, Funck-Brentano C. Assessment of CYP 2D6 activity in very elderly healthy subjects. Fund Clin Pharmacol 1996; 10:158–159.

3
Drug Interactions

Bruce G. Pollock
University of Pittsburgh Medical Center, Pittsburgh, Pennsylvania

Patients older than age 65 represent 12% of the U.S. population, yet they receive from 25 to 35% of all prescription drugs (1). Studies from a variety of settings have estimated that those over 65 years of age receive from two to six prescription drugs (2). Moreover, those patients who reside in the community consume additional quantities of over-the-counter medicines, for which estimates range from one to four items (3,4). The health problems of older patients may lead not only to increased use of medication, but also may cause physiological alterations (e.g., reduced renal function), that will also lower the threshold for a drug interaction. Nonetheless, the incidence of adverse drug reactions increases exponentially with the number of medications prescribed; this is most clearly due to the increased likelihood of drug–drug interactions (5).

A drug–drug interaction occurs when the coadministration of a second drug alters the pharmacological effect of one or both drugs. The consequences of an interaction could be either an increase or a decrease in the magnitude or duration of a drug's action. There are two general categories of interactions: pharmacokinetic and pharmacodynamic; the former affects drug concentration and the latter impacts on the relationship of drug concentration to response.

It is important to appreciate the limits of achieving knowledge of drug interactions. Much of this information is derived from uncontrolled observations in one or two patients who were treated with complicated medication regimens, and whose renal and hepatic function were not characterized. When a formal pharmacokinetic interaction study is done, typically in young, healthy volunteers, single doses or short-term dosing strategies are utilized. This leaves open the question of chronic treatment in medically compromised older patients. Even when a statistically significant interaction is found in a rigorous pharmacokinetic study, the underlying clinical implications must always be clarified. One schema attempts to reserve the term "established" only for those rare interactions that have been substantiated by well-controlled studies. More common designations range from "probable," through "suspected" and "possible," to "doubtful."

Recently, information has been gleaned from both in vitro and in vivo studies concerning metabolism of psychotropics by specific P450 isozymes and their inhibition by commonly prescribed medications. This has permitted the development of a rudimentary structure for rationalizing and anticipating some drug–metabolic interactions, but here it is also important to discern the sources of information (i.e., whether in vitro microsomal experiments, case reports, or pharmacokinetic experiments in well-characterized subjects) (6,7).

The intention of this chapter is to provide an organizing framework toward understanding psychopharmacological drug interactions in an older population, rather than an exhaustive list of potential interactions. For more detailed information, the reader is encouraged to consult several excellent texts (8,9). Moreover, the Medical Letter and Physicians GenRx have very helpful computerized compendia of interactions.

I. PHARMACOKINETIC INTERACTIONS

Pharmacokinetics provides a way of describing and predicting drug concentrations in plasma and various tissues over time. A pharmacokinetic drug interaction is said to occur when the absorption, distribution, metabolism, or elimination of one drug is affected by another, with a resulting significant change in drug concentration. In general, interactions that reduce the clearance of medications with narrow therapeutic indices, such as cardiac antiarrhythmics, anticoagulants, lithium, or tricyclic antidepressants, are of greatest concern.

A. Absorption

Clinicians should be aware of the potential for antacids, high-fiber supplements, and the cholesterol binding resin, cholestyramine, to diminish significantly the absorption of some medications. A notable exception is warfarin absorption, which is enhanced by magnesium- but not aluminum-containing antacids. Drugs with anticholinergic properties may decrease absorption of L-dopa, due to delayed gastric emptying in conjunction with the gastric metabolism of L-dopa (10). Food has variable effects on the bioavailability of psychotropics, but these are rarely of clinical significance (11). A possible exception is sertraline, whose bioavailability is increased by 20 to 40% when taken concomitantly with food (12). Given the propensity of older patients to develop Parkinsonism at higher doses of sertraline, this enhanced bioavailability may be relevant.

B. Distribution

The majority of psychotropics are transported in the blood extensively bound to plasma proteins such as albumin, alpha-1-acidglycoprotein and lipoproteins. Typically, more than 90% of the total drug in plasma is bound. Fluvoxamine and venlafaxine are notable exceptions to this general rule, being 80% and 27% bound, respectively. Drug displacement interactions were previously the subject of considerable concern because the protein-bound drug acts as an enormous, pharmacologically inactive reservoir. It is not recognized that not only is free drug pharmacologically active, but also is more available for metabolism and tissue distribution. An increase in the absolute concentration of free drug, such as by reduction in plasma proteins, or a displacement interaction would be immediately buffered and a new equilibrium rapidly established (13,14). Thus, it is now considered unlikely that protein-binding-mediated changes alone are responsible for clinically important interactions. However, when plasma drug monitoring is used to adjust tricyclic antidepressant or anticonvulsant doses, it should be appreciated that the total drug concentrations (free plus protein bound) are usually reported. Although a change in absolute drug concentration caused by a change in protein binding is transient, the new equilibrium in the proportion of bound and free drug may appear as an alteration in the drug's plasma level. In practice, this might be of concern if a severe intercurrent illness resulted in increased alpha-1-acidglycoprotein in patients who were well maintained on a monitored medication. In these circumstances, an increase in bound drug might be interpreted as an increase in the drug's plasma level (15). The use of unbound drug levels in these situations has been found to be useful for lidocaine, theophylline, phenytoin, and digitoxin.

C. Metabolism

The purpose of drug metabolism is to transform lipid-soluble compounds into more water-soluble derivatives that can be more effectively eliminated and may be less active pharmacodynamically. Biotransformation of drugs is categorized as belonging to either phase I (oxidation or reduction) or phase II (conjugation). A large group of heme-containing enzymes, collectively called cytochrome P450, is responsible for oxidative (phase 1) drug metabolism.

Cytochrome P450 is really a family of enzymes that vary in substrate preferences. With the use of monoclonal antibodies and molecular biological techniques, our capacity to identify unique forms of these enzymes has vastly outstripped knowledge of substrate metabolism. Moreover, utilization of this knowledge is still on the periphery of clinical application. At least 16 human P450 isoenzymes have been identified, each with distinct, although partly overlapping, substrate specificity. There are four families defined by a 40% amino acid sequence homology in the peptide chains of the isoenzyme protein molecules; a subfamily is determined by a 60% sequence homology (16). As more is learned about both the diversity and specificity of the cytochrome P450 enzymes, a structure is emerging for categorizing potential drug–drug interactions.

A drug may act as a substrate for one cytochrome P450 at a time or simultaneously for more than one. A drug can act as both a substrate and a competitive inhibitor for the same isozyme or it can act as a noncompetitive inhibitor for a different enzyme. Individual, genetically mediated variation in baseline metabolic capacity may be an important, currently unexplored variable affecting interactions. For example, among 90% of the population with active CYP 2D6, the range of activity can vary 40-fold.

Some inhibitors such as quinidine, cimetidine, fluoxetine, or sertraline are not necessarily metabolized by the P450s they inhibit. Conversely, if a drug inhibits the P450 predominantly responsible for its own metabolism (e.g., paroxetine, perphenazine, or desipramine), it is a good candidate for nonlinear pharmacokinetics. This means that the reaction ceases to be "first order" and that the proportionality between therapeutic doses and plasma levels will be lost, making dosage adjustments according to plasma level monitoring unpredictable. For example, if the dose of desipramine is tripled, its plasma level may increase 14-fold (17).

Quantitatively, most of the hepatic P450 is made up of isozymes of the 3A and 2C families, which account for 30% and 20%, respectively, of the total P450 content (18). Although cytochrome P450 (CYP) 2D6 comprises only 2% of the total P450 content, it is essential for the metabolism of antidepressants, neuroleptics, and several antiarrhythmics (Table 1). To date, there are few substrates associated with CYP 2E1, although it is inducible by alcohol and may play a role in alcoholic and acetaminophen-induced liver disease (19). Chronic, but not acute, alcohol intake will increase the metabolism of several psychotropics possibly through its inductive effects on CYP 2E1 (20).

CYP 2D6

About 5–10% of the population are genetically poor 2D6 metabolizers, who completely lack CYP 2D6 activity and will be unaffected by inhibitors of this enzyme. Older patients who are poor 2D6 metabolizers have been shown to be at increased risk of neuroleptic side effects when treated with fixed doses of perphenazine (21). In the rest of the population who are extensive metabolizers, many commonly used drugs will competitively or noncompetitively inhibit this enzyme. Table 2 identifies inhibitors or inducers of P450; it should be noted that CYP 2D6 is a high-affinity/low-capacity enzyme. This means that it is particularly likely to be saturated and inhibited by higher concentrations of a drug or by multiple substrates. Patients taking antidepressants, neuroleptics, quinidine, diltiazem, diphenhydramine, cimetidine, and fluoxetine have been shown to have significantly slower 2D6 metabolism. All selective serotonin reuptake inhibitors (SSRIs) (excepting fluvoxamine and venlafaxine) may also inhibit 2D6. Conversely, the SSRIs differ in their capacity to inhibit the other important drug-metabolizing enzymes (7). For example, fluoxetine and fluvoxamine may cause substantial inhibition of CYP 3A4. One study found that 2D6 inhibition is significant in patients prescribed neuroleptic drugs (i.e., 40% of subjects taking antipsychotics were found to be poor 2D6 metabolizers) (22). Another report noted that the combination of SSRIs with tricyclics may result in toxic elevations in tricyclic blood levels (23).

Although CYP 2D6 itself is noninducible, sometimes the induction of other isoenzymes such as 3A4, 1A2, or 2E1 will result in enhanced clearance of substrates that are usually more specifically metabolized by 2D6. For example, phenobarbital treatment will reduce desipramine bioavailability by approximately 40% (24).

While work so far suggests 2D6 is not affected by age alone, the fact that drug concentrations for many antidepressants and antipsychotics are clearly tied to 2D6 function, coupled with the fact that this enzyme is so potently inhibited by many drugs prescribed in later life, makes this enzyme a key locus for interactions in geriatric psychopharmacology (25). Although inhibition of 2D6 may increase the risk of drug toxicity, there are also examples of therapeutic potentiation when tricyclics and SSRIs are combined (26).

An interesting example of loss of therapeutic effect, caused by metabolic inhibition, is provided by codeine. The metabolism of codeine to morphine by o-demethylation is dependent on CYP 2D6. Codeine exerts its analgesic action predominantly through morphine and has been rendered an ineffective analgesic when 2D6 is selectively inhibited by quinidine (27).

CYP 2C9 and 19

CYP 2C19 contributes to the demethylation of tertiary tricyclic antidepressants and diazepam as well as the oxidation of desmethyldiazepam, omeprazole, propranolol, and several barbiturates. Phenytoin, tolbutamide, and warfarin are metabolized by CYP 2C9. Metabolic interactions are theoretically possible among combinations of these medications. Of particular importance are possible interactions with warfarin involving the 2C9 isozyme.

TABLE 1 Oxidative Metabolism Associated with Specific P450s

P450 2D6	P450 1A2
Antidepressants	Antidepressants
Desipramine	Fluvoxamine
Nortriptyline	Amitriptyline } Demethylation
Amitriptyline } Hydroxylation	Clomipramine } Demethylation
Clomipramine } Hydroxylation	Imipramine } Demethylation
Imipramine } Hydroxylation	
Fluoxetine/norfluoxetine	Antipsychotics
Maprotiline	Clozapine
Mianserin	Haloperidol
Paroxetine	
Trazodone	Miscellaneous
m-CPP (metabolite of Trazodone and nefazodone)	Tacrine
Venlafaxine	Caffeine
	Theophylline
	Phenacetin
Antipsychotics	Warfarin (R-enantiomer)
Haloperidol	
Perphenazine	
Risperidone	
Thioridazine	
Cardiovascular	
Type 1C antiarrhythmics: (encainide, flecainide, propafenone)	
β-Blockers: (alprenolol, metoprolol, propranolol, timolol)	
Miscellaneous	
Codeine	
Dextromethorphan	

P450 3A3-4		P450 2C19/9	
Antidepressants		Antidepressants	
Nefazodone		Citalopram	
Sertraline		Moclobemide	
Amitriptyline		Amitriptyline	
Clomipramine	Demethylation	Clomipramine	Demethylation
Imipramine		Imipramine	
Benzodiazepines		Benzodiazepines	
Alprazolam		Diazepam	
Midazolam		Desmethyldiazepam	
Triazolam			
Zolpidem		Anticonvulsants	
		Phenytoin	
Antihistamines		Mephenytoin	
Astemizole		Methobarbital	
Loratadine		Hexobarbital	
Terfenadine			
		Miscellaneous	
Cardiovascular		Omeprazole	
Amiodarone		Proguanil	
Diltiazem		Propranolol	
Lidocaine		Tolbutamide	
Nifedipine		Warfarin (S-enantiomer)	
Nimodipine			
Quinidine			
Verapamil			
Endocrine			
Dexamethasone			
Estrogens			
Tamoxifen			
Testosterone			
Anticonvulsants			
Carbamazepine			
Ethosuximide			
Immunosuppressants			
Cyclosporine			
Tacrolimus			
Miscellaneous			
Cisapride			
Erythromycin			
Lovastatin			
Vinblastine			

TABLE 2 Potent Inhibitors or (Inducers) of Specific P450s

P450 2D6	P450 1A2	P450 3A3-4	P450 2C19/2C9
Chlorpromazine	Clozapine	Barbiturates (inducers)	Fluvoxamine
Desipramine	Fluvoxamine	Carbamazepine (inducer)	Fluoxetine
Diltiazem	Theophylline	Cimetidine	Norethindrone
Fluoxetine/norfluoxetine	Smoking (inducer)	Desmethylsertraline	Omeprazole
Fluphenazine	Criciferous vegetables (inducers)	Dexamethasone (inducer)	Proguanil
Haloperidol	Omeprazole (inducer)	Clarithromycin	Sertraline
Labetalol		Diltiazem	Tenoposide
Lobeline		Erythromycin	
Methadone		Fluconazole	
Moclobemide		Fluoxetine	
Paroxetine		Fluvoxamine	
Perphenazine		Grapefruit juice	
Propafenone		Itraconazole	
Quinidine		Ketoconazole	
Sertraline/desmethylsertraline		Nefazodone	
Thioridazine		Norfluoxetine	
		Oral contraceptives	
		Phenytoin-acute	
		Phenytoin-chronic (inducer)	
		Rifampicin (inducer)	
		Sertraline	
		Trazodone	
		Troleoandomycin	
		Verapamil	
		Vinca alkaloids	

CYP 3A3/4

CYP 3A3 and 3A4 have been found to be essentially homologous and are therefore referred to as CYP 3A3/4. CYP 3A3/4 is responsible for the metabolism of numerous medications including lidocaine, diltiazem, verapamil, quinidine, erythromycin, triazolam, alprazolam, cisapride, and terfenadine (28). Interestingly, grapefruit juice is a potent inhibitor of CYP 3A3/4 and has been shown to raise triazolam plasma levels (29).

There has been substantial recent interest in the effects of the new serotonergic antidepressants on 3A3/4. Venlafaxine has no appreciable effects on this isoenzyme (30). Paroxetine, sertraline, fluoxetine (via its demethylated metabolite), and fluvoxamine have modest effects on 3A3/4, with increasing inhibition in the order shown (31). It is unclear if the magnitude of these effects is sufficient to be clinically significant. There are as yet only two case reports of interactions of fluoxetine or sertraline with terfenadine (32,33). von Moltke and colleagues have estimated the effects of the SSRIs on terfenadine clearance based on their in vitro affinity for 3A3/4 and their concentrations at different doses (34). Paroxetine 30 mg/day is estimated to decrease terfenadine clearance 21%, fluoxetine 20 mg/day and sertraline 100 mg/day decrease clearance 44%, and fluvoxamine 300 mg/day results in a 48% decrease. Because terfenadine reaches dangerous levels after a 93% decrease in clearance, von Moltke suggests the SSRIs are not likely to cause a significant interaction with terfenadine. Nonetheless, serious events have occurred when CYP 3A4-mediated clearance of terfenadine, astemizole, and cisapride is diminished (35). This would suggest the need for considerable caution when coprescribing these medications with known inhibitors of CYP 3A3/4. Nefazodone is a more potent inhibitor of CYP 3A3/4 than the SSRIs, but is still less potent than ketoconazole (36). Estimates of the effects of nefazodone on terfenadine have not yet been reported and, until they are, it would be prudent to avoid their concomitant use.

Psychiatrists are likely to encounter the concurrent use of the SSRIs with the triazolo benzodiazepines (alprazolam, triazolam, and midazolam). Clinical effects will depend on the magnitude of the interaction. The SSRIs have modest effects on the plasma concentrations of these rapidly metabolized benzodiazepines in the order described above (venlafaxine < paroxetine < sertraline < fluoxetine (via its demethylated metabolite) < fluvoxamine) (31). Nefazodone will have a greater effect. In one report, nefazodone at 200 mg b.i.d. raised steady-state alprazolam levels twofold (37).

If one of the 3A3/4-inhibiting antidepressants is used, loratidine may be a safer alternative for the nonsedating antihistamines, and metocopramide may be used instead of cisapride. An active metabolite of trazodone and nefazodone, generated by 3A3/4, is metachlorophenylpiperazine (m-CPP) which has anxiogenic properties. Since m-CPP undergoes further metabolism by CYP 2D6, potential interactions at this locus may be of concern.

Carbamazepine is both a substrate and an inducer of CYP 3A3/4 and will thus increase its own metabolism, a process referred to as autoinduction. If two inducers of the same isozyme are coprescribed (e.g., phenytoin and phenobarbital), the inducer that undergoes more rapid metabolism (i.e., phenobarbital) will induce the metabolism of the other drug. Since induction involves the synthesis of a new enzyme, its effects evolve more slowly than with inhibitory interactions and may persist even longer. When an inhibitor is prescribed, its effects are usually apparent in 3 to 5 days, roughly corresponding to attainment of its steady-state concentration. In contrast, the effects of an inducing drug, such as carbamazepine, may not become maximal for 10 days. Moreover, carbamazepine's induction of 3A4 may persist for 3 to 4 weeks after its discontinuation.

CYP 1A2

Fluvoxamine is unusual among antidepressants in that it inhibits CYP 1A2, raising the potential for significant interactions with theophylline and tacrine. CYP 1A2, which also contributes to tertiary tricyclic antidepressant demethylation, readily undergoes induction by cigarette smoking, cruciferous vegetables, and charcoaled meats. Smoking has recently been shown to reduce levels of fluvoxamine (38).

D. Excretion

Age-associated decline in renal clearance may affect excretion of drug metabolites and lithium in older patients (25). The accumulation of active hydroxylated metabolites of antidepressants has been observed in older patients with putative adverse consequences (39,40). Risperidone is metabolized by 2D6 to a 9-OH metabolite that possesses dopamine antagonism comparable to risperidone (41). Given that this metabolite may accumulate in older patients, unanticipated extrapyramidal side effects may occur because of variable renal as well as hepatic function.

Since there is often a decline in muscle mass, the major source of creatinine, with age and debilitation, serum creatinine may not appear elevated in the face of declining renal function. It is therefore preferable to do a creatinine clearance from an abbreviated, timed urine collection aided by computer programs such as Creat Comp (Kallen RJ, Computac Associates, Mt. Sinai Medical Center, Cleveland, OH) or approximate from nomograms. The fact that nonsteroidal antiinflammatory drugs may reduce lithium's clearance (possibly through effects on renal tubular prostaglandin) deserves particular emphasis given their widespread use by the elderly and their over-the-counter availability. An interesting and important example of an age-related interaction, putatively mediated by diminished renal clearance, was provided by Guven and colleagues (42). They noted that 1 mg of alprazolam caused dramatic increases in serum digoxin levels in those older, but not younger, than age 65. Low-salt diets and the possibility that SSRIs may cause inappropriate antidiuretic hormone secretion with concomitant hyponatremia, particularly in older patients, may be additional sources of interactive complications with lithium (43).

II. PHARMACODYNAMIC INTERACTIONS

Pharmacodynamic interactions produce a change in drug action in the absence of a change in drug concentrations. Pharmacodynamic drug interactions are not as amenable to study as are kinetic interactions, and they resist an easy classification. One scheme is to sort them into direct and indirect interactions. Direct interactions occur clearly at a key receptor (e.g., drugs with anticholinergic properties may have cumulative effects at muscarinic receptors). Indirect interactions may be as obvious as two medications with sedative properties engendered by different mechanisms combining in effect. Alternatively, the serotonergic actions of SSRIs may combine therapeutically with lithium's facilitation of serotonergic transmission or result in severe toxicity in combination with dextromethorphan-induced serotonin release or when combined with an irreversible inhibitor of serotonin metabolism (i.e., a monoamine oxidase inhibitor). In practice, interactions can be labeled pharmacodynamic only after controlling for plasma concentrations.

As patients age, there is a general reduction in homeostatic mechanisms (e.g., postural control, orthostatic circulatory responses, thermoregulation, visceral muscle function, higher cognitive function). This may interfere with the ability to adapt to changes in the environment and may be manifest as an adverse drug reaction. For instance, all psychotropics may increase the risk of falls and hip fracture in the elderly (44) and may increase cognitive impairment (45).

A. Anticholinergic Interactions

Two groups of drugs cause anticholinergic effects: those used therapeutically for their anticholinergic properties (e.g., oxybutynin [Ditropan], benztropine), and those that have anticholinergic effects that are incidental to their main actions (e.g., amitriptyline). Tune and colleagues (46) quantified the antimuscarinic potential of 25 of the most commonly used medications in older patients. Ten of these medications, usually not thought to be especially anticholinergic (ranitidine, codeine, dipyridamole, warfarin, isosorbide, theo-

TABLE 3 Selected Interactions of Concern to Geriatric Psychopharmacology

Tricyclic Antidepressants (TCAs)
Carbamazepine (increases TCA metabolism)
SSRIs (decreases TCA metabolism)
Quinidine (marked decrease in TCA metabolism)
Procainamide, disopyramide (excessive decrease in cardiac conduction)
Clonidine (reduction of antihypertensive effect)
Epinephrine or norepinephrine (increased pressor effect)
Selective Serotonin Reuptake Inhibitors (SSRIs)
Codeine (loss of analgesic effect)
Coumadin (may potentiate)
Cisapride (inhibition of cisapride clearance by CYP 3A3/4 may trigger cardiac arrhythmias)
MAOIs (risk of lethal serotonergic syndrome)
Monoamine Oxidase Inhibitors (MAOIs)
Meperidine (demerol) (cardiovascular instability, hyperpyrexia)
Dextromethorphan
Lithium
Nonsteroidal antiinflammatory drugs (reduction of lithium clearance)
Thiazide diuretics (reduction of lithium clearance)
Methyldope (reduction of lithium clearance)
Acetazolamide (increase in lithium clearance)
Theophylline, caffeine (increase in lithium clearance)
Calcium channel blockers; ACE inhibitors (variable and unpredictable effects on lithium clearance)
Succinylcholine, pancuroniuim (prolongation of neuromuscular blockade)

phylline, nifedipine, digoxin, Lanoxin, and prednisolone), were found to demonstrate antimuscarinic potencies that have been associated with cognitive impairments in healthy elderly subjects. Peripheral manifestations of anticholinergicity include dry mouth, tachycardia, blurring of vision, urinary retention, and constipation. In pharmacodynamic studies, the elderly have been shown to be very sensitive to central nervous system (CNS) effects of anticholinergic medications (47). This CNS toxicity may range from subtle changes, such as apparent worsening of depression, mild confusion, and impairment of recent memory to frank delirium (48). Tachycardia, in patients with preexisting myocardial ischemia, is an additional concern with the use of many psychotropics; secondary to their anticholinergic effects, these effects appear not to be ameliorated by time (49).

B. Anticoagulant Interactions

Older patients have been found to require smaller doses of anticoagulants to achieve the same degree of anticoagulation (50). Although confounded by effects of other medications and hepatic dysfunction, the increased sensitivity of the elderly to anticoagulants is believed possible. Fluvoxamine and sertraline cause increased warfarin serum levels (51). However, increased bleeding times when paroxetine and fluoxetine were combined with warfarin were found not to be due to a pharmacokinetic interaction (52). Concurrent therapy need not be avoided, but close monitoring is advisable whenever an SSRI is combined with warfarin.

C. Antiarrhythmic Interactions

Membrane-stabilizing (quinidinelike) properties of some psychotropics may delay cardiac conduction and seriously interact with either underlying pathophysiology or antiarrhythmic medication. EKG changes have been noted most frequently for the tricyclic antidepressants and antipsychotics of the diphenylbutylpiperidine (i.e., pimozide) and piperidine (e.g., thioridazine) type. The risk of antipsychotic and tricyclic antidepressant–cardiovascular drug interactions is considerably amplified since many of these medications intersect both metabolically and dynamically. For example, quinidine and diltiazem will not only inhibit cardiac conduction, but CYP 2D6 as well. In patients with preexisting conduction disturbance, there is a clear need for increased watchfulness. In older patients who are chronically treated with antipsychotics, the prevalence of obesity, poor nutritional status, and increased triglycerides may contribute additional cardiovascular risk factors (53). In rare instances, SSRIs may induce bradycardia (54). Caution is therefore urged when patients whose pretreatment heart rate is less than 60 beats per minute or in those treated with beta-blockers.

D. Antihypertensive Interactions

Specific age-associated changes have been most extensively investigated for autonomic receptor-mediated effects (47). Reductions in α_2 (but not α_1) adrenoceptor responsiveness may occur with age and could contribute to the increased risk of orthostatic hypotension in elderly patients. Orthostatic hypotension is a major risk in the elderly, and the possibility of an indirect dynamic interaction suggests caution against the use of monoamine oxidase inhibitors (MAOIs), lower potency antipsychotic drugs, tricyclic antidepressants, trazodone (at antidepressant dosages), and nefazodone in combination with antihypertensives. In hypertensive patients treated with venlafaxine, the possibility that this antidepressant has some potential for raising blood pressure at higher doses should be considered. The classic dynamic interaction is between guanethidine-type drugs and phenothiazines or tricyclic antidepressants and occurs because of blockade of drug entry into adrenergic neurons. Another dynamic interaction that can cause loss of efficacy or significant rebound hypertension has been found when patients treated with clonidine are coprescribed clomipramine, desipramine, or imipramine (55). Although interactions between ACE inhibitors and psychotropics have not been reported, careful and regular assessment is mandatory whenever an antihypertensive drug is combined with a psychotropic.

E. Serotonergic Interactions

The serotonin syndrome has been recognized since 1960; however, since the introduction of clomipramine and the SSRIs, it has been seen more frequently. The increased use of SSRIs in medically compromised older patients mandates that there be particular vigilance for serotonergic interactions. This toxic hyperserotonergic condition is characterized by mental status changes (agitation, restlessness, cognitive impairment, hypomania), altered muscle tone (myoclonus, hyperreflexia, incoordination, tremor), and autonomic instability (diaphoresis, shivering, hyper or hypotension, tachycardia, diarrhea) (56). The serotonin syndrome has been seen when MAOIs (including selegiline) are combined with SSRIs or when either class of drug is combined with serotonin agonists such as clomipramine, dextromethorphan, meperidine, lithium, and L-tryptophan. In Parkinsonian patients, it should be appreciated that dopamine agonists (i.e., bromocriptine, levodopa/carbidopa) will indirectly cause serotonin release, raising the potential of the serotonin syndrome when these medications are coadministered with serotonin agonists (57).

III. CONCLUSION

The most severe drug interactions associated with psychopharmacotherapy in older patients may be contained by education followed by surveillance. High-risk medications, including anticoagulants, antihypertensives, and antiarrhythmics including digitalis have been consistently emphasized in long-term, comprehensive surveys of adverse drug reactions in older patients (58,59). Physicians need to be particularly vigilant and knowledgeable when one of these high-risk medications is prescribed. The study by Hale and colleagues (59), for example, found that 40% of patients taking quinidine were also taking digitalis and that 30% of patients taking warfarin were coprescribed a drug that could cause an interaction. Since most interactions are infrequent and unexpected, geriatric psychiatrists should employ a set of routinized procedures as follows:

1. Be knowledgeable about drug actions and clearance.
2. Identify patient risk factors, such as medical status, use of high-risk medications, diet, and alcohol use.

3. Take a thorough drug history, involving the primary caregiver, and be sure to include over-the-counter medications and update regularly in a prominent place in the patient's record.
4. Use lowest effective doses and avoid unnecessary polypharmacy.
5. In the face of a potential inhibitor, lower the dose of existing therapy before beginning low doses of the potential inhibitor and, whenever possible, monitor plasma levels and pharmacodynamic effects.
6. Careful monitoring is also essential when a drug that induces metabolism or otherwise diminishes the bioavailability of a second drug has been discontinued.
7. Educate patients and caregivers about their medications and dosing regimens and monitor compliance.
8. If there is a deterioration in a patient's physical or cognitive state, always suspect an adverse drug interaction.

REFERENCES

1. Helling DK, Lemke JH, Semla TP, Wallace RB, Lipson DP, Cononi-Huntley J. Medication use characteristics in the elderly. J Am Geriatr Soc 1987; 35:4–12.
2. Stewart RB, Cooper JW. Polypharmacy in the aged. Drugs Aging 1994; 4:449–461.
3. Stoller EP. Prescribed and over-the-counter medicine use by the ambulatory elderly. Med Care 1988; 26:1149–57.
4. Benrimoj SI, Langford JH, Bowden MG, Triggs EJ. Switching drug availability from prescription only to over-the-counter status. Are elderly patients at increased risk? Drugs Aging 1995; 7:255–265.
5. Nolan L, O'Malley K. Adverse drug reactions in the elderly. Br J Hosp Med 1989; 41:452–457.
6. Pollock BG. Recent developments in drug metabolism of relevance to psychiatrists. Harv Rev Psychiatry 1994; 2:204–213.
7. Nemeroff CB, DeVane CL, Pollock BG. Newer antidepressants and the cytochrome P450 system. Am J Psychiatry 1996; 153:311–320.
8. Ciraulo DA, Shader RI, Greenblatt DJ, Creelman W. Drug Interactions in Psychiatry. Baltimore: Williams & Wilkins, 1995.
9. Stockley I. Drug Interactions, 3rd ed. Oxford: Blackwell Scientific Publications, 1994.
10. Algeri S, Cerletti C, Curcio M, Morselli PL, Bonollo L, Buniva M, Minazzi M, Minoli G. Effect of anticholinergic drugs on gastrointestinal absorption of L-dopa in rats and man. Eur J Pharmacol 1976; 35:293–299.
11. Vesell ES. Complex effects of diet on drug disposition. Clin Pharmacol Ther 1984; 36:285–296.
12. van Harten J. Clinical pharmacokinetics of selective serotonin reuptake inhibitors. Clin Pharmacokinet 1993; 24:203–220.

13. Greenblatt DJ, Sellers EM, Shader RI. Drug disposition in old age. N Engl J Med 1982; 306;1081–1088.
14. Rolan PE. Plasma protein binding displacement interactions - Why are they still regarded as clinically important? Br J Clin Pharmacol 1994; 37:125–128.
15. Pollock BG, Perel JM. Tricyclic antidepressants: Contemporary issues for therapeutic practice. Can J Psychiatry 1989; 34:609–617.
16. Guengerich FP. Human cytochrome P-450 enzymes. Life Sci 1992; 50:1471–1478.
17. Nelson JC, Jatlow PI. Nonlinear desipramine kinetics: prevalence and importance. Clin Pharmacol Ther 1987; 41:666–670.
18. Shimada T, Yamazaki H, Mimura M, Inui Y, Guengerich FP. Interindividual variations in human liver cytochrome P-450 enzymes involved in the oxidation of drugs, cacinogens and toxic chemicals: studies with liver microsomes of 30 Japanese and 30 Caucasians. JPET 1994; 270:414–423.
19. Ingelman-Sundberg M, Johansson I, Yin H, Terelius Y, Eliasson E, Clot P, Albano E. Ethanol-inducible cytochrome P450 2E1: Genetic polymorphism, regulation, and possible role in the etiology of alcohol-induced liver disease. Alcohol 1993; 10:447–452.
20. Lieber CS. Hepatic, metabolic, and toxic effects of ethanol. Alcohol Clin Exp Res 1991; 15:573–592.
21. Pollock BG, Mulsant BH, Sweet RA, Rosen J, Altieri LP. Prospective P450 2d6 phenotyping for neuroleptic treatment in dementia. Psychopharmacol Bull 1995; 31:327–331.
22. Syvälahti EKG, Lindberg R, Kallio J, DeVocht M. Inhibitory effects of neuroleptics on debrisoquine oxidation in man. Br J Clin Pharmacol 1986; 22:89–92.
23. Westermeyer J. Fluoxetine-induced tricyclic toxicity: Extent and duration. J Clin Pharmacol 1991; 31:388–392.
24. Spina E, Avenoso A, Campo GM, Caputi AP, Perucca E. Phenobarbital induces the 2-hydroxylation of desipramine. Ther Drug Monit 1996; 18:60–64.
25. Pollock BG. Issues in psychotropic drug development for the elderly. In: Bergener M, Brocklehurst JC, Finkel SI, eds. Aging, Health and Healing. New York: Springer Publishing, 1995: 235–242.
26. Nelson JC, Mazure CM, Bowers MB, Jatlow PI. A preliminary, open study of the combination of fluoxetine and desipramine for rapid treatment of major depression. Arch Gen Psychiatry 1991; 48:303–307.
27. Sindrup SH, Brøsen K, Bjerring P, Arendt-Nielsen L, Larsen U, Angelo HR. Codeine increases pain thresholds to copper vapor laser stimuli in extensive but not poor metabolizers of sparteine. Clin Pharmacol Ther 1991; 49:686–693.
28. Ketter TA, Flockhart DA, Post RM, Denicoff K, Pazzaglia PJ, Marangell LB, George MS, Callahan AM. The emerging role of cytochrome P450 3A in psychopharmacology. J Clin Psychopharmacol 1995; 15:387–398.
29. Hukkinen SK, Varhe A, Olkkola KT, Neuvonen PJ. Plasma concentrations of triazolam are increased by concomitant ingestion of grapefruit juice. Clin Pharmacol Ther 1995; 58:127–131.
30. Ball S, Ahern D, Kao J, Scatina J. Venlafaxine (VF): effects on CTO2D6 dependent imipramine (IMP) and desipramine (DMP) 2-hydroxylation; comparative

studies with fluoxetine (FLU) and effects on CYP1A2, 3A4, and 2C9. Clin Pharmacol Ther 1996; 59:171.
31. von Moltke LL, Greenblatt DJ, Court MH, Duan SX, Harmatz JS, Shader RI. Inhibition of alprazolam and desipramine hydroxylation in vitro by paroxetine and fluvoxamine: Comparison with other selective serotonin reuptake inhibitor antidepressants. J Clin Psychopharmacol 1995; 15:125–131.
32. Swims MP. Potential terfenadine-fluoxetine interaction (letter). Ann Pharmacother 1993; 27:1404–1405.
33. Rosenblatt JE, Rosenblatt NC. Sertraline-terfenadine interaction? Curr Affect Ill 1996; 15:14.
34. von Moltke LL, Greenblatt DJ, Duan SX, Harmatz JS, Wright CE, Shader RI. Inhibition of terfenadine metabolism in vitro by azole antifungal agents and by selective serotonin reuptake inhibitor antidepressants: relation to pharmacokinetic interactions in vivo. J Clin Psychopharmacol 1996; 16:104–112.
35. Honig PK, Wortham DC, Zamani K, Conner DP, Mullin JC, Cantilena LR. Terfenadine-ketoconazole interaction pharmacokinetic and electrocardiographic consequences. J Am Med Assoc 1993; 269:1513–1518.
36. von Moltke LL, Greenblatt DJ, Schmider J, Harmatz JS, Shader RI. Nefazodone in vitro: metabolic conversions and inhibition of P450-3A isoforms. Clin Pharmacol Ther 1996; 59:176.
37. Greene DS, Dockens RC, Salazar DE, Barbhaiya RH. Coadministration of nefazodone (NEF) and benzodiazepines I: pharmacokinetic assessment. Clin Pharmacol Ther 1994; 55:141.
38. Spigset S, Carleborg L, Hedenmalm K, Dahlqvist R. Effect of cigarette smoking on fluvoxamine pharmacokinetics in humans. Clin Pharmacol Ther 1995; 58:399–403.
39. Young RC, Alexopoulos GS, Shamoian CA, Kent E, Dhar AK, Kutt H. Plasma 10-hydroxynortriptyline and ECG changes in elderly depressed patients. Am J Psychiatry 1985; 142:866–868.
40. Sweet RA, Pollock BG, Wright B, Kirshner M, DeVane C. Single and multiple dose bupropion pharmacokinetics in elderly patients with depression. J Clin Pharmacol 1995; 35:876–884.
41. Ereshefsky L, Lacombe S. Pharmacological profile of risperidone. Can J Psychiatry 1993; 38 (Suppl 3):S80–S88.
42. Guven H, Tuncok Y, Guneri S, Cavdar C, Fowler J. Age-related digoxin-alprazolam interaction. Clin Pharmacol Ther 1993; 54:42–44.
43. Druckenbord R, Mulsant BH. Fluoxetine-induced syndrome of inappropriate antidiuretic hormone secretion. J Geriatr Psychiatry Neurol 1994; 7:255–258.
44. Tinetti ME, Speechley M, Ginter SF. Risk factors for falls among elderly persons living in the community. New Engl J Med 1988; 319:1701–1707.
45. Larson EB, Kukull WA, Buchner D, Reifler BV. Adverse drug reactions associated with global cognitive impairment in elderly persons. Ann Intern Med 1987; 107:169–173.
46. Tune L, Carr S, Hoag E, Cooper T. Anticholinergic effects of drugs commonly prescribed for the elderly: Potential means for assessing risk of delirium. Am J Psychiatry 1992; 149:388–392.

47. Pollock BG, Perel JM, Reynolds CF. Pharmacodynamic issues relevant to geriatric psychopharmacology. J Geriatr Psychiatry Neurol 1990; 3:221–228.
48. Schor JD, Levkoff SE, Lipsitz LA, Reilly CH, Cleary PD, Rowe JW, Evans DA. Risk factors for delirium in hospitalized elderly. J Am Med Assoc 1992; 267:827–831.
49. Pollock BG, Perel JM, Paradis CF, Fasicka AL, Reynolds CF. Metabolic and physiologic consequences of nortriptyline treatment in the elderly. Psychopharmacol Bull 1994; 30:145–150.
50. Shepherd AMM, Hewick DS, Moreland TA, Stevenson IH. Age as a determinant of sensitivity to warfarin. Br J Clin Pharmacol 1977; 4:315–320.
51. Benfield P, Ward A. Fluvoxamine, a review of its pharmacodynamic and pharmacokinetic properties and therapeutic efficacy in depressive illness. Drugs 1986; 32:313–334.
52. Bannister SJ, Houser VP, Hulse JD, Kisicki JC, Rasmussen JGC. Evaluation of the potential interactions of paroxetine with diazepam, cimetidine, warfarin and digoxin. Acta Psychiatr Scand 1989; 80 (suppl 350):102–106.
53. Martinez JA, Velasco JJ, Urbistondo MD. Effects of pharmacological therapy on anthropometric and biochemical status of male and female institutionalized psychiatric patients. J Am Coll Nutrition 1994; 13:192–197.
54. Buff DD, Brenner R, Kirtane SS, Gilboa R. Dysrhythmia associated with fluoxetine treatment in an elderly patient with cardiac disease. J Clin Psychiatry 1991; 52:174–176.
55. Hui KK. Hypertensive crisis induced by the interaction of clonidine with imipramine. J Am Geriatr Soc 1983; 31:164–165.
56. Sternbach H. The serotonin syndrome. Am J Psychiatry 1991; 148:705–713.
57. Sandyk R. L-dopa induced "serotonin syndrome" in a parkinsonian patient on bromocriptine. J Clin Pharmacol 1986;. 6:194–195.
58. May FE, Stewart RB, Cluff LE. Drug interactions and multiple drug administration. Clin Pharmacol Ther 1977; 22:322–328.
59. Hale WE, May FE, Marks RG. Drug-drug and drug-disease interactions in the elderly. J Geriatric Drug Ther 1989; 3:67–86.

4

Treatment of Major Depression in the Elderly

J. CRAIG NELSON
YALE UNIVERSITY SCHOOL OF MEDICINE, AND YALE-NEW HAVEN HOSPITAL, NEW HAVEN, CONNECTICUT

I. SIGNIFICANCE OF DEPRESSION

A. Prevalence

Depression is a common disorder in the elderly, particularly among medically ill and institutionalized patients; yet, its prevalence varies considerably in different settings. Depressive symptoms occur in about 15% of community-dwelling elders, but the prevalence of major depression is estimated to be less than 3% (1,2). This rate is lower than that for nonelderly adults (2), a finding that contradicts the myth that depression is merely an attribute of old age.

Depression is more common in medical settings. In nursing homes, reported rates of depression range from 9 to 38% (3). In medical inpatients and outpatients, rates from 10% to 42% have been reported (3), although the prevalence of well-defined major depression may be lower. Magni and associates (4) interviewed 220 geriatric patients hospitalized on medical units. Eight percent met criteria for major depression, 22% had dysthymic disorder, and 6% had atypical depression.

Suicide is an important adverse outcome in depressed patients. Rates of completed suicide in the elderly are twice those of younger patients, and are especially high in elderly white males (5,6). The importance of these findings takes on even greater significance because the elderly, particularly those over 85, are the most rapidly growing segment of our population.

B. Depression and Functioning

Recent studies by Wells and associates (7,8) have emphasized the effect of depression on functioning. In mixed-age samples, major depression had a more marked effect on role functioning and physical functioning than several other common medical disorders such as hypertension, diabetes, and arthritis. Only heart disease caused greater functional impairment. Depression had the greatest effect on the patients' perception of well-being. This finding may not surprise mental health professionals, but is particularly important with respect to treatments aimed at improving quality of life. Few treatments in medicine address more directly the symptoms affecting quality of life such as loss of interest, loss of enjoyment or sense of well-being, than does the treatment of depression.

In the elderly, functional impairment is frequently expressed as a decline in the ability to perform the activities of daily living (ADLs). Depression significantly affects these abilities. In one prospective study of patients over 70 (9), individuals depressed at the start of the study were significantly more likely to demonstrate impairment in their ADLs during the 2.5 years of the study. Gait and hygiene were most affected. Because the ability to perform ADLs so directly relates to independent living, depression may lead to nursing home placement.

C. Depression and Medical Illness

Depression is commonly associated with medical illness. Although the studies of this relationship have usually not been restricted to the elderly, medical comorbidity is high in the elderly. In a study of a consecutive series of 168 patients 60 years and older admitted to a psychiatric inpatient setting, Conwell and associates found 78% suffered from at least one major medical illness (10). Among the 94 patients with unipolar major depression in this sample, 89% had at least one medical illness (11). Medical illness is common in the elderly, and its presence may increase the risk for depression. In three studies (10, 12,13), medical illness was the most common apparent precipitant for the major depressive episode in older patients.

Although rates of major depression in patients with medical illness are variable among medical illnesses, rates of 20 to 25% are common (14,15). Depression in heart disease, stroke, cancer, and dementia has been well studied, is common, and may influence the course of the medical illness. For these reasons, it is discussed in more detail in subsequent chapters.

Depression has a deleterious effect on the morbidity and mortality of patients with medical illness. For example, in a 13-year follow-up study of patients participating in the Baltimore Epidemiological Catchment Area (ECA) survey, patients with a history of major depression had a fourfold increase in their risk of myocardial infarction (16). In another study, postmyocardial infarction patients had an increased risk of major depression, and those with major depression had a fivefold increase in their risk of death during the 6 months post-MI (17). In elderly patients with a variety of medical illnesses, depression can further impair ADL functioning and can increase pain and mortality. In patients receiving home care after hospitalization, depression is common and associated with impaired functioning and increased pain (18). Patients depressed on admission to a nursing home are significantly more likely to die in the first year of their placement, with mortality rates of 47.4% in depressed patients vs. 29.8% in nondepressed residents reported (19). In a follow-up study of patients participating in the ECA study, Bruce and associates (20) found those depressed at the outset had a 2.0-fold greater risk of death during a 9-year follow-up. Patients with depression and medical illness were even more likely to succumb.

The relationship of depression and medical illness underscores the importance of recognizing depression, not only in traditional mental health settings, but in primary care and general medicine. Demonstration of the benefits of treating depression would help to emphasize the importance of the association. Data of this sort are limited. One retrospective study suggested that adequate antidepressant treatment may decrease the rate of myocardial infarction (21) but these are questions that beg further exploration.

II. DIAGNOSIS OF DEPRESSION IN THE ELDERLY

A. Diagnosis of Depression

The preceding discussion emphasized the importance of recognizing depression in elderly patients with and without medical illness. One of the first steps in this process is to recognize that demoralization and depressive symptoms are not an expected outcome of normal aging. As the ECA data demonstrate, rates of depression are not higher in community-dwelling elders.

The diagnosis of major depression in older patients is based on the same criteria as used in younger patients. Some investigators have questioned whether this practice underestimates depression in elders, yet there is no commonly accepted alternative. Older patients, however, report more somatic symptoms than younger patients and this may also complicate assessment of depressive symptoms (22,23). For example, older patients are more likely to experience sleep disturbance. Their appetite and level of energy may be reduced. As a result, the use of these symptoms as diagnostic criteria is complicated. When assessing these symptoms, it is especially useful to determine if there has been a recent change during which the cluster of symptoms characteristic of major depression developed.

Because medical illness is common in elders, some symptoms, which are common in medical illness, may be less useful for the diagnosis of depression. For example, loss of energy, loss of appetite, and insomnia may be associated with many medical conditions. Clark and associates (24) found that the affective and psychological symptoms of depression are more specific for depression and more useful for diagnosis when medical illness is present. For example, anhedonia, preoccupation with guilt, feelings of worthlessness or hopelessness, and thoughts of suicide are not likely to be the result of medical illness and are more specific for depression.

In medical settings, it is important for clinicians to be aware that many patients with depression do not present with a primary complaint of depressed mood. In fact, two studies (25,26) suggest that in primary care settings more than 50% of depressed patients will present with somatic symptoms. These patients are likely to be dysophoric but describe this feeling state as pain, lack of energy, or as other somatic complaints. On questioning, they will confirm the presence of lack of interest or enjoyment, as well as other symptoms of major depression. The older literature emphasized concepts of "masked depression" and "depressive equivalents," and assumed that patients were denying their sad or depressed mood. A simpler explanation is that some individuals who are depressed in fact do not experience typical sadness or they do not label their discomfort as sadness. They do experience and recognize the physical symptoms of depression, and use those terms to describe their feeling state. Sifneos refers to the tendency to experience symptoms in somatic rather than psychological terms as "alexithymia" (27). These patients seek treatment from medical clinicians both because of established relationships and because they believe they have a physical illness. It is also possible that patients assume that their primary clinician expects them to report physical symptoms.

It seems unlikely that older individuals would be any more able to recognize depressed mood than younger persons. Public awareness of depression as a medical disorder is a relatively recent phenomenon. Patients over 65 grew up during a period when depression was less well understood, when ideas about etiology differed, and the stigma of psychiatric illness was even greater. It might be expected that the current cohort of elderly patients would be less likely to identify symptoms of major depression than would younger patients.

For researchers, the question of whether to "count" symptoms, which could be explained by medical illness, toward the diagnosis of major depression has stirred much debate. Chapter 12 provides a detailed discussion of inclusive and restrictive approaches to the diagnosis of depression and dementia. The basic issues are the same whether the second illness is dementia or another medical illness. The clinician would best be suspicious of the diagnosis of depression when the symptoms are present regardless of whether each symptom is explained by the depression. Other considerations, such as recent change, the development of the cluster of symptoms typical of depression, and the presence of "positive" psychological symptoms will be most useful in establishing the diagnosis. Finally, the clinician should consider whether an antidepressant trial might help to resolve the diagnostic issue. Of course, when the diagnosis is less clear, active participation of the patient in the decision to begin a therapeutic trial is especially important, but the clinician plays a crucial role in laying out the risks, and most important, explaining the odds that a trial would be successful. The primary caveat in this situation is that if the diagnosis is unclear, the clinician should be especially careful to consider whether active medical illness is present, and if it requires other treatment.

B. Differential Diagnosis

Numerous medical disorders have been associated with depression (3). Clinical lore has emphasized the need to "rule out" medical causes of depression. This emphasis may be misplaced. It is clear that the incidence of depression is increased in many medical disorders (14,15) and that medical inpatients and outpatients have increased rates of depression (3); however, almost all these data show an *association* between depression and medical illness, but seldom has a *causal link* been made. Clinicians seeing an individual patient will have a particularly difficult time trying to establish a causal link. For example, it is well established that rates of depression are increased following stroke and myocardial infarction. These are good examples because the onset of the medical illness can be identified, but the cause of the depression may remain elusive. If the patient develops depression 3 months after a stroke, is the depression caused by the stress of paralysis or aphasia or by the loss of independence or is it a psychophysiological manifestation of the neuroanatomic injury? When faced with such an individual patient, it is usually impossible to determine etiology. Further, even in the case of poststroke or post-MI depression, where the index of suspicion may be high, treatment of the medical condition will not ameliorate the depression. There are some exceptions. Hypothyroidism may present with depressive features that may improve with treatment of the medical disorder.

Even in a general hospital setting, it is uncommon to see a patient for whom a medical cause of depression *can be firmly established*. In two studies (10,28), we reviewed the diagnoses of 300 patients hospitalized on a psychiatric unit in a general hospital, of whom 214 were 60 or older and for whom medical illness was common. Yet, even in these "high-risk" patients, it was rare that we could confirm a medical *cause* for depression. The most frequent cause that could be confirmed was medication, partly because the onset of symptoms occurred shortly after beginning medication, and partly because symptoms abated shortly after it was discontinued. As a result of the difficulty in establishing causality, the Diagnostic and Statistical Manual (DSM-IV) category "depression due to . . . (the medical cause)" is uncommon. It is more useful to retain a multifactor, final common pathway model in which the medical illness is viewed as one factor increasing the likelihood of depression.

This does not mean that evaluation of medical illness is not important. Careful assessment of concurrent medical illness remains an essential task. Management of the medical illness may change as the depression is treated. For example, insulin requirements may increase as the severely depressed patient regains his or her appetite and starts to eat more. These requirements may be further affected by changes in activity level. Management of the medical disorder may be affected by antidepressant medications regardless of change in the depression. For example, antihypertensive treatments may need to be decreased during tricyclic treatment. Finally, drug interactions may occur among both the drugs used to treat the depression and those used to treat the medical disorder.

C. Depression and Dementia

The relationship of depression and dementia is of special relevance for elderly patients, and is discussed in detail in Chapter 12. A few major points are worth summarizing. The concept of *pseudodementia* was introduced over 30 years ago (29), as a result of the observation that some depressed patients can present with confusion suggesting dementia. When introduced, the concept was important for reminding clinicians that the apparent dementia might be reversed with successful treatment of the depression (30). Subsequently, as clinicians became familiar with the concept, the term became less useful and, to some extent, misleading. The cognitive deficits associated with depression are not merely subjectively reported symptoms, and the impairment of memory and concentration is very real (31). Further, the concept of pseudodementia tends to encourage an "either or" approach to diagnosis that can be misleading. In fact, in the elderly, depression and dementia are both very common disorders that frequently coexist (32). It is likely, just on a statistical basis, that a certain percentage of elderly depressed patients will be demented. In a series of elderly depressed inpatients, we found 14% (19/135) also had dementia (33). Depression also is increased in demented patients, with rates of 2 to 23% reported (34–38). The geriatric psychiatrist needs to know that depression can be associated with cognitive deficits, that the cognitive deficits are real, and that these deficits will often improve with antidepressant treatment; however, the clinician also needs to know that dementia may also be present and that both disorders need to be assessed independently.

D. Depression and Medications

Another potential risk factor for the development of depression are the medications given for medical conditions. Many medications, reviewed elsewhere (39), have been associated with depression. Because the timing of the initiation of medication can usually be established and the medication can sometimes be discontinued, a causal link may be more easily established. Even then, the relationship of the medication to the depressive syndrome may be complicated. There has been debate whether drugs cause a true or full syndrome of depression, whether they cause some symptoms, such as apathy or lethargy, which are similar to depression, or whether they act as precipitants in vulnerable individuals. Reserpine is a good example. Reserpine was one of the first drugs suggested to *cause* depression and this association, coupled with the observation that reserpine depletes catecholamines, was, in part, the basis for the catecholamine depletion hypothesis of depression (40). Yet, even for reserpine, there was debate about whether the drug caused a full syndrome of depression in the absence of vulnerability. Goodwin and Bunney (41), in reviewing the data, noted that the development of a syndrome similar to endogenous depression was uncommon with reserpine, and only occurred after months of treatment. It was their impression that a full syndrome of endogenous depression was more likely to develop in individuals vulnerable to depression. Thus, even reserpine, a drug whose mechanism of action directly relates to the catecholamine hypothesis of depression, may act more as a trigger in vulnerable individuals than as an etiologic agent.

With these considerations in mind, the clinician or researcher needs to consider the temporal association of the administration of a medication with the onset of depression, and then consider whether the medication in question can be discontinued. The onset and relief of depression with changes in the medication will help to establish an association, but a full understanding of etiology will also need to consider the individual's vulnerability to recurrent depression.

E. Subtypes of Depression

Most of our knowledge about the predictive value of subtypes comes from studies of nongeriatric adults; however, in the absence of other data, subtyping distinctions from younger patients provide the basis for treatment decisions in older patients. Studies of some subtypes common in the elderly (e.g., psychotic depression and melancholia) have included older patients in the samples. In other cases (e.g., atypical depression), older patients have seldom been studied.

Depressed patients with delusions or hallucinations who have psychotic depression respond less well to antidepressants alone (42,43), require combined neuroleptic–antidepressant treatment (44,45) or electroconvulsive therapy (ECT), and are discussed elsewhere in this text. Some patients can present with distorted ruminative thinking that is not clearly delusional but comes close. These near-delusional patients respond less well to antidepressant agents (46,47), but sometimes do respond to the addition of a neuroleptic (47). Although little has been written about this group of patients, this is not an uncommon presentation in the elderly.

Bipolar patients with a history of mania or hypomania require other treatment. Because antidepressants may provoke mania or rapid cycling in these patients, mood-stabilizing agents are usually employed from the beginning of treatment (48). Sometimes a mood stabilizer will be sufficient. Other patients require the addition of an antidepressant. Studies of specific antidepressants in bipolar depression are limited and have been conducted in nongeriatric adults. Himmelhoch et al. (49), in a prospective blind comparison study, found tranylcypromine, a monoamine oxidase inhibitor (MAOI), more effective than imipramine. Another study (50) found bupropion as effective as desipramine but less likely to induce mania. Although the selective serotonin reuptake inhibitors (SSRIs) have not been well studied in bipolar patients, induction of mania appeared to be infrequent in the early clinical trials with these agents.

In patients with nonpsychotic unipolar major depression, the subtype predictors for pharmacological treatment are atypical depression and melancholia. In nongeriatric adults with atypical depression, the MAOIs are superior to the tricyclic antidepressants (TCAs) (51). The SSRIs are also effective in this group, although their efficacy is not as well established (52,53). Atypical depression is not well described in geriatric patients and it appears to be less prevalent in the elderly.

Melancholia is common in the elderly and studies of melancholia have often included older patients. The best treatment for severe melancholia has been a matter of debate. Roose and associates (54) have suggested that the SSRIs may be less effective than the TCAs in this group. In a systematic comparison of nortriptyline and fluoxetine, they found the TCA more effective, but this was not a blind parallel design study. The Danish University group conducted two double-blind parallel comparison studies of an SSRI and TCA in severely depressed melancholic inpatients (55,56). They found that paroxetine and citalopram were less effective than clomipramine. Alternatively, analyses of outpatient samples treated with SSRIs have generally found no difference in response between more severe and less severe patients on the basis of Hamilton Depression Rating Scale (HAM-D) scores, or between melancholic and nonmelancholic patients (57). In part, this issue may have to do with characterization of the subtype. The patients in question have melancholic features and are severely depressed; however, HAM-D scores, which can be greatly influenced by patient-reported anxiety, may not capture the nature of the severity. These are patients with greater functional impairment who, in the past, have usually been treated in inpatient settings. Among the elderly, these are patients who spend the day on their bed, may be extremely ruminative, and for whom maintaining adequate nutrition can be a problem. These are patients for whom electroconvulsive therapy may be considered. The best pharmacological treatment for these severe melancholic patients remains unsettled. The clinician treating such patients will want to consider the status of the agent they are using with respect to its established efficacy in severe melancholic patients. The efficacy of the TCAs has been well studied in melancholic inpatients and, as a result, is best established in this patient group. The selective serotonin uptake inhibitors have not been well studied in inpatients and thus their effectiveness in this group is less clear.

It has been hypothesized that venlafaxine may be a more effective agent in severe depression because of its combined serotonergic–noradrenergic effects (58). Its efficacy in the elderly has not been well studied, but European studies of inpatients with melancholia suggest that the drug is more effective than placebo (59), more effective than fluoxetine (60), and comparable to imipramine (61). Venlafaxine is currently being studied in the United States in elderly patients and melancholic inpatients.

Recently the diagnosis of dysthymia in the elderly has received attention (62). It appears to be a common disorder (2), and successful treatment has been described with imipramine (63), fluoxetine (64), and sertraline (65), in nongeriatric adults. The data from nongeriatric samples do not suggest that one class of drugs is better than another, but demonstrate the value of active treatment over placebo. Little has been published about the treatment of dysthymia in the elderly. In a recent report, Nobler et al. (66) described open-label treatment of 23 elderly dysthymic patients with fluoxetine. Their mean age was 67 years and they had been ill on average for 18.5 years. Twelve of the patients (52%) responded. Treatment with a mean maximum dose of 35 mg/day of fluoxetine was tolerated well.

In addition to subtypes, other symptom predictors have been explored. Anxious depressives respond less well to TCAs than do less anxious patients (47,67,68), and some studies suggest that MAOIs may be more effective in anxious patients (69–71). Agitation and retardation have frequently been examined as predictors (72,73), but it is not clear that one class of antidepressants is more effective than another for patients with these symptoms. The studies of symptom predictors have primarily been conducted in nongeriatric samples.

Finally, there has been interest in whether late onset helps to identify a distinct subtype of depression in elderly patients. DSM-IV does not include late onset as a subtype but the literature suggests this distinction has predictive value. Patients with late-onset depression are less likely to have a family history of depression (11,74–76). They are more likely to have neuropsychological test findings or brain imaging findings suggestive of dementia or degenerative changes in the brain (77–82). Patients with late-onset depression respond less well to treatment and appear more likely to have residual symptoms after acute treatment (11). They have a worse prognosis (77,83) and increased mortality (79, 80). There has been some debate as to whether late-onset patients are more likely to have delusions. Meyers and Greenberg (84) found that delusions were associated with late-onset depression but Nelson et al. did not (85).

Clinically, the diagnosis of late-onset depression helps to predict the course of the illness, but is not helpful for selection of antidepressant treatment. There are currently no data that suggest that one antidepressant is any better than another for late-onset depression. All conventional antidepressants are likely to be somewhat less effective in this group. It is interesting to consider whether the study of degenerative changes associated with late onset might lead to more effective alternative treatments.

III. TREATMENT OF GERIATRIC DEPRESSION

A. Predictors for Drug Treatment

There are now an array of antidepressant medications that can be used for treatment of depression. In addition, psychotherapy may be effective for some patients (86,87). The predictors of which patients respond best to psychotherapy or drug treatment are not firmly established, but severity appears to be one of the most important (88,89). In nongeriatric samples, psychotherapy appears most useful in depressions that are mild to moderate, and is less effective in severe depression. Other predictors of the need for drug treatment have been described by the AHCPR guidelines (90), and include depressions that are bipolar, psychotic, melancholic, severe, and recurrent. Of course, history of response to an antidepressant in the past may argue for that treatment, and the patient may have strong opinions about the type of treatment they prefer.

There are several general questions pertaining to the treatment of elderly depressed patients. Are antidepressants effective in the depressed elderly? Are the elderly more sensitive to treatment? Do they respond to low doses and low blood levels? Are they more resistant to treatment? Do they take longer to respond? Is there one class of agents that is better than another in this group?

B. Efficacy

In 1988, Gerson et al. reviewed the available antidepressant drug studies conducted in elderly patients prior to 1986 (91). Their careful description of these studies highlights both the nature of the findings and the limitations of these studies. They found 25 double-blind studies; however, several serious problems were noted. Six studies included younger patients. Eleven did not limit the sample to major depression (although it should be noted that some of the studies were conducted before criteria for major depression were developed or were in common use). Thirteen of these studies employed placebo. Six of the studies investigated drugs—nomifensine, mianserin, and gerovital—that are not currently marketed in the U.S. The majority of the studies employed imipramine, amitriptyline, or doxepin, TCAs which are the most anticholinergic and antihistaminic, and are most likely to cause side effects.

The reviewers concluded that the antidepressant drugs were effective—the mean improvement in patients with major depression was 51% (range 35 to 68%) on the HAMD, which was essentially twice that seen with placebo. They concluded that the drugs were relatively comparable in efficacy but differed with respect to side effects. This review also called attention to the paucity of studies of TCAs, such as nortriptyline and desipramine, which are preferred for use in older patients. They found only one placebo-controlled trial of nortriptyline in patients over age 60 (92), but none for desipramine. They also noted one placebo-controlled trial of trazodone (93) and two with bupropion (94,95).

Subsequent to that review, three other placebo-controlled trials have been reported. Tollefson (96) described the results of a large study of 671 patients over the age of 60, with unipolar major depression, who were randomly assigned to fluoxetine 20 mg or placebo for 6 weeks of treatment. The mean age of those studied was 67.7 years, and 78.5% of the fluoxetine group and 80.7% of the placebo group completed the study. Using an intent-to-treat analysis, 36% of the fluoxetine and 27% of the placebo-treated patients achieved response defined as 50% improvement on the HAMD ($p = 0.014$). Discontinuations because of adverse events occurred in 11.6% of patients receiving fluoxetine and 8.6% of those receiving placebo. Although all patients assigned to fluoxetine began treatment with a dose of 20 mg/day, only 6.6% of the patients required a reduction to 20 mg every other day.

Wakelin (97) described a comparison of fluvoxamine, imipramine, and placebo in patients aged 60 to 71. Some patients began the study as inpatients. In 33 patients receiving fluvoxamine, the mean dose was 161 mg/day. In 29 patients receiving imipramine, the mean dose was 160 mg/day. Fourteen patients received placebo. Response was rated at 4 weeks. The adverse event discontinuation rate was 15% for fluvoxamine, 21% for imipramine, and 14%

for placebo. The study demonstrated that both active compounds were significantly more effective than placebo. On a CGI scale, the completer response rate was 79% for fluvoxamine, 65% for imipramine, and 25% for placebo. The respective intent-to-treat rates were 61%, 39%, and 23%.

The studies reviewed demonstrated the efficacy of antidepressants in elderly patients, although the findings apply primarily to medically stable, young–old patients (i.e., patients in the 60- to 75-year age range). Salzman et al. (98) called attention to the limited number of studies in the frail elderly. In their review, they found only four reports of antidepressant treatments in patients over 75 years of age: three of these were case reports with a total of seven patients; the fourth was the study described below.

Katz et al. (99) conducted a placebo-controlled study of nortriptyline in nursing home residents. Their average age was 84 years. Thirty patients entered the double-blind phase of the trial. The mean change in the HAM-D was 39.6% in the drug-treated patients and 10.5% in the placebo-treated patients, a significant and meaningful difference. Among patients completing treatment, 7/12 (58%) drug-treated patients were judged much or very much improved on the CGI scale, while 1/11 (9%) placebo-treated patients were similarly rated ($p = 0.009$). However, because of the drop-out rate, the intent-to-treat response rates among all patients who began treatment were low, 39% for drug and 8% for placebo. Six patients in the drug-treatment group dropped out because of side effects that included rapid ventricular rate (1), orthostatic hypotension (1), falls (3), and gait disturbance (1). These investigators also treated 14 patients on an open basis either before the study or after placebo treatment. Five of these 14 developed adverse events. Overall 11 of the 32 (34%) patients who received nortriptyline had a serious adverse reaction that interrupted treatment. In this sample of frail elderly, slightly more than one-third responded to treatment, one-third dropped out because of adverse effects, and one-third failed to respond.

The screening process, which the investigators carefully described, was quite informative. Of the 141 patients identified as possible candidates for the study, 79 were judged to have depression sufficient to warrant drug treatment. Of these 79, 23% either refused treatment or were uncooperative with procedures, 22% had an unstable medical condition or a contraindication to nortriptyline, 7.6% had psychotic symptoms, 5.1% were deemed too severe and needed urgent treatment, and 3.8% spontaneously improved during evaluation. Only 44% (35/79) of those with depression in need of treatment actually entered the study. These data suggest that the findings of this study pertain primarily to the less complicated patients. It seems likely that inclusion of uncooperative, medically unstable, psychotic, or extremely impaired patients would have adversely affected outcome.

C. Sensitivity to Treatment

The adage "start low, go slow" is familiar to all geriatric psychiatrists. The reason for caution is based on the relatively well-established sensitivity of elderly patients to side effects (100). In a study of 84 inpatients treated with comparable doses of desipramine, we found a fivefold increase in major adverse reactions that interrupted treatment in patients over 60 compared to younger patients (39% vs. 7%; $p < 0.001$) (101). Medical illness also predicted an increase in side effects and was more common in older patients. Multiple regression analysis indicated age was the more predictive variable, but it seemed likely that medical illness explained part of the effect of age. In this study, the other variable that predicted an increase in side effects was concomitant neuroleptic treatment. Thirty-two percent of patients who received desipramine with a neuroleptic developed a major adverse reaction vs. 8% in patients on desipramine alone ($p = 0.01$). The effect of neuroleptics was independent of the effect of age, yet older patients were more likely to receive a neuroleptic. Major side effects were not explained by higher desipramine plasma levels in this study, in part because the most common side effect, orthostatic hypotension, frequently occurred at low blood levels.

In another series of 99 consecutive patients with a psychotic depressive syndrome (28), we examined the incidence of major adverse reactions which interrupted treatment during administration of desipramine and a neuroleptic. No patient was excluded because of medical illness and the age range was broad (53 patients were younger than 60; 46 were 60 or older). Although adverse rates were higher overall because of combined neuroleptic–TCA treatment, all patients received a relatively similar neuroleptic dose of perphenazine or its equivalent (25 mg/day) and a standard dose of desipramine (2.5 mg/kg/day). In this study, medical illness was defined as an active symptomatic illness.

Both age and medical illness resulted in higher rates of adverse reactions (Table 1). The adverse reaction rate in patients aged 60 and over was 37% vs. 17% in younger patients. Among those with any active medical illness, the major adverse event rate was 50% vs. 18% in other patients. If patients were older and had medical illness, the rate increased slightly to 53%. In this study, active medical illness had a more profound effect than age on adverse effects.

There are two factors to consider when evaluating the risk for side effects in elders—the frequency of the physiological effect itself and the consequences of that effect. For example, both younger and older patients can develop orthostatic hypotension, but older patients are more likely to fall because of it, and if they fall, they are more likely to fracture their hips. There is little question that the frail elderly will have more serious consequences from a side effect.

TABLE 1 Rates of Major Adverse Reactions in 99 Inpatients Receiving Desipramine and a Neuroleptic by Age and Active Medical Illness

		Active medical illness	
		Absent	Present
Age	< 60 years	6/46 (13%)	3/7 (43%)
	≥ 60 years	7/27 (26%)	10/19 (53%)

Source: Ref. 28.

Few studies have examined side effects under similar conditions across the age range, but not all side effects are more frequent in the elderly. For example, tachycardia during TCA therapy appears to be more pronounced in younger patients, perhaps because of increased autonomic sensitivity (102, 103). The elderly appear to be more sensitive to side effects involving gait, tremor, and confusion or delirium. They also appear more sensitive to anticholinergic effects, which result in bowel problems, urinary retention, or blurred vision.

Response to Low Dose or Low Blood Levels

Another correlate of the start low, go slow adage is the suggestion that the elderly may respond to low doses. This was suggested by two earlier studies of low-dose tricyclic therapy (104,105). In the first study of 32 outpatients, with a mean age of 67 years, 25 to 75 mg/day of imipramine or doxepin was more effective than placebo (104). In the second study of 24 depressed patients over 70 years of age receiving treatment on a medical rehabilitation unit, 10 to 20 mg/day of doxepin was more effective than placebo (105).

Yet recent studies of nortriptyline and desipramine do not support this view. In two studies with desipramine (106,107), we examined relationships of dose, plasma level, and response in patients between 60 and 75, and in patients 75 or older, and compared our findings with those for younger patients (108). We found patients over 60 years of age required blood levels above 115 ng/ml, the threshold needed in younger patients for response. In a subsequent study of patients over 75 years of age, again similar blood levels were required for response. In both the young–old and old–old groups, patients required doses similar to those of younger patients to reach the desired blood levels. These data are similar to other reports (109,110) that found no effect of age on desipramine plasma concentrations.

Our data are relatively consistent with those for nortriptyline. Katz et al. (111) in their study of nursing home elders, adjusted dose to achieve a blood level in the 50 to 150 ng/ml range. Although this study was not designed to relate levels to response, they found that the mean dose necessary to achieve a level of 100 ng/ml was 80 mg/day. This dose was similar to that required in younger patients to reach this level, and is also nearly identical to the mean dose obtained in the only other placebo-controlled study of nortriptyline in elderly patients (92). In that study of 90 patients over 55 years, nortriptyline was dosed to achieve a level between 50 and 180 ng/ml. The average nortriptyline dose administered was 79 mg/day. Other studies that have examined the relationship of age with nortriptyline plasma concentration have reported variable results. Two studies found nortriptyline concentrations increased with age (112, 113), but four others found no relationship between age and nortriptyline levels (114–117). Even if there is a modest effect of age on nortriptyline clearance, the variability in rates of metabolism between individual patients is much greater.

The findings of similar blood level to dose relationships for nortriptyline and desipramine in younger and older patients are also supported by pharmacokinetic studies. Abernathy et al. (118) examined the pharmacokinetics of desipramine in normal volunteers. They found no effect of age on the clearance of desipramine. Similar results were obtained in another kinetic study of CYP 2D6 activity in very elderly healthy subjects (119). Both desipramine and nortriptyline are primarily metabolized by the 2D6 pathway. These findings suggest that the clearance of drugs metabolized by 2D6 may be unaffected by age.

These relationships are different for the hydroxy metabolites of desipramine and nortriptyline. Concentrations of these metabolites are more dependent on renal clearance, which decreases with age. As a result, these metabolites are elevated. Hydroxydesipramine, an active metabolite (120), is usually present at levels of about 40 to 50% of the parent compound (121). In the elderly it may be increased 50%, but this still represents only a 15% in crease in the total concentration of the drug present and is not likely to be a clinically meaningful difference (122). These relationships are different for nortriptyline. Hydroxynortriptyline is usually present at levels slightly exceeding the parent (116,117). In the elderly, hydroxynortriptyline levels are even higher. In one study, they were twice as high as the parent compound (117). Hydroxy levels of both desipramine and nortriptyline correlate with EKG abnormalities (123–125) and thus contribute disproportionately to the development of cardiac arrhythmias. Hydroxynortriptyline levels have been implicated in at least one case of heart failure (126); however, the actual frequency of this potential problem is not well established. Unlike hydroxydesipramine, which appears comparable to desipramine in reuptake potency (127), hydroxynortriptyline has about half the potency of the parent compound (116). At high levels it may interfere with the action of nortriptyline, reduce response (128), and explain in part the therapeutic window described for nortriptyline.

For both desipramine (129) and nortriptyline (112,130), methods have been described for adjusting dose using a single blood sample obtained 24 h after an initial test dose. For both drugs, this method is relatively effective especially since the target is a relatively broad range. However, in many settings this method may not be feasible. First the laboratory must be ready to do the assay quickly, otherwise the advantage of rapid adjustment is lost. In addition, because calculations are based on the 24-h level, errors in the drug assay may be magnified. Most laboratories set their internal standards in order to obtain precision in the therapeutic range. Levels that are well below the range usually do not need to be precise. Yet, 24-h levels, which are low, do need to be precise if they are the basis of dose adjustment. For many clinicians, a simpler method is to obtain one sample after 5 to 7 days of drug treatment on a constant dose, and then adjust dose on that basis. The practical reasons for obtaining a level are twofold—to identify slow metabolizers with high levels who may be at increased risk for adverse effects and to avoid empirical trials at blood levels that are usually ineffective.

The metabolism of other antidepressants varies. Venlafaxine is metabolized, at least in part, by the 2D6 pathway. It might be expected to show similar pharmacokinetics in younger and older patients. The possibility that fluoxetine levels are elevated in the elderly has been reported (131); however, this suggestion was based on a prior report of steady-state levels in four elderly patients (132). Yet mean concentrations from small samples can be very misleading because blood level distributions can be grossly skewed depending on the number of slow metabolizers included. In a pharmacokinetic study of healthy elders, Lemberger et al. (133) found no effect of age on fluoxetine clearance. In the largest study of fluoxetine in a geriatric sample (96), 6-week steady-state fluoxetine and norfluoxetine concentrations were determined in 235 patients aged 65 or older (data on file, Eli Lilly). The final mean steady-state concentrations of fluoxetine, norfluoxetine, and the total were 96.2 ng/ml, 127.0 ng/ml, and 223.2 ng/ml, respectively. These values were compared with those obtained in 615 nongeriatric patients receiving fluoxetine 20 mg/day in the acute treatment phase of a maintenance study (134). Mean fluoxetine, norfluoxetine, and total concentrations were 97 ng/ml, 128 ng/ml, and 225 ng/ml, respectively. These values were nearly identical to those of the geriatric sample. Both the pharmacokinetic study and the population data from these large samples indicate that fluoxetine and norfluoxetine levels were not higher in older patients.

Limited information is available for paroxetine and sertraline beyond that provided in the product information (135). This information indicates that during chronic administration at doses of 20, 30, and 40 mg/day, drug concentrations of paroxetine in elderly patients were 70 to 80% higher than in younger patients. For sertraline, plasma clearance was 40% less in elderly patients than in younger patients, but an estimated effect on plasma concentration was not provided. This information suggests that lower doses of paroxetine and sertraline should be used when starting treatment; however, as discussed below, the question of whether lower doses of these drugs are effective in the elderly has not been tested.

Clearance of imipramine and amitriptyline is reduced in the elderly (136) but the demethylation of these agents is not dependent on 2D6. Other data suggest that the activity of the 3A4 pathway does decrease with age (137,138). Sertraline and nefazodone are metabolized by 3A4 and their blood levels might be expected to be higher in elderly patients. In one study with nefazodone (139), elderly women had the higher levels than younger patients, both with chronic dosing and after single doses. Older men had intermediate levels.

In summary, there are two aspects of the low-dose issue. The first is pharmacodynamic and has to do with whether elderly patients respond to low doses or levels. The second is pharmacokinetic and has to do with whether low doses produce higher blood levels. The second question is more easily answered. The data currently suggest that for several antidepressants, specifically nortriptyline, desipramine, and fluoxetine, low doses result in low blood levels. The doses required to reach a given level will be relatively similar in younger and older patients. Exceptions are the tertiary tricyclics, such as amitriptyline and imipramine, and drugs metabolized by the 3A4 pathway, such as nefazodone. The initial product information suggests levels of paroxetine and sertraline may be higher in elderly patients, but population data are lacking.

The answer to the pharmacodynamic question of whether elderly patients respond to lower doses or blood levels is more complicated. First, there are no fixed-dose studies in the elderly that establish the minimal effective dose for any antidepressant, although plasma level–response relationships for nortriptyline and desipramine have been examined in the elderly. Tertiary TCAs may be effective at lower doses, but the two studies reporting efficacy (104,105) used very low doses. No subsequent work has replicated these findings. This may be a moot point since other drugs, with fewer side effects, are now available. The existing data for nortriptyline and desipramine suggest the elderly require plasma concentrations similar to those in younger adults for response (92,106,107,111).

For the SSRIs, two placebo-controlled (96,97) and 19 double-blind comparison studies of SSRIs (97,132,140–156) have been conducted in elderly patients. None of these studies systematically investigated the effectiveness of a lower dose. In fact, the minimum dose in all studies was the minimum dose used in nongeriatric adults (20 mg/day for fluoxetine, 50 mg/day for sertraline, and 20 mg/day for paroxetine). The only exceptions were two flexible dosing studies of paroxetine that allowed starting doses of 10 and 15 mg/day (148, 149). In the largest single study of 671 elderly patients, fluoxetine was started at 20 mg/day (96). Dose reduction was allowed, but only required in 7% of the patients.

In summary, there are no data supporting the efficacy of low-dose SSRI treatment in the elderly and few data suggesting that a low dose is necessary. These findings do not necessarily argue against starting with a lower dose to test tolerance, but if there are no adverse effects, the dose can be raised fairly quickly. Although there are few empirical data to support the need for this practice, many geriatric psychiatrists prefer this approach. In practice, clinicians see patients who are less enthusiastic about treatment than patients who volunteer for clinical trials. These patients may have more medical comorbidity. They may have had prior adverse effects. Starting with a low dose to assess tolerance may help to minimize side effects and keep the patient in treatment. Alternatively, the data reviewed above suggest that the final dose will be within the usual effective range for the drug.

D. Resistance to Treatment

Although elderly patients are more sensitive to certain types of side effects, they are not necessarily more sensitive to primary treatment effects. In fact, the elderly may be more resistant to treatment. In our studies of response to desipramine across the age range, we found lower response rates in patients over 75 years of age, even when they achieved adequate blood levels, than in patients between 60 to 75 years of age, or under 60 years of age (Fig. 1) (106–108). The difference in the two groups under age 75 was minimal.

Another data set addressing this issue is the review of controlled trials published by the AHCPR (90). Fourteen efficacy trials of tricyclics in elderly patients and 102 trials in nonelderly outpatient samples were reviewed. There were more efficacy trials for the TCAs than for any other drug class by a wide margin. The overall mean intent-to-treat response rate was lower in the elderly samples than in younger adults (40.4% vs. 51.5%). Yet the drug–placebo differences in these two groups were very similar, 22% and 21.3%. These findings indicate that both drug response rates and placebo rates are lower in the elderly, but that actual drug–placebo differences are relatively similar.

The data for the SSRIs are less clear. In the 20 placebo-controlled or comparison studies reviewed above, eight reported intent-to-treat response rates, with response defined as 50% improvement on the HAM-D (96,132, 141–143,146,153,156). Response rates ranged from 36% to 60%, with a mean of 44.3% for the 785 patients who received SSRIs. This mean intent-to-treat rate is relatively similar to that for the TCAs in the elderly patients described above.

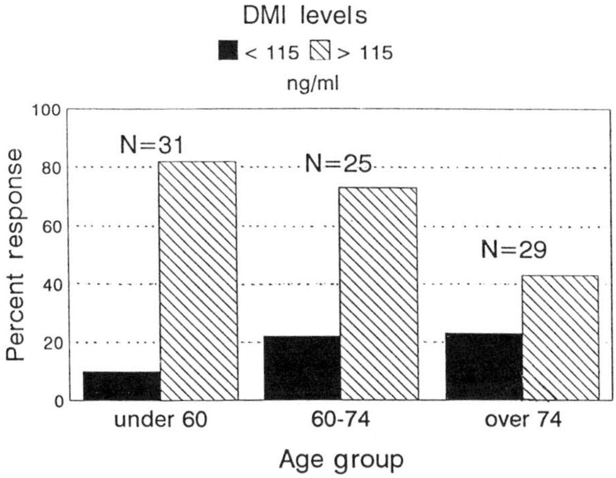

FIGURE 1 Response to desipramine by age group. Response = HAM-D ≤ 10 and ≥ 50% improvement. Each age group is divided by the plasma desipramine concentration of 115 ng/ml.

Reynolds has asserted that the elderly are responsive to treatment, citing a 78% response rate in the acute treatment phase of a maintenance treatment study (157). Patients in this study, however, also received psychotherapy, were treated for 16 weeks, and a portion of the sample also received augmentation with lithium or a neuroleptic. Further, a prior history of remission between episodes was required for patients to enter the study and this might predict a more favorable outcome. Finally, the average age was 70, and most of the patients were between the ages of 65 and 75, so that this was a "young–old" sample. Nevertheless, the findings do indicate that in patients capable of responding, treatment with adequate dose or blood levels, for adequate duration, and with adjunctive treatments if needed, will be successful in four out of five patients.

Another aspect of treatment resistance is the time-to-response. Georgotas and McCue reported that the elderly take longer to respond (158). Because their report is often cited, it is worth describing the actual data. They noted that at the end of a 7-week controlled drug trial, 54% of the patients had responded. The patients were followed for another 2 weeks on an open basis and the cumulative rate rose to 70% (Fig. 2). Yet recent clinical trials of the SSRIs in nongeriatric adults, which have been of longer duration than earlier TCA trials, suggest that the cumulative response rate may continue to increase for a longer period than previously appreciated. Unfortunately, there are no

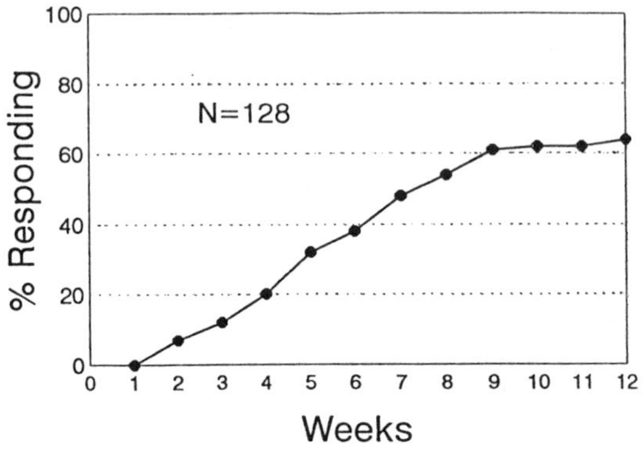

FIGURE 2 Cumulative percent responding each week during antidepressant drug treatment.

data comparing time-to-response in younger and older patients treated under similar conditions.

From a theoretical perspective, it is not surprising that the elderly might be sensitive to side effects but resistant to treatment effects. Many side effects including anticholinergic effects, antihistamine effects, anti-α_1 adrenergic effects result from receptor blockade. If the effectiveness of neurotransmission in the brain is declining (see Chap. 1), these systems may be more vulnerable to receptor blockade. Alternatively, antidepressant drugs act by facilitating serotonergic or noradrenergic transmission. If these systems are declining, it may be more difficult to enhance neurotransmission. For example, a study of the noradrenergic system found that higher doses of isoproterenol were required in the elderly to produce the same increase in heart rate manifested in younger patients (159).

E. The Effect of Medical Illness on Antidepressant Response

Another possible explanation of resistance to treatment is the effect of medical illness on response. This question has not been well studied. Usually medically ill patients are excluded from controlled trials. In a study of patients with major depression identified on a medical consultation service, Popkin (160) described response to TCA treatment in 58 patients. Twenty patients (34%) discontinued treatment because of adverse effects, and 40% of the dropouts had delirium. Thirty-four completed treatment, and 20 responded. The completer response rate was 59%, but the intent-to-treat rate was 34%. In other words, of those beginning treatment, one of three responded and one of three had adverse effects that interrupted treatment.

In the retrospective review of patients with a psychotic depressive syndrome described above (28), all patients received relatively similar combined neuroleptic-TCA treatment. In this study, active medical illness was associated with a high rate of adverse reactions, but had little effect on response. Although the overall rate of response was low, 29.3% (29/99), response rates were similar for patients with and without active medical illness, 8 of 26 (31%) vs. 21 of 73 (29%).

Giakis et al. (161) reported the results of a double-blind comparison of fluoxetine and bupropion in medically ill patients. Patients ranged in age from 51 to 92. Fluoxetine was dosed up to 40 mg/day, bupropion to 450 mg/day. Of the 18 patients receiving fluoxetine, 6 responded (33%) and 3 dropped out with adverse effects. Of the 16 bupropion patients, 2 responded (12.5%) and 2 dropped out with adverse effects. This study suggested that second-generation antidepressants might be better tolerated in medically ill patients, but the efficacy of the two drugs differed. The intent-to-treat rate for fluoxetine was similar to the rate previously reported in a large study of fluoxetine in the elderly (96); however, bupropion was not effective.

These limited data suggest that medical illness results in a higher adverse event discontinuation rate, especially for the tricyclics. Response rates, however, appear to be less affected by medical illness.

IV. SELECTION OF AN ANTIDEPRESSANT

The tricyclic antidepressants have been the mainstay of treatment of depression for nearly three decades. They are clearly effective in the elderly. Because of side effects, however, the tertiary TCAs—imipramine, amitriptyline, and doxepin—are no longer recommended. Amitriptyline is the most anticholinergic of the TCAs; doxepin is one of the most potent H_1 antihistaminic compounds available (162). Imipramine is intermediate but more anticholinergic and antihistaminic than desipramine or nortriptyline. Of the TCAs, nortriptyline and desipramine have become the drugs of choice in the elderly. Nortriptyline has the least orthostatic hypotension (163,164) but has modest anticholinergic effects. Desipramine has the least anticholinergic effects but does cause orthostatic hypotension (101). Both can increase heart rate, delay ventricular conduction, be dangerous in overdose, and may pose a long-term hazard for patients with ischemic heart disease (165) (see Chap. 8).

The SSRIs have become popular in the treatment of elderly patients just as they have become first-line drugs for nongeriatric patients (166). In the 19 SSRI comparison studies in depressed elders described above, 13 provided a comparison with a TCA. In these 13 studies, antidepressant effectiveness was very similar for the SSRI and TCA. In 11 of the SSRI–TCA comparison studies for which adverse event discontinuation rates were reported, drop-out rates were higher for the TCA than the SSRI in seven studies, equal in two, and higher for the SSRI in two [both paroxetine (149,156)]. Unfortunately, all but one of the studies used a tertiary TCA as the comparator. In the one study using nortriptyline (155), the adverse event drop-out rate was higher for nortriptyline, 13 of 104 (12.5%), than for sertraline, 8 of 104 (7.6%). Because of safety and tolerability, an SSRI will often be the drug of choice. In addition, dosing of the SSRIs is relatively simple. They are given once a day and often can be started at an effective dose. Even if a lower dose is given to test tolerance, dose adjustment is less complicated than for the TCAs.

Another concern in elderly patients is the effect of antidepressants on cognition. Fairweather et al. (150) compared the effects of 20 mg/day fluoxetine and 75 mg/day amitriptyline on a variety of cognitive measures in elderly depressed patients. The two drugs had similar effects on depression, but as the depression improved, fluoxetine was associated with greater improvement in information processing and reaction time than was amitriptyline. Fluoxetine was also associated with less drowsiness than amitriptyline.

There are concerns to be aware of using the SSRIs in elderly patients. The common side effects are similar to those described in younger patients—nausea, diarrhea, anxiety, insomnia, nervousness, and tremor. In elderly patients for whom maintaining adequate nutrition has been a problem, anorexia and weight loss associated with the SSRIs can be of particular concern. In a retrospective review of elderly depressed patients who were medically ill or frail, Brymer and Winograd (167) found that fluoxetine was associated with significant anorexia and a mean weight loss of 10 pounds in 15 patients who were 75 years of age or older. Another less common problem is hyponatremia. Among all patients treated with SSRIs, this is an uncommon occurrence; however, it is more frequent in the elderly. Liu et al. (168) reviewed 736 cases of hyponatremia or SIADH reported for the SSRIs. Over three-quarters of the cases occurred in patients over 65 years of age.

The other issue of concern for the SSRIs is their pharmacokinetic drug interactions. Fluoxetine and paroxetine are potent inhibitors of 2D6 (169,170), and serious adverse interactions have been observed when these drugs are combined with conventional doses of the tricyclics (171). Nefazodone is a moderately potent inhibitor of 3A4 (172), and serious interactions with terfenadine or astemizole could potentially occur. These interactions are discussed in detail in Chapter 3. Usually these interactions do not prohibit treatment, but they may require dose adjustment of other drugs, and in some cases blood level monitoring.

Hazardous pharmacodynamic interactions can also occur when the SSRIs are combined with the MAOIs (173). For this reason, the combined use of these drugs is absolutely contraindicated. A 2-week washout period should be allowed when switching from one drug class to the other, with the exception that fluoxetine will require a 5-week washout because of its long elimination half-life.

Other antidepressants have also been employed in the elderly. Placebo-controlled trials support the efficacy of trazodone (93), bupropion (94,95), fluvoxamine (97), and phenelzine (92). Phenelzine is an effective agent and relatively well tolerated except for orthostatic hypotension. Georgotas (92) found that, with reasonable attention to dietary restrictions, hypertensive reactions were rare. Because of these restrictions, the MAOIs are used infrequently; yet many experienced psychopharmacologists find them very effective agents, especially in patients who have failed other drug classes. Trazodone is more effective than placebo in the elderly (93); however, its use has decreased as less sedating compounds have become available. Sedation can be a particular problem in the elderly and can prevent an adequate dose from being attained. Yet this potent secondary effect of trazodone can be used to advantage in some patients when the drug is used as an hypnotic (174,175).

Bupropion is also effective in the elderly (95) and appears to have a relatively benign side-effect profile, but its place in an algorithm for treatment of the elderly is somewhat unclear. Two early placebo-controlled studies of bupropion employed small samples. In one of the studies, bupropion was not significantly more effective than placebo and appeared to be less effective than imipramine (94). In a study of medically ill older patients (161), it was not effective. Another drawback is the lack of published information about its pharmacokinetics, its use in the elderly, and its potential drug interactions.

The three newest agents—venlafaxine, nefazodone, and mirtazepine—have not been well studied in the elderly. There is some evidence in nongeriatric patients that venlafaxine may be an effective agent in severe depression (59–61), especially at higher doses; but at these doses side effects may increase. An unusual side effect of venlafaxine is supine hypertension. Increased supine blood pressure is dose-dependent and is uncommon at doses up to 225 mg/day (176). Patients already on antihypertensive agents do not appear to be affected, an important observation for treatment of the elderly. Nefazodone appears to have antianxiety and antiagitation effects that occur early in treatment (177), but it can be sedating in elderly patients. Because of higher blood levels, especially in older women beginning treatment (139), initiation at a low dose is important. Less is known about mirtazepine in the elderly. Its secondary effects, sedation and weight gain, may be advantageous in some elderly patients.

V. AUGMENTATION STRATEGIES

In mixed-age samples, augmentation strategies have become widely used as a mechanism for enhancing response and have been reviewed elsewhere (178, 179). If the elderly are more resistant to treatment, augmentation strategies might be particularly helpful. Published reports of the use of these strategies in elderly patients are quite limited, although a modest literature exists on the use of lithium augmentation in the elderly. Between 1982 and 1992, 10 reports described 17 patients over 60 years of age who were successfully treated with lithium augmentation after failing prior treatments (180–189). The patients described suffered from both psychotic and nonpsychotic major depression. Four larger series of elderly cases have also been described. Lafferman and associates found lithium augmentation effective in 7 of 14 older patients resistant to prior treatment (190). Reynolds et al. found lithium addition effective in 11 of 16 (69%) older patients who had failed at least 8 weeks of nortriptyline and psychotherapy (191). The largest study was a retrospective review of 51 elderly depressed patients who received lithium augmentation (192). Eighteen patients (35%) had a complete response, another 15 patients (30%) were partial responders. These rates of response are very similar to those observed in nongeriatric samples (178). Not all studies have been positive. A systematic study of lithium augmentation in 15 elderly patients reported disappointing results (193). Patients entering the trial had failed 4 weeks of nortriptyline at adequate blood levels. Lithium was then added for 3 weeks in an open trial. Two partial responders to nortriptyline had a complete response when lithium was added, but only one of the nonresponders to nortriptyline had a complete response after the addition of lithium. Lithium is a difficult drug to use in older patients both because of reduced renal clearance and because of apparent increased sensitivity to lithium (see Chapter 15). Three groups have observed the development of neurotoxicity during lithium augmentation (190,192,194).

The relationship of lithium levels to response during augmentation has not been well studied in older patients. In nongeriatric patients, lithium levels above 0.4 meq/L appear to be necessary for response (195), and lacking other information this threshold appears reasonable for elderly patients. Levels of 1.0 meq/L, however, are not necessary for augmentation and, given the sensitivity of the elderly to lithium, lower levels would be advised. With these considerations, a level between 0.4 to 0.7 meq/L would appear to be ideal for augmentation. In elderly patients, lower doses may be sufficient to achieve this level because of reduced renal clearance. There are no data in the lithium augmentation literature to suggest that the use of lithium will allow the clinician to use lower doses of the primary antidepressant.

Another question is whether to continue lithium in patients who respond to augmentation. In the Reynolds et al. study (191), lithium augmentation was administered for 4 to 6 weeks and then gradually withdrawn. Relapse occurred after withdrawal in 5 of 11 (45.5%) patients. These data, while limited, pose a clinical dilemma—50% of the patients responding to lithium augmentation will continue to require its administration, but the other 50% will not. The clinician will have to make a judgment weighing the hazards of continued lithium against the consequences of relapse in that patient.

The use of the combination of a TCA, usually nortriptyline, and an SSRI was described by Seth et al. in eight elderly depressed patients refractory to other treatments (196). The combination was useful even in patients refractory to ECT. In our experience in mixed-age samples (197) this is an effective combination for refractory patients, but it may be associated with more side effects than some augmentation strategies, and the SSRI–TCA drug interactions need to be considered. Fluoxetine and paroxetine will raise desipramine levels about threefold (197), thus the desipramine dose is reduced to one-third that usually administered. The actual desipramine dose required to achieve an adequate blood level will usually be between 75 and 125 mg/day. The effect of 2D6 inhibitors on nortriptyline is less clear, but an interaction would be expected. The average dose of nortriptyline given alone will be about 75 mg/day (92,99). If given with fluoxetine or paroxetine, one-third of this amount, or 25 mg/day, would be a reasonable starting dose for nortriptyline. Blood level monitoring can then be used to further adjust the dose.

A number of open studies, which have been reviewed elsewhere (178, 198) describe the adjunctive use of stimulants. Although use in the elderly has not been specifically addressed, the samples described included older patients. Although controlled studies are lacking, the open studies and experience suggest this may be a useful approach, particularly in retarded or anergic patients. Stimulants, at the doses used, are safe agents, even in medically ill patients (199). At low doses, they do not usually affect blood pressure. The common side effects are behavioral (e.g., agitation, irritability, or paranoid thinking). A number of other agents have been used for augmentation, including T_3, tryptophan, busperione, pindolol, and other antidepressant combinations, but have not been reported in the elderly.

VI. SUMMARY

Treatment of elderly depressed patients remains a challenge. Comorbid medical conditions complicate diagnosis and treatment. Adverse reactions appear to be more common, and can have more serious consequences when they occur. The tradition of starting treatment cautiously appears justified by the concern for safety; yet, doses and blood levels comparable to younger adults will usually be required for response. Even with adequate treatment, the elderly may be resistant to treatment and less likely to respond. Augmentation strategies would appear to offer one approach to treatment resistance but have seldom been studied in older patients. More effective treatments that are safe are still needed. Although there is a growing body of literature describing the use of the SSRIs in elderly patients, to my knowledge there are no controlled or systematic studies of these agents in patient samples over 75 years of age. Thus, regrettably, while the very old are the most frail and most challenging patients, there are few empirical data to guide the clinician when treating these patients.

REFERENCES

1. NIH Consensus Development Panel on Depression in Late Life. Diagnosis and treatment of depression in late life. JAMA 1992; 268:1018–1024.
2. Robins LN, Helzer JE, Weissman MM, Orvaschel H, Gruenberg E, Burke D Jr, Regier DA. Lifetime prevalence of specific psychiatric disorder in three sites. Arch Gen Psychiatry 1984; 41:949–958.
3. Fitten LJ, Morley JE, Gross PL, petry SD, Cole KD. Depression: UCLA Geriatric Grand Rounds. J Am Geriatr Soc 1989; 37:459–472.
4. Magni G, Schifano F, de Leo D. Assessment of depression in an elderly medical population. J Affect Disord 1986; 11:121–124.
5. Conwell Y. Suicide in elderly patients. In: Schneider LS, Reynolds CF, Leibowitz BD, Friedhoff A, eds. Diagnosis and Treatment of Depression in Late Life: Results of the NIH Consensus Development Conference. Washington DC: American Psychiatric Press, 1994; 397–418.
6. Blazer DG, Bachar JR, Manton KG. Suicide in late life: review and commentary. J Am Geriatr Soc 1986; 34:519–525.
7. Wells KB, Stewart A, Hays RD, Burnam MA, Rogers W, Daniels M, Berry S, Greenfield S, Ware J Jr. The functioning and well being of depressed patients: results from the Medical Outcomes Study. JAMA 1989; 262:914–919.
8. Hays RD, Wells KB, Sherbourne CD, Rogers W, Spritzer K. Functioning and well-being outcomes of patients with depression compared with chronic general medical illnesses. Arch Gen Psychiatry 1995; 52:11–19.
9. Bruce ML, Seeman TE, Merrill SS, Blazer DG. The impact of depressive symptomatology on physical disability: MacArthur studies of successful aging. Am J Publ Health 1994; 84:1796–1799.
10. Conwell Y, Nelson JC, Kim KM, Mazure CM. Elderly patients admitted to the psychiatric unit of a general hospital. J Am Geriatr Soc 1989; 37:35–41.
11. Conwell Y, Nelson JC, Kim KM, Mazure CM. Depression in late life: age of onset as a marker of a subtype. J Affect Disord 1989; 17:189–195.
12. Giaturo DT, Busse EW. Psychiatric problems encountered during a long-term study of normal aging volunteers. In: Isaacs AD, Post F, eds. Studies in Geriatric Psychiatry. New York: John Wiley and Sons, 1978.

13. Murphy E. Social origins of depression in old age. Br J Psychiatry 1982; 141:135–142.
14. Rodin G, Voshart K. Depression in the medically ill: an overview. Am J Psychiatry 1986; 143:696–705.
15. Katon W, Sullivan MD. Depression and chronic medical illness. J Clin Psychiatry 1990; 51(Suppl 6):3–11.
16. Pratt LA, Ford DE, Crum RM, Armenian HK, Gallo JJ, Eaton WW. Depression, psychotropic medication, and risk of myocardial infarction. Circulation 1996; 94: 3123–29.
17. Frazure-Smith N, Lesperance F, Talajic M. Depression following myocardial infarction: impact on 6-month survival. JAMA 1993; 270:1819–1825.
18. Bruce ML, Baker DI. Depressive symptoms in medical homecare patients: a pilot study. Presented at the Claude D. Pepper Older Americans Independence Center Meetings, May 1996, Washington DC.
19. Rovner BW, German PS, Brant LJ, Clark R, Burton L, Folstein MF. Depression and mortality in nursing homes. JAMA 1991; 265:993–996.
20. Bruce ML, Leaf PJ, Rozal GPM, Florio L, Hoff RA. Psychiatric status and 9-year mortality data in the New Haven epidemiologic catchment area study. Am J Psychiatry 1994; 151:716–721.
21. Avery D, Winokur G. Mortality in depressed patients treated with electroconvulsive therapy and antidepressants. Arch Gen Psychiatry 1976; 33:1029–1037.
22. Raskin A. Signs and symptoms of psychopathology in the elderly. In: Raskin A, Jarvik LF, eds. Psychiatric Symptoms and Cognitive Loss in the Elderly Evaluation and Assessment Techniques. Washington, DC: Hemisphere Publishing Corporation, 1979:3–18.
23. Caine ED, Lyness JM, King DA. Reconsidering depression in the elderly. Am J Geriatric Psychiatry 1993; 1:4–20.
24. Clark DC, Cavanaugh SV, Gibbons RD. The core symptoms of depression in medical and psychiatric patients. J Nerv Ment Disord 1983; 171:705–713.
25. Wilson DR, Widmer RB, Cadoret RJ, et al. Somatic symptoms: a major feature of depression in a family practice. J Affect Disord 1983; 5:199–207.
26. Bridges KW, Goldberg DP. Somatic presentation of DSM III psychiatric disorders in primary care. J Psychosomatic Res 1985; 29:563–569.
27. Sifneos PE. Short-term psychotherapy and emotional crisis. Cambridge: Harvard University Press, 1972.
28. Nelson JC, Mennesson M, Levinson J. Age, medical illness, and response to combined antipsychotic/antidepressant treatment in psychotic depression. Annual Meeting of Am Assoc Geriatr Psychiatry, San Diego, CA, Feb 18, 1990.
29. Kiloh LG. Pseudo-dementia. Acta Psychiatr Scand 1961; 37:336–351.
30. McAllister TW. Overview: pseudodementia. Am J Psychiatry 1983; 140:528–533.
31. Burt D, Zembar M, Niederehe G. Depression and memory impairment: a meta-analysis of the association, its pattern, and specificity. Psychol Bull 1995; 117:285–305.
32. Devanand D, Nelson JC. Concurrent depression and dementia: implications for diagnosis and treatment. J Clin Psychiatry 1985; 46:389–392.

33. Nelson JC, Conwell Y, Kim K, Mazure CM. Concurrence of dementia in inpatients with affective disorder. Abstract. Annual meeting of the American Association of Geriatric Psychiatry, San Diego, CA, 1990.
34. Reifler BV, Larson E, Hanley R. Coexistence of cognitive impairment and depression in geriatric outpatients. Am J Psychiatry 1982; 139:623–626.
35. Reding M, Haycox J, Blass J. Depression in patients referred to a dementia clinic. Arch Neurol 1985; 42:894–896.
36. Rovner BW, Broadhead J, Spencer M, Carson K, Folstein MF. Depression and Alzheimer's disease. Am J Psychiatry 1989; 146:1239.
37. Greenwald BS, Kramer-Ginsberg G, Martin DB, Laidman LB, Hermann CK, Mohs R, Davis KL. Dementia with coexistent major depression. Am J Psychiatry 1989; 146:1472–1478.
38. Weiner MF, Bruhn M, Svetlik D, Tintner R, Hom J. Experiences with depression in a dementia clinic. J Clin Psychiatry 1991; 52:234–238.
39. Wood KA, harris MJ, Morreale AN, Rizos AL. Drug-induced psychosis and depression in the elderly. Psychiatric Clin N Am 1988; 11:167–193.
40. Schildkraut J. Catecholamine hypothesis of affective disorders. Am J Psychiatry 1965; 122:509–522.
41. Goodwin FK, Bunney WE Jr. Depressions following reserpine: a re-evaluation. Semin Psychiatry 1971; 3:435–448.
42. Glassman A, et al. Depression, delusions and drug response. Am J Psychiatry 1975; 132:716–719.
43. Chan CH, Janicak PG, Davis JM. Response of psychotic and nonpsychotic depressed patients to tricyclic antidepressants. J Clin Psychiatry 1987; 48:197–200.
44. Nelson JC, Bowers MB. Delusional unipolar depression: description and drug response. Arch Gen Psychiatry 1978; 35:1321–1328.
45. Spiker DG, Weiss JC, Dealy RS, et al. The pharmacologic treatment of delusional depression. Am J Psychiatry 1985; 142:430–436.
46. Janicak PG, Pandey GN, Davis JM, Boshes R, Bresnahan D, Sharma R. Response of psychotic and nonpsychotic depression to phenelzine. Am J Psychiatry 1988; 145:93–95.
47. Nelson JC, Mazure CM, Jatlow PI. Characteristics of tricyclic refractory depression. J Clin Psychiatry 1994; 55:12–19.
48. American Psychiatric Association. Practice guideline for the treatment of patients with bipolar disorder. Am J Psychiatry 1994; 151(Suppl):1–35.
49. Himmelhoch JM, Thase ME, Mallinger AG, Houck P. Tranylcypromine versus imipramine in anergic bipolar depression. Am J Psychiatry 1991; 148:910–916.
50. Sachs GS, Lafer B, Stoll A, Banov M, Thibault AB, Tohen M, Rosenbaum JF. A double-blind trial of bupropion versus desipramine for bipolar depression. J Clin Psychiatry 1994; 55:391–393.
51. Quitkin FM, Stewart JW, et al. Antidepressant specificity in atypical depression. Arch Gen Psychiatry 1988; 45:129–137.
52. Reimherr FW, Wood DR, Byerley B, Brainard J, Grosser VI. Characteristics of responders to fluoxetine. Psychopharmacol Bull 1984; 20:70–72.
53. Pande AC, Haskett RF, Greden JF. Fluoxetine treatment of atypical depression. Presented at the APA Annual Meeting, Washington, D.C., May 5, 1992.

54. Roose SP, Glassman AH, Attia E, Woodring S. Comparative efficacy of selective serotonin reuptake inhibitors and tricyclics in the treatment of melancholia. Am J Psychiatry 1994; 151:1735–1739.
55. Danish University Antidepressant Group: Citalopram: clinical effect profile in comparison with clomipramine. A controlled multicenter study. Psychopharmacology 1986; 90:131–138.
56. Danish University Antidepressant Group: Paroxetine: a selective serotonin reuptake inhibitor showing better tolerance, but weaker antidepressant effect than comipramine in a controlled multicenter study. J Affect Disord 1990; 18:289–299.
57. Montgomery SA. The efficacy of fluoxetine as an antidepressant in the short and long term. Int Clin Psychopharmacol 1989; 4(Suppl):113–119.
58. Nelson JC. The synergistic benefits of serotonin and noradrenaline reuptake inhibition. Eur Psychiatry 1996; 11:253s.
59. Guelfi JD, White C, Hackett D, et al. Effectiveness of venlafaxine in patients hospitalized for major depression and melancholia. J Clin Psychiatry 1995; 56:450–458.
60. Clerc GE, Ruimy P, Verdeau-Pailles J. A double-blind comparison of venlafaxine and fluoxetine in patients hospitalized for major depression and melancholia. Int Clin Psychopharmacol 1994; 9;138–143.
61. Benkert O, Hackett D, Realini R, et al. A randomized, double-blind comparison of a rapidly escalating dose of venlafaxine and imipramine in inpatients with major depression and melancholia (abstract). Neuropsychopharmacology 1994; 10 (Suppl):165S.
62. Devanand DP, Nobler MS, Singer T, Kiersky JE, Turret N, Roose SP, Sackeim HA. Is dysthymia a different disorder in the elderly? Am J Psychiatry 1994; 151: 1592–99.
63. Kocsis JH, Frances AJ, Voss CB, Mann JJ, Mason BJ, Sweeney J. Imipramine for treatment of chronic depression. Arch Gen Psychiatry 1988; 45:253–257.
64. Hellerstein DJ, Yanowitch P, Rosenthal J, Samstag LW, Maurer M, Kasch K, Burrows L, Poster M, Cantillon M, Winston A. A randomized double-blind study of fluoxetine versus placebo in the treatment of dysthymia. Am J Psychiatry 1993; 150:1169–1175.
65. Thase ME, Fava M, Halbreich U, Kocsis JH, Koran L, Davidson J, Rosenbaum J, Harrison W. A placebo-controlled, randomized clinical trial comparing sertraline and imipramine for the treatment of dysthymia. Arch Gen Psychiatry 1996; 53: 777–784.
66. Nobler MS, Devanand DP, Kim MK, Fitzsimons LM, Singer TM, Turret N, Sackeim HA, Roose SP. Fluoxetine treatment of dysthymia in the elderly. J Clin Psychiatry 1996; 57:254–256.
67. Kupfer DJ, Spiker DG. Refractory depression: prediction of nonresponse by clinical indicators. J Clin Psychiatry 1981; 42:307–312.
68. Roose SP, Glassman AH, Walsh BT, Woodring S. Tricyclic nonresponders, phenomenology and treatment. Am J Psychiatry 1986; 143:345–348.
69. Davidson JRT, Giller EL, Zisook S, Overall JE. An efficacy study of isocarboxizid and placebo in depression and its relationship to depressive nosology. Arch Gen Psychiatry 1988; 45:120–127.

70. Robinson DS, Nies A, Ravaris L, Lamborn KR. The monoamine oxidase inhibitor, phenelzine, in the treatment of depressive-anxiety states. Arch Gen Psychiatry 1973; 29:407–413.
71. Paykel ES, Rowan PW, Parker RR, Bhat AV. Response to phenelzine and amitriptyline in subtypes of outpatient depression. Arch Gen Psychiatry 1982; 39:1041–1049.
72. Joyce PR, Paykel ES. Predictors of drug response in depression. Arch Gen Psychiatry 1989; 46:89–99.
73. Nelson JC, Charney DS. The symptoms of major depressive illness. Am J Psychiatry 1981; 138:1–12.
74. Mendlewicz J. The age factor in depressive illness: some genetic considerations. J Gerontol 1976; 31:300–303.
75. Winokur G, Behar D, Schlesser M. Clinical and biological aspects of depression in the elderly. In: Cole JO, Bennett JE, eds. Psychopathology in the Aged. New York: Raven Press, 1980:145–153.
76. Brown RP, Sweeney J, Loutsch E, Kocsis J, Frances A. Involutional melancholia revisited. Am J Psychiatry 1984; 141:24–28.
77. Cole M, Hicking H. Frequency and significance of minor organic signs in elderly depressives. Can Psychiatr Assoc J 1976; 21:7–12.
78. Davies G, Hamilton S, Hendrickson DE, Levy R, Post F. Psychological test performance and sedation thresholds of elderly dements, depressives, and depressives with incipient brain damage. Psychol Med 1978; 8:103–109.
79. Kay DWK. Outcome and cause of death in mental disorders of old age: a long-term follow-up of functional and organic psychoses. Acta Psychiatr Scan 1962; 38:249–276.
80. Jacoby RJ, Levy R, Bird JM. Computed tomography and the outcome of affective disorder: a follow-up study of eldelry patients. Br J Psychaitry 1981; 139:288–292.
81. Shima S, Shikano T, Kitamura T, Masuda Y, Tsukumo T, Kanbu S, Asai. Depression and ventricular enlargement. Acta Psychiatr Scan 1984; 70:275–277.
82. Rossi A, Stratta P, Petruzzi C, DeDonatis M, Nistico R, Casacchia M. A computerized tomographic study in DSM-III affective disorders. J Affect Disord 1987; 12:259–262.
83. Post F. The management and nature of depressive illnesses in late life: follow-through study. Br J Psychiatry 1972; 121:393–404.
84. Meyers BS, Greenberg R. Late-life delusional depression. J Affect Disord 1986; 11:133–137.
85. Nelson JC, Conwell Y, Kim KM, Mazure CM. Age of onset in late-life delusional depression. Am J Psychiatry 1989; 146:785–786.
86. Thompson LW, Gallagher D, Breckenridge JS. Comparative effectiveness of psychotherapies for depressed elders. J Consult Clin Psychol 1987; 55:385–390.
87. Scogin F, McElreath I. Efficacy of psychosocial treatments for geriatric depression: a quantitative review. J Consult Clin Psychol 1994; 62:69–74.
88. Elkin I, Shea T, Watkins JT, et al. NIMH treatment of depression collaborative research program: general effectiveness of treatments. Arch Gen Psychiatry 1989; 46:971–982.

89. Klein DF, Ross DC. Reanalysis of the NIMH Treatment of Depression Collaborative Research Program General Effectiveness report. Neuropsychopharmacology 1993; 8:241–251.
90. Agency for Health Care Policy and Research. Clinical Practice Guideline: Depression in Primary Care: Treatment of Major Depression. Vol 2. Rockville, MD: U.S. Government Printing Office, 1993.
91. Gerson SC, Plotkin DA, Jarvik LF. Antidepressant drug studies, 1964 to 1986: empirical evidence for aging patients. J Clin Psychopharmacol 1988; 8:311–322.
92. Georgotas A, McCue RE, Hapworth W, Friedman E, Kim OM, Welkowitz J, Chang I, Cooper TB. Comparative efficacy and safety of MAOIs versus TCAs in treating depression in the elderly. Biol Psychiatry 1986; 21:1155–1166.
93. Gerner R, Estabrook W, Steuber J, Jarvik L. Treatment of geriatric depression with trazodone, imipramine, and placebo: a double-blind study. J Clin Psychiatry 1980; 41:216–220.
94. Branconnier RJ, Cole JO, Ghazvinian S, Spera KF. Oxenkrug GF, Bass JL. Clinical pharmacology of bupropion and imipramine in elderly depressives. J Clin Psychiatry 1983; 44(Suppl 5):130–133.
95. Kane JM, Cole K, Sarantakos S, Howard A, Borenstein M. Safety and efficacy of bipropion in elderly patients: preliminary observations. J Clin Psychiatry 1983; 44(Suppl 5):134–136.
96. Tollefson GD, Holman SL. Analysis of the hamilton depression rating scale factors from a double-blind, placebo-controlled trial of fluoxetine in geriatric major depression. Int Clin Psychopharmacol 1993; 8:253–259.
97. Wakelin JS. Fluvoxamine in the treatment of the older depressed patient; double-blind, placebo-controlled data. Int Clin Psychopharmacol 1986; 1:221–230.
98. Salzman C, Schneider L, Lebowitz B. Antidepressant treatment of very old patients. Am J Ger Psychiatry 1993; 1:21–29.
99. Katz IR, Simpson GM, Curlik SM, Parmelee PA, Muhly C. Pharmacologic treatment of major depression for elderly patients in residential care settings. J Clin Psychiatry 1990; 51(Suppl 7):41–48.
100. Holister LE. Drug therapy. N Engl J Med 1978; 299:1168–1172.
101. Nelson JC, Jatlow PI, Bock J, Quinlan DM, Bowers MN Jr. Major adverse reactions during desipramine treatment: relationship to drug plasma concentrations, concomitant antipsychotic treatment and patient characteristics. Arch Gen Psychiatry 1982; 39:1055–1061.
102. Rosenstein DL, Nelson JC. Heart rate during desipramine treatment as an indicator of $beta_1$-adrenergic function. Society of Biological Psychiatry Scientific Program. Biol Psychiatry 1991; 29:132A.
103. Walsh T, Hadigan CM, Wong LM. Increased pulse and blood pressure associated with desipramine treatment of bulimia nervosa. J Clin Psychopharmacol 1992; 12:163–168.
104. Jarvik LF, Mintz J, Steuer J, Gerner R. Treatment geriatric depression: a 26-week interim analysis. J Am Geriatr Soc 1982; 30:713–717.
105. Lakshmanan M, Mion LC, Frengley JD. Effective low dose tricyclic antidepressant treatment for depressed geriatric rehabilitation patients: a double-blind study. Am Geriatr Soc 1986; 34:421–426.

106. Nelson JC, Jatlow PI, Mazure CM. Desipramine plasma levels and response in elderly melancholics. J Clin Psychopharmacol 1985; 217–220.
107. Nelson JC, Mazure CM, Jatlow PI. Desipramine treatment of major depression in patients over 75 years of age. J Clin Psychopharmacol 1995; 15:99–105.
108. Nelson JC, Jatlow PI, Quinlan DM, et al. Desipramine plasma concentrations and antidepressant response. Arch Gen Psychiatry 1982; 39:1419–1422.
109. Cutler NR, Zavadil AP, Eisdorfer C, Ross RJ, Potter WZ. Concentrations of desipramine in elderly women. Am J Psychiatry 1981; 138:1235–1237.
110. Amsterdam JD, Brunswick DJ, Potter L, Winokur A, Rickels K. Desipramine and 2-hydroxydesipramine plasma levels in endogenous depressed patients. Arch Gen Psychiatry 1985; 42:361–364.
111. Katz IR, Simpson GM, Jethanandani V, Cooper T, Muhly C. Steady state pharmacokinetics of nortriptyline in the frail elderly. Neuropsychopharmacology 1989; 2:229–236.
112. Dawling S, Crome P, Heyer EJ, Lewis RR. Nortriptyline therapy in elderly patients: dosage prediction from plasma concentration at 24 hours after a single 50 mg dose. Br J Psychiatry 1981; 139:413–416.
113. Kragh-Sorensen P, Larsen NE. Factors influencing nortriptyline steady-state kinetics: plasma and salva levels. Clin Pharmacol Ther 1980; 28:796–803.
114. Smith RC, Reed K, Leelavathi DE, et al. Pharmacokinetics and the effects of nortriptyline in geriatric depressed patients. Psychopharmacol Bull 1980; 16:54–57.
115. Zeigler VE, Biggs JT. Tricyclic plasma levels: effect of age, race, sex, and smoking. JAMA 1977; 238:2167–2169.
116. Bertilsson L, Mellstrom B, Sjoqvist P. Pronounced inhibition of noradrenaline uptake by 10-hydroxy metabolites of nortriptyline. Life Sci 1979; 25:1285–1292.
117. Young RC, Alexopoulos GS, Shamolan CA, Manley MW, Dhar AK, Kutt H. Plasma 10-hydroxy-nortriptyline in elderly depressed patients. Clin Pharmacol Ther 1984; 35:540–544.
118. Abernethy DR, Greenblatt DJ, Shader RI. Imipramine and desipramine disposition in the elderly. J Pharmacol Exp Ther 1985; 232:183–188.
119. Laurent-Kenesi MA, Jacqz-Aigrain E, LeJouc JL, Jaillon P, Funck-Brentano C. Assessment of CYP 2D6 activity in very elderly healthy subjects. Fundam Clin Pharmacol 1996; 10:158–159.
120. Nelson JC, Mazure C, Jatlow PI. Antidepressant activity of 2-hydroxy-desipramine. Clin Pharmacol Ther 1988; 44:283–288.
121. Nelson JC, Bock JL, Jatlow PI. The clinical implications of 2-hydroxy desipramine in plasma. Clin Pharmacol Ther 1983; 33:183–189.
122. Nelson JC, Mazure CM, Attilasoy E, Jatlow PI. Hydroxy-desipramine in the elderly. J Clin Psychopharmacol 1988; 8:428–433.
123. Kutcher SP, Reid K, et al. ECG changes and therapeutic desipramine and 2-OH-DMI concentrations in elderly depressives. Br J Psychiatry 1986; 14:676–679.
124. Young RC, Alexopoulos GS, Shamoian CA, et al. Plasma 10-hydroxynortriptyline and ECG changes in elderly depressed patients. Am J Psychiatry 1985; 142:866–868.
125. Schneider LS, Cooper TB, Severson JA, et al. Electrocardiographic changes with nortriptyline and 10-hydroxynortriptyline in elderly depressed outpatients. J Clin Psychopharmacol 1988; 8:402–408.

126. Young RC, Alexopoulos GS, Shamoian CA, Dhar AK, Kutt H. Heart failure associated with high plasma 10-hydroxynortriptyline levels. Am J Psychiatry 1984; 141:432–3.
127. Potter QZ, Calil HM, Manian AA, Zavadil AP, Goodwin FK. Hydroxylated metabolites of tricyclic antidepressants: preclinical assessment of activity. Biol Psychiatry 1979; 14:601–613.
128. Young RC, Alexopoulos GS, Shindledecker R, et al. Plasma 10-hydroxynortriptyline and therapeutic response in geriatric depression. Neuropsychopharmacology 1988; 1:213–215.
129. Nelson JC, Jatlow PI, Mazure CM. Rapid desipramine dose adjustment using 24-hour levels. J Clin Psychopharmacol 1987; 7:72–77.
130. Schneider LS, Cooper TB, Staples FR, Sloane RB. Prediction of individual dosage of nortriptyline in depressed elderly outpatients. J Clin Psychopharmacol 1987; 7:311–314.
131. Preskorn SH. Recent pharmacologic advances in antidepressant therapy for the elderly. Am J Med 1993; 94(Suppl. 5A):2S–12S.
132. Feighner JP, Cohn JB. Double-blind comparative trials of fluoxetine and doxepin in geriatric patients with major depressive disorder. J Clin Psychiatry 1985; 46(3, Sec 2):20–25.
133. Lemberger L, Bergstrom RF, Wolen RL, Farid NA, Enas GG, Aronoff GR. Fluoxetine: clinical pharmacology and physiologic disposition. J Clin Psychiatry 1985; 46(Suppl 3):14–19.
134. Amsterdam JD, Hornig-Rohan M, Fawcett J, Quitkin FM, Reimherr FW, Rosenbaum JF, Michelson D, Beasley CM. Fluoxetine and norfluoxetine plasma concentrations in major depression: a multi-center study. Am J Psychiatry (in press).
135. Physicians Desk Reference. Montvale, NJ: Medical Economics Data, 1995.
136. von Moltke LL, Greenblatt DJ, Harmatz JS, Shader RI. Psychotropic drug metabolism in old age: principles and problems of assessment. In: Bloom FE, Kupfer DJ, eds. Psychopharmacology: The Fourth Generation of Progress. New York: Raven Press, 1995:1461–1469.
137. von Moltke LL, Greenblatt DJ, Shader RI. Clinical pharmacokinetics of antidepressants in the elderly: therapeutic implications. Clin Pharmacokinet 1993; 24: 141–160.
138. George J, Byth K, Farrell C. Age but not gender selectively affects expression of individual cytochrome P450 proteins in human liver. Biochem Pharmacol 1995; 50:727–730.
139. Barahaiya RH, Buch AB, Greene DS. A study of the effect of age and gender on the pharmacokinetics of nefazodone after single and multiple doses. J Clin Psychopharmacol 1996; 16:19–25.
140. Altamura AC, DeNovellis F, Guercetti G, Invernizzi G, Percudani M, Montgomery SA. Fluoxetine compared with amitriptyline in elderly depression: a controlled clinical trial. Int J Clin Pharmacol Res 1989; IX(6):391–396.
141. Falk WE, Rosenbaum JF, Otto MW. Fluoxetine versus trazodone in depressed geriatric patients. J Geriatr Psychiatry Neurol 1989; 2:208–214.
142. Guillibert E, Pelicier Y, Archambault JC, Chabannes JP, Clerc G, Desvilles M, Guibert M, Pagot R, Poisat JL, Thobie Y. A double-blind, multicentre study of

paroxetine versus clomipramine in depressed elderly patients. Acta Psychiatr Scand 1989; 80(Suppl 350):132–134.
143. Cohn CK, Shrivastava R, Mendels J, Cohn JB, Fabre LF, Claghorn JL, Dessain EC, Itil TM, Lautin A. Double-blind, multicenter comparison of sertraline and amitryptyline in elderly depressed patients. J Clin Psychiatry 1990; 51(Suppl B12):28–33.
144. Rahman MK, Akhtar MJ, Savla NC, Sharma RR, Kellet JM, Ashford JJ. A double-blind, randomised comparison of fluvoxamine with dothiepin in the treatment of depression in elderly patients. Br J Clin Pharmacology 1991; 45:255–258.
145. Samuelian JC. Comparison of efficacy and safety of increasing doses of paroxetine and clomipramine in elderly patients. Biol Psychiatry 1991; 29:635S.
146. Hutchinson DR, Tong S, Moon CAL, Vince M, Clarke A. Paroxetine in the treatment of elderly depressed patients in general practice: a double-blind comparison with amitriptyline. Br J Clin Research 1991; 2:43–57.
147. Phanjoo AL, Wonnacott S, Hodgson A. A double-blind comparative multicentre study of fluvoxamine and mianserin in the treatment of major depressive episode in elderly people. Acta Psychiatr Scand 1991; 83:476–479.
148. Dorman T. Sleep and paroxetine: a comparison with mianserin in elderly depressed patients. Int Clin Psychopharmacol 1992; 4:53–58.
149. Dunner DL, Cohn JB, Walshe T, Cohn CK, Feighner JP, Fieve RR, Halikas JP, Hartford JT, Hearst ED, Settle EC Jr, Menolascino FJ, Muller DJ. Two combined, multicenter double-blind studies of paroxetine and doxepin in geriatric patients with major depression. J Clin Psychiatry 1992; 53(Suppl 2):57–60.
150. Fairweather DB, Kerr JS, Harrison DA, Moon CA, Hindmarch I. A double-blind comparison of the effects of fluoxetine and amitriptyline on cognitive functioning in elderly depressed patients. Human Psychopharmacol 1993; 8:41–47.
151. La pia S, Georgio D, Ciriello R, Sannino A, De Simone L, Paoletti C, Colonna CV. Evaluation of the efficacy, tolerability, and therapeutic profile of fluoxetine versus mianserin in the treatment of depressive disorders in the elderly. Current Ther Res 1992; 52:847–858.
152. Pelicier Y, Schaeffer P. Etude multicentrique en double aveugle comparant l'efficacite et la tolerance de la paroxetine et de la clomipramine dans la depression reactionnelle du suet age. L'Encephale 1993; 19:257–261.
153. Schone W, Ludwig M. A double-blind study of paroxetine compared with fluoxetine in geriatric patients with major depression. J Clin Psychopharmacol 1993; 13(Suppl 2):34S–39S.
154. Linden RD, Newhouse PA, Krishnan RR, Farmer M, Goldstein BJ, Lazarus LW. Sertraline and fluoxetine in geriatric depression. Presented at the Annual Meeting of the American Psychiatric Association, Miami, FL, 1995.
155. McEntee WJ, Coffey DJ, Bondareff W, Alpert M, Raj AB, Rappaport SA, Finkel SI, Rosenthal MH, DuBoff EA, Jenkyn L, Friedhoff A, Heiser J, Weiner M, Richter EM. A double-blind comparison of sertraline and nortriptyline in the treatment of depressed geriatric outpatients. Presented at the 148th annual meeting of the American Psychiatric Association, Miami, FL, 1995.
156. Geretsegger C, Stuppaeck CH, Mair M, Platz T, Fartacek, Heim M. Multicenter double blind study of paroxetine and amitriptyline in elderly depressed inpatients. Psychopharmacology 1995; 119:227–281.

157. Reynolds CF, Frank E, Perel JM, Imber SD, Cornes C, Morycz RK, Mazumdar S, Miller MD, Pollock BG, Rifai AH, Stack JA, George CJ, Hourck PR, Kupfer DJ. Combined pharmacotherapy and psychotherapy in the acute and continuation treatment of elderly patients with recurrent major depression: a preliminary report. Am J Psychiatry 1992; 149:1687–1692.
158. Georgotas A, McCue RE. The additiional benefit of extending an antidepressant trial past seven weeks in the depressed elderly. Int J Geriatr Psychiatry 1989; 4:191–195.
159. Montamat SC, Davies AO. Physiologic response to isoproterenol and coupling of beta-adrenergic receptors in young and elderly human subjects. J Gerontol Med Sci 1989; 44:M100–105.
160. Popkin MK, Callies AL, Mackenzie TB. The outcome of antidepressant use in the medically ill. Arch Gen Psychiatry 1985; 42:1160–63.
161. Giakas WJ, Miller HL, Hensala JD, Rohrbaugh R, Salomon RM, Licinio J, Charney DS, Delgado PL. Fluoxetine versus bupropion in geriatric depression. Presented at the Annual Meeting of the American Psychiatric Association, San Francisco, CA, 1993.
162. Richelson E. Synaptic effects of antidepressants. J Clin Psychiatry 1996; 16(Suppl 2):1S–9S.
163. Roose SP, Glassman AH, Siris SG, Walsh BT, Bruno RL, Wright LB. Comparison of imipramine and nortriptyline-induced orthostatic hypotension: a meaningful difference. J Clin Psychopharmacol 1981; 1:316–319.
164. Thayssen P, Bjerre M, Kragh-Sorenson P, et al. Cardiovascular effects of imipramine and nortriptyline in elderly patients. Psychopharmacology 1981; 74:360–364.
165. Glassman AH, Roose SP, Bigger JT Jr. The safety of tricyclic antidepressants in cardiac patients: risk/benefit reconsidered. JAMA 1993; 269:2673–2675.
166. Nelson JC, Docherty JP, Henschen GM, Kasper S, Nierenberg AA, Ward NG. Algorithms for the treatment of subtypes of unipolar major depression. Psychopharmacol Bull 1995; 31:475–482.
167. Brymer C, Winograd CH. Fluoxetine in elderly patients: is there cause for concern? J Am Geriatr Soc 1992; 40:902–905.
168. Liu BA, Mittmann N, Knowles SR, Shear NH. Hyponatremia and the syndrome of inappropriate secretion of antidiuretic hormone associated with the use of selective serotonin reuptake inhibitors: a review of spontaneous reports. Can Med Assoc J 1996; 155:519–527.
169. Preskorn SH, Alderman J, Chung M, et al. Pharmacokinetics of desipramine coadministered with sertraline or fluoxetine. J Clin Psychopharmacol 1994; 14:90–98.
170. von Moltke L, Greenblatt DJ, Court MH, Duan SX, Harmatz JS, Shader RI. Inhibition of alprazolam and desipramine hydroxylation in vitro by paroxetine and fluvoxamine: comparison with other selective serotonin reuptake inhibitor antidepressants. J Clin Psychopharmacology 1995; 15:125–131.
171. Preskorn SH, Beber JH, Faul JC, Hirschfeld RMA. Serious adverse effects of combining fluoxetine and tricyclic antidepressants. Am J Psychiatry 1990; 147: 532.

172. von Moltke L, Greenblatt DJ, Schmider J, Harmatz JS, Shader RI. Nefazodone in vitro: metabolic conversions, and inhibition of P450-3A isoforms. Clin Pharmacol Ther 1996; 55:176.
173. Feighner JP, Boyer WF, Tyler DL, et al. Adverse consequences of fluoxetine-MAOI combination therapy. J Clin Psychiatry 1990; 51:222–225.
174. Jacobsen FM. Low dose trazodone as a hypnotic in patients with MAOIs and other psychotropics: a pilot study. J Clin Psychiatry 1990; 51:298–302.
175. Nierenberg AA, Adler LA, Peselow E, Zornberg G, Rosenthal M. Trazodone for antidepressant-associated insomnia. Am J Psychiatry 1994; 151:1069–1972.
176. Feignher JP. Cardiovascular safety in depressed patients: focus on venlafaxine. J Clin Psychiatry 1995; 56:574–579.
177. Fawcett J, Marcus RN, Anton SF, O'Brien K, Schwiderski U. Response of anxiety and agitation synptoms during nefazodone treatment of major depression. J Clin Psychiatry 1995; 56(Suppl 6):37–42.
178. Nelson JC. Augmentation strategies for treatment of unipolar major depression. In: Rush AJ, ed. Modern Problems of Pharmacology. New York: Basel Karger, 1996.
179. Thase ME, Rush AJ. Treatment-resistant depression. In: Bloom FE, Kupfer DJ, eds. Psychopharmacology: The Fourth Generation of Progress. New York: Raven Press Ltd, 1995.
180. Nelson JC, Byck R. Rapid response to lithium in phenelzine nonresponders. Br J Psychiatry 1982; 141:85–86.
181. Price LH, Conwell Y, Nelson JC. Lithium augmentation of combined neuroleptic-tricyclic treatment in delusional depression. Am J Psychiatry 1983; 140:318–322.
182. Weaver KEC. Lithium for delusional depression. Am J Psychiatry 1983; 140:962–963.
183. Pande AD, Max P. A lithium-tricyclic combination for treatment of depression. Am J Psychiatry 1985; 142:1228–1229.
184. Schrader GD, Levien HE. Response to sequential administration of clomipramine and lithium carbonate in treatment-resistant depression. Br J Psychiatry 1985; 147:573–575.
185. Pai M, White AC, Deane AG. Lithium augmentation in the treatment of delusional depression. Br J Psychiatry 1986; 148:736–738.
186. Kushnir SL. Lithium-antidepressant combinations in the treatment of depressed, physically ill geriatric patients. Am J Psychiatry 1986; 143:378–379.
187. Fein S, Paz V, Rao N, LaGrassa J. The combination of lithium carbonate and an MAOI in refractory depression. Am J Psychiatry 1988; 145:249–250.
188. Lieff A, Herrmann N. Combined drug therapy for an elderly depressed patient. Am J Psychiatry 1988; 145:1034–1035.
189. Schreiber S, Shalev A. Lithium augmentation for mianserin-resistant depression in the elderly. Harefuah 1992; 123:250–251.
190. Lafferman J, Solomon K, Ruskin P. Lithium augmentation for treatment-resistant depression in the elderly. J Geriatr Psychiatry Neurol 1988; 1:49–52.
191. Reynolds CF, Frank E, Perel JM, et al. High relapse rate after discontinuation of adjunctive medication for elderly patients with recurrent major depression. Am J Psychiatry 1996; 153:1418–1422.

192. van Marwijk HWJ, Bekker FM, Nolen WA, Jansen PAF, van Nieuwkerk JF, Hop WCJ. Lithium augmentation in geriatric depression. J Affect Disord 1990; 20: 217–223.
193. Zimmer B, Rosen J, Thornton JE, Perel JM, Reynolds CF III. Adjunctive lithium carbonate in nortriptyline-resistant elderly depressed patients. J Clin Psychopharmacol 1991; 11:254–256.
194. Austin LS, Arana GW, Melvin JA. Toxicity resulting from lithium augmentation of antidepressant treatment in elderly patients. J Clin Psychiatry 1990; 51:344–345.
195. Stein G, Bernadt M. Lithium augmentation therapy in tricyclic-resistant depression: a controlled trial using lithium in low and normal doses. Br J Psychiatry 1993; 162:634–640.
196. Seth R, Jennings AL, Bindman J, et al. Combination treatment with noradrenaline and serotonin reuptake inhibitors in resistant depression. Br J Psychiatry 1992; 161:562–565.
197. Nelson JC, Mazure CM, Bowers MB, Jatlow PI. A preliminary open study of the combination of fluoxetine and desipramine for rapid treatment of major depression. Arch Gen Psychiatry 1991; 48:303–307.
198. Ayd FJ Jr, Zohar J. Psychostimulant (amphetamine or methylphenidate) therapy for chronic and treatment-resistant depression. In: Zohar J, Belmaker RH, eds. Treating Resistant Depression. New York: PMA Publishing, 1987:343–355.
199. Satel SL, Nelson JC. Stimulants in the treatment of depression: a critical overview. J Clin Psychiatry 1989; 50:241–249.

5
Treatment of Psychotic Depression

Barnett S. Meyers
Cornell University Medical College, and The New York Hospital–Cornell Medical Center, White Plains, New York

I. INTRODUCTION

The parallel developments in psychiatric phenomenology and antidepressant treatments over the past three decades has contributed profoundly to the elucidation and definition of subtypes of psychiatric disorders. The distinction of delusional from the more prevalent nondelusional form of depression is a direct consequence of these studies. This chapter will review the evolution of our knowledge about delusional depression (DD) that derived, initially, from studies of course and treatment response. The importance and complexity of arriving at an accurate diagnosis will be discussed. The limited information available on the course and treatment response of DD specifically in elderly patients will be described. Finally, studies indicating a relationship between disturbed dopaminergic functioning in DD and the relationship of these findings to more recent treatment approaches will be discussed.

II. HISTORICAL OVERVIEW

Studies of the course of severe depressive illness in the period preceding antidepressant pharmacotherapy recognized that patients with depression associated with delusions had a poorer short-term prognosis and lower rates of spontaneous recovery than patients with nondelusional depression (ND) (1,2).

Early antidepressant studies conducted in the 1960s and early 1970s mixed DD with ND subjects; furthermore, interpretation of these studies is limited by the absence of information on the relationship between antidepressant concentrations and therapeutic response. However, post hoc analyses of early antidepressant trials suggested that subjects with DD were less responsive to standard antidepressant therapies (3,4). The demonstration that DD patients who fail to respond to high doses of imipramine recover after treatment with electroconvulsive therapy (ECT) (5) contributed to the impression that ECT is the preferred treatment for this condition (2).

The seminal study of Glassman et al. (6,7) profoundly influenced our understanding of both the treatment of severe major depression and of the relevance of delusions to response. A post hoc analysis of concentration:response relationships demonstrated that hospitalized major depressives with imipramine plasma levels above the sample's median level of 180 ng/ml were significantly more likely to meet stringent criteria for recovery. However, this concentration effect did not apply for patients with DD; fewer than 40% of the subsample of DDs remitted, regardless of blood levels; furthermore, after excluding these patients, 19 of 20 NDs (95%) met rigorous response criteria to high imipramine concentrations. These results demonstrated the contribution of both plasma concentrations and the presence of delusions to responsiveness to antidepressant monotherapy.

Despite persistent controversy over whether the use of imipramine (8) and either inadequate dosage or too brief a treatment trial (9) contributed to the results reported by Glassman, subsequent antidepressant studies have generally recognized the potential effect of delusions on response and assessed subjects for fixed irrational thoughts prior to instituting treatment. Furthermore, reports that patients with DD respond to pharmacotherapy when antipsychotics are combined with a standard antidepressant (10) provided an additional rationale for establishing whether major depression is accompanied by delusions.

III. DIAGNOSIS OF DELUSIONAL DEPRESSION

A. Phenomenological and Temporal Factors

Interest in delusional depression has led to studies comparing DD to ND for associated phenomenological and historical features. Using items on the Hamilton Depression Rating Scale (Ham-D) (11), patients with DD have been shown to have higher total scores (12–14) and both greater agitation (12,13,15) and increased pyschomotor retardation (12,14). These studies contributed to the suggestion that depressed patients with psychomotor disturbance should be assessed especially carefully for the presence of delusions (12).

The finding of higher Ham-D scores in DD (12–14) has been interpreted as indicating that DD is simply an expression of greater severity (13). However, retrospective studies of hospitalized major depressives suggests an alternative explanation. In both mixed-age (15) and elderly samples (16), the association between delusions and depression appears to be consistent through repeated episodes; that is, patients suffering from DD at index have a significantly greater likelihood of having had previous delusional episodes than patients with an index episode of ND. Recent prospective studies have expanded on these findings (17,18). Patients who have psychotic depression at their index episode are at least five times more likely to have psychotic recurrences, an association that continues through the fifth episode (17). The finding that nonpsychotic recurrences in the initially psychotic group were of a significantly shorter duration than nonpsychotic recurrences in consistently nonpsychotic patients (18) suggests that psychotic depression is an expression of a lifelong vulnerability acting in concert with a particularly severe depressive episode (18).

The conceptualization of an underlying individual vulnerability to psychotic episodes is consistent with reports that young adults (19) and elderly patients (20) with DD have lower activity of dopamine beta hydroxylase, a heritable enzyme that converts dopamine into norepinephrine. Thus, an interaction between genetic vulnerability and the psychobiological stress of a severe depression may result in psychotic phenomenology. Such an explanation has important treatment implications that can be assessed empirically. Thus, nonpsychotic recurrences of patients with previous DD should be less severe and respond to antidepressants alone, while psychotic recurrences should be associated with greater depressive symptoms and require the use of either ECT or one of the aggressive pharmacotherapies described below. This underscores both the importance of ongoing postrecovery monitoring of DD patients and of rapidly treating newly evolving episodes.

B. Differential Diagnosis from Other Major Psychoses

The differential diagnosis of patients with clear-cut psychotic features accompanying a major depression must consider schizoaffective schizophrenia and delusional disorder associated with depression. Both phenomenological and historical/temporal criteria are relevant to distinguishing these conditions.

The diagnosis of schizoaffective disorder requires meeting criterion A for schizophrenia in addition to the criteria for major depression. Because loss of capacity for pleasure can accompany dementia, depressed mood from the A criteria for major depression must be present (21). Temporal criteria are crucial; specifically, delusions or hallucinations must have been present for at least 2 weeks in the absence of a prominent mood disturbance and criteria for the mood disorder must be present for a substantial portion of the present illness.

Delusional disorder requires the presence of a nonbizarre delusion for a minimum for 1 month without the full symptom presentation of criterion A for schizophrenia (21). Importantly, delusional disorder can be accompanied by a major depression as long as the duration of mood symptoms is brief relative to the duration of the delusional period. Delusional content does not have diagnostic relevance because somatic and persecutory delusions can occur in both delusional disorder and DD. In the absence of the criteria for schizophrenia, the clinician must rely on information about the pattern of symptom evolution and the relative dominance of mood versus psychotic symptoms to make an accurate diagnosis. Delusional disorder is related to descriptions of late-life paraphrenia and late paranoia (22), syndromes described prior to the introduction of contemporary nosology. The phenomenology of late-life paraphrenia, once thought to account for upward of 10% of geriatric inpatient admissions, included prominent delusions, usually associated with hallucinations, and preservation of the personality and the capacity for emotional responses (23). The Diagnostic and Statistical Manual (DSM-IV) criteria would classify most of these individuals as suffering from either late-onset schizophrenia or late-onset paranoia, an insidious illness that is frequently chronic as well (21,22).

Patients diagnosed as having delusional disorder, schizophrenia, or schizoaffective disorder can have a concurrent major depression that requires treatment. Although controlled studies comparing the efficacy of various pharmacotherapies for these diagnoses to that in DD are lacking, the more protracted course and dominance of psychotic symptoms in the primarily nonaffective psychoses suggest that these patients would require more aggressive and prolonged neuroleptic treatment.

In young adults, diagnosis is further confounded by the possibility that an individual meeting criteria for DD at baseline will later meet criteria for another Axis I psychiatric disorder. Thus, a second-wave assessment of individuals from the New Haven site of the Epidemiologic Catchment Area (ECA) study found that 10.1% of individuals who met criteria for psychotic depression were reclassified as having schizophrenia 1 year later, compared to 1.5% of individuals with nonpsychotic major depression (24). Interestingly, only 3.3% of psychotic and 3.0% of initially nonpsychotic depressives met criteria for bipolar illness at the second assessment; however, the strong association between DD in probands and bipolar disorder in family members (25) and the markedly higher frequency of DD in bipolar as compared to unipolar depressives (26) suggests that a higher proportion of individuals initially diagnosed as unipolar DD would meet criteria for bipolar depression over a longer follow-up period. These data bear on the diagnosis and treatment of late-life depression; because elderly individuals have passed the peak risk periods for onset of both schizophrenia and bipolar disorders, geriatric patients with DD are generally presumed to be suffering from a unipolar depression.

Reversible cognitive impairment and psychotic features during an episode of late-life major depression have been associated with an increased risk for developing a frank dementia during a 3-year follow-up (27). These findings build on the report that DD associated with cognitive impairment at index is associated with irreversible dementia at follow-up (28). Thus, the presence of cognitive impairment, like that of psychomotor disturbance, requires careful assessment for the presence of delusional ideation because of the effect of DD on responsiveness to standard antidepressant therapy.

C. Establishing the Presence of Delusions

The absence of both a standardized assessment instrument and a method for validation are major obstacles to establishing the diagnosis of DD. A recent NIMH workshop on DD highlighted this problem by giving high priority to the development of a sensitive delusional rating instrument (29). Existing scales mix ratings of different dimensions (e.g., subjective feeling of certainty, acting on the belief, ability to consider alternative possibilities, etc.) in determining an overall severity level; furthermore, these measures do not assess or quantify "near delusional" ideation (30) or the severity of unrealistic preoccupations that fall short of classification as fixed false beliefs. A relationship between near-delusional ideation and responsiveness to antidepressants is supported by the finding that patients who demonstrate exaggerated depressive ideas or who report brief periods of apparently delusional ideation earlier in their illness are significantly less likely to respond to therapeutic concentrations of desipramine (30).

Indirect evidence for the prognostic importance of near-delusional preoccupations comes from studies of anxiety as a predictor of treatment response. A secondary analysis of predictors of nonresponse to therapeutic tricyclic concentrations demonstrated that nonresponders had significantly higher scores on the Ham-D psychic anxiety item at baseline (31). Of note, this item is itself multidimensional; thus, higher scores may reflect different aspects of anxiety (e.g., subjective tension and irritability, worrying over minor matters, apprehensive attitude/worrying, fears expressed without questioning) rather than greater severity. We have reported that the specific anxiety factors of subjective anxiety and excessive worrying, which are different scores of the same Ham-D item, each predicted time to recurrence in elderly major depressives after the completion of continuation treatment; in contrast, total scores on Ham-D and the psychic anxiety item did not predict course (32). Geriatric depression is particularly associated with anxiety about physical health status. One report found that 40% of depressed elderly inpatients had exaggerated somatic complaints with these concerns reaching delusional proportions in 12% (33). Because this study did not assess the extent to which somatic preoccupations were fixed and/or influenced behavior, information on the relationship between near-delusional somatic anxiety and outcome is unavailable. Furthermore, focused studies are needed to determine relationships between both the degree of preoccupation with and implausibility of excessive worrying and the response to adequate trials of antidepressant monotherapy.

IV. PHARMACOTHERAPY OF GERIATRIC DELUSIONAL DEPRESSION: CONTEMPORARY APPROACHES

A. Combination Therapy with Tricyclic Antidepressants

Despite the high reported prevalence of delusional depression in elderly psychiatric admissions (34,35), information on the effectiveness of antidepressant treatment for DD is based largely on retrospective studies of mixed-aged samples that included relatively few geriatric patients. Therefore, the treatment response and ability to tolerate side effects in older and more complicated samples of geriatric patients can be expected to differ from those in published studies. This section will review recent studies of antidepressant treatments of DD in mixed-age samples and the available literature bearing on the pharmacotherapy of late-life DD.

Contemporary pharmacotherapies of DD have arisen out of a hypothesized catecholamine pathogenesis of DD (36–38) and findings from the 1970s supporting this conceptualization. Consistent with the theory that excess dopamine contributes to the presence of delusions, early reports and chart review studies indicated that patients with DD had a better response to combination therapy using a tricyclic with an antipsychotic medication than to monotherapy with the antidepressant alone (10,39,40); furthermore, systematic reviews of combination therapy studies demonstrated an effectiveness comparable to that reported for ECT (41,42).

Evidence favoring combination therapy based on retrospective studies is supported by a single published prospective controlled study (43). Fifty-eight systematically assessed patients with DD were randomized to perphenazine alone, amitriptyline plus perphenazine or amitriptyline monotherapy. Importantly, high doses of medication were used, with average amitriptyline doses exceeding 200 mg/day in monotherapy patients and 170 mg/day in those assigned to combination treatment; furthermore, combination therapy patients received average daily doses of 54.2 ± 16.8 mg of perphenazine. Results demonstrated that 78% of combination treatment patients met strict criteria for recovery, compared to 41% for those assigned to amitriptyline alone and only 19% for perphenazine. Of note, a concentration:response relationship was noted in amitriptyline monotherapy subjects; in this group, blood levels of >250 ng/ml of amitriptyline were associated with a significantly better response (44).

Systematic studies of neuroleptic dosage requirements for effective combination pharmacotherapy of DD are lacking. However, a retrospective analysis has demonstrated a dose–response relationship (45); of patients treated with desipramine plus perphenazine, the combination of high antidepressant concentrations and doses of neuroleptic greater than the median of 32 mg/day of perphenazine equivalents was associated with a significantly greater response rate.

We have reported the results of a chart review study comparing the treatment responses of elderly delusional depressives to geriatric patients with ND (46,47). Fifty-one patients with ND met criteria for adequate intensity of acute therapy with various antidepressants, given as monotherapy or combination treatment, compared to 33 patients with DD. The average age of these hospitalized patients was 71.7 ± 7. Overall, 69% of patients with ND were rated as having marked improvement or recovery, compared to 36% of those with DD ($p < 0.01$). Only 35% of the subgroup of 17 DD patients who received combination therapy responded. A comparison of the eight patients in this subgroup treated with ≥ 32 mg perphenazine equivalents a day to nine treated with lower antipsychotic dosages demonstrated comparably low response rates in the two groups (38.5% and 33%, respectively) (47). Interestingly, ECT was highly effective whether given as an initial treatment or after failure to respond to pharmacotherapy, with 91% of the 21 DD patients who received ECT initially responding compared to 86% of the 21 patients treated with ECT after nonresponse to medication.

The demonstration that combination therapy with a secondary amine tricyclic may be efficacious (47) has obvious relevance to the treatment of geriatric DD. Patients described in earlier reports and in the prospective study of Spiker et al. (43) were, for the most part, treated with amitriptyline. The notion that use of amitriptyline may increase the antidepressant responsiveness of DD (8) has particular relevance to geriatric patients, because this population is unlikely to tolerate high doses of this strongly anticholinergic and antihistaminic agent (48).

It is also unclear whether elderly patients with DD can tolerate the intensive treatment with antipsychotics found to be efficacious in younger adults. Geriatric patients are considered more vulnerable to developing extrapyramidal symptoms (48) and are at increased risk for falls during neuroleptic treatment (49). Although increased age is associated with a higher prevalence of tardive dyskinesia in association with antipsychotic treatment (50,51), the relevance of this finding to short-term combination therapy is uncertain.

The only prospective study of combination therapy of late-life delusional depression has used the secondary amine nortriptyline plus perphenazine. Preliminary results from this ongoing investigation (52) suggest that this combination therapy may be less effective for geriatric DD than the combination therapy strategy reported in young adults (43).

B. New Generation Antidepressants and Other Antidepressant Strategies

Amoxapine, a tetracyclic antidepressant and metabolite of the neuroleptic loxapine, has neuroleptic properties as well; these are contributed to, in part, by amoxapine's 7-hydroxy metabolite (53). A controlled study in patients with psychotic depression comparing high doses of amitriptyline plus perphenazine with amoxapine alone at average daily doses of over 400 mg/day demonstrated high response rates for both treatments; 50% reduction in Ham-D scores was achieved by 76% and 75% of subjects, respectively (54). Amoxapine subjects were significantly less likely to develop extrapyramidal side effects, perhaps because 5HT-2 blockade appears to contribute to amoxapine's antipsychotic effects (55).

The suggestion that serotonin may have a role in the pathogenesis of DD (56) has direct relevance to studies of both serotonin-reuptake inhibitors (SSRIs) and novel antipsychotics that block the 5HT-2 receptor. An open study combining 20 mg of fluoxetine with 32 mg of perphenazine reported a 73% response rate, although 40% of the subjects demonstrated mild to moderate rigidity (57). A trial combining paroxetine with a neuroleptic treatment found similar results, with 57% of 14 subjects demonstrating a 50% improvement in Ham-D scores and significant decreases in Ham-D "delusional" items during treatment (58). However, the association between SSRI treatment and extrapyramidal side effects (59) may limit their usefulness as a combination therapy in geriatric patients with DD.

The most striking SSRI findings were reported in a recent study of fluvoxamine monotherapy (60). Forty-eight of 57 (84.2%) hospitalized delusional depressives who completed a trial of 300 mg/day of fluvoxamine achieved the stringent response criteria of an end-point Ham-D score of <8. Five of the nonresponders subsequently responded to imipramine plus haloperidol, and another three responded to ECT. These findings, suggestive of a breakthrough in the treatment of DD, require replication; furthermore, studies of high-dose fluvoxamine treatment in elderly patients is needed.

Systematic studies of monotherapy or combination therapy using other classes of antidepressants to treat DD are largely lacking. A prospective study of the monoamine oxidase inhibitor phenelzine found a relationship similar to that reported with tricyclics: 68% of ND patients responded compared to

43% of those rated as probably psychotic and only 21% of individuals classified as definitely psychotic (61).

Although the efficacy of lithium as an acute antidepressant remains controversial, existing evidence suggests that lithium is more effective in bipolar than unipolar depression (62,63). The relevance of data demonstrating the efficacy of lithium augmentation in refractory nondelusional unipolar depression (64) to the treatment of unipolar DD is unclear. A retrospective study of lithium augmentation for DD found that 8 of 9 bipolar patients responded compared to only 3 of 12 patients with unipolar DD (65). In contrast, our ongoing study of maintenance pharmacotherapy has found that the four geriatric unipolar patients who suffered depressive relapses during post-ECT nortriptyline continuation therapy had remissions after lithium was added at concentrations below 0.6 meq/L (66).

V. COURSE OF DELUSIONAL DEPRESSION AND POST-RECOVERY PHARMACOTHERAPY

Naturalistic studies of mixed-age samples have consistently demonstrated poor short-term outcomes for DD. One-year follow-up data from a mixed-age epidemiological sample demonstrated that individuals with DD at index were significantly more likely to be depressed and on welfare or disability at 1 year than those with ND (24); of note, this report did not reanalyze the data after controlling for the DD cases that were later rediagnosed as having first-onset schizophrenia. Retrospective data from clinical samples have demonstrated a similar pattern; patients with DD were found to have lower recovery rates in the 2 years following hospital discharge, with this difference disappearing over a longer follow-up (67,68). Results from a 10-year prospective study demonstrated that patients with psychotic depression at intake had significantly greater impairment in both social and recreational functioning at follow-up (18). From a clinical perspective, psychotic depression was associated with a longer persistence of symptoms and shorter periods of wellness. These results build on clinical studies demonstrating that 80% of patients with DD relapsed within a year of hospital discharge (69), and that DD is associated with an increased frequency of rehospitalization (70).

Importantly, type of acute treatment does not appear to influence the long-term prognosis; responders to ECT and pharmacotherapy have comparable relapse rates with reports ranging from 50 to 95% in the year following recovery (71,72).

Results from studies of the effectiveness of postrecovery pharmacotherapy are discouraging. Although naturalistic studies suggest that the intensity of postrecovery antidepressant therapy does not predict wellness (72,73), there are no prospective studies of a systematically applied treatment. The finding that failure to respond to an initial course of pharmacotherapy strongly predicted relapse in ECT responders did not control the intensity of either antidepressants or neuroleptics prescribed during the postrecovery period (73).

Few studies have assessed the course of late-life DD. Post's follow-up study did not distinguish the presence of delusions from severity of depression at baseline as a predictor of course (74). The seminal prospective investigation of Murphy demonstrated a particularly poor outcome for late-life delusional depression, with only 10% of these patients recovering and remaining well for 1 year, compared to 44% of elderly patients with ND depression (75). Furthermore, DD was associated with a greater risk for the group of poor outcomes particularly relevant to geriatric psychiatry: death, dementia, and chronicity. A retrospective study of the course of late-life DD failed to replicate Murphy's finding of poorer short-term outcomes but did find that late-life DD was associated with a 2.5 times greater frequency of readmission over a 3- to 5-year follow-up (76).

Systematic studies on the relationship of postrecovery pharmacotherapy to the course of late-life delusional depression are lacking. Prophylactic studies of elderly patients with ND depression demonstrate that most of these patients can tolerate long-term treatment with therapeutic concentrations of nortriptyline (77,78). However, data indicating that ongoing antidepressants have limited effectiveness in preventing relapses of DD (71,72) and an apparent temporal association between decreases in antipsychotic dosage and relapses (79) suggest that combination continuation therapy could improve the course of DD (80).

The potential benefit of low-dose lithium to augment the prophylactic response of a standard antidepressant also merits consideration. Although geriatric patients have an increased sensitivity to the neurological side effects of this medication (e.g., tremor) (81), case reports with ND geriatric patients (82) and our own experience with DD described earlier suggest that elderly depressives may respond to combination therapy using lithium concentrations below 0.6 meq/L.

Studies of appropriate combination strategies are needed, but they must consider the vulnerability of elderly patients to side effects from both antipsychotics and lithium. Thus, 1-year incidences of tardive dyskinesia approximating 30% have been found in prospective studies of geriatric patients treated with neuroleptics (83,84); furthermore, a history of 3 months of neuroleptic treatment has been associated with a 16% prevalence (85). Thus, systematic studies of prophylaxis must carefully assess risks versus benefits in order to establish an optimal long-term treatment strategy for a disorder associated with poor psychiatric and physical health outcomes.

Finally, maintenance ECT has been found to improve the course of patients apparently resistant to pharmacotherapy (86). Retrospective data have demonstrated that patients with DD maintained on ECT had significantly lower relapse rates than historical controls treated with continuation pharmacotherapy prior to the initiation of the maintenance ECT program (87). Nevertheless, the initiation and continuation of postrecovery ECT in geriatric patients have obvious difficulties, including the likelihood that aging-related medical morbidities will limit the ability of patients to tolerate prolonged ECT prophylaxis. The optimal approach to preventing recurrences of late-life DD will require the identification of a safe and effective pharmacotherapeutic strategy.

VI. TREATMENT GUIDELINES: INTEGRATING RESEARCH LITERATURE WITH CLINICAL PRACTICE

It is apparent from the preceding discussion that empirical studies have not delineated a clear algorithm for the optimal treatment of late-life DD. In young adults, aggressive combination pharmacotherapy with high doses of neuroleptics (over 32 mg/equivalents of perphenazine) appears to be effective in most cases. However, some patients with DD suffer life-threatening forms of the illness (e.g., delusional guilt can lead to suicidal behavior and paranoid delusions can lead to refusal of food). In these cases, ECT is frequently the preferred initial treatment.

The treatment of late-life DD is further complicated by the difficulty elderly patients have tolerating high neuroleptic doses. Although some older patients with DD may respond to doses of neuroleptics below those found effective in studies of young adults, clinicians implementing less intensive combination therapy for geriatric DD should be aware of the dearth of empirical data bearing on this issue.

Despite an early report suggesting the contrary (88), mood-congruence of delusions does not appear to increase responsiveness to antidepressant monotherapy (41). Furthermore, the potential effectiveness of monotherapy must be balanced with the report that psychotic symptoms are worsened when antidepressants are administered alone (89). The latter phenomenon has been thought to explain the high frequency of a so-called drug-induced delirium reported in early antidepressant studies of older patients (90).

Thus, data available from the limited number of controlled studies and clinical reports must be integrated to maximize the effectiveness of treatment. Good judgment and practice dictate considering both the urgency of the clinical situation and the patient's health status in choosing among treatment approaches that include antidepressant monotherapy, low neuroleptic dose combination therapy, aggressive combination pharmacotherapy, and ECT. The potential effectiveness of recently introduced pharmacotherapies, including 5HT-2 blockers and fluvoxamine, in the treatment of late-life DD requires further study.

REFERENCES

1. Lewis A. Melancholia: Prognostic study and case material. J Ment Sci 1936; 82: 488–558.
2. Kantor SJ, Glassman AH. Delusional depressions: Natural history and response to treatment. Br J Psychiatry 1977; 131:351–360.
3. Friedman C, Mowbray MS, Hamilton VJ. Imipramine (tofranil) in depressive states. J Ment Sci 1961; 107:948–953.
4. Hordern A, Nol NF, Burt CG, Gordon WF. Amitriptyline in depressive states: Phenomenology and prognostic considerations. Br J Psychiatry 1963; 109:815–825.
5. Avery D, Lubrano A. Depression treated with imipramine and ECT: The De Carolis study reconsidered. Am J Psychiatry 1979; 136:559–562.
6. Glassman A, Kantor S, Shostak M. Depression, delusions, and drug response. Am J Psychiatry 1975; 132:716–719.
7. Glassman AH, Perel JM, Shostak M, Kantor SJ, Fleiss JL. Clinical implications of imipramine plasma levels for depressive illness. Arch Gen Psychiatry 1977; 34:197–204.
8. Ziegler VE, Clayton JC, Biggs JT. More of the treatment of delusional depressed patients (lett). Am J Psychiatry 1975; 132:1332–1333.
9. Quitkin F, Rifkin A, Klein DF. Imipramine response in deluded depressed patients. Am J Psychiatry 1978; 135:806–811.
10. Nelson CJ, Bowers MB. Delusional unipolar depression: Description and drug response. Arch Gen Psychiatry 1978; 35:1321–1328.
11. Hamilton M. A rating scale for depression. J Neurol Neurosurg Psychiatry 1960; 23:56–62.
12. Glassman AH, Roose SP. Delusional depression: A distinct clinical entity? Arch Gen Psychiatry 1981; 38:424–427.
13. Frances A, Brown RG, Kocsis JH, Mann JJ. Psychotic depression: A separate entity? Am J Psychiatry 1981; 138:831–833.
14. Lykouras E, Malliaras D, Christodoulou GN, Papakostas Y, Vougari A, Tzonou A, Stefanis C. Delusional depression: Phenomenology and response to treatment. Acta Psychiatr Scand 1986; 73:324–329.
15. Charney DS, Nelson CJ. Delusional and nondelusional unipolar depression: Further evidence for a distinct subtype. Am J Psychiatry 1981; 138:382–333.
16. Baldwin RC. Delusional and non-delusional depression in late life: Evidence for distinct subtypes. Br J Psychiatry 1988; 152:39–44.
17. Coryell W, Winokur G, Shea T, Maser JD, Endicott J, Aksiskal HS. The long-term stability of depressive subtypes. Am J Psychiatry 1994; 151:199–204.

18. Coryell W, Elon A, Winokur G, Endicott J, Keller M, Aksiskal H, Solomon D. Importance of psychotic features to long-term course in major depressive disorder. Am J Psychiatry 1996; 153:483–489.
19. Meltzer HY, Cho HW, Carroll BJ, Russo P. Serum dopamine-B-hydroxylase activity in the affective psychoses and schizophrenia. Arch Gen Psychiatry 1976; 33: 585–591.
20. Meyers BS, Gabriele M, Kakuma T. Correlates of late-life delusional depression. Annual meeting of the American Psychiatric Association, San Francisco, CA, 1993.
21. American Psychiatric Association. Diagnostic and Statistical Manual of Mental Disorders. 4th ed. Washington, DC: American Psychiatric Press, 1994.
22. Roth M. The natural history of mental disorders in old age. J Ment Sci 1955; 101: 281–301.
23. Roth M. Late paraphrenia: Phenomenologic and etiologic factors and their bearing upon problems of the schizophrenic family of disorders. In: Miller NE, Cohen GD, eds. Schizophrenia and Aging. New York: Guilford Press, 1987:217–234.
24. Johnson J, Horwath E, Weissman EE. The validity of major depression with psychotic features based on a community study. Arch Gen Psychiatry 1991; 48:1075–1081.
25. Weissman MM, Prusoff BA, Merikangas KR. Is delusional depression related to bipolar disorder? Am J Psychiatry 1984; 141:892–893.
26. Goodwin FK, Jamison KR. Manic-Depressive Illness. New York: Oxford University Press, 1990:266–268.
27. Alexopoulos GS, Meyers BS, Young RC, Mattis S, Kakuma T. The course of geriatric depression with "reversible dementia": A controlled study. Am J Psychiatry 1993; 150:1693–1699.
28. Rabins P, Merchant A, Nestadt G. Criteria for diagnosing reversible dementia caused by depression: Validation by two-year follow-up. Br J Psychiatry 1984; 144: 488–492.
29. Martinez RA, Mulsant BH, Meyers BS, Lebowitz BD. Delusional and psychotic depression in late-life: Clinical research needs. Am J Geriatr Psychiatry 1996; 4: 77–84.
30. Nelson JC, Mazure CM, Jatlow PI. Characteristics of desipramine-refractory depression. J Clin Psychiatry 1994; 55:12–19.
31. Roose SP, Glassman AH, Walsh TB, Woodring S. Tricyclic nonresponders: Phenomenology and treatment. Am J Psychiatry 1986; 143:345–348.
32. Meyers BS, Gabriele M, Kakuma T, Ippolito L, Alexopoulos GS. Anxiety and depression as predictors of recurrence in geriatric depression: A preliminary report. Am J Geriatr Psychiatry 1996; 4:252–257.
33. Kramer-Ginsberg E, Greenwald BS, Aisen PS, Brod-Miller C. Hypochondriasis in the elderly depressed. J Am Geriatr Soc 1989; 37:507,510.
34. Post F. The Significance of Affective Symptoms in Old Age. London: Oxford University Press, 1962.
35. Meyers BS, Greenberg R. Late-life delusional depression. J Affect Disord 1986; 11:133–137.
36. Exstein I. Bowers MB. The pharmacological meaning of successful antipsychotic-antidepressant combinations. Comprehensive Psychiatry 1975; 16:427–434.

37. Schatzberg AF, Rothschild AJ, Langlais PJ, Bird ED, Cole JO. A corticosteroid/dopamine hypothesis for psychotic depression and related states. J Psychiatr Res 1984; 18:217–223.
38. Sweeney D, Nelson C, Bowers M, Maas J, Heninger G. Delusional versus nondelusional depression: Neurochemical differences. Lancet 1978; ii:100–101.
39. Kaskey GB, Nasr S, Meltzer H. Drug treatment of delusional depression. Psychiatr Res 1980; 2:267–277.
40. Chan CK, Janicak PG, Davis JM, Altman E, Andriukaitis S. Response of psychotic and nonpsychotic depressed patients to tricyclic antidepressants. J Clin Psychiatry 1987; 48:197–200.
41. Kroessler D. Relative efficacy rates for therapies of delusional depression. Convuls Ther 1985; 1:173–182.
42. Parker GD, Hadzi-Pavlovic I, Hickie P, Mitchell K. Wilhelm H. Psychotic depression: A review and clinical experience. Aust NZ J Psychiatry 1991; 25:169–180.
43. Spiker DG, Weiss JC, Dealy RS, Griffin SJ, Hanin I, et al. The pharmacological treatment of delusional depression. Am J Psychiatry 1985; 142:430–436.
44. Spiker DG, Dealy RS, Hanin I, Cofsky-Weiss J, Kupfer D. Treating delusional depressives with amitriptyline. J Clin Psychiatry 1986; 47:243–245.
45. Nelson JC, Price LH, Jatlow PI. Neuroleptic dose and desipramine concentrations during combined treatment of unipolar delusional depression. Am J Psychiatry 1986; 143:1151–1154.
46. Meyers BS, Greenberg R, Mei-Tal V. Delusional depression in the elderly. In: Treatment of Affective Disorders in the Elderly. Washington DC: American Psychiatric Press, 1985.
47. Meyers BS, Alpert S, Kalayam B, Kakuma T, Alexopoulos GS, Young RC. Geriatric delusional depression and ECT. Annual Meeting of the American Psychiatric Association, Washington, DC, 1992.
48. Young RC, Meyers BS. Psychopharmacology. In: Sadavoy J, Lazarus LW, Jarvik LF, Grossberg GT, eds. Comprehensive Review of Geriatric Psychiatry-II. Washington, DC: American Psychiatric Press, 1996:755–818.
49. Tinetti ME, Speechley M, Ginter SF. Risk factors for falls among elderly persons living in the community. N Engl J Med 1988; 319:1701–1707.
50. Smith JM, Baldessarini MD. Changes in prevalence, severity and recovery in tardive dyskinesia with age. Arch Gen Psychiatry 1980; 37:1368–1375.
51. Jeste DV, Wyatt RJ. Aging and tardive dyskinesia. In: Miller NE, Cohen CD, eds. Schizophrenia and Aging. New York: Guilford, 1987.
52. Mulsant BH, Sweet RA, Perel JM, Zubenko GS, Reynolds, III CF. Pharmacotherapy of psychotic major depression. Annual Meeting of the American Psychiatric Association, San Francisco, CA, 1993.
53. Cohen BM, Harris PQ, Altesman RI, Cole JO. Amoxapine: Neuroleptic as well as antidepressant? Am J Psychiatry 1982; 139:1165–1167.
54. Anton RF, Burch EA. Amoxapine versus amitriptyline combined with perphenazine in the treatment of psychotic depression. Am J Psychiatry 1990; 147:1203–1208.
55. Anton RF, Sexauer JD. Efficacy of amoxapine in psychotic depression. Am J Psychiatry 1983; 140:1244–1347.

56. Schatzberg AF, Rothschild AJ. Serotonin activity in psychotic (delusional) depression. J Clin Psychiatry 1992; 53(S):52–55.
57. Rothschild AJ, Samson JA, Bessette MP, Carter-Campbell JT. Efficacy of combination fluoxetine and perphenazine in the treatment of psychotic depression. J Clin Psychiatry 1993; 54:338–342.
58. Wolfserdorf M, Barg T, Konig F, Liebfarth M, Grunewald I. Paroxetine as antidepressant in combined antidepressant-neuroleptic therapy in delusional depression: Observation of clinical use. Pharmacopsychiatry 1995; 28:56–60.
59. Coulter DM, Pillans PI. Fluoxetine and extrapyramidal side effects. Am J Psychiatry 1995; 152:122–125.
60. Gatti F, Bellini L, Gasperini M, Perez J, Zanardi R, Smeraldi E. Fluvoxamine alone in the treatment of delusional depression. Am J Psychiatry 1996; 153:414–416.
61. Janicak PG, Pandey GN, Davis JM, Boshes R, Bresnahan D, Sharma R. Response of psychotic and nonpsychotic depression to phenelzine. Am J Psychiatry 1988; 145:93–95.
62. Goodwin FK, Murphy DL, Dunner DL, Bunney Jr WE. Lithium response in unipolar versus bipolar depression. Am J Psychiatry 1972; 129:44–47.
63. Mendels J, Secunda SK, Dyson WL. A controlled study of the antidepressant effects of lithium carbonate. Arch Gen Psychiatry 1972; 26:154–157.
64. Joffe RT, Singer W, Levitt AJ, MacDonald C. A placebo-controlled comparison of lithium and triiodothyronine augmentation of tricyclic antidepressants in unipolar refractory depression. Arch Gen Psychiatry 1993; 50:387–393.
65. Nelson JC, Mazure CM. Lithium augmentation in psychotic depression refractor to combined drug treatment. Am J Psychiatry 1986; 143:363–366.
66. Meyers BS. Geriatric delusional depression: diagnosis, treatment, and course. Annual Meeting of the American Association for Geriatric Psychiatry, Tucson, AZ, 1996.
67. Coryell WH, Tsuang MT. Primary unipolar depression and the prognostic significance of delusions. Arch Gen Psychiatry 1981; 139:1181–1184.
68. Coryell W, Endicott J, Keller M. The importance of psychotic features to major depression: Course and outcome during a 2-year follow-up. Acta Psychiatr Scand 1987; 75:78–85.
69. Robinson DG, Spiker DG. Delusional depression: A one year follow-up. J Affect Disord 1985; 9:79–83.
70. Parker GD, Hadzi-Pavlovic I, Hickie P, Mitchell K, Wilhelm H. Psychotic depression: A review and clinical experience. Aust NZ J Psychiatry 1991; 25:169–180.
71. Spiker DG, Stein J, Rich CL. Delusional depression and electroconvulsive therapy: One year later. Convuls Ther 1985; 1:167–172.
72. Aronson TA, Shukla S, Hoff A. Continuation therapy after ECT for delusional depression: A naturalistic study of prophylactic treatments and relapse. Convuls Ther 1987; 3:251–259.
73. Sackeim HA, Prudic J, Devanand DP, Decina P, Kerr B, et al. The impact of medication resistance and continuation pharmacotherapy on relapse following response to electroconvulsive therapy in major depression. J Clin Psychopharm 1990; 10:96–104.

74. Post F. The management and nature of depressive illness in late life: A follow-through study. Br J Psychiatry 1972; 121:393–404.
75. Murphy E. The prognosis of depression in old age. Br J Psychiatry 1983; 142: 111–119.
76. Baldwin RC, Jolley DJ. The prognosis of depression in old age. Br J Psychiatry 1986; 149:574–583.
77. Reynolds CF, Perel JM, Cornes C, Kupfer DJ. Open-trial maintenance pharmacotherapy of late-life depression: Survival analysis. Psychiatr Res 1989; 27:225–231.
78. Reynolds CF, Frank E, Perel JM, Mazumdar S, Kupfer DJ. Maintenance therapies for late-life recurrent major depression: Research and review circa 1995. Int Psychogeriatr 1995; 7(S):27–39.
79. Aronson T, Shukla S, Gujavarty K, Hoff A, DiBuono M, et al. Relapse in delusional depression: A retrospective study of the course of treatment. Comprehensive Psychiatry 1988; 29:12–21.
80. Meyers BS. Late-life delusional depression: Acute and long-term treatment. Int Psychogeriatr 1995; 7(S):113–124.
81. Kushnir SL. Lithium-antidepressant combinations in the treatment of depressed, physically ill geriatric patients. Am J Psychiatry 1986; 143:378–379.
82. Murray N, Hopwood S, Balfour JK. The influence of age on lithium efficiency and side effects in out-patients. Psychol Med 1983; 13:53–60.
83. Saltz BL, Worener MG, Kane JM, Lieberman JA, Alvir JMJ, Bergmann KJ, Blank K, Koblenzer J, Kahaner K. Prospective study of tardive dyskinesia incidence in the elderly. J Am Med Assoc 1991; 266:2402–2406.
84. Jeste DV, Caligiuri MP, Paulsen JS, Heaton RK, Lacro JP, harris MJ, Bailey A, Fell RL, McAdams LA. Risk of tardive dyskinesia in older patients: a prospective longitudinal study of 266 outpatients. Arch Gen Psychiatry 1995; 52:756–765.
85. Sweet RA, Mulsant BH, Gupta B, Rifai AH, Pasternak RE, McEachran A, Zubenko GS. Duration of neuroleptic treatment and prevalence of tardive dyskinesia in late life. Arch Gen Psychiatry 1995; 52:478–486.
86. Thornton JE, Mulsant BH, Dealy R, Reynolds III CF. A retrospective study of maintenance electroconvulsive therapy in a university-based psychiatric practice. Convuls Ther 1990; 6:121–129.
87. Petrides G, Dhossche D, Fink M, Francis A. Continuation ECT: Relapse prevention in affective disorders. Convuls Ther 1995; 10:189–194.
88. Minter RE, Mandel MR. The treatment of psychotic major depressive disorder with drugs and electroconvulsive therapy. J Nerv Ment Disord 1979; 167:726–733.
89. Nelson JC, Bowers MB. Exacerbation of psychosis by tricyclic antidepressants in delusional depression. Am J Psychiatry 1979; 136:574–576.
90. Meyers BS, Mei-Tal V. Psychiatric reactions during tricyclic treatment of the elderly reconsidered. J Clin Psychopharmacol 1983; 3:2–6.

6
Treatment of Major Depressions During Bereavement

Selby Jacobs
Yale University School of Medicine, New Haven, Connecticut

Sidney Zisook
University of California, San Diego, La Jolla, California

I. INTRODUCTION

In this chapter, we discuss the psychopharmacological treatment of major depressions that occur due to bereavement in late life. Special consideration is devoted to this topic for several reasons. First, treatment decisions during acute bereavement are often overshadowed by philosophical attitudes about the delineation of normal states from psychopathology. Second, differential diagnosis in the circumstances of bereavement is more challenging than ordinary. Third, a nascent literature of systematic studies on this topic is available but, perhaps, not well known. Finally, there are interesting questions about the nature of major depressions during bereavement, the treatment of these depressions, and their relationship of the phenomenology of grief, which deserve particular attention on the research agenda.

The literature on psychopharmacological treatments for complications of bereavement is in its infancy. A search of the literature reveals two early, anecdotal reviews by noted psychopharmacologists. One review published in 1969 encourages treatment for "abnormal emotional states," including depressions (1), and the other review, published in 1972, discusses treatment in a conservative vein (2). These represent different points on a spectrum of attitudes about treatment of the complications of bereavement. Little else appears until the publication in 1987 and 1991 of two open trials of antidepressants for the depressions of bereavement (3,4). These are discussed in more detail below, along with a third trial that is still unpublished (5). In 1991, an NIH Consensus Development Conference on the Diagnosis and Treatment of Depression in Late Life included a section on the diagnosis and indications for treatment of depression associated with late-life bereavement (6) and recommended more research in this area.

II. A PHILOSOPHY OF TREATMENT

A background philosophical question about the treatment of depressions that occur during bereavement must be addressed as a fundamental, first step in our discussion. The question is whether it is wise to treat depressions with pharmacological agents during acute bereavement under any conditions. Strong philosophical attitudes prevail in the medical community and society in general to the effect that we should not "medicalize" and interfere with the natural, healing process of grief. Moreover, as part of medical education, all physicians are taught the professional dictum of "primum non nocere," which lends itself to conservative treatment. These concerns must be taken seriously.

We believe the debate about whether to treat should hinge on scientific studies of depressions that occur during bereavement. We anchor our position in studies that define and validate the depressive syndromes of bereavement as clinical complications. That is, the depressions of bereavement ought to be verified as disorders associated with a typical syndrome, which is stable over time and associated with functional impairment, potential for disability, and medical or psychiatric comorbidity (see Section III for a summary of these data). The depressions of bereavement may not only qualify as disorders by standard, scientific criteria but also may contribute to maladaptive, pathological patterns of grief (7). The latter view is reflected among many clinicians who specialize in seeing complications of bereavement and believe that depressive syndromes in the circumstances of bereavement can interfere with the expression and course of normal grief.

In addition to scientific evidence, there are philosophical arguments that serve as a counterpoint to entrenched cultural attitudes against treatment during bereavement. For example, we believe it is reasonable to ask how much a bereaved person needs to suffer and to consider the responsibility of professionals to alleviate excessive pain and to attenuate, if not prevent, complications. The metaphor of inflammation after an injury is useful as an analogy for loss and grief (8). The analogy provides concepts for understanding how a knowledge of normal physiology can be applied to monitor the natural process of grief, and how medical interventions can be used to help bereaved persons without compromising the normal physiological process.

In this chapter, we argue that the nature of depressions that occur during bereavement justifies treatment. Careful differential diagnosis is necessary. In our view, major depressions during bereavement are underdiagnosed and antidepressants are underutilized in their treatment. Also, we believe the risks of using antidepressants are small. Therefore, we advocate more active consideration of the place of antidepressants in treatment for this patient population.

III. THE NATURE OF DEPRESSIVE SYNDROMES IN THE CIRCUMSTANCES OF BEREAVEMENT DURING LATE LIFE

By several criteria, the depressive syndromes that occur after a loss qualify as clinically significant disorders rather than variations of uncomplicated bereavement. For example, while there are some conflicting data (9), in two studies these syndromes are associated with positive personal and family histories of depression, which increase risk of depression during bereavement about twofold (10,11). Also, the depressive syndromes of bereavement often include severe and malignant symptoms such as feelings of worthlessness, suicidal ideation, and melancholic symptoms (12,13). Moreover, these depressive syndromes have a prolonged and unrelenting course, substantial and protracted psychosocial impairment, and help-seeking by those afflicted by the syndrome (13). About 20% of acutely bereaved persons develop chronic depressions, which are probably preventable (14).

The studies from which these conclusions are drawn include many elderly persons; however, they are not based exclusively on elderly samples. Still, there is little reason to suspect that the depressions of bereavement in late life differ from those at a younger age. For example, studies of elderly bereaved persons reveal more similarities than differences between depressions experienced by older versus younger individuals (6). Also, although the rate of major depressions in elderly bereaved individuals (> 65 years) is somewhat lower than the rate in their younger (< 65 years) counterparts during the first year of bereavement, by the end of the second year of bereavement 14% of bereaved persons in late life will report symptoms of major depressive disorder and many more will experience ongoing depressive symptoms which do not fully meet criteria for major depression (15). Thus, given the large number of elderly individuals who lose spouses, other relatives, and close friends each year, the depressions associated with bereavement represent a substantial public health problem.

IV. DIAGNOSIS OF DEPRESSIONS DURING BEREAVEMENT

In the circumstances of bereavement, the challenge to the clinician is to make a judgment about normal and abnormal states in the midst of a natural healing process. For this purpose, a thorough knowledge of normal grief is fundamental so as not to misconstrue the ubiquitous, ordinarily transient depressive phenomena of normal grief as major depression.

In contrast to major depression, the essence of normal grief is separation distress (14,16–18). The concept of separation distress incorporates the classic pang of grief (19) and searching behavior (14,17). There are also depressive, neurovegetative, and dissociative dimensions of normal grief that ordinarily have a transient natural history (14).

The Diagnostic and Statistical Manual of Mental Disorders, Fourth Edition (DSM-IV), recommends that physicians diagnose major depression if (1) a depressive syndrome is present for more than 2 months after a loss or (2) a depressive syndrome includes marked functional impairment, morbid preoccupation with worthlessness, morbid guilt, suicidal ideation, psychotic symptoms, or psychomotor retardation (20). The face validity of the symptomatic criteria in the second part of this guideline strongly indicate the need for treatment whenever they are encountered after a loss.

A more detailed consideration of the time threshold for pharmacological treatment given in the first part of the DSM-IV guideline leads to a refinement of the manual's recommendations. In the absence of the symptomatic indications for treatment, the critical issue for deciding when to treat is not the time since bereavement (i.e., 2 months or whatever), but rather other factors. Clinicians should ask themselves two questions. The first is what factors predict who, among acutely bereaved persons meeting criteria for major depression, will get better on their own (and who will not) in the first 6 months of bereavement. We know from one study that the symptoms of depression will remit spontaneously in about two-thirds of sufferers (21). It is important to emphasize the question we are posing here is not the same question as who among the acutely bereaved will develop a major depressive syndrome in the first year, for which a small literature exists (for review and discussion, see Refs. 12, 22, 23).

Based on our combined experiences over the past several years, we suggest that the risk factors for unrelenting major depressions during acute bereavement are the following: (1) the presence of the depressive symptoms already itemized above; (2) symptoms that are severe, impair function, and lead to marked subjective distress; (3) prolonged duration of depressive symptoms (symptoms may have started even before the loss itself); and (4) a past personal history of major depression. The more of these four factors that are present, the more likely it is that antidepressant medications are indicated.

In contrast, we believe that the psychopharmacological treatment of mildly to moderately severe, first-time depressions, starting after the loss and during the first few months of bereavement, is premature. Most of these patients will respond to tincture of time, support, and perhaps psychosocial interventions alone.

In considering the time threshold for pharmacological treatment, the second question that clinicians must pose is when is spontaneous recovery accomplished from the depressive syndromes that occur early in bereavement. Unfortunately, there are little data to help answer this question, as it requires multiple observations in the first 6 months of bereavement, and no one has carried out these difficult studies. Again, based on our clinical experience, we believe that early occurring major depressive syndromes that do not remit by 6 months or have not responded to psychosocial interventions warrant psychopharmacological treatment at that point.

Additionally, major depressions arising late in the first year of bereavement (after the first few months) are unlikely to heal on their own (21) and warrant prompt treatment. In these cases, the clinician might begin with a psychosocial intervention rather than psychopharmacology if the severity is mild or moderate. As in other forms of major depression, combined pharmacotherapy and psychotherapy may often be better than either treatment alone. The natural history of late-occurring depressions needs more study, including a more precise definition of "late."

A final caveat is that all these clinical guidelines should be tested by systematic observation and studies. For example, our 6-month boundary for remission is not empirically determined at present and might be 4 months or 7 months. It is a time boundary drawn from our clinical experience to serve as a working guideline until studies document the natural history of depressions that occur during bereavement.

V. STUDIES OF TREATMENT WITH ANTIDEPRESSANT DRUGS

No one has completed randomized clinical trials of antidepressant drug treatment for major depressions associate with acute bereavement. Two open trials with desipramine and nortriptyline, and a third study using fluoxetine have been reported or completed, and are the basis for our discussion. All the open trials demonstrate an apparent response of depressive symptoms in bereaved persons to treatment.

The first study reported on treatment response during a 4-week, open trial of desipramine (one case was treated with nortriptyline) among 10 persons ranging in age from 36 to 65 (3). The participants were bereaved 12 months earlier and met SCID-DSM-III criteria for major depression. The average dosage of desipramine was 119 mg and ranged from 75 to 150 mg. Seven of the 10 persons had moderate to marked improvement of depressive symptoms on the Hamilton Depression Rating Scale (Ham-D). One person who had minimal change at the end of 4 weeks was considerably improved 1 month later after the Christmas holidays. One person had no response and one person dropped out of the trial after 1 week because of anticholinergic side effects. In responders, improvement was noted in appetite, sleep patterns, mood, and cognition. Of interest, despite improvement in depressive symptoms, grief intensity remained at least moderately intense 1 year after the loss for most of the participants.

A second study reported on treatment response during a 16-week, open trial of nortriptyline among 13 elderly persons (4). The subjects ranged in age from 61 to 78. They were bereaved on the average 11.9 months earlier and met Research Diagnostic Criteria (RDC) for stable, major depression. The mean dose of nortriptyline at the time of response was 49.2 ± 13.5 mg/day with a mean steady-state plasma level of 68.1 ± 19.4 ng/ml. Depressive symptoms were moderately to markedly improved in all 13 persons, with a decrease in Ham-D scores of 67.9% from pretreatment (22.1 ± 3.6) to posttreatment (7.2 ± 2.8) assessments for the sample. The median response time was 6.4 weeks (mean = 9.6 ± 82). This treatment study incorporated sleep assessments into its design and demonstrated improvement in sleep quality, REM percent, REM latency, REM density, and delta sleep ratio during remission of symptoms while on nortriptyline (24). When the nortriptyline was discontinued, REM percent, REM latency, and delta ratio reverted to pretreatment levels. Notably similar to the previous study, the Texas Revised Inventory of Grief, a measure of grief intensity, was the only measure that showed little or no response to antidepressant treatment and remained high throughout the study. As part of this ongoing study of late-life, bereavement-related depression, the authors have observed a response of intensive grief symptoms to paroxetine at a dosage of 20 mg in two persons (Reynolds CF, personal communication). One of these was a nonresponder to nortriptyline for depression. These pilot observations open up a potentially important new avenue for future clinical trials.

Another study, which is still unpublished, observed 48 HIV seropositive men with major depression who were treated with a combination of group treatment and either fluoxetine or placebo medications (5). About half the men in this study had experienced the death of at least one close friend or lover during the year preceding the study. Although the sample is small, it appeared that fluoxetine was more efficacious than placebo in relieving depressive symptoms for both the nonbereaved and bereaved samples. The group whose major depressive episodes followed bereavement did at least as well as the group who had not experienced bereavement. In no instances did it appear that fluoxetine treatment interfered with or worsened grief.

In summary, these studies, including some subjects over 65 years of age, provide preliminary evidence for the use of either tricyclic antidepressants or serotonergic agents in the treatment of major depressions during bereavement.

VI. CHOICE OF MEDICATION, DOSAGE, AND DURATION OF TREATMENT

No data indicate that a particular class of medications is more effective than others for the treatment of depressions occurring in the circumstances of bereavement. The choice of antidepressant, the dosage, and the duration of use in treating this patient population are clinical decisions that do not differ systematically from those made in the general psychiatric clinic. In short, selection of a medication should be based on past personal or family history of response and, to a lesser extent, on the subtype of depression. In the absence of this information, side effects and toxicity guide the choice. Newer antidepressant agents such as the serotonin uptake blockers, buproprion, venlofaxine, and nefazodone have the advantage of more tolerable side effects for the elderly person and are less lethal in overdose than the older tricyclics and monoamine oxidase inhibitors.

VII. OTHER TREATMENTS FOR THE DEPRESSIONS OF BEREAVEMENT

Brief psychotherapy offers an alternative strategy for treating mild to moderately severe major depressions in the circumstances of bereavement. For mild to moderately severe depressions, psychotherapy is often the first choice. For severe depressions, it is supplemental and better if integrated into a multimodal treatment plan.

Brief psychotherapies developed and tested for major depression seem to hold equal promise in the circumstances of bereavement. There is some evidence that this is true for elderly patients as well as younger persons (25). In particular, interpersonal psychotherapy (26) and brief, dynamic psychotherapy (27) may be well suited for depressions of bereavement, since the problems posed by a loss figured prominently in their development. Indeed, one small series of case reports found interpersonal psychotherapy effective in late-life spousal bereavement (28).

Two newly reported approaches to the psychotherapeutic treatment of the complications of bereavement may prove useful as well. Biologically informed psychotherapy assumes as a starting point that the major depressions of bereavement are biomedical illnesses. This psychotherapy emphasizes that the cognitive distortions, psychological conflict, repressed anger, and impaired self-esteem are the consequences, not the causes, of depression (29). Problem-focused psychotherapy emphasizes psychoeducational intervention as part of integrated, multimodal treatment (14,30). Both of these psychotherapies integrate therapeutic strategies from interpersonal psychotherapy, cognitive behavioral therapy, and brief, dynamic psychotherapy with specific innovations for the circumstances of bereavement. They may be particularly well suited for treating depressions of bereavement as they emphasize symptom relief, strategies for coping with illness, and the importance of treating severe major depressions with antidepressants when they are diagnosed.

VIII. THE NATURE OF THE PSYCHOPATHOLOGY ASSOCIATED WITH BEREAVEMENT

A loss exposes acutely bereaved persons to a higher risk for several types of psychiatric disorders (14) including major depressions (11–13,31), panic and generalized anxiety disorders (32), posttraumatic stress disorders (33), and increased alcohol use and abuse (34). Furthermore, there is renewed and current interest in pathological grief, either as a disorder of separation distress (14) or a variant of posttraumatic stress disorder (35,36).

With the exception of the information on the treatment of major depressions summarized above, little from systematic studies is known about the treatment of most of these disorders in the circumstances of bereavement. The multiple ramifications of psychopathology raises the possibility that specific psychopharmacological agents may prove useful for specific target symptoms and syndromes.

IX. FUTURE STUDIES

Two small, uncontrolled medication trials and one psychotherapy report noted above suggest that the major depressive episodes associated with bereavement are treatable. As a next step, these pilot studies need to be followed up by rigorously designed, randomized, controlled, double-blind studies.

At least four basic questions about antidepressant treatment in the circumstances of bereavement remain unanswered. First, what is the time threshold after a loss for psychopharmacological treatment? On the one hand, treating too early exposes individuals to needless time, expense, adverse effects, and possible toxicity for syndromes that might dissipate spontaneously. On the other hand, treating too late needlessly exposes depressed individuals to the suffering, disability, interpersonal difficulties, role dysfunctions, and possibly even suicidal risk of depression. Thus, the natural history and risk factors for persistence or worsening of the early depressions of bereavement need to be better delineated by carefully designed prospective studies. Such studies would require serial observations during follow-up over the first 6 months of bereavement. Alternatively, the question of "when to treat" might be answered by a series of random, double-blind trials in depressed, bereaved individuals where treatment is initiated at different points postbereavement and subjects are followed longitudinally. Unfortunately, such a study would be extraordinarily difficult to complete and would involve larger numbers of subjects than any one center could provide.

Second, what is the appropriate symptom threshold for psychopharmacological treatment? Depressive symptoms during bereavement, which are diagnostically subthreshold, are common and persistent (6,37). It is important to determine if subthreshold depression (or minor depression) during bereavement is associated with disability and comorbidity as it is in other populations (38,39). If so, guidelines for treatment deserve attention.

Third, how long should treatment last? Major depression, even in late life, tends to be a chronic and/or recurrent condition (40). Thus, guidelines for the duration of treatment generally suggest continuation of treatment for at least 6 months, with maintenance treatment for a much longer period of time in certain circumstances (41). However, it is not known whether these guidelines apply for major depressions associated with severe life stress, such as bereavement. Some early data from the University of Pittsburgh suggest that if antidepressant medications are discontinued too soon after symptomatic response in the depression of bereavement, relapse is likely (42).

Fourth, which medication is best for the depressions of bereavement? The open studies reviewed above suggest that tricyclic antidepressives (TCAs) reduce depressive symptomatology but have little impact on grief intensity. It would be useful to know if the serotonin reuptake inhibitors (SSRIs), or other newer medications, might simultaneously treat separation distress while executing their antidepressant effects. This is especially important in late life where the side effect profiles of the newer medications offer such advantages over the older TCAs (43).

The same series of questions can be asked of psychotherapy. That is, what is the optimal time after bereavement, symptom threshold, duration of treatment, and type of psychotherapy for managing the depressions of bereavement? Perhaps even more important might be a study addressing the issue of whether (or when) combination treatment is indicated. A randomized, four-cell study comparing medication alone, psychotherapy alone, medication plus psychotherapy, and no active treatment would go a long way toward establishing the ideal treatment for the depressions of bereavement.

X. CONCLUSIONS

Depressions which occur during bereavement in late life can be severe, persistent, and disabling for a substantial minority of persons. Major depressions during bereavement are underdiagnosed and antidepressants are underutilized in their treatment as a result of philosophical conservatism, misunderstanding of normal grief, lack of confidence in differential diagnosis, and inadequate understanding of the natural history of depressive states after a loss. As the risks of using antidepressants are small, we advocate active consideration of antidepressants, along with psychotherapy and other interventions, in multimodal treatment for patients with major depressions in the circumstances of a loss.

REFERENCES

1. Klein DF, Blank HR. Psychopharmacological treatment of bereavement and its complications. In: Death and Bereavement, Kutcher AH, ed. Springfield, IL: Charles C Thomas, 1969.
2. Hollister L. Psychotherapeutic drugs in the dying and bereaved. J Thanatol 1972; 2:623–29.
3. Jacobs SC, Nelson JC, Zisook S. Treating depressions of bereavement with antidepressants: a pilot study. Psychaitric Clin North Am 1987; 10:501–510.
4. Pasternak RE, Reynolds CF, Schlernitzauer M, Hoch CC, Buysse DJ, Houck PR, Perel JM. Acute open-trial nortriptyline therapy of bereavement-related depression in late life. J Clin Psychiatry 1991; 52:307–310.
5. Zisook S, Shuchter SR, Summers J, Grant I, Hutchin S, Burns K. Adult bereavement and depression. Syllabus and Proceedings of the 148th American Psychiatric Association Annual Meeting, Miami, FL, 1995.
6. Zisook S, Shuchter SR, Sledge P. Diagnostic considerations in depression associated with late-life bereavement. In: Diagnosis and Treatment of Depression in the Elderly: Results of the NIH Consensus Development Conference. Washington, DC: American Psychiatric Association Press, 1994.
7. Prigerson HG, Bierhals AJ, Kasl SV, Reynolds CF, Shear MK, Day N, Newsome JT, Jacobs SC. Mental and physical consequences of complicated grief. Am J Psychiatry, in press.
8. Engel GL. Is grief a disease? A challenge for medical research. Psychosomatic Med 1961; 23:18–22.
9. Bruce ML, Kim K, Leaf PJ, Jacobs SC. Depressive episodes and dysphoria resulting from conjugal bereavement in a prospective community sample. Am J Psychiatry 1990; 147:608–611.
10. Richards JG, McCallum J. Bereavement in the elderly. NZ Med J 1979; 89:201–204.
11. Zisook S, Shuchter SR. Depression through the first year after a death of a spouse. Am J Psychiatry 1991; 148:1346–1352.
12. Jacobs SC, Hansen FF, Berkman L, et al. Depressions of bereavement. Comprehensive Psychiatry 1989; 30:218–24.
13. Zisook S, Shuchter SR. Uncomplicated bereavement. J Clin Psychiatry 1993; 54: 365–72.

14. Jacobs S. Pathologic Grief: Maladaptation to Loss. Washington, DC: American Psychiatric Press, 1993:43–44.
15. Zisook S, Shuchter SR. Major depression associated with widowhood. Am J Geriatr Psychiatry 1993; 1:316–26.
16. Bowlby J, Parkes CM. Separation and loss. In: The International Yearbook for Child Psychiatry and Allied Disciplines, Vol. 1: The Child and His Family. New York: Wiley, 1970.
17. Parkes CM. Bereavement: Studies of Grief in Adult Life. New York: International Universities Press, 1972.
18. Bowlby J. Attachment and Loss, Vol. III: Loss, Sadness and Depression. New York: Basic Books, Inc., 1980.
19. Lindeman E. Symptomatology and management of acute grief. Am J Psychiatry 1944; 101:141–148.
20. Diagnostic and Statistical Manual of Mental Disorders, Fourth Edition. Washington, DC: American Psychiatric Association, 1994:326, 684.
21. Bornstein PE, Clayton PJ. The anniversary reaction. Dis Nervous System 1972; 33: 470–711.
22. Clayton PJ. Preventing depression: the symptom, the syndrome, or the disorder. In: Depression Prevention: Research Directions, Munoz R, ed. Washington, DC: Hemisphere Publishing Co., 1988:31–43.
23. Zisook S, Shuchter SR, Summers J. Bereavement risk and preventive intervention. In: The Handbook of Preventive Psychiatry, Raphael B, Burrows GD, eds. (in press).
24. Pasternak RE, Reynolds CF, Houck PR, Schlernitzauer M, Buysse DJ, Hoch CC, Kupfer DJ. Sleep in bereavement-related depression during and after pharmacotherapy with nortriptyline. J Geriatr Psychiatry Neurol 1994; 7:69–73.
25. Scogin F, McElreath L. Efficacy of psychosocial treatments for geriatric depression: a quantitative review. J Consult Clin Psychol 1994; 62:69–74.
26. Klerman GL, Weissman MM, Rounsaville BJ, Chevron ES. Interpersonal Psychotherapy of Depression. New York: Basic Books, 1984.
27. Horowitz M, Marmar C, Krupnick J, Wilner N, Kaltreider N, Wallerstein R. Personality Styles and Brief Psychotherapy. New York: Basic Books, 1984.
28. Miller MD, Frank E, Carnes C, et al. Applying interpersonal psychotherapy to bereavement-related depression following loss of a spouse in late-life. J Psychother Pract Res 1994; 3:149–162.
29. Zisook S, Shuchter SR. Psychotherapy of the depressions of bereavement. In: Session: Psychotherapy in Practice, in press.
30. Jacobs SC, Prigerson HG. Problem-focused, integrated psychotherapy for a woman with complicated grief. In: Session: Psychotherapy in Practice, in press.
31. Bornstein PE, Clayton PJ, Halikas JA, Maurice WL, Robins E. The depression of widowhood after thirteen months. Br J Psychiatry 1973; 122:561–566.
32. Jacobs SC, Hansen FF, Kasl SV, et al. Anxiety disorders during acute bereavement: risk and risk factors. J Clin Psychiatry 1990; 51:269–274.
33. Schut HAW, de Keijser J, van den Bout J. Incidence and prevalence of post-traumatic symptomatology in conjugally bereaved (abs). Proceedings of the Third

International Conference on Grief and Bereavement in Contemporary Society, Sydney, Australia, 1991.
34. Zisook S, Shuchter SR, Mulvihill M. Alcohol, Cigarette, and Medication Use During the First Year of Widowhood. Psychiatr Ann 1990; 20:318–326.
35. Horowitz MJ. Stress Response Syndromes. New York: Jason Aronson, Inc., 1976.
36. Prigerson HG, Frank E, Kasl SV, Reynolds CF, Anderson B, Zubenko GS, Houck PR, George CJ, Kupfer DJ. Complicated grief and bereavement related depression as distinct disorders: preliminary empirical validation in elderly bereaved spouses. Am J Psychiatry 1995; 152:22–30.
37. Zisook S, Shuchter SR, Sledge P, Paulus M, Judd LL. The spectrum of depressive phenomena after spousal bereavement. J Clin Psychiatry 1994; 55(4, suppl):29–36.
38. Wells KB, Stewart A, Hays RD, Burnam MA, Rogers W, Daniels M, Berry S, Greenfield S, Ware J. The functioning and well being of depressed patients: results from the Medical Outcomes Study. J Am Med Assoc 1989; 262:914–919.
39. Spitzer RL, Kroenke K, Linzer M, Hahn SR, Williams JBW, Verloin deGruy F, Brody D, Davies M. Health-related quality of life in primary care patients with mental disorders. J Am Med Assoc 1995; 274:1511–1517.
40. Keller MB, Levori RW, Meueller TI, et al. Time to recovery, chronicity, and levels of psychopathology in major depression: A 5 year prospective follow-up of 431 subjects. Arch Gen Psychiatry 1992; 419:809–816.
41. Hirschfeld RMA. Guidelines for the long-term treatment of depression. J Clin Psychiatry 1994; 55(12, suppl):61–69.
42. Pasternak R, Fasiczka A, Reynolds CF III. The post-treatment course of depression in bereaved elders. Proceedings of the 2nd International Conference on New Directions in Affective Disorders, Jerusalem, Israel, 1995.
43. Dunner DL. Therapeutic considerations in treating depression in the elderly. J Clin Psychiatry 1994; 55(12, suppl):48–58.

7

Maintenance Therapies for Late-Life Recurrent Major Depression: Research and Review Circa 1996

Charles F. Reynolds III, Ellen Frank, James M. Perel, and David J. Kupfer
University of Pittsburgh Medical Center, Pittsburgh, Pennsylvania

Sati Mazumdar
University of Pittsburgh, Pittsburgh, Pennsylvania

I. INTRODUCTION

The objectives of this chapter are (1) to define what we currently know, or think we know, about the efficacy and safety of maintenance therapies in elders with recurrent unipolar major depression (nonbipolar and nondelusional); (2) to review the main methodological and ethical challenges encountered in carrying out maintenance therapies protocols enrolling elderly subjects, together with our responses to these challenges; and (3) to identify unresolved questions in the field and to suggest directions for further research. This chapter is an updated version of a recent review by the authors (1), but with an expanded reference section on course of illness in late-life depression, as well as expanded data from our own ongoing studies and data on maintenance treatment with selective serotonin reuptake inhibitors (SSRIs) in nongeriatric populations (for possible extrapolation to elderly patients).

Related to the first broad objective ("current knowledge and belief"), we review the scope of the problem, as suggested by naturalistic follow-up studies from the United Kingdom and from Europe and as reviewed by the NIH Consensus Conference on the Diagnosis and Treatment of Depression in Late Life (2,3). This section also summarizes data from Georgotas et al. (4,5) on continuation and maintenance therapy with nortriptyline and phenelzine; the UK data on dothiepin and placebo (6); and the Pittsburgh data on acute, continuation, and maintenance therapy with nortriptyline, interpersonal psychotherapy, and placebo (7,8).

Related to the methodological and ethical challenges of conducting maintenance therapies clinical trials in the elderly, we discuss issues of recruitment, retention, compliance (enforcement and measurement), selection of outcomes, and informed consent. In each area we summarize our response to these challenges.

Finally, with respect to unresolved questions and research direction, we examine several needs: (1) to develop predictive models of long-term course that factor in type and intensity of treatment, as well as their interaction with medical illness and psychosocial variables, including life events, that can affect onset and offset of illness; (2) to examine other types of mood disorders in the elderly, particularly bipolar, delusional, and dementia-related; and (3) to define more accurately the risks and benefits of long-term therapy with other classes of agents, such as SSRIs, in special populations.

II. CURRENT KNOWLEDGE AND BELIEF

A. Scope of Problem

The development of cost-effective maintenance programs to help elderly depressed patients maintain gains achieved during acute treatment and to minimize relapse and recurrence rates is clearly valuable from a clinical and public health perspective. That compliance with effective maintenance treatment could also be, literally, a matter of life and death is highlighted by psychological autopsies of elderly suicides which have revealed a high prevalence of major mood disorders and contact with a physician during the last month of the patient's life (9). We believe that it is reasonable to hypothesize that compliance with long-term treatment will probably reduce suicide rates in the elderly (10).

Although the short-term treatment response of depressed elders to either pharmacotherapy or psychotherapy is good, the long-term prognosis for depression in old age is generally believed to be poor, with only one-quarter to one-half of patients showing a good outcome at 1–3 year follow-up (11–15). In addition, older age at first onset of illness is associated with an increased risk for recurrence (particularly after the second episode) (16). Among unipolar depressed patients aged 60 and older, the probability of a recurrence within 24 months from the onset of the first episode was found to be 70% (16). Cycle length also decreases as a function of episode number—from 20 months after episode 2 to 16 months after episode 3. Thus the major concern of maintenance therapies research is to identify treatments that can maintain wellness and diminish the costs associated with subsequent affective morbidity, including chronic psychosocial invalidism, poor compliance with other concurrent medical therapies, cognitive impairment, and suicide.

It is our view that most elderly patients would probably benefit from continuation and maintenance therapy; and that it therefore behooves the clinician to review the indications for such therapy in each elderly patient with a major mood disorder. More specifically, the purpose of continuation therapy (i.e., that phase of treatment administered 4–6 months after symptomatic resolution of the index episode) is to prevent return of depressive symptoms and relapse back into the index episode. Maintenance therapy is the phase of treatment that begins after full remission of the index episode is achieved and sustained for 4–6 months; its objective is to preserve recovery and to prevent recurrence of new episodes of major depression. We believe also that psychotherapeutic approaches should be evaluated in conjunction with pharmacotherapies in maintenance research, because the availability of psychotherapeutic modalities for use in the elderly would be particularly important for those who either cannot, or will not, take antidepressant medication.

B. Open-Trial Findings

With respect to maintenance pharmacotherapy, Kragh-Sorensen et al. (17) have reported high recurrence rates among older patients with recurrent depression (aged 50 and above) who discontinued nortriptyline maintenance, in contrast to patients maintained on adequate plasma levels of nortriptyline. In the experience of the Danish investigators, 71% of 19 older endogenous depressed patients suffered recurrence of depression after discontinuation of nortriptyline over a period of 2 years, while none of the 14 older patients followed up from 5 to 48 months who maintained plasma concentrations in the therapeutic range of 50–150 ng/ml had recurrences. Our open-trial pilot work with elderly patients prescribed nortriptyline (steady-state 50–150 ng/ml) yielded a similar observation, with only 4 of 27 patients suffering recurrence over a follow-up period of 18 months (18).

C. Controlled Data

Georgotas et al. (4) reported relapse rates of 17% for nortriptyline and 20% for phenelzine in elderly depressed patients during 4–8 months of continuation therapy. The Old Age Depression Interest Group (OADIG) in the United Kingdom (6) have reported that elders with major depression are 2.5 times less likely to suffer recurrence of major depression on dothiepin maintenance (75 mg/day for 2 years) than on placebo. In our ongoing maintenance therapy study (described below), we reported a relapse rate of 24% during 4-week tapering of nortriptyline after 16 weeks of continuation therapy and double-blind substitution of placebo, but no relapse among patients randomly assigned to continue full-dose nortriptyline (7).

In a subsequent placebo-controlled comparison of nortriptyline and phenelzine in maintenance therapy (1 year) of elderly depressed patients, Georgotas et al. (5) reported that "patients administered phenelzine (n = 15) did significantly better with 13.3% recurrences than patients administered either nortriptyline (n = 13; 53.8% recurrences) or placebo (n = 23, 65.2% recurrences)" (p. 783). A nortriptyline window of 190–684 nmol/L (50–170 ng/ml) was used in this study. It is our view that this window may be too broad, and that patients taking either lower or higher doses of nortriptyline may demonstrate a curvilinear long-term response with respect to recurrence. For this reason, we chose a narrower nortriptyline level of 80–120 ng/ml in the University of Pittsburgh maintenance therapies study.

D. The University of Pittsburgh Maintenance Therapies Trial in Late-Life Recurrent Major Depression ("MTLLD"): Study Description and Preliminary Outcome Data

In 1989, with the support of the National Institute of Mental Health, the authors undertook a randomized, placebo-controlled, double-blind clinical trial of maintenance nortriptyline (NT) and interpersonal psychotherapy (IPT) in elders with recurrent major depression. The study is still ongoing, with a targeted enrollment of 200 patients (intake to be completed by early 1996). Briefly, the "MTLLD" protocol enrolls patients aged 60 and older who are minimally in their second life-time episode of major depression (unipolar, nondelusional). An interepisode wellness interval of at least 2 months but no longer than 3 years between the index and prior episodes is required, together with a Hamilton depression rating of 17 or higher and the absence of any medical contraindications to nortriptyline. During the initial, open phases of acute and continuation therapy, patients are treated with combined full-dose nortriptyline (to produce a steady-state blood level of 80–120 ng/ml) and weekly 50-min sessions of IPT. After clinical response (defined as a Hamilton depression rating of 10 or lower for 3 consecutive weeks), maintained for 16 weeks of continuation therapy, patients are then randomly assigned to one of four maintenance therapy cells: (1) NT with supportive medication clinic (but without a specific psychotherapy); (2) NT with IPT; (3) placebo (PBO) with medication clinic; and (4) placebo with IPT. The transition from continuation to maintenance therapy lasts 6 weeks in order to allow for the gradual tapering of NT and substitution of PBO in the 50% of remitted patients who are randomly assigned to a PBO condition (with or without the continuation of IPT).*

*We increased the duration of NT taper from 4 to 6 weeks after experiencing a 24% relapse rate during the 4-week taper of NT and gradual substitution of placebo (Ref. 7).

During maintenance therapy, patients come to the clinic monthly for 3 years, or until recurrence of major depression, whichever is first. It should be understood that NT-randomized subjects continue to receive "full-dose" NT (i.e., the same dose used during acute and continuation therapy, associated with levels of 80–120 ng/ml; on average 80–90 mg/day of NT, but with a very broad range of 20–200 mg/day), whereas IPT-randomized subjects receive IPT only on a once-a-month basis. It should also be understood that the experimental protocol (with randomized, double-blind, placebo control) begins on average 28 weeks after patients have entered treatment, allowing for about 12 weeks to achieve remission and an additional 16 weeks of continuation therapy to assure stability of response. The design of the protocol is shown in Figure 1.

E. Preliminary Outcome Data

As of December, 1995, 182 patients have entered treatment and are thus eligible for intent-to-treat analyses. Of these, 123 (67.6%) have responded and

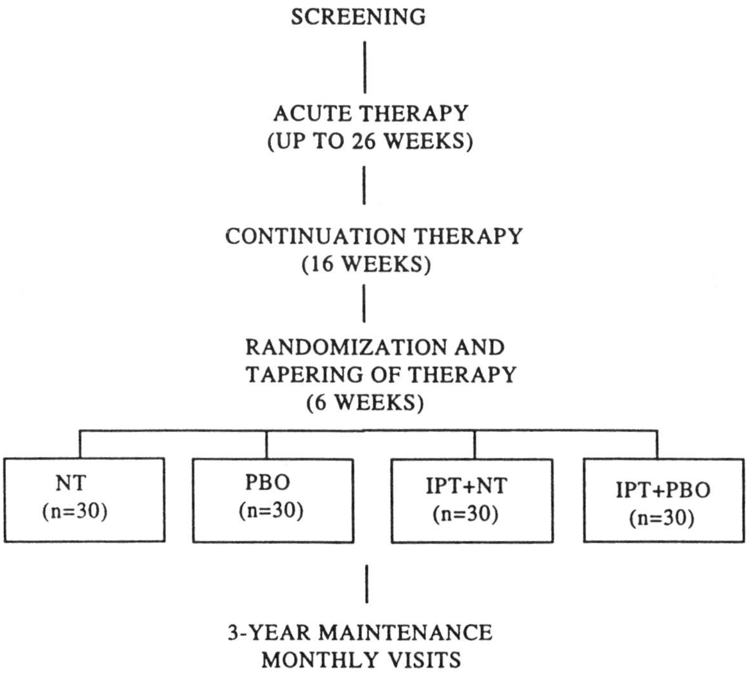

FIGURE 1 Maintenance therapies in late-life depression.

109 (59.9%) have been randomly assigned to one of the four maintenance therapy cells described above.

Interim descriptive analysis (without inferential analysis) of first-year maintenance therapy outcomes reveals that approximately 80% of patients randomly assigned to a nortriptyline condition (with or without interpersonal psychotherapy) show continued absence of major depression after 1 year of maintenance treatment (8). About 50% of patients randomized to IPT with placebo continue to show absence of major depression 1 year into maintenance treatment. Only 20% of patients randomized to a maintenance PBO condition without IPT continue to be well after 1 year. The IPT finding of 50% continued absence of major depression at 1 year is remarkable, considering that IPT is administered only *once* a month during the maintenance phase, while nortriptyline is continued at full dose. To our knowledge, if this finding holds, it will be the first demonstration of maintenance efficacy of psychotherapy in the treatment of major depression in later life. Although the combination of IPT and NT does not appear to be superior to NT alone in preventing recurrence, other outcome measures relating to quality of life should also be examined before making inferences about clinical practice. The other comment that appears warranted is the similarity of these 1-year outcomes to those reported by Frank et al. (19) in their study of maintenance therapies in midlife patients with recurrent major depression treated with imipramine and interpersonal psychotherapy. As we emphasize below, the overall pattern of similar treatment response in the midlife and late-life samples is both reassuring and exciting. At this time, however, the authors caution that no inferences be drawn from these preliminary analyses until the study is complete and survival analyses have examined differences in both primary and secondary outcome measures.

F. Safety and Tolerability

Our additional analyses have supported the continued safety and tolerability of full-dose maintenance nortriptyline during acute and continuation therapy (20) and during the first year of double-blind, placebo-controlled maintenance therapy (21). For example, our placebo-controlled observation is that nortriptyline is not a strong promoter of weight gain or orthostasis, and residual somatic complaints (which might be mistaken for side effects) covary strongly with residual depressive symptoms *regardless* of random assignment to nortriptyline or placebo (21).

G. Summary

In a review of long-term prevention of recurrences in elderly patients conducted for the NIH Consensus Conference (22), a consensus gleaned from existing data suggested that "long-term prevention of new episodes of unipolar disorder in both elderly and younger patients appears to be best achieved by maintaining patients on the same dose of antidepressant medication that was used successfully to treat the acute episode" (p. 318). Furthermore, "there is some evidence that maintenance psychotherapy can extend the well interval in patients who cannot or will not take maintenance medication" (p. 318). These conclusions still appear valid but await definitive confirmation from the MTLLD trial.

III. METHODOLOGICAL AND ETHICAL ISSUES

A. Recruitment

Recruitment of elderly depressed patients into the MTLLD trial has been challenging, averaging an intake rate of two patients per month since the start of the study. Of the initial 518 subjects identified through media announcements, clinician referrals, and word of mouth, 128 (24.7%) eligible patients gave informed consent to protocol participation. Of the 390 ineligible patients, 315 (80.8%) failed to meet psychiatric inclusion criteria [such as a previous episode of depression within 3 years ($n = 150$)], and 39 (10%) were excluded due to medical contraindications to NT. The remaining patients did not want to make the time commitment involved with protocol participation and/or did not wish to change their current psychiatric care. Of the patients who began active treatment, 48.7% were clinically referred, 42.6% were solicited through media and community presentations, and 8.7% learned of the program by word of mouth. Our examination of recruitment method (clinical referral vs. solicitation via media announcements) has shown that pathway into treatment did not affect retention in the study, time to clinical response in the treatment of the acute episode, or rate of treatment response (23). However, we have observed a greater proportion of black patients among subjects who were clinically referred as compared with those who were solicited. Given the scientific and ethical imperative to include appropriate proportions of minority subjects, this finding is particularly interesting and timely because it suggests that recruitment efforts might be productively focused on clinicians who see minority patients.

B. Retention and Treatment Compliance

The most important obstacle to adequate treatment of late-life depression (and hence to treatment research) is patient compliance. As many as 70% of elderly patients take only 50–75% of their prescribed dose (2). Thus, we have made a strenuous and ongoing effort to minimize attrition rates due to treatment refusal or noncompliance in the MTLLD trial. In our database, dropouts are highest during acute treatment (20/150; 13.3%) and lower during continuation therapy (5/116; 4.3%) and maintenance treatment (2.5%) (24).

Several factors may promote retention and long-term treatment compliance in elderly patients with recurrent major depression. In order to increase credibility and acceptance of treatment, we stress the importance of compliance during clinic visits and educate patients about the rationale for long-term therapy. We attempt to convey to patients and family members alike the message that "getting well is not enough—it's staying well that counts." We believe that compliance is also enhanced by attention to side effects and by the use of appropriate countermeasures to improve the quality of life. The creation and maintenance of an alliance with family members, through educational workshops, monthly telephone calls, and family support groups, is useful in this regard. Finally, collaboration with primary care physicians serves to enhance awareness about the challenge and treatment of depression in late life and usually elicits support for participation in long-term treatment.

We have developed the use of a biological measure, constancy of level-to-dose (L:D) ratios, as a means of providing an objective assessment of compliance. A larger variability in L:D ratios is associated with behavioral measures of noncompliance and poorer clinical outcome (25). For example, two L:D values exceeding the mean by 1.5 standard deviations provides a useful indicator of probable noncompliance with nortriptyline (25).

C. Choice of Outcome Measures: Quality of Life

In addition to recurrence of major depressive episodes (vs. their absence), we believe that it is important to attempt to measure quality of life during acute, continuation, and maintenance treatment. The choice of an appropriate measure for quality of life is not a trivial problem, partly because of the tendency of such measures to covary strongly with measures of depressive symptoms (in other words, not to convey more information than depression rating scale). While we do not claim to have solved the problem, our data suggest that the General Life Functioning (GLF) scale is promising. The GLF scale was developed in the context of the NIMH Treatment of Depression Collaborative Research Program to measure overall symptomatology and functioning (26). In the MTLLD study, therapists administer the GLF at pretreatment and then subsequently at each office visit throughout all phases of treatment.

Results of a factor analysis conducted on the first 110 MTLLD patients at baseline revealed the emergence of three distinct clusters of items, which we termed "coping," "well-being," and "interpersonal closeness" (27). We examined changes in GLF scores in 91 recovered and 19 nonrecovered patients, observing significant improvements in GLF scores in both groups, but greater and faster improvement among fully recovered subjects. Similar trajectories were seen in the measures provided by the "coping" and "well-being" factors. Importantly, effects were significant after adjusting for the level of depression (i.e., using Hamilton depression ratings as time-dependent covariates in the repeated measures analysis of covariance). The shared variance between Hamilton and GLF measures was modest, as suggested by an overall correlation of –.47 at baseline, –.68 at week 12 of treatment, and –.77 at week 24 of treatment.

D. Ethical Issues

Although we assert our belief that the risk–benefit ratio of participation in the MTLLD study remains extremely favorable, we must also acknowledge that this is a complex judgment based upon several considerations, not the least of which is a comparison with the usual care that such patients would receive if they were not in an NIMH-supported maintenance therapies protocol. The demands of a rigorous maintenance therapies trial, particularly the ongoing surveillance of patients (including their medical conditions and nortriptyline levels) and regular communication with families and primary care physicians, result in a level of care that far exceeds that which is usually achievable or affordable. In essence, our view is that patients are better off and safer in the study than they would be in usual care. We summarize below the data that form the basis of our belief.

First, Reynolds et al. (28) have recently performed intent-to-treat analyses of acute responses and relapse rates during continuation therapy comparing MTLLD subjects with those in the midlife maintenance therapies studies conducted by Frank et al. (19). Remission rates were similar in the two groups [116/148 (78.4%) in the elderly; 149/214 (69.6%) in midlife patients], but the time course of treatment response was somewhat slower in the elderly (9.3-point vs. 11.4-point drop in Hamilton rating over the first 8 weeks), and rates of relapse were higher among the elderly [18/116 (15.5%) vs. 10/149 (6.7%)] during continuation therapy. However, notwithstanding the slower treatment response and greater tendency to relapse during continuation therapy, intent-to-treat analyses showed comparable rates of recovery and subsequent randomization to maintenance therapy in the two studies: 67.3% in the MTLLD study and 56.9% in the midlife study. These observations are important in our view because they run counter to the widely held opinion that depression is less treatable in the elderly and that clinicians are justified in expecting a less favorable outcome. In essence, the fact that patients participate in this study makes them our "partners" in, as well as the direct beneficiaries of, an important discovery that would never have occurred in routine clinical practice.

Second, an examination of the temporal course of recovery from major depressive episodes in the elderly treated with NT and IPT has shown clinically and statistically reliable discrimination of recovering from nonrecovering patients at 4–5 weeks of treatment. A discriminant function model using early Hamilton ratings, age, duration of episode, and personality pathology scores was 80% accurate by 5 weeks of treatment (29). These findings have implications for clinical decision making (i.e., risk–benefit ratio), assuming that rigorous treatment has been conducted. The findings specifically underscore the importance of continuous, systematic treatment for at least 4–5 weeks before deciding whether or not a given approach is likely to be helpful. Again, our patients were our partners in, and the direct beneficiaries of, this finding.

The crux of the ethical issue arising out of the use of placebo is illuminated by the fate of patients who suffer recurrence of major depression after having been randomly assigned to a placebo condition in the maintenance phase of therapy. Our examination of treatment success rates in such patients has shown that 90% can be successfully treated to robust recovery using the same dose of NT (combined with weekly IPT) employed in the treatment of the index episode, and that time to recovery is shortened (from a median of 12–13 weeks in the index episode, to a median of 7–8 weeks in the subsequent or recurrent episode) (30). Very similar outcomes were reported by Kupfer et al. (31) in the midlife study. Again, the convergence of these two separate studies strongly supports our inference that recurrent major depression is as treatable in the elderly as in midlife patients. Our patients participate in, and benefit from, this conclusion.

Thus, we are reassured by the high success rate for restabilizing patients who have suffered a recurrence of major depression after having been assigned to a maintenance placebo condition. In addition, once patients have completed participation in the research protocol, we offer them continuing care (on a fee-for-service basis) through our Benedum Geriatric Clinical Center with the same study psychiatrist and psychotherapist/clinician. We thereby maintain a long-term commitment to our study patients, and they to us, ensuring that the demands of good science, good clinical practice, and ethical treatment of human subjects coincide.

We have never felt it necessary to utilize proxy consent (by next of kin or primary caregiver) in the MTLLD study, but we nonetheless make an effort to inform families of the demands of the protocol, its objectives, and its risk–benefit considerations. We practice "informed consent" on an ongoing basis, rather than simply at the start of the study, based upon the belief that patients' decision-making capacities improve as their depression is treated and remits.

IV. FUTURE DIRECTIONS

The MTLLD protocol incorporates two additional substudies designed to address important unresolved issues in maintenance therapies research in late-life mood disorders. One such substudy, known locally as the "full-dose/half-dose study," compares the maintenance efficacy of nortriptyline at full dose (associated with steady-state levels of 80–120 ng/ml) vs. half-dose (with steady-state levels of 40–60 ng/ml). To date we have recruited 45 patients into the study, with a target sample size of 60 or 30 subjects per cell. The second substudy aims to address 4- and 5-year outcomes in full-dose NT- vs. PBO-randomized "survivors" of the main study (i.e., patients who have remained depression-free for 3 years in the main study while in a nortriptyline condition, who are then rerandomized to continue nortriptyline or placebo for years 4 and 5). Studies such as these will generate data needed to illuminate further the long-term risks and benefits of maintenance therapy, as well as the "intensity" parameters of such treatment (e.g., maintenance "dose" of medication or psychotherapy).

Data sets such as those being acquired through the MTLLD protocols will also provide the means for building models of long-term course, including correlates of response and nonresponse, as well as models that show the interaction of different maintenance treatments with supervening medical and psychosocial variables, such as severe life events or other "provoking agents" (e.g., see Ref. 32).

The MTLLD protocol deals with only one type of recurrent depressive illness in the elderly. It is clear to us, however, that other types of mood disorders in later life also require systematic, controlled investigation, including bipolar mood disorders, delusional depression, and depression associated with neurodegenerative disorders such as Alzheimer's dementia (AD). In addition, we need a better definition of the benefits and risks of long-term therapy with other classes of agents, including the SSRI antidepressants.

As an illustrative case example of these issues, our group has a particular interest in the treatment of depression associated with Alzheimer's dementia. In our view, data are needed to determine whether antidepressant medication is superior to placebo in the acute, continuation, and maintenance treatment of depression in AD patients, in order to enhance both the scientific and ethical basis of clinical practice. The questions are whether depression can be effectively and safely treated in AD, and whether its recurrence can be prevented. However, relevant outcome measures must include not only resolution of depressive symptoms, but also effects of intervention on cognitive impairment, change in ADL and IADL functional capacity, impact on caregiver strain, duration of community tenure, and utilization of health and social service resources.

In order to assess *both* short- and long-term benefits of antidepressant medication in depressed AD patients (in this case, paroxetine), we have proposed a double-blind, variable discontinuation design because it permits an assessment of *both* acute and chronic efficacy in the same trial. In our view, the ethical conduct of such research necessarily incorporates a provision for proxy consent by next of kin (due to the impaired decision-making capacity of AD patients, particularly those who are psychiatrically impaired by depression), the use of placebo to further define with precision the risks and benefits of active treatment, a safety net for managing the risks associated with suicidal ideation, delirium, and psychosis; and an ongoing process of informed consent that builds partnership and trust with patients and their families.

V. SUMMARY

Currently available data suggest that recurrent unipolar depression can be as successfully treated on a long-term basis in the "young elderly" as in midlife patients, using either an antidepressant medication (nortriptyline) at full dose (i.e., the same dose employed during acute therapy to bring out remission of symptoms) or a psychosocial intervention (interpersonal psychotherapy) administered once a month. The success of these approaches depends upon consistent compliance with treatment, but this is not easily assured in the elderly. Maintenance treatment with nortriptyline or interpersonal psychotherapy appears to be acceptable to most patients and safe, with due cognizance of the medical contraindications to nortriptyline. Given current and developing practice patterns, however, the field would benefit from additional data bearing upon the comparative long-term efficacy, tolerability, and safety of nortriptyline versus the newer selective serotonin reuptake inhibitors, such as sertraline, paroxetine, or citalopram. There is good reason to think that the SSRIs may be safer and better tolerated in the old old or frail elderly, with more benign effects on measures of neuropsychological function, but whether they are as effective on a short- and long-term basis is not known. The prophylactic efficacy and tolerability of sertraline over 44 weeks (33), paroxetine over 1 year (34), and fluoxetine over 1 year (35) in younger patients is promising in this regard.

Clinical practice also needs to be informed by data from clinical trials enrolling "tough" patients at very high risk for severe, chronic illness and suicide, such as those with delusional or bipolar forms of illness, as well as mood disorders associated with neurodegenerative illnesses. The role of psychosocial interventions with such disorders, particularly in assuring compliance with treatment and easing the burden of caregiving, deserves special attention.

Finally, researchers need to develop and test treatment approaches to such patients that are transferable from university-based laboratory settings ("efficacy") to other community-based settings dealing with more diverse, heterogeneous populations than those enrolled in controlled clinical trials ("effectiveness").

ACKNOWLEDGMENTS

This chapter is an updated version of a review published in *International Psychogeriatrics* (7:27–40, 1995), entitled "Maintenance Therapies for Late-Life Recurrent Major Depression: Research and Review Circa 1995," by the same authors. This work was supported by MH43832, MH00295, MH52247, and MH30915.

REFERENCES

1. Reynolds CF, Frank E, Perel JM, Mazumdar S, Kupfer DJ. Maintenance therapies for late-life recurrent major depression: Research and Review Circa 1995. Int Psychogeriatr 1995; 7(suppl):27–40.
2. NIH Consensus Conference. Diagnosis and Treatment of Depression in late life. J Am Med Assoc 1992; 268:1018–1024.
3. Schneider LS, Reynolds CF, Lebowitz BD, Friedhoff AJ, eds. Diagnosis and Treatment of Depression in Late Life: Proceedings of the NIH Consensus Development Conference. Washington, DC: American Psychiatric Press, 1994.
4. Georgotas A, McCue RE, Cooper TB, Nagachandran N, Chang I. How effective and safe is continuation therapy in elderly depressed patients? Factors affecting relapse rate. Arch Gen Psychiatry 1988; 45:939–932.
5. Georgotas A, McCue RE, Cooper TB. A placebo-controlled comparison of nortriptyline and phenelzine in maintenance therapy of elderly depressed patients. Arch Gen Psychiatry 1989; 46:783–786.
6. Old Age Depression Interest Group (OADIG). How long should the elderly take antidepressants? A double-blind, placebo-controlled study of continuation/prophylaxis therapy with dothiepin. Br J Psychiatry 1993; 162:175–182.
7. Reynolds CF, Frank E, Perel JM, et al. Combined pharmacotherapy and psychotherapy in the acute and continuation treatment of elderly patients with recurrent major depression: A preliminary report. Am J Psychiatry 1992; 149(12):1687–1692.
8. Reynolds CF, Frank E, Perel JM, Imber S, Kupfer DJ. Maintenance therapies in late-life depression. Neuropsychopharmacology 1994; 10:61S.
9. Conwell Y, Rotenberg M, Caine ED. Completed suicide at age 50 and older. J Am Geriatr Soc 1990; 38:640–644.
10. Reynolds CF, Zubenko GS, Pollock BG, et al. Depression in Late Life: A Review for Current Opin Psychiatry 1994; 7:18–21.
11. Post F. The management and nature of depressive illnesses in late life: a follow-through study. Br J Psychiatry 1972; 121:393–404.

12. Murphy E. The prognosis of depression in old age. Br J Psychiatry 1983; 142:111–119.
13. Baldwin RC, Folly DJ. The prognosis of depression in old age. Br J Psychiatry 1986; 149:574–583.
14. Cole MG. The prognosis of depression in the elderly. Can Med Assoc J 1990; 43:633–639.
15. Burvill PW, Hall WD, Stampfer HG, Emmerson JP. The prognosis of depression in old age? Br J Psychiatry 1991; 162:75–182.
16. Zis AP, Grof P, Webster M, Goodwin FK. Prediction of relapse in recurrent affective disorder. Psychopharmacol Bull 1980; 16:47–49.
17. Kragh-Sorensen P, Hvidberg EF, Hansen CE, Baestrup PC. Therapeutic control of plasma concentrations and long-term effect of nortriptyline in recurrent affective disorders. Pharmacopsychiatry 1976; 9:178–182.
18. Reynolds CF, Perel JM, Frank E, et al. Open-trial maintenance pharmacotherapy in late-life depression: Survival analysis. Psychiatry Res 1989; 27:225–231.
19. Frank E, Kupfer DJ, Perel JM, et al. Three-year outcomes for maintenance therapies in recurrent depression. Arch Gen Psychiatry 1990; 47:1093–1099.
20. Miller MD, Pollock BG, Rafai AH, Paradis CF, Perel JM. Longitudinal analysis of nortriptyline side effects in elderly depressed patients. J Geriatr Psychiatry Neurol 1991; 4:226–230.
21. Reynolds CF, Frank E, Perel JM, et al. Nortriptyline side effects during double-blind randomized placebo-controlled maintenance therapy in elderly depressed patients. Am J Geriatr Psychiatry 1995; 3:170–175.
22. Frank E. Long-term prevention of recurrences in elderly patients. In: Schneider LS, Reynolds CF, Lebowitz BD, Friedhoff AJ, eds. Diagnosis and Treatment of Depression in Late Life: Results of the NIH Consensus Development Conference. Washington, DC: American Psychiatric Press, 1994:317–329.
23. Stack JA, Paradis CF, Reynolds CF, et al. Does recruitment method make a difference? Effects on protocol retention and treatment outcome in elderly depressed patients. Psychiatry Res 1995; 56:17–24.
24. Reynolds CF. Treatment of depression in late life. Am J Med 1994; 97(suppl 6A): 39S–46S.
25. Perel JM. Geropharmacokinetics of therapeutics, toxic effects, and compliance. In: Schneider LS, Reynolds CF, Lebowitz BD, Friedhoff AJ, eds. Diagnosis and Treatment of Depression in Late Life: Results of the NIH Consensus Development Cofnerence. Washington, DC: American Psychiatric Press, 1994:245–247.
26. Elkin I, Shea MT, Watkins JT, et al. National Institute of Mental Health Treatment of Depression Collaborative Research Program: General effectiveness and treatments. Arch Gen Psychiatry 1989; 46:971–983.
27. Mazumdar S, Reynolds CF, Houck P, et al. Quality of life in elderly patients with recurrent major depression. Psychiatr Res 1996; 63:183–190.
28. Reynolds CF, Frank E, Perel JM, et al. Treatment outcome in recurrent major depression: a post-hoc comparison of elderly and mid-life patients. Am J Psych 1996; 153(10):1288–1292.

29. Reynolds CF, Frank E, Dew MA, et al. Discrimination of recovery in the treatment of elderly patients with recurrent major depression: Limits of prediction. Depression 1995; 2:218–222.
30. Reynolds CF, Frank E, Perel JM, et al. Treatment of consecutive episodes of major depression in the elderly. Am J Psychiatry 1994; 151(12):1740–1743.
31. Kupfer DJ, Frank E, Perel JM. The advantage of early treatment intervention in recurrent depression. Arch Gen Psychiatry 1989; 46:771–775.
32. Frank E, Anderson B, Reynolds CF, Ritenour A, Kupfer DJ. Life events and the RDC endogenous subtype: A confirmation of the distinction using the Bedford College Methods. Arch Gen Psychiatry 1994; 51:519–524.
33. Doogan DP, Caillard V. Sertraline in the prevention of depression. Br J Psychiatry 1991; 160:217–222.
34. Montgomery SA, Dunbar G. Peroxetine is better than placebo in relapse prevention and the prophylaxis of recurrent depression. Int Clin Psychopharmacol 1993; 8:189–195.
35. Montgomery SA, Dufour H, Brion S, et al. The prophylactic efficacy of fluoxetine in unipolar depression. Br J Psychiatry 1988; 153(Suppl 3):69–76.

8
Depression and Cardiac Disease

Steven P. Roose
Columbia University, New York, New York

It is appropriate that a volume on geriatric psychopharmacology includes a chapter on depression and cardiac disease because these conditions frequently coexist in the older population. Any clinician treating this population, whether psychiatrist, cardiologist, or primary care physician, will encounter a patient with these concurrent conditions and there is a significant body of data that can guide the clinician to a safe and effective treatment for the depressed patients with cardiac disease. Such data are available because of concerns related to the observation that tricyclic antidepressant (TCA) overdose could result in a cardiac death (1). These concerns led a number of research groups to pursue the systematic investigation of the cardiovascular effects of TCAs in depressed patients with and without cardiac disease. These studies not only established the adverse effects associated with antidepressant use in cardiac patients, but also illuminated the complex multidimensional relationship that exists between affective disorder and cardiac disease.

This chapter will review (1) the cardiovascular safety of antidepressant medication; (2) the observation that depressed patients have a higher than expected rate of sudden cardiovascular death; (3) the finding that depression in the postmyocardial infarction (MI) period is associated with increased cardiac mortality; (4) a possible physiological explanation for the increased mortality rate in depressed patients; and (5) data that suggest that the cardiovascular effects of tricyclics are age-dependent.

I. THE CARDIOVASCULAR EFFECTS OF ANTIDEPRESSANT MEDICATION

The most studied antidepressants with respect to cardiovascular effects are the TCAs. A number of studies have established TCA effects on (1) blood pressure; (2) left ventricular function; (3) cardiac conduction; and (4) cardiac rate and rhythm.

A. Orthostatic Hypotension

One of the most frequent and potentially serious side effects of TCA treatment is orthostatic hypotension; fractures, lacerations, myocardial infarctions, and sudden deaths have all been reported as a consequence of this effect (2,3). Though the data would suggest that the orthostatic effect of the TCAs is comparable in younger and older patients, the adverse events associated with orthostatic hypotension are clearly more significant in the geriatric depressed patient (2,4). For example, a Michigan study of patients over the age of 65 reported a twofold increase in the risk of hip fracture in patients taking tricyclic antidepressants (odds ratio 1.9; $p < .001$) (5).

The orthostatic effects of imipramine, desipramine, amitriptyline, and doxepin are comparable and these medications induce symptomatic orthostatic hypotension in approximately 10% of otherwise medically healthy, depressed patients (2,6–8). Nortriptyline is the only tricyclic that is significantly different in its orthostatic effect (9,10). A number of studies have reported that (1) nortriptyline caused significantly less orthostatic hypotension than the other TCAs, and (2) patients who were forced to discontinue a TCA other than nortriptyline because of intolerable symptoms of orthostatic hypotension could subsequently be treated with nortriptyline without the same problem (9).

Both the frequency of orthostatic hypotension and the magnitude of clinical difference between nortriptyline and the other TCAs increase dramatically when treating depressed patients with cardiac disease. For example, in a series of 25 depressed patients with congestive heart failure treated with imipramine, the rate of orthostatic hypotension requiring discontinuation of drug was approximately 50% (11), but in a comparable group of 21 patients treated with nortriptyline, the rate of orthostatic hypotension was only 5% (12). Furthermore, 19 of the 21 nortriptyline patients had received a previous trial of another tricyclic, most often imipramine, and 8 had sustained falls while on the other tricyclic. Thus, even in depressed patients with congestive heart failure, nortriptyline is the least problematic tricyclic with respect to orthostatic hypotension. This lack of orthostatic effect is the singular reason that nortriptyline has become the TCA of preference for the geriatric depressed patient.

Although the mechanism of tricyclic-induced orthostatic hypotension is unclear, two studies suggest that the diagnosis of depression itself may be a significant risk factor. Constantino et al. reported a series of patients who experienced intolerable orthostatic hypotension on tricyclics and who were subsequently treated with electroconvulsive therapy (13). Following a successful course of treatment, the patients were restarted on the tricyclic but did not develop the same problems with orthostatic hypotension (i.e., the development of orthostatis was in part state-dependent, the state being depression itself). Another source of data that suggests that depression is a critical variable in TCA-induced orthostatic hypotension comes from studies where tricyclics are used to suppress ventricular arrhythmias. Giardina et al. reported that in nondepressed cardiac patients with congestive heart failure treated with imipramine for arrhythmia control, the rate of orthostatic hypotension was only 4% (14). This result contrasts with the approximately 50% rate of orthostatic hypotension in *depressed* patients having congestive heart failure treated with imipramine. These data suggest that the development of symptomatic orthostatic hypotension may represent a drug–diagnosis interaction, not just an inherent capacity of the drug itself.

The mechanism by which tricyclics induce orthostatic hypotension is unclear. It has been suggested that this effect is a result of α_1-adrenergic blockade. However, U'Prichard et al. (15) have shown that nortriptyline and imipramine have equivalent α_1-adrenergic blocking effects, whereas desipramine has significantly less. If orthostatic hypotension were a direct function of α_1-blockade, it would suggest that nortriptyline and imipramine should cause the same degree of orthostatic hypotension and desipramine should induce substantially less. This does not appear to be the case; in a crossover design study Giardina et al. showed that imipramine and desipramine have essentially equivalent orthostatic effects (6).

Furthermore, the observation that depressed patients with congestive heart failure have an increased frequency of orthostatic hypotension raises the possibility that norepinephrine has a role in the development of this side effect. Patients with congestive heart failure and depression have high circulating plasma levels of norepinephrine that may result in decreased beta-receptor sensitivity with the consequent inability to mount a compensatory tachycardia in response to an orthostatic drop. In summary, tricyclic-induced orthostatic hypotension is likely the result of a complex interaction of multiple factors, and any theory of mechanism must explain not only the difference in the orthostatic potential between the tricyclics, but also the difference in the effect of a single drug in different patient populations as well.

B. Left Ventricular Function

Shortly after TCAs began to be widely used, a number of studies concluded that the tricyclics directly impair cardiac muscle (16–18). However, these studies used the same flawed method to assess ventricular function, thereby making the results misleading. The advent of radionuclide angiography made available a more reliable means of assessing TCA effect on cardiac output, and subsequently a number of studies in depressed patients with left ventricular impairment have consistently demonstrated that the TCAs, whether imipramine, nortriptyline, or doxepin, do not appear to have a deleterious effect on left ventricular function (8,11,12). However, the studies to date include no more than 100 patients, and therefore it would be premature to conclude that the tricyclics are always "safe" in patients with congestive heart failure. A case in point is the report of a 79-year-old man with mild congestive heart failure who had a marked decrement in his ejection fraction and a significant deterioration in his clinical condition when treated with either nortriptyline or doxepin (19). Nonetheless it is reasonable to conclude that direct impairment of cardiac contractility is not a routine effect of the TCAs.

C. Cardiac Conduction

One of the most well-established cardiovascular effects of the TCAs is their propensity to slow cardiac conduction which is manifest on the electrocardiogram by significant increases in the PR, QRS, and QTc intervals (20,21). Electrophysiological studies have established that the TCAs cause primarily intraventricular rather than atrioventricular (AV) nodal conduction prolongation, an effect which is comparable to that of quinidine (22–24). In depressed patients with normal cardiac conduction, as reflected by a normal pretreatment electrocardiogram (ECG), the effect of tricyclics on conduction is not clinically significant in terms of causing conduction complications. However, the fact that tricyclics reliably slow cardiac conduction, coupled with the observation that in TCA overdose atrioventricular block is a frequent complication, led to the concern that patients with preexisting cardiac conduction disease, such as bundle branch block, would have a significantly increased risk of conduction complications if treated with a tricyclic. This concern was proved correct by a study that found that depressed patients with bundle branch block treated with a tricyclic had a 20% rate of significant conduction complication, either the development of 2:1 AV block or greater than 50% widening of the QRS (25). To date there is no evidence to suggest that one tricyclic is safer than another if given to depressed patients with preexisting bundle branch disease.

D. Antiarrhythmic Effect

Perhaps the most unexpected and striking finding that emerged from the studies of the cardiovascular effects of tricyclics is that the TCAs have a significant antiarrhythmic effect. When taken in overdose, tricyclics cause significant ventricular arrhythmias (1), and so it is understandable that for a long time it was believed that the TCAs were potentially arrhythmogenic in healthy patients or, at the very least, were contraindicated in patients with preexisting arrhythmias. However, a clinically significant antiarrhythmic effect has now been documented for imipramine, nortriptyline, and doxepin and, although the antiarrhythmic effect of the other tricyclics have not been studied to the same extent, it is likely that these TCAs also have antiarrhythmic activity to a significant degree (8,26–29).

In vitro studies have established that imipramine has a major effect on the initial inward sodium current of the Purkinje fiber (23,24) and, taken together with the studies that show a reduction of intraventricular conduction velocity (20), these data support the conclusion that the TCAs have an electrophysiological profile that is characteristic of type I antiarrhythmic compounds such as quinidine, encainide, flecainide, and moricizine (30). This electrophysiological profile is also a characteristic of the metabolites of the parent tricyclic (e.g., for imipramine, desipramine, and the hydroxy metabolites) (31,32). In fact, 2-hydroxy imipramine is equivalent to imipramine with respect to slowing conduction velocity in isolated Purkinje fibers and suppressing ouabain-induced arrhythmia. In the clinical setting two studies of nortriptyline (33,34) and one of desipramine (35) all found an association between the level of hydroxy metabolite and slowing of cardiac conduction as evidenced by an increase in conduction intervals. This is especially significant because it has been reported that the hydroxy metabolites of desipramine (36) and nortriptyline (37) are increased in patients over 60. This implies that we must consider the effect of the hydroxy metabolites when assessing cardiovascular safety, something which is of special importance in both the elderly and the rapid metabolizer in whom there is a high level of metabolites.

II. THE SAFETY OF TRICYCLIC ANTIDEPRESSANTS IN CARDIAC PATIENTS RECONSIDERED

A knowledge of the adverse cardiac effects of the tricyclics which forewarn the clinician when to expect trouble, combined with the robust efficacy of the TCAs, led our group to conclude that in most circumstances there was a favorable risk/benefit ratio to tricyclic treatment in depressed patients with heart disease. Specifically, the depressed patient with ventricular arrhythmias would especially benefit from the combined antidepressant and antiarrhythmic effect of the TCAs. Unfortunately, recent studies from the field of cardiology strongly indicate that these conclusions on the relative safety and clinical usefulness of tricyclics in patients with cardiac disease need to be significantly revised (38).

The impetus for this revision comes from studies that attempted to establish that suppression of ventricular premature depolarizations (VPDs) would decrease the risk of mortality in the post-MI patient. Though it has been well established that VPDs are a risk factor for sudden death after MI, a 1983 meta-analysis of all available data did not support the assumption that pharmacological suppression of VPDs would reduce mortality in the post-MI patient (39). This report prompted the National Heart Lung and Blood Institute to initiate a series of multicenter studies to determine whether the common practice of suppressing VPDs post-MI is in fact beneficial. The first of these studies, known as the CAST I (Cardiac Arrhythmic Suppression Trial), was prematurely discontinued after only 2 years because treatment with two of the three antiarrhythmic drugs being tested, encainide and flecainide, was associated with a significant excess of deaths compared with placebo-treated controls (40). Since encainide and flecainide are both type IC antiarrhythmics, it was hoped that this finding might not apply to the third drug in the trial, moricizine, a drug with type IA antiarrhythmic action. Therefore, a second study (CAST II) was initiated comparing only moricizine to placebo (41). Unfortunately, this study had to be prematurely discontinued when it became clear that moricizine also induced an increase in mortality comparable to encainide and flecainide.

CAST I and CAST II were done in patients who had asymptomatic or minimally symptomatic ventricular arrhythmias post-MI. Other studies further imply that antiarrhythmic drugs may carry a risk of increased mortality not only in patients with ventricular arrhythmias post-MI, but also when these compounds are used to suppress atrial fibrillation (42–44). If the mechanism by which type IA and IC antiarrhythmic drugs cause increased mortality were determined, it could help define the range of cardiac patients at increased risk when treated with these drugs. It is clear that the reason for the increased mortality is not conventional proarrhythmia, which is a paradoxical response to antiarrhythmic medication that occurs in 5–10% of patients with VPDs treated with antiarrhythmics and which, by definition, must occur within 30 days of initiating therapy. In the CAST studies patients were excluded if they had a proarrhythmic response and the difference in mortality rates between treatment with type IC antiarrhythmics and placebo continued to increase as exposure to the drugs lengthened. Recently, suspicion has focused on an interaction between the antiarrhythmic drug and ischemic myocardia, which results in an increased probability of ventricular fibrillation as the mechanism for the increased risk of mortality (45–47). If this suspicion proves correct, it would imply that the risk of using type IA or IC antiarrhythmic drugs increases proportionately with the severity of the ischemic heart disease.

The critical connection between the results of the CAST studies and the TCAs is that the tricyclics have type IA antiarrhythmic action similar to quinidine and moricizine. Again, data from the CAST studies are the most informative available when trying to quantify the magnitude of risk associated with these medications in the clinical setting. During the initial 2 weeks of moricizine treatment in the CAST II trial, 665 patients received moricizine and 17 died or had a cardiac arrest, while 660 patients were given placebo and only three died or had a cardiac arrest ($p < .001$) (41). Thus, an excess of approximately two patients out of each 100 treated with moricizine after MI either had a cardiac arrest or died. Unless more specific information to the contrary becomes available, it would be prudent to assume that the TCAs carry a similar risk of increased mortality if given to depressed patients with ischemic heart disease.

III. THE CARDIOVASCULAR EFFECTS OF NONTRICYCLIC ANTIDEPRESSANTS

Given that it would be preferable to avoid the use of tricyclics in depressed patients with ischemic heart disease, the obvious question is whether there is a proven safe and effective alternative. Data are available on the cardiovascular effects of two nontricyclic antidepressants in depressed patients with heart disease. The first is bupropion, which was studied in 36 patients with serious cardiac illness (48). This study concluded that bupropion (1) did not affect heart rate, (2) caused an elevation in supine systolic blood pressure in a number of patients, (3) did not adversely affect left ventricular function, (4) induced symptomatic orthostatic hypotension in only 1 of 36 patients, and (5) did not significantly prolong cardiac conduction or induce higher degrees of AV block in patients with preexisting bundle branch block. Intriguingly, there was some evidence that bupropion has antiarrhythmic activity, but if that effect does exist it would not appear to be the result of type IA action as with the tricyclics. Though in this study bupropion appeared to be relatively safe in patients with heart disease, only 36 patients were studied, and consequently there may be important cardiovascular effects that were not detected in this relatively small sample. Nonetheless, there do appear to be patients who cannot tolerate a TCA because of adverse cardiovascular effects who can be treated with bupropion. However, it should be noted that the efficacy of bupropion has not been satisfactorily established in either the elderly or the melancholic depressed patient.

Perhaps a more important issue is whether the selective serotonin reuptake inhibitors (SSRIs) carry less cardiovascular risk than the tricyclics. Despite their widespread use, the information on the cardiovascular effects of the SSRIs has been limited to data collected as addendum to efficacy studies that included primarily younger depressed patients free of significant medical disease (49–51). As a group, the SSRIs do not appear to prolong conduction intervals on the ECG, nor do they seem to induce changes in systolic, diastolic, or orthostatic blood pressure. There has been a repeated finding that the SSRIs induce a small, but statistically significant, decrease in heart rate on the average of 3 beats per minute. However, all these findings are compromised by the limitations inherent in the method of data collection.

Recently, data were presented from the first systematic study of the use of an SSRI, fluoxetine, in the treatment of depressed patients with cardiac disease (52). Twenty-seven patients with heart failure and/or conduction disease and/or ventricular arrhythmias were treated with fluoxetine for 7 weeks with a mean dose of 55 mg per day. The mean age of the patients was 73 ± 9 years, 74% of the patients were male, and 45% had a history of documented MI. Fluoxetine induced a 5 beat per minute decrease in heart rate, which was statistically significant. There were no significant effects on blood pressure, cardiac conduction, and no evidence of any effect on ventricular ectopic activity. Surprisingly, there was a statistically significant increase in the ejection fraction of patients with preexisting left ventricular impairment. However, this is the first study of fluoxetine's effect on left ventricular function and included only 12 patients. Therefore, it would be prudent to defer concluding that SSRIs have a beneficial effect on left ventricular function until this finding is replicated.

In this study, cardiovascular effects were assessed at week 2 and at week 7; there were no significant findings that emerged at week 7 that were not evident at week 2, despite the fact that the mean plasma level of fluoxetine plus nor-fluoxetine was 4 times greater at week 7 than at week 2. Most significantly, although 30% of the fluoxetine-treated patients did not complete the medication trial, there were no dropouts due to adverse cardiac events. Thus fluoxetine appears to be a benign treatment in depressed patients with cardiac disease and has fewer adverse cardiovascular effects than reported for the tricyclics, including nortriptyline.

Preliminary data are now available from the first prospective randomized control trial comparing an SSRI, paroxetine, to a tricyclic, nortriptyline, in depressed patients with ischemic heart disease (53). The study included 81 patients with a mean age of 58 ± 13 years, 33% of whom had a prior myocardial infarction, 37% were status postangioplasty, and 37% status postcoronary artery bypass surgery. Patients were randomized to a 6-week trial of either a therapeutic plasma level of nortriptyline or paroxetine up to 30 mg per day.

Nortriptyline treatment induced the expected cardiovascular effects, specifically an increase in heart rate and orthostatic blood pressure drop. Most striking was the difference between the medication groups with respect to documented cardiac events that required an intervention by the cardiologist and discontinuation of drug. Such an event occurred in one of the 41 patients treated with paroxetine and 8 of 40 patients treated with nortriptyline (chi square = 4.60 $p < .05$). Therefore, despite the relatively small number of patients in this study, the tricyclic was associated with a higher rate of significant adverse cardiac effects compared to the SSRI. Unfortunately, the apparent cardiovascular safety of the SSRIs may be somewhat mitigated by data that suggest that the SSRIs may not be effective as a tricyclic in both severely depressed patients and in the elderly (54).

IV. SUDDEN CARDIAC DEATH AND DEPRESSION

The systematic study of the cardiovascular effects of antidepressant medication also produced a new understanding of the clinical observation that medically healthy depressed patients have a higher than expected rate of sudden cardiovascular death. The first and still most definitive study supporting this clinical observation was published in 1937 by Malzberg et al. (55). In this study the mortality rate of patients hospitalized for involutional melancholia was compared to the death rate of the general population. In order to control for the effect of age, patients with melancholia and the general population were separated into 5-year age groups: e.g., the death rate of patients aged 60–64 was compared to the death rate in a comparable age group in the general population. Overall, the death rate was six times greater in patients with melancholia compared to the general population, and this was consistent in all age groups. Cardiac disease accounted for almost 40% of all deaths reported in these patients, and the rate of cardiac death in patients was eight times greater than the corresponding rate in the general population. This study remains unique because the data were collected in an era when there were no specific somatic treatments for affective disorder; thus, the findings represent the natural course of the illness.

The Malzberg study has been replicated, in part or completely, by a number of subsequent studies (56–59). One of the most informative studies compared mortality rates in adequately vs. inadequately treated depressed patients (60). In a sample of 519 patients, 328 patients received adequate treatment (defined as a certain minimum dose of tricyclic or ECT) and 191 received inadequate treatment. The rates of overall mortality, nonsuicidal mortality, and, specifically, cardiac mortality were significantly greater in the inadequately treated as compared to the adequately treated patients.

The mechanism underlying the increased cardiac mortality in depressed patients is unclear, but recent data suggest that changes in the ratio between sympathetic and parasympathetic tone make depressed patients more vulnerable to ventricular fibrillation (61–63). Ventricular fibrillation occurs when the heart receives an electrical stimulus during the brief vulnerable period of the cardiac cycle (repolarization) that is significantly greater than the threshold required to cause electrical instability of the myocardium (64). Central nervous system activity can significantly affect electrophysiological properties of the heart so as to decrease the threshold for ventricular fibrillation, an effect that is presumably mediated through the autonomic nervous system (65). It has been established that increased sympathetic neuronal input to the heart can lower the threshold for ventricular fibrillation whereas increased parasympathetic tone, which is generally transmitted through vagal activity, raises the threshold and therefore reduces the risk of ventricular fibrillation (66).

The measurement of heart rate variability can illuminate a possible relationship between depression, autonomic tone, and ventricular fibrillation. Heart rate variability is the standard deviation of successive R to R intervals in sinus rhythm and reflects the interplay and balance between sympathetic and parasympathetic input on the cardiac pacemaker. It has been demonstrated that a high degree of heart rate variability is present in compensated hearts with good cardiac function whereas heart rate variability can be significantly decreased in patients with severe coronary artery disease or congestive heart failure. In fact, decreased heart rate variability, specifically a decrease in the high-frequency component that most directly reflects vagal tone may be the strongest predictor of cardiac mortality in post-MI patients (67). There have been a number of studies assessing heart rate variability measurements in depressed patients but so far they have produced inconsistent findings (61–63). However, one result that has repeatedly emerged is that depressed patients have a decrease in the high-frequency component, which represents vagally driven (i.e., parasympathetic tone) respiratory sinus arrhythmia. This finding implies that depressed patients have decreased parasympathetic activity compared with normal controls. Insofar as decreased parasympathetic tone lowers the threshold for ventricular fibrillation, it is possible, although as yet unproven, that the decreased high-frequency variability may reflect the mechanism that underlies the increased rate of cardiovascular mortality in depressed patients.

V. THE INFLUENCE OF DEPRESSION ON THE PROGNOSIS OF CARDIAC DISEASE

It is now well documented that both the depressive symptoms and the full depressive syndrome occur frequently in patients with ischemic heart disease and, specifically, in the post-MI period. For example, Carney et al. found that in a series of 50 patients with a diagnosis of coronary artery disease documented by coronary angiography, 18% met Diagnostic and Statistical Manual, 3rd ed., (DSM-III) criteria for current major depression (61). In one of the most methodologically rigorous studies to date, Schleifer et al. interviewed a series of 283 patients in the immediate post-MI period (68). Eighteen percent of patients met Research Diagnostic Criteria for current major depression, and, in addition, 27% met criteria for minor depression. In follow-up interviews 3 months post-MI, 44% of the patients who were initially diagnosed as having current major depression still met criteria.

Importantly, both the Schleifer and Carney studies noted that even when the presence of depression was recognized by the treating physician, the illness was invariably untreated. This occurred despite the fact that the deleterious impact of depression in the post-MI period has been highlighted by studies that found that depressive symptoms have a negative impact on the maintenance of healthy behavior changes during rehabilitation post-MI and contribute to difficulties and delays in returning to an appropriate level of function (69,70). Other studies have emphasized that depression is one of several psychological characteristics that predict poor compliance with medical therapy and follow-up (71).

A recent study by Frasure-Smith et al. emphasizes another and perhaps the most important implication of depression post-MI (72). This study evaluated 222 consecutive MI patients and found that the rate of DSM-III major depressive illness was 18%. Most striking was that the depressed patients had a significantly higher rate of mortality in the 6 months post-MI compared to their nondepressed counterparts who had cardiac disease of comparable severity. It was further determined that patients who did not meet criteria for major depression, but who did have symptoms of depression as reflected by a Beck depression score of 10 or more, were also at greater risk for cardiac mortality than comparable cardiac patients with no depressive symptoms. After 18 months follow-up post-MI, approximately 17% of patients with a diagnosis of major depression or depressive symptoms had died a cardiac death compared to only 3% of comparable cardiac patients without depressive symptomatology (73).

Not only did the Frasure-Smith study conclusively demonstrate the deleterious effect of depression on cardiac prognosis, but it also suggested a possible pathophysiological mechanism responsible for it. Further data analysis examined the relationship between depression, cardiac death, and ventricular irritability and found that although ventricular irritability was no more common in the depressed compared to the nondepressed post-MI patient, the highest mortality rate occurred in patients who had both depression and ventricular ectopic activity. This result is compatible with the finding previouslydiscussed that depressed patients have a decrease in high-frequency heart rate variability which implies an increased vulnerability to ventricular fibrillation.

Though the data come from different studies and different patient populations, a compelling story is emerging that describes changes in parasympathetic tone in the depressed patient, which creates a vulnerability to ventricular fibrillation that results in an increased rate of sudden cardiac death, particularly in the depressed patient with ischemic heart disease. It is further suggested that treatment of depression will reduce cardiac mortality; therefore, it is imperative to find a safe and effective treatment for depression in the post-MI patient. It is a cruel disappointment that the tricyclics, which are robustly effective antidepressants in this patient population, also carry such a significant cardiovascular risk.

VI. THE RELATIONSHIP BETWEEN AGE AND CARDIOVASCULAR EFFECTS OF TRICYCLICS

Most of the data on the cardiovascular effects of antidepressants, in particular tricyclics, have been collected in an adult population, specifically, a geriatric population, when considering the adverse events in patients with preexisting cardiac disease. However, tricyclics are also used extensively in children and adolescents, and recently collected cardiovascular data suggest that there may be an important association between age and the effect of the tricyclic. In a study by Walsh et al. the cardiovascular effects of a therapeutic plasma level of desipramine (DMI) was assessed in patients with a mean age of 17.5 ± 6.4 years (74). In this group of patients, DMI induced an increase in heart rate of approximately 20 beats per minute, and an increase in lying systolic and diastolic blood pressure of approximately 10 mmHg. The effect of DMI on heart rate and increased supine blood pressure reported by Walsh is consistent with previous reports in children (75–77), and all available data suggest the tricyclic effect on blood pressure and pulse are substantially different in children compared to adults. There was also a substantial reduction in the high-frequency component of heart rate variability. Walsh has suggested that the tricyclic effect on heart rate in children is mediated by the blockade of parasympathetic input via the anticholinergic properties of the TCAs. It is established that parasympathetic input to the heart declines substantially with age and, therefore, the significant anticholinergic effect of the TCAs will produce a greater decrease in parasympathetic tone in younger, as compared to older, patients, not because of a differential effect of the drug, but because parasympathetic tone is greater in the younger patient. This explanation may also account for the rise in blood pressure.

These data on the differential effects of tricyclics on blood pressure and heart rate in young vs. old patients illustrate that whether the potential side effects of a drug are expressed depends in part on the interaction between the drug and the physiological state of the patient. Two variables that affect the physiology of the patient are age and diagnosis. As was discussed previously, the diagnosis of depression is a risk factor for the expression of TCA-induced orthostatic hypotension and now it is apparent that younger age predisposes the patient to increased heart rate and increased supine blood pressure when treated with a TCA. Therefore, in the clinical setting we should not simply think of a tricyclic as having cardiovascular effects. Rather, we must ask what cardiovascular effects can be anticipated when this drug is given to this patient who is this age with this diagnosis?

VII. CONCLUSION

The treatment of the depressed patient with cardiac disease is a commonly occurring dilemma for the clinician, and unfortunately we do not have all of the information that we need to make an informed decision. The situation is most problematic and clinically most pressing for depressed patients with ischemic heart disease. Currently the clinical approach of our group is that if a pharmacological treatment is indicated in a patient with mild or moderate depression and ischemic heart disease, we initiate treatment with an SSRI, and consider a TCA only if the patient fails to respond. In a patient with a comparable degree of ischemic disease, but a more severe melancholic depression, we initiate treatment with a TCA in spite of our concerns about the cardiovascular risk. This decision is reached after balancing the documented efficacy of the TCAs in this population and the morbidity and mortality associated with severe major depressive disorders against the magnitude of increased risk of mortality suggested by the CAST studies. However, we further believe that the risk of sudden death from tricyclic treatment increases proportionately to the severity of the ischemic disease and the consequent risk of infarction, and therefore at some point the risk/benefit ratio would weigh against a tricyclic in favor of alternatives, such as SSRI or electroconvulsive therapy, even in the patient with a melancholic depression. Unfortunately, the information necessary to define the gradient of risk is not available and, consequently, even within our own group, we cannot always reach consensus on how to treat the severely depressed patient with serious ischemic heart disease.

The prevalence of depressive disorders and ischemic heart disease in the geriatric population, coupled with the clear indication that depressive illness has a negative impact on the prognosis for the cardiac patient, means that new research that helps establish the parameters of safety and efficacy in treating this patient group will have a significant and immediate clinical impact.

REFERENCES

1. Williams RB Jr, Sherter C. Cardiac complications of tricyclic antidepressant therapy. Ann Intern Med 1971; 74:395–398.
2. Glassman AH, Bigger JT Jr, Giardina EGV, Kantor SJ, Perel JM, Davies M. Clinical characteristics of imipramine-induced orthostatic hypotension. Lancet 1979; 1:468–472.
3. Muller OF, Goodman N, Bellet S. The hypotensive effect of imipramine hydrochloride in patients with cardiovascular disease. Clin Pharmacol Ther 1961; 2:300–307.
4. Hayes JR, Born GF, Rosenbaum AH. Incidence of orthostatic hypotension in patients with primary affective disorders treated with tricyclic antidepressants. Mayo Clin Proc 1977; 52:509–512.
5. Ray WA, Griffin MR, Schaffner W, Baugh DK, Melton LJ III. Psychotropic drug use and the risk of hip fracture. N Engl J Med 1987; 316:363–369.
6. Giardina EGV, Bigger JT Jr, Glassman AH, et al. Desmethylimipramine and imipramine on left ventricular function and the ECG: A randomized crossover design. Int J Cardiol 1983; 2:375–385.
7. Kopera H. Anticholinergic and blood pressure effects of mianserin, amitriptyline and placebo. Br J Clin Pharmacol 1978; 5(suppl 1):29s–34s.
8. Roose SP, Dalack GW, Glassman AH, Woodring S, Walsh BT, Giardina EGV. Is doxepin a safer tricyclic for the heart? J Clin Psychiatry 1991; 52:338–341.
9. Roose SP, Glassman AH, Siris SG, Walsh BT, Bruno RL, Wright LB. Comparison of imipramine- and nortriptyline-induced orthostatic hypotension: A meaningful difference. J Clin Psychopharmacol 1981; 1:316–319.
10. Thayssen P, Bjerre M, Kragh-Sorensen P, et al. Cardiovascular effects of imipramine and nortriptyline in elderly patients. Psychopharmacology 1981; 74:360–364.
11. Glassman AH, Johnson LL, Giardina EGV, et al. The use of imipramine in depressed patients with congestive heart failure. J Am Med Assoc 1983; 250:1997–2001.
12. Roose SP, Glassman AH, Giardina EGV, et al. Nortriptyline in depressed patients with left ventricular impairment. J Am Med Assoc 1986; 256:3253–3257.
13. Constantino EA, Roose SP, Woodring S. Tricyclic-induced orthostatic hypotension: Significant difference in depressed and non-depressed states. Pharmacopsychiatry 1993; 26:125–127.
14. Glassman AH, Roose SP, Giardina EGV, Bigger JT Jr. Cardiovascular effects of tricyclic antidepressants. In: Meltzer HY, ed. Psychopharmacology: The Third Generation of Progress. New York: Raven Press, 1987:1437–1442.
15. U'Prichard DC, Greenberg DA, Sheehan PP, Snyder SH. Tricyclic antidepressants: Therapeutic properties and affinity for alpha-noradrenergic receptor binding sites in the brain. Science 1978; 199:197–198.

16. Raeder EA, Burckhardt D, Neubauer H, Walter R, Gastpart M. Long-term tri- and tetra-cyclic antidepressants, myocardial contractility, and cardiac rhythm. Br Med J 1978; 2:666–667.
17. Burkchardt D, Raeder EA, Muller V, Imhof P, Neubauer H. Cardiovascular effects of tricyclic and tetracyclic antidepressants. J Am Med Assoc 1978; 239:213–216.
18. Taylor DJE, Braithwaite RA. Cardiac effects of tricyclic antidepressant medication: A preliminary study of nortriptyline. Br Heart J 1978; 40:1005–1009.
19. Dalack GW, Roose SP, Glassman AH. Tricyclics and heart failure (Letter). Am J Psychiatry 1991; 148:1601.
20. Kantor SJ, Glassman AH, Bigger JT Jr, Perel JM, Giardina EGV. The cardiac effects of therapeutic plasma concentrations of imipramine. Am J Psychiatry 1978; 135:534–538.
21. Glassman AH, Bigger JT Jr. Cardiovascular effects of therapeutic doses of tricyclic antidepressants. A review. Arch Gen Psychiatry 1981; 38:815–820.
22. Vohra J, Burrows GD, Hunt D, Sloman G. The effect of toxic and therapeutic doses of tricyclic antidepressant drugs on intracardiac conduction. Eur J Cardiol 1975; 3:219–227.
23. Weld FM, Bigger JT Jr. Electrophysiological effects of imipramine on ovine cardiac Purkinje and ventricular muscle fibers. Circ Res 1980; 46:167–175.
24. Rawling DA, Fozzard HA. Effects of imipramine on cellular electrophysiological properties of cardiac Purkinje fibers. J Pharmacol Exp Ther 1979; 209:371–375.
25. Roose SP, Glassman AH, Giardina EGV, Walsh BT, Woodring S, Bigger JT Jr. Tricyclic antidepressants in depressed patients with cardiac conduction disease. Arch Gen Psychiatry 1987; 44:273–275.
26. Bigger JT Jr, Giardina EGV, Perel JM, Kantor SJ, Glassman AH. Cardiac antiarrhythmic effect of imipramine hydrochloride. N Engl J Med 1977; 296:206–208.
27. Giardina EGV, Barnard JT, Johnson LL, Saroff AL, Bigger JT Jr, Louie M. The antiarrhythmic effect of nortriptyline in cardiac patients with ventricular premature depolarizations. J Am Coll Cardiol 1986; 7:1363–1369.
28. Giardina EGV, Bigger JT Jr, Glassman AH, Perel JM, Kantor SJ. The electrocardiographic and antiarrhythmic effects of imipramine hydrochloride at therapeutic plasma concentrations. Circulation 1979; 60:1045–1052.
29. Raeder EA, Zinsli M, Burckhardt D. Effect of maprotiline on cardiac arrhythmias. Br Med J 1979; 2:102.
30. Hoffman BF, Bigger JT Jr. Antiarrhythmic drugs. In: DiPalma JR, ed. Drill's Pharmacology in Medicine, 4th ed. New York: McGraw-Hill, 1971:824–852.
31. Muir WW, Strauch SM, Schaal SF. Effects of tricyclic antidepressant drugs on the electrophysiological properties of dog Purkinje fibers. J Cardiovasc Pharmacol 1982; 4:82–90.
32. Wilkerson RD. Antiarrhythmic effects of tricyclic antidepressant drugs in ouabain-induced arrhythmias in the dog. J Pharmacol Exp Ther 1978; 205:666–674.
33. Young RC, Alexopoulos GS, Shamoian CA, Kent E, Dhar AK, Kutt H. Plasma 10-hydroxynortriptyline and ECG changes in elderly depressed patients. Am J Psychiatry 1985; 142:866–868.

34. Schneider LS, Cooper TB, Severson JA, Zemplenyi T, Sloane RB. Electrocardiographic changes with nortriptyline and 10-hydroxynortriptyline in elderly depressed outpatients. J Clin Psychopharmacol 1988; 8:402–408.
35. Kutcher SP, Reid K, Dubbin JD, Shulman KI. Electrocardiogram changes and therapeutic desipramine and 2-hydroxy-desipramine concentrations in elderly depressives. Br J Psychiatry 1986; 148:676–679.
36. Young RC, Alexopoulos GS, Shamoian CA, Manley MW, Dhar AK, Kutt H. Plasma 10-hydroxynortriptyline in elderly depressed patients. Clin Pharmacol Ther 1984; 35:540–544.
37. Nelson JC, Atillasoy E, Mazure CM, Jatlow PI. Hydroxydesipramine in the elderly. J Clin Psychopharmacol 1988; 8:428–433.
38. Glassman AH, Roose SP, Bigger JT Jr. The safety of tricyclic antidepressants in cardiac patients: Risk/benefit reconsidered. J Am Med Assoc 1993; 269:2673–2675.
39. Furberg CD. Effect of antiarrhythmic drugs on mortality after myocardial infarction. Am J Cardiol 1983; 52:32C–36C.
40. Cardiac Arrhythmia Suppression Trial (CAST) Investigators. Preliminary report: Effect of encainide and flecainide on mortality in a randomized trial of arrhythmia suppression after myocardial infarction. N Engl J Med 1989; 321:406–412.
41. Cardiac Arrhythmia Suppression Trial II Investigators. Effect of the antiarrhythmic agent moricizine on survival after myocardial infarction. N Engl J Med 1992; 327:227–233.
42. Selzer A, Wray HW. Qunidine syncope: Paroxysmal ventricular fibrillation occurring during treatment of chronic atrial arrhythmias. Circulation 1964; 30:17–26.
43. Falk RH. Flecainide-induced ventricular tachycardia and fibrillation in patients treated for atrial fibrillation. Ann Intern Med 1989; 111:107–111.
44. Coplen SE, Antman EM, Berlin JA, Hewitt P, Chalmers TC. Efficacy and safety of quinidine therapy for maintenance of sinus rhythm after cardioversion: A meta-analysis of randomized control trials. Circulation 1990; 82:1106–1116.
45. Bigger JT Jr. Implications of the Cardiac Arrhythmia Suppression Trial for antiarrhythmic drug treatment. Am J Cardiol 1990; 65:3D–10D.
46. Echt DS, Liebson PR, Mitchell LB, et al. Mortality and morbidity in patients receiving encainide, flecainide, or placebo. The Cardiac Arrhythmia Suppression Trial. N Engl J Med 1991; 324:781–788.
47. Greenberg HM, Dwyer EM Jr, Hochman JS, Steinberg JS, Echt DS, Peters RW. Interaction of ischaemia and encainide/flecainide treatment: a proposed mechanism for the increased mortality in CAST I. Br Heart J 1995; 74:631–635.
48. Roose SP, Dalack GW, Glassman AH, Woodring S, Walsh BT, Giardina EGV. Cardiovascular effects of bupropion in depressed patients with heart disease. Am J Psychiatry 1991; 148:512–516.
49. Cooper GL. The safety of fluoxetine—an update. Br J Psychiatry 1988; 153 (suppl 3):77–86.
50. Kuhs H, Rudolf GAE. Cardiovascular effects of paroxetine. Psychopharmacology 1990; 102:379–382.
51. Fisch C. Effect of fluoxetine on the electrocardiogram. J Clin Psychiatry 1985; 46 (3, pt 2):42–44.

52. Roose SP, Glassman AH, Attia E, Woodring S, Giardina EGV, Bigger JT Jr. Cardiovascular effects of fluoxetine in depressed patients with heart disease. 1997, submitted for publication.
53. Finkel MS, Gaffney A, Laghrissi-Thode F, et al. Randomized trial of antidepressants in patients with ischemic heart disease. (Abstract). J Am Coll Cardiol 1996; 27(suppl A):186A.
54. Roose SP, Glassman AH, Attia E, Woodring S. Comparative efficacy of selective serotonin reuptake inhibitors and tricyclics in the treatment of melancholia. Am J Psychiatry 1994; 151:1735–1739.
55. Malzberg B. Mortality among patients with involution melancholia. Am J Psychiatry 1937; 93:1231–1238.
56. Black DW, Warrack G, Winokur G. The Iowa record-linkage study: III. Excess mortality among patients with "functional" disorders. Arch Gen Psychiatry 1985; 42:82–88.
57. Weeke A, Vaeth M. Excess mortality of bipolar and unipolar manic-depressive patients. J Affect Disord 1986; 11:227–234.
58. Murphy JM, Monson RR, Olivier DC, Sobol AM, Leighton AH. Affective disorders and mortality. A general population study. Arch Gen Psychiatry 1987; 44:473–480.
59. Rabins PV, Harvis K, Koven S. High fatility rates of late-life depression associated with cardiovascular disease. J Affect Disord 1985; 9:165–167.
60. Avery D, Winokur G. Mortality in depressed patients treated with electroconvulsive therapy and antidepressants. Arch Gen Psychiatry 1976; 33:1029–1037.
61. Carney RM, Rich MW, Tevelde A, Saini J, Clark K, Freedland KE. The relationship between heart rate, heart rate variability and depression in patients with coronary artery disease. J Psychosom Res 1988; 32:159–164.
62. Yeragani VK, Pohl RB, Balon R, et al. Heart rate variability in patients with major depression. Psychiatry Res 1991; 37:35–46.
63. Roose SP, Dalack GW. Treating the depressed patient with cardiovascular problems. J Clin Psychiatry 1992; 53(Suppl):25–31.
64. Lown B, DeSilva RA, Reich P, Murawski BJ. Psychophysiologic factors in sudden cardiac death. Am J Psychiatry 1980; 137:1325–1335.
65. Lown B. Sudden cardiac death: biobehavioral perspective. Circulation 1987; 76 (1, pt 2):I186–I196.
66. Kliks BR, Burgess MJ, Abildskov JA. Influence of sympathetic tone on ventricular fibrillation threshold during experimental coronary occlusion. Am J Cardiol 1975; 36:45–49.
67. Kleiger RE, Miller JP, Bigger JT Jr, Moss AJ, Multicenter Post-Infarction Research Group. Decreased heart rate variability and its association with increased mortality after acute myocardial infarction. Am J Cardiol 1987; 59:256–262.
68. Schleifer SJ, Macari-Hinson MM, Coyle DA, et al. The nature and course of depression following myocardial infarction. Arch Intern Med 1989; 149:1785–1789.
69. Kennedy GJ, Hofer MA, Cohen D, Shindledecker R, Fisher JD. Significance of depression and cognitive impairment in patients undergoing programed stimulation of cardiac arrhythmias. Psychosom Med 1987; 49:410–421.

70. Finnegan DL, Suler JR. Psychological factors associated with maintenance of improved health behaviors in postcoronary patients. J Psychol 1985; 119:87–94.
71. Blumenthal JA, Williams RS, Wallace AG, Willaism RB Jr, Needles TL. Physiological and psychological variables predict compliance to prescribed exercise therapy in patients recovering from myocardial infarction. Psychosom Med 1982; 44:519–527.
72. Frasure-Smith N, Lesperance F, Talajic M. Depression following myocardial infarction: Impact on 6-month survival. J Am Med Assoc 1993; 270:1819–1825.
73. Frasure-Smith N, Lesperance F, Talajic M. Depression and 18-month prognosis after myocardial infarction. Circulation 1995; 91:999–1005.
74. Walsh BT, Giardina EGV, Sloan RP, Greenhill L, Goldfein J. Effects of desipramine on autonomic control of the heart. J Am Acad Child Adolesc Psychiatry 1994; 33:191–197.
75. Biederman J. Sudden death in children treated with a tricyclic antidepressant. J Am Acad Child Adolesc Psychiatry 1991; 30:495–498.
76. Fletcher SE, Case CL, Sallee FR, Hand LD, Gillette PC. Prospective study of the electrocardiographic effects of imipramine in children. J Pediatr 1993; 122:652–654.
77. Geller B. Commentary on unexplained deaths of children on Norpramin. J Am Acad Child Adolesc Psychiatry 1991; 30:682–684.

9

Treatment of Poststroke Psychiatric Disorders

Robert G. Robinson, Susan K. Schultz, and Sergio Paradiso
University of Iowa, Iowa City, Iowa

Cerebrovascular disease represents a major health problem facing the geriatric population in the United States, as its prevalence increases steadily with each decade of life (1). The neuropsychiatric complications of cerebrovascular disease include a wide range of emotional and cognitive disturbances. These disturbances have substantial clinical importance warranting prompt recognition and treatment for a number of reasons. First, poststroke syndromes such as depression or apathy occur relatively frequently (2,3). Second, the presence of poststroke depression has been shown to adversely impact on physical recovery (4) and to increase the risk of mortality following stroke (5). This chapter presents an overview of the major affective syndromes known to occur following cerebrovascular injury and discusses the treatment of these conditions.

I. POSTSTROKE DEPRESSION

Depression is the most common poststroke psychiatric syndrome, occurring in 20–50% of patients following acute stroke (6–8). Poststroke depression has been demonstrated to be phenomenologically similar to major depression in the absence of stroke (as discussed below), yet it also has unique features, such as its relationship to lesion location, which suggest that poststroke depression arises from a distinct mechanism related to cerebrovascular injury. Indeed, one study has shown a striking association between the presence of vascular disease in patients with late-life-onset depression compared to patients with onset of depression early in life (9). This reflects the biological nature of depressive symptoms associated with cerebral ischemic injury (as opposed to a greater degree of genetic influences in depression not associated with brain injury, i.e., functional depression), and highlights the status of poststroke depression as a distinct clinical entity.

A. Diagnosis

Most recent studies of poststroke depression have used structured interviews and diagnostic criteria as defined by Diagnostic and Statistical Manual (DSM-III-R) (10) or Research Diagnostic Criteria (11),(3,5,12). The latest criteria published in DSM-IV now categorizes poststroke depression as "mood disorder due to a general medical condition (i.e., stroke)" specifically with (1) depressive features; (2) major depressivelike episode; (3) manic features; or (4) mixed features (13). Two types of depressive disorders associated with cerebral ischemia have been identified. One type is major depression, which occurs in about 20% of patients (6). The other type is minor depression, which has been defined for research purposes using DSM-III symptom criteria for dysthymic depression (excluding duration criteria) or by DSM-IV research criteria. Minor depression occurs in approximately 20% of patients following stroke, and appears to have a more variable clinical course than major depression.

B. Phenomenology

Two studies have suggested that the phenomenology of poststroke depression contains the core features associated with major depression in the absence of stroke (14,15). In the first study (16), the frequency of depressive symptoms was compared between patients with poststroke major depression and patients with "functional" (i.e., no known brain pathology) depression. The two groups were found to display nearly identical symptom profiles. In the second study (15), depressive symptoms among stroke patients were assessed in relationship to physical impairment. The study found that, except for early morning awakening, all of the affective and autonomic symptoms of depression occurred more frequently among stroke patients with a depressed mood than among patients without a depressed mood. Moreover, the presence of nonspecific symptoms of depression in the absence of depressed mood occurred in only 3% of patients (representing possible false-positive cases), and only 5% of patients displayed symptoms necessary for a diagnosis of major depression in the absence of depressed mood (i.e., possible false-negative cases). Therefore, the use of DSM criteria in an acutely medically ill population does not appear to produce significant numbers of false-positive or false-negative cases.

The assessment of symptomatology in patients with language impairment is another aspect of the stroke patient that may impact on phenomenology.

Virtually all studies of patients with depression following stroke have excluded patients with impaired language comprehension. Our studies have utilized either reliability in responses to the Zung Depression Rating Scale or the ability to perform the tasks on Part 1 of the Token Test as standardized measures of comprehension. Patients with nonfluent aphasia (Broca's aphasia) can be examined for symptoms of depression if their verbal comprehension is intact. These patients have been included in many of our studies and have been found (17) to have more severe depressive symptoms than patients with mild comprehension deficit and fluent (Wernicke's) aphasia or global aphasia.

The obvious question raised by the exclusion of patients with comprehension deficits from systematic studies of poststroke depression is whether the exclusion of these patients significantly affects the clinical or lesion correlates of poststroke depression. Although this question cannot be definitively answered, from the available evidence in patients with mild comprehension deficits, these patients do not appear to have a high frequency of depression. Although one might expect that the existence of a language impairment could lead to depression, the available evidence (18) suggests that depression and language impairment are parallel processes that frequently co-occur (since Broca's area is in the dominant hemisphere frontal lobe and the area associated with depression is also in the dominant hemisphere frontal lobe) but are not usually related to one another. For example, the frequency of depression among patients with aphasia who can be examined is not significantly greater than the frequency of depression among patients with dominant hemisphere lesions but without aphasia (18). In addition, among patients with nonfluent (Broca's) aphasia, the most severely impaired patients are not the most depressed. There are patients, however, who cannot be examined using verbal or written interviews and therefore we cannot definitively measure the frequency of depression in this population. Although clinical impressions (19) and the findings in patients with mild comprehension deficits (17) do not suggest that these patients have a high frequency of depression, other methods for the assessment and diagnosis of depression in these patients need to be developed.

In summary, the phenomenology of depressive disorder in stroke patients appears to be extremely similar to that found in patients with functional mood disorders. The existence of aphasia with comprehension deficits has led to the exclusion of a number of patients from studies of poststroke depression. Although aphasia does not appear to be a cause of depression in most patients, alternate means of assessment of patients with comprehension deficits need to be developed for thoroughness of examination of this population. Finally, the presence of an acute medical illness such as stroke does not appear to lead to a significant increase in the number of nonspecific depressive symptoms. Thus, the use of DSM-IV symptom criteria for major depression does not lead to a significant increase in the number of incorrectly diagnosed cases of depression.

C. Prevalence

Following the demonstration of poststroke depression as a clinical syndrome distinguishable by diagnostic criteria, a number of groups have assessed the prevalence of this disorder. One study of 103 patients with acute cerebrovascular lesions found that 26% had the symptom cluster of major depression, while 20% showed the symptom cluster of minor (dysthymic) depression (6). Others have reported a similar prevalence of depression in stroke patients in a variety of settings, such as rehabilitation centers, general hospitals, outpatient clinics, and community surveys (5,7,12,20). Thus, about 20–40% of patients may develop depression within the first few months after an acute stroke. Approximately half will show the symptom cluster of major depression, while half will show the symptom cluster of minor depression.

D. Duration of Illness

A number of studies have assessed the duration of poststroke depression (5, 21–23). The majority of patients with major depression experienced remission within the first year, with a minority of cases becoming chronic major depression persisting up to 3 years following stroke. On the other hand, minor depression appeared to be more variable, with both short-term and long-term duration of symptoms (5,24). Two factors have been identified that can influence the natural course of poststroke depression. One is active treatment of the depression with antidepressant medication and the second is the location of stroke lesion. Findings related to lesion location will be briefly discussed before addressing treatment issues.

E. Lesion Correlates

The first study to report a significant clinical–pathological correlation in poststroke depression found a significant inverse correlation between the severity of depression and the distance from the left frontal pole to the anterior border of the lesion ($r = -.76$) using CT imaging (23). This surprising finding led to a number of subsequent investigations of this phenomenon. One such investigation demonstrated a significant correlation between left frontal proximity and presence of depression in 10 patients who were right-handed and had no known risk factors for depression ($r = -.92$; $p < .05$) (25). Several further studies have provided evidence supporting that both left-sided lesions and proximity of the lesion to the frontal pole appear to increase the likelihood of depression (23,26). Other work has supported the correlation with frontal proximity without the association with left-hemisphere lesions (27,28). In summary, several studies conducted by different investigators support the hypothesis that depression severity following stroke increases with proximity to the frontal pole and that left-hemisphere lesions may be more likely to show this relationship. Thus the location of the lesion along the anterior–posterior dimension appears to be an important variable in the severity of depression following stroke.

Subsequent work has addressed the distinction between cortical and subcortical stroke in terms of severity and presence of depressive symptoms following stroke. One study noted that patients who had lesions in the left hemisphere had significantly higher rates of depression than patients with right-hemisphere lesions, regardless of the cortical or subcortical location of the lesion (Fig. 1). In addition, correlations between depression scores and the distance of the lesion from the frontal pole were significant for patients with both left cortical and subcortical lesions. These relationships were not significant for patients with right-hemisphere lesions.

Further attempts to identify lesion correlates have taken a variety of approaches including assessments of specific brain nuclei and vascular distributions. These studies have implicated lesions in the left basal ganglia (29), the middle cerebral artery distribution (30), and right parietal white matter (31). The mechanisms underlying the relationship between these lesion locations

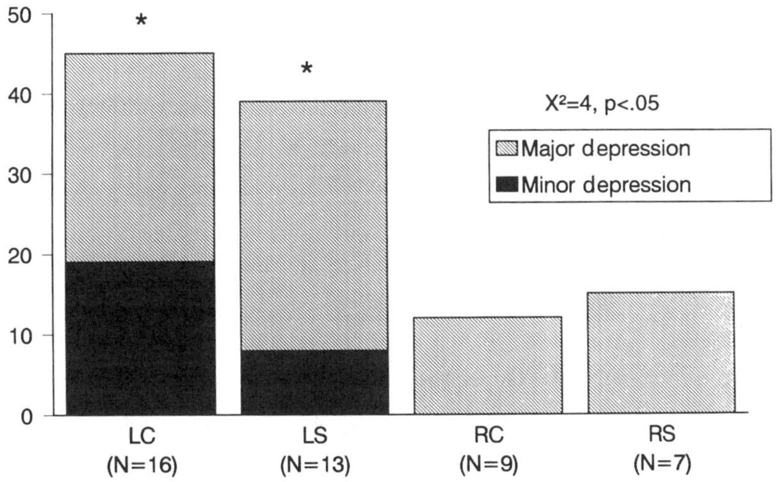

Figure 1 Percent of patients with single-stroke lesions visualized on CT scan and localized to left cerebral cortex (LC), right cerebral cortex (RC), left subcortical nuclei (LS), or right subcortical nuclei (RS) who have major or minor depression. There was a significant increase in the frequency of major depression among patients with LC or LS lesions compared to patients with RC or RS lesions.

and the development of poststroke depression remain unclear, although the preponderance of evidence continues to associate left frontal lesions with the presence of depression.

F. Mechanisms of Poststroke Depression

Although the underlying mechanism of poststroke depression remains unknown, dysfunction of biogenic amine regulation has been hypothesized to play an etiological role. Noradrenergic and serotonergic cell bodies within the brain stem send ascending projections through the median forebrain bundle to the frontal cortex. These axons then run longitudinally through the deep layers of the cortex (32). Lesions that disrupt these pathways in the frontal cortex or the basal ganglia may affect many downstream fibers. Based on these neuroanatomical facts and the clinical findings that the severity of depression correlates with the proximity of the lesion to the frontal pole, Robinson et al. (25) suggested that poststroke depression may be the consequence of severe depletion of norepinephrine and/or serotonin resulting from left frontal or left basal ganglia lesions. Investigations in rats have supported this hypothesis through demonstration of a lateralized response to ischemic lesions. Right-hemisphere lesions produced depletion of norepinephrine, whereas comparable lesions of the left hemisphere did not (33). More recently, a lateralized biochemical response to ischemia in human subjects was reported by Mayberg et al. (34). Right-hemisphere lesions resulted in significantly higher rates of ipsilateral spiperone binding [presumably 5HT-2 (serotonin) receptor binding] in noninjured temporal and parietal cortex compared to patients with left-hemisphere strokes. Patients with left-hemisphere lesions, on the other hand, showed a decrement in serotonin binding in the left temporal cortex, which inversely correlated with depression scores. These findings are intriguing, suggesting that the left hemisphere may be in some way more vulnerable to biogenic amine dysregulation than the right hemisphere, perhaps involving impaired compensatory upregulation of receptors in the face of ischemic injury.

G. Treatment of Poststroke Depression

Despite early anecdotal reports suggesting the clinical utility of tricyclic antidepressants or stimulant medications in the treatment of poststroke depression, only a few randomized double-blind treatment studies of the efficacy of antidepressant treatment have been published. One such study (14) involved 14 poststroke patients treated with nortriptyline and 20 patients given placebo. In the group treated with nortriptyline, 11 who completed the 6-week study showed significantly greater improvement in their scores on the Hamilton Rating Scale for Depression (Ham-D) (35) compared to 15 placebo study completers (Fig. 2). Nortriptyline levels in the treated group were between 50 and 150 ng/ml. Notably, six patients experienced side effects (including delirium, dizziness, and sedation), which precipitated discontinuation from the study.

Another study utilizing tricyclics during poststroke recovery was conducted by Balunov et al. (36). In this study, 90 subjects were recruited following stroke, and although no specific diagnostic criteria were used, the mean Hamilton Depression Scale Score was 13 (SD = 1), suggesting that mild-to-moderate depressive symptoms were present (perhaps minor depression). The subjects were assigned to three treatment groups. One group ($n = 30$) received amitriptyline titrated to 75 mg per day over 4 weeks. Another group ($n = 30$) received a benzodiazepine (valium), and the third group ($n = 30$) received placebo. At the end of the 4-week trial, the group receiving amitriptyline had significantly lower Ham-D scores compared to the other two groups. This study suggests that tricyclics are of greater benefit than anxiolytics following stroke: depressive symptoms are not secondary to anxiety but respond to treatment of depression.

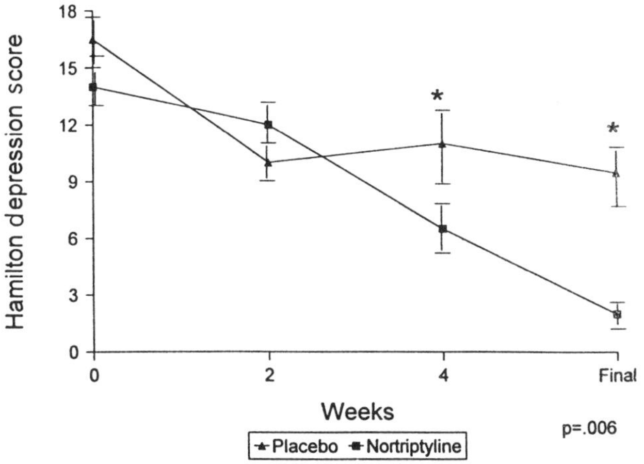

FIGURE 2 Hamilton depression scores during 6 weeks of double-blind treatment with nortriptyline or placebo for post-stroke depression. The study included 11 nortriptyline and 15 placebo-treated patients. At 4 and 6 weeks after beginning treatment, the nortriptyline-treated patients had significantly lower depression scores than placebo patients. Error bars represent ± SEM. p values shown are derived from repeated measures analysis of variance of treatment and time interaction. (reprinted with permission)

In addition to tricyclic antidepressants, the heterocyclic agent trazodone has been investigated in poststroke depression in a double-blind placebo-controlled manner. Reding et al. (37) reported that patients receiving trazodone (target dosage of 200 mg/day) with either a clinical diagnosis of depression or elevated Zung depression scores showed greater improvement in activities of daily living as measured by the Barthel Index compared to patients receiving placebo. This study also measured dexamethasone suppression tests (DST), and found that the trazodone-treated group, which displayed significant improvement in activity of daily living (ADL) scores had a greater association with an abnormal DST compared to the placebo group. Reding et al. had previously shown that the presence of an abnormal DST correlated with elevated depression ratings in poststroke patients, and was 87% specific and 47% sensitive to the clinical diagnosis of depression (38). However, this group was not able to find a relationship between DST and outcome measures in terms of measures of rehabilitation and improvement in self-care function. Subsequent studies have suggested that the DST is not adequately sensitive in the diagnosis of depression following stroke (39); thus the clinical assessment remains the optimal diagnostic tool in this population as it is with the vast majority of psychiatric syndromes.

Other tetracyclic medications have been investigated as possible adjunctive agents for use with tricyclic therapy. One such agent is mianserin. The mechanism of action of mianserin is primarily through serotonin receptor antagonism, although it also inhibits norepinephrine reuptake (40). Mianserin displays unique receptor binding activity in contrast to tricyclic antidepressants, which suggests that it may be particularly efficacious for the poststroke patient. For example, in rat studies, lesions of presynaptic serotonergic fibers in the dorsal and medial raphe have substantial effects on [3H]-imipramine binding of serotonergic receptors, but do not appear to affect [3H]-mianserin binding of serotonergic receptors (41). A controlled study of combined treatment of poststroke depression with either imipramine plus mianserin or desipramine plus mianserin showed that the imipramine combination was superior to the desipramine combination (42). Criteria for the diagnosis of depression in this study involved a Ham-D rating of 15 or greater. Dosages used in this investigation included a mean dose of 75 mg of imipramine, 66 mg of desipramine, and 25–27 mg of mianserin. One may speculate that the effect of mianserin on serotonin receptors contributed to its antidepressant efficacy in conjunction with imipramine, although the underlying mechanisms remain unclear.

Another agent that has been investigated in poststroke depression is the selective serotonin reuptake inhibitor (SSRI) citalopram. A recent double-blind controlled trial by Andersen et al. (43) using citalopram found that Ham-D scores were significantly improved over 6 weeks in patients receiving active drug (n = 27) compared with placebo (n = 32) treatment. At both 3 and 6 weeks, the active group had significantly lower Ham-D scores than the placebo group. Interestingly, this effect was primarily accounted for by subjects who became depressed 7 or more weeks after the stroke, as those who became depressed early after the acute stroke had a substantial rate of spontaneous recovery. This highlights the importance of placebo control, stringent diagnostic criteria, and close longitudinal follow-up in making determinations of antidepressant response following stroke. Most importantly, this study was instrumental in establishing the efficacy of SSRIs in the treatment of poststroke depression in a placebo-controlled fashion. Newer agents such as nefazodone and venlafaxime also hold promise but await investigation through controlled trials to establish efficacy in this population.

H. Potential Adverse Effects

Placebo-controlled trials comparing tricyclics, SSRIs, and the new atypical antidepressants will be of great value in distinguishing the relative efficacy of these agents. Clinical experience suggests that these agents have the advantage of fewer anticholinergic side effects, which may be particularly problematic in this population. Impairment in sensorium associated with anticholinergic side effects may interfere with assessment of cognitive impairment during stroke recovery. In more severe cases, anticholinergic effects may result in disorientation, confusion, dysarthria, incoherent speech, and anxiety (44,45). Clearly, as some of these symptoms may already be present secondary to the cerebrovascular lesion, treatment with tricyclics should be performed cautiously with careful assessment of other concomitant medications for the presence of anticholinergic agents. Often a patient may be using an over-the-counter antihistamine or hypnotic agent containing diphenhydramine that may compound the problem. Further, gait instability and urinary dysfunction resulting from stroke may be exacerbated by the effects of orthostatic hypotension and urinary retention associated with anticholinergic effects.

Another potential adverse event that may be exacerbated by the use of antidepressant medications is the development of seizures following stroke. Stroke is the most common cause of new-onset seizures in adults and poststroke seizures are most likely to develop early after the cerebrovascular event (46,47). It has been shown that poststroke seizures occur in approximately 3–10% of patients (47–49). Interestingly, it has also been shown that among poststroke patients who develop seizures, cortical lesions are more common than other lesion locations (49). This has clinical relevance, as some antidepressant medications such as bupropion (50) or tricyclics have a tendency to lower the seizure threshold, particularly maprotiline and clomipramine (51).

In summary, the clinical considerations discussed above all necessitate that clinicians must closely monitor medications in poststroke patients for possible adverse side effects. Nevertheless, antidepressant medications have established efficacy in treating depression following stroke and may confer benefit not only in resolution of depressive symptoms, but in improvement of overall stroke recovery (3,4).

I. Stimulant Treatment of Poststroke Depression

A few studies have evaluated the use of stimulants such as methylphenidate in the treatment of poststroke depression, although placebo-controlled double-blind trials have not been completed to date (52–54). One open trial of methylphenidate involved 25 poststroke patients diagnosed with major depression using DSM-III criteria (52). The subjects received 15–40 mg of methylphenidate per day for a clinically determined period of time with individual variation. Only two subjects dropped out due to side effects. Fifty-two percent of the group were identified as experiencing clinically significant improvement, and a substantial response was often noted within the first 2 days of treatment. Another study examined rehabilitation patients referred for psychiatric evaluation (53). Ten subjects meeting DSM-III-R criteria for major depression underwent a 3-week open trial of methylphenidate with assessment of Ham-D scores. In this sample, 80% displayed significant improvement with only minimal side effects. Another study of methylphenidate for poststroke depression retrospectively evaluated the medical records of 10 patients treated for depression while participating in a stroke rehabilitation program (54). Similarly, 70% were clinically improved in terms of depressive symptoms with no notable adverse effects based on chart review. Notably these studies are limited to small open trials and chart reviews, but they suggest that future controlled trials may demonstrate clinical benefit from the use of stimulants. As suggested in the study below, stimulants may have a nonspecific beneficial effect in rehabilitation measures regardless of diagnosis of depression.

One interesting study combined the treatment effects of physical therapy with the effects of dextroamphetamine. In a group of hemiplegic patients (n = 10), dextroamphetamine (10 mg) or placebo was administered in conjunction with physical therapy sessions over a 1-year follow-up period. The group receiving active drug showed accelerated motor recovery that was most pronounced and sustained *after* the end of the study period. This suggests that the improvement in motor recovery was not a transient effect of the stimulant. It is important to note, however, that depression was not assessed in this study, so whether alleviation of depression played a role in treatment response is not known. Further studies such as this one, which combine various rehabilitation modalities with treatment of depressive disorders, are likely to yield interesting results.

Electroconvulsive therapy (ECT) has also been demonstrated to be a potentially effective treatment for poststroke depression. In a retrospective study, Murray et al. (55) reviewed the clinical course of 14 patients receiving ECT following stroke. Twelve of the 14 experienced substantial clinical improvement in depression. Similarly, Currier et al. (56) evaluated 20 medically ill patients with poststroke depression treated with ECT: 19 subjects improved and no patient displayed an exacerbation of preexisting neurological deficits. However, 37% relapsed (typically 4 months after completing ECT), despite maintenance treatment with antidepressant medication. The role of continuance or maintenance of ECT in the treatment of poststroke depression has not yet been investigated.

In summary, a variety of antidepressants have been shown to be potentially efficacious in the treatment of poststroke depression, including tricyclics, SSRIs, stimulants, and ECT. Further research will better distinguish the relative advantages of each of these antidepressant agents and delineate their role in the poststroke population. At present, except in the case of hemorrhagic strokes, SSRIs appear to be a wise clinical choice with fewer side effects. In addition, these agents may correct the possible serotonergic dysregulation involved in the development of poststroke depression. Further, a number of novel agents have become available recently (e.g., venlafaxime, nefazodone, fluxovamine, etc.) and the potential benefits of these agents have yet to be explored.

II. DEPRESSION AND COGNITIVE IMPAIRMENT

It has been demonstrated that patients with poststroke major depression display a greater degree of cognitive impairment than nondepressed patients with comparable lesions (30,57). One study compared the severity of cognitive impairment in 13 stroke patients with major depression paired with 13 nondepressed stroke patients matched for size and location of brain lesion (30). The depressed patients had significantly lower Mini-Mental State Exam (MMSE) scores, suggesting that the presence of depression may confer a vulnerability to greater cognitive impairment.

Another study assessed the relationship between poststroke depression and cognitive impairment using a neuropsychological approach (57). Among patients with left-hemisphere lesions, those with major depression demonstrated greater overall cognitive impairment (including impairment in orientation, language, visuoconstruction, executive function, and frontal lobe functioning) compared to nondepressed patients. In contrast, among patients with right-hemisphere lesions, overall severity of cognitive impairment did not differ significantly between depressed and nondepressed patients. These findings suggest that depression following left-hemisphere strokes may be associated with an underlying mechanism distinct from depression following right-hemisphere strokes.

A. Treatment of Cognitive Impairment in Poststroke Depression

The findings noted above suggest that cognitive impairment may in some cases be related to the presence of depression (57). This suggests that treatment of depression may result in improvement in cognitive functioning. This issue was addressed in the treatment study discussed above by Lipsey et al. (14). Although cognitive function was not the principal outcome variable in this study, MMSE scores were examined before and after treatment. This study did not show a significant difference in MMSE scores between the nortriptyline and placebo-treated patients. These negative findings may have been partially attributed to inclusion of patients with both major and minor depression, as minor depression has not been shown to be associated with cognitive impairment following stroke (58).

Another group has recently assessed cognitive function following treatment of poststroke major and minor depression (59). This study involved 6 weeks of open-label treatment with nortriptyline or fluoxetine during the first 3 months following stroke. This study demonstrated that both antidepressants were associated with improvement in MMSE scores compared to placebo. In this study, patients were given nortriptyline 20–100 mg ($n = 11$) or fluoxetine 20 mg ($n = 26$). When the treated group was compared to a matched group of nondepressed patients, the depressed patients showed a greater rate of improvement over time, such that at the end of the 6-week period, there was no longer a significant difference between the groups. While there are no controlled trials specifically addressing the effect of antidepressant treatment on cognitive function, preliminary evidence suggests that during the first few months following stroke, cognitive impairment may improve with treatment of depression.

III. POSTSTROKE MANIA

Manic symptoms following stroke occur much less frequently than depressive symptoms. One center observed only three cases among a consecutive series of more than 300 stroke patients (58). It is notable that most studies utilize patients with multiple sources of cerebral injury in addition to stroke in investigations of lesion-induced mania. One such study examined a series of 12 consecutive patients who met DSM-III criteria for an organic affective syndrome, manic type (60). These patients developed mania after a variety of cerebral insults (stroke, traumatic brain injury, or tumors) and were compared with patients with functional (i.e., no known neuropathology) mania. Both groups of patients showed similar frequencies of elation, pressured speech, flight of ideas, grandiose thoughts, insomnia, hallucinations, and paranoid delusions. Thus the secondary mania had the same phenomenological appearance as primary mania, although, as will be discussed later, treatment response appears less predictable in the former group.

A. Lesion Location

Like poststroke depression, it has been suggested that lesion location may influence the manifestation of mania. In a case series, Cummings and Mendez (61) described two patients who developed mania following right-thalamic lesions. Similarly, Robinson et al. (58) reported on 17 patients with secondary mania. The majority of the patients had right-hemisphere lesions involving either cortical limbic areas (such as the orbitofrontal cortex and the basotemporal cortex) or subcortical nuclei (such as the head of the caudate and the thalamus). The frequency of right-hemisphere lesions in patients with poststroke mania was significantly greater than in patients with major depression (n = 25), who tended to have left frontal or left basal ganglia lesions, or in patients with no mood disorder following stroke (n = 36) (Fig. 3).

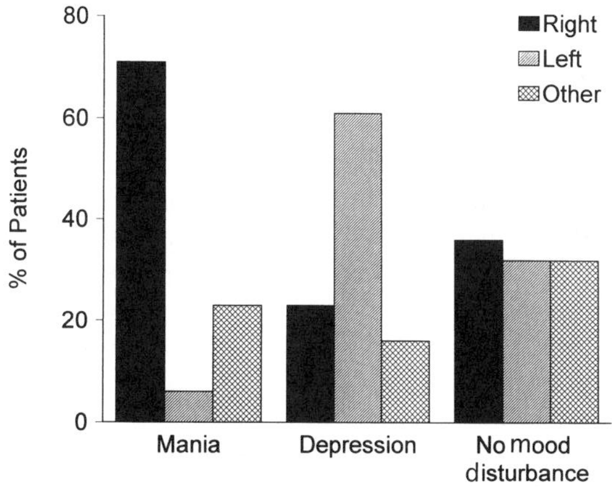

FIGURE 3 The percent of patients with mania (N = 17), major depression (N = 31), or no mood disorder (N = 28), following stroke divided by hemispheric lesion location. Mania was strongly associated with right hemisphere lesions and major depression with left hemisphere injury. (reprinted with permission)

An evaluation of lesion location in another series of eight patients with secondary mania supported similar findings (60). All eight patients had right-hemisphere lesions (seven unilateral and one bilateral injury). Lesions were either cortical (basotemporal cortex in four cases and orbitofrontal cortex in one case) or subcortical (frontal white matter, head of the caudate, and anterior limb of the internal capsule, respectively, in three cases).

In summary, several studies have found that secondary mania is associated with a greater frequency of right-hemisphere lesions compared to major depression or no mood disturbance. The right-hemisphere lesions associated with mania frequently involve brain regions with connections to the limbic system, particularly the right basotemporal cortex.

B. Poststroke Bipolar Disorder

Occasionally secondary mania has been followed by recurrent manic episodes, while in other instances the mania has been followed or preceded by episodes of depression. In an effort to determine which factors affect whether patients have associated manic or depressive episodes, Starkstein et al. (60) examined 19 patients with the diagnosis of secondary mania. Subjects were divided into two groups, one with bipolar disorder (both mania and depression) and the other with mania only, using DSM-III-R criteria for organic mood syndrome, manic and depressive types. All of the patients had CT scan evidence of vascular, neoplastic, or traumatic brain lesion, and no history of other neurological, toxic, or metabolic conditions.

The group with both manic and depressive episodes was found to have greater cognitive impairment as measured by MMSE scores. Six of the seven patients had lesions restricted to the right hemisphere and, of these, five were subcortical lesions. Similarly, eight of twelve patients with recurrent mania had lesions restricted to the right hemisphere, but eleven of the twelve had cortical lesions and only one patient had a subcortical lesion ($p < .05$). These interesting findings suggest that subcortical mechanisms in the right hemisphere may play a role in poststroke bipolar syndromes, while cortical mechanisms may be associated with a unipolar manic syndrome.

FIGURE 4 Top: Longitudinal evolution of mood disorder for individual patients with bipolar disorder. The length of follow-up is indicated by the length of the bar which shows duration of episode and pharmacological treatment. Bottom: Longitudinal evolution of mood disorder for individual patients with unipolar mania. Tr = tricyclic antidepressant; Ne = nortriptyline; Li = lithium; Ca = carbamazepine. (reprinted with permission)

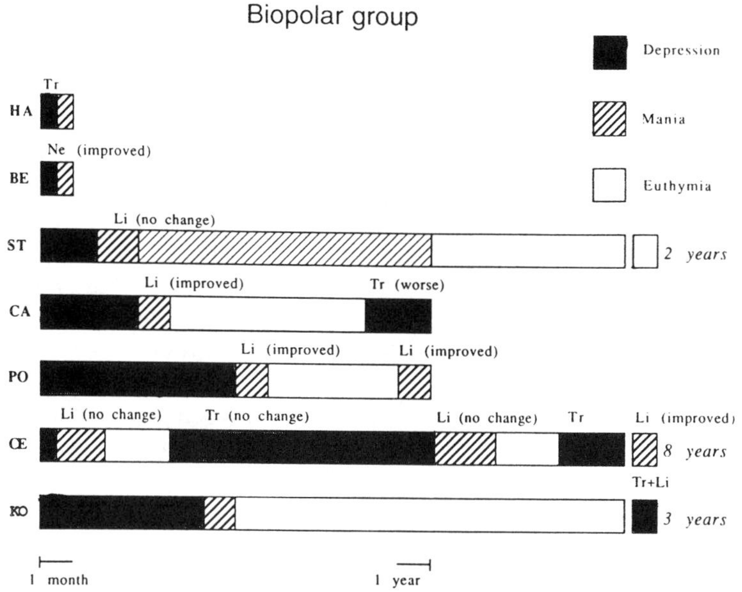
Biopolar group
Depression
Mania
Euthymia
Tr
HA
Ne (improved)
BE
Li (no change)
ST
2 years
Li (improved)
Tr (worse)
CA
Li (improved)
Li (improved)
PO
Li (no change)
Tr (no change)
Li (no change)
Tr
Li (improved)
ŒE
8 years
Tr+Li
KO
3 years
1 month
1 year

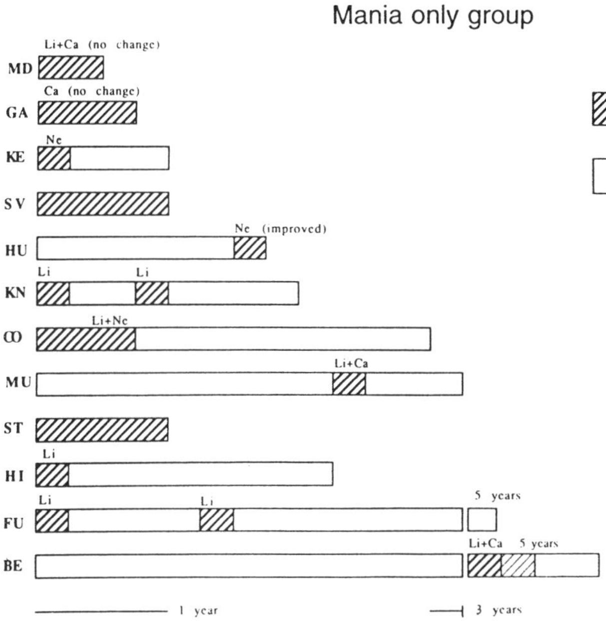
Mania only group
Mania
Euthymia
Li+Ca (no change)
MD
Ca (no change)
GA
Ne
KE
SV
Ne (improved)
HU
Li
Li
KN
Li+Ne
CO
Li+Ca
MU
ST
Li
HI
Li
Li
5 years
FU
Li+Ca
5 years
BE
1 year
3 years

C. Treatment of Poststroke Mania

There are no systematic studies on the treatment of mania following brain injury, and the existing case reports reflect a variety of treatments and responses (Fig. 4). Overall the consensus appears to be that secondary manic states are characteristically more difficult to treat than primary mania (62). Bakchine et al. (63) reported on the treatment of a single patient with mania following brain injury. In this case, clonidine (600 mg/day), rapidly reversed the manic symptoms, whereas carbamazepine (1200 mg/day) had no effect and L-dopa (375 mg/day) resulted in an increase in manic symptoms. Some reports have also suggested that patients who develop secondary mania (particularly those associated with seizure disorders) may not be as responsive to lithium as patients with primary mania (64). Anecdotal reports in the literature have indicated that some patients with secondary mania may respond to treatment with anticonvulsant drugs such as carbamazepine or valproate (64).

In summary, the pharmacological treatment of secondary manic syndromes following stroke is clinically quite variable, but typically relies on the same regimens used for primary mania. If lithium is not effective, carbamazepine, clonidine, valproate, verapamil, or neuroleptic augmentation may be useful alternatives. The anticonvulsants such as carbamazepine and valproate may be particularly beneficial for stroke patients due to the risk of seizures in this population. It should be noted that the use of antipsychotics warrants close monitoring, as the aging patient with neurological compromise is particularly vulnerable to the development of tardive dyskinesia as well as drug-induced parkinsonism (65). Controlled therapeutic trials in secondary mania, however, are needed to provide an empirical basis for managing these disorders and establishing a basis for further therapeutic advances.

D. Poststroke Anxiety Disorder

Studies of patients with functional depression have demonstrated that it is important to distinguish depression associated with significant anxiety symptoms (i.e., agitated depressions) from depression without these symptoms (i.e., retarded depressions). Evidence suggests that the underlying pathophysiology and clinical course may be different (66). The clinical implications of these studies for the treatment of stroke patients may have significant importance, as this population is uniquely vulnerable both to affective syndromes as well as to prominent anxiety symptoms.

Starkstein et al. (67) systematically examined anxiety disorders following stroke. A consecutive series of 98 patients with acute stroke lesions were examined for the presence of both anxiety and depressive symptoms. Modified DSM-III criteria for generalized anxiety disorder (GAD) (i.e., excluding 6-month duration criteria) were used for the diagnosis of anxiety disorder. Of 98 patients with first episode stroke, only six met the criteria for generalized anxiety disorder in the absence of any other mood disorder. Notably, these patients had a significantly higher frequency of alcohol abuse than the other groups. On the other hand, 23 out of 47 patients with major depression also met the criteria for generalized anxiety disorder. Examination of CT scans revealed that anxious-depressed patients had a significantly higher frequency of cortical lesions compared to depressed patients without anxiety or to nondepressed, nonanxious patients. In contrast, patients with depression *without anxiety* were noted to have significantly higher frequency of subcortical lesions compared with the anxious-depressed group.

Castillo et al. (68,69) found that 27% of a group of 309 patients hospitalized with an acute stroke met DSM-III-R criteria for generalized anxiety disorder (excluding the 6-month duration criteria). The majority of patients with GAD also had major or minor depression (i.e., 58 of 78 GAD patients had depression). Depression plus anxiety was associated with left cortical lesions, while anxiety alone was associated with right-hemisphere lesions. A 2-year follow-up in a subgroup of 142 patients found that 23% of patients developed GAD after the initial in-hospital evaluation (i.e., 3–24 months poststroke). Early- but not late-onset GAD was associated with a prior history of psychiatric disorder, including alcohol abuse. In addition, the early-onset anxiety disorder had a shorter mean duration (1.5 months) compared to delayed-onset GAD (3.0 months) (69).

E. Treatment of Poststroke Anxiety Disorders

There have been no systematic studies of the treatment of anxiety disorders following stroke. For guidance, the clinician must look to studies performed in patients with anxiety disorders not associated with brain injury. However, even in these studies the efficacy of pharmacological agents in the management of generalized anxiety has been particularly difficult to characterize for a variety of reasons, including small sample sizes and difficulties in diagnostic certainty (70). Benzodiazepines are the most commonly used medications in generalized anxiety disorders, although, as mentioned above, controlled trials have been problematic and there are no studies addressing the poststroke population. Short-acting benzodiazepines are a prudent choice, as longer acting agents may place the patient at greater risk for adverse effects. The clinician must always remain cognizant of the potential vulnerability of the poststroke patient to benzodiazepine side effects such as sedation, ataxia, disinhibition, and confusion. As with tricyclics, very conservative dosage and careful monitoring must be employed. In light of the comorbidity of anxiety and depression, tricyclics may also be of benefit for the poststroke GAD patient.

It has been demonstrated that tricyclics may be efficacious in the treatment of GAD even in the absence of depression (although, again, the specific needs of the poststroke patient have not been investigated). In one multicenter trial that excluded patients with comorbid depression, both chlordiazepoxide and imipramine were found to be superior to placebo in treatment of GAD over an 8-week period (71). Finally, busipirone may be useful in reducing anxiety without many of the adverse side effects, such as sedation, and without the risk of developing tolerance. In summary, anxiety disorders are a frequent consequence of stroke. Treatment of these disorders may include tricyclics, benzodiazepines, busipirone, or SSRIs, with the recognition that the majority of poststroke anxiety disorders occur comorbidly with depression. Optimal treatment of this condition awaits definition through controlled trials.

F. Apathy

Another condition accounting for psychiatric morbidity following stroke is apathy. Apathy is the absence or lack of feeling, emotion, interest, or concern and has been reported frequently among patients with brain injury including stroke. Using an apathy scale, one study examined a consecutive series of 80 patients with single stroke lesions (2). Of the 80 patients, 11% showed apathy as their only psychiatric symptom while another 11% displayed apathy and depression. In this study, it was noted that patients with apathy were significantly older than patients without apathy, but otherwise there were no sociodemographic differences between groups. It is of clinical importance that this study found that apathetic patients had more severe deficits in activities of daily living (ADL) than nonapathetic patients. Also, there was a significant interaction between depression and apathy as measured by ADL scores (i.e., the presence of both depression and apathy was associated with even greater impairment in ADLs than depression or apathy alone). There have been no controlled trials addressing the treatment of apathy, although treatment trials utilizing SSRI or tricyclic antidepressants or stimulants (methylphenidate or amphetamines) have been tried as well as optimization of the social milieu to minimize social withdrawal and isolation.

G. Pathological Emotions

Emotional lability is another common complication of stroke. This phenomenon is characterized by sudden, easily provoked episodes of crying or laughing which are typically precipitated by appropriately emotional stimuli. This type of lability may occur with diffuse or focal cerebral disease and its manifestations are usually congruent with the physical expressions of the patient and the emotional context of the situation. In contrast, *pathological* laughing and crying represents a more severe form of emotional lability and is characterized by episodes of laughing and/or crying that often are not appropriate to the context. They may appear spontaneously or may be elicited by nonemotional events and do not correspond to underlying emotional feelings or physical expressions. Other terms for these disorders have included emotional incontinence, pseudobulbar affect, or forced spasmotic lability. This type of pathological emotional display has frequently been observed in lacunar vascular disease, demyelinating diseases, and amyotrophic lateral sclerosis (72).

The clinical correlates and treatment of pathological laughter and crying have been examined in 28 patients with either acute or chronic stroke (73). A Pathological Laughter and Crying Scale (PLACS) was developed to assess the existence and severity of emotional lability. PLACS scores did not correlate with either Ham-D scores, MMSE scores, ADL scores, or Social Ties scores, suggesting that the PLACS was assessing a factor other than those measured by these instruments.

In the same study, a double-blind drug trial of nortriptyline versus placebo was conducted to determine the responsiveness of this condition to tricyclic antidepressants. The dose of nortriptyline was titrated to 100 mg over 4 weeks and 28 patients completed the 6-week protocol. Patients on nortriptyline showed significant improvement in PLACS scores compared with placebo-treated controls (Fig. 5). These group differences were statistically significant at weeks 4 and 6. Although a significant improvement in depression scores was

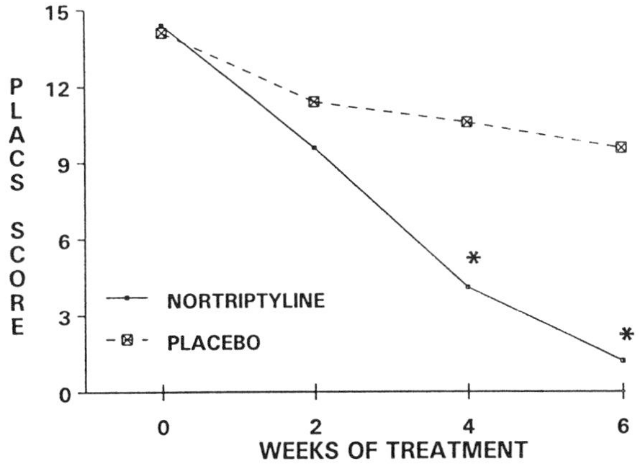

FIGURE 5 Mean pathological laughter and crying scale (PLACS) scores during 6 weeks of double-blind treatment. The nortriptyline-treated group had significantly lower (more improved) PLACS scores at 4 and 6 weeks of treatment compared with the placebo-treated group (N = 14). (reprinted with permission)

also observed, improvements in PLACS scores were significant for both depressed and nondepressed patients with pathological laughing and crying, suggesting that treatment response was not related to treatment of depression.

Like poststroke major depressive syndrome, disruption of serotonergic mechanisms has also been implicated in the mechanism of pathological crying. Citalopram (an SSRI) has been evaluated in the treatment of this phenomenon (74). In a double-blind placebo-controlled crossover study, 16 patients were evaluated. Citalopram was noted to have a rapid and substantial effect by decreasing crying frequency in 73% of the patients. Additionally, depressive symptoms were also noted to be significantly decreased in subjects who were receiving citalopram.

In conclusion, poststroke depression and pathological laughing and crying appear to be independent phenomena, although they may coexist. Moreover, both depression and pathological laughing and crying have been shown to respond to treatment with nortriptyline or citalopram.

IV. SUMMARY

There are numerous emotional and behavioral disorders that occur following cerebrovascular lesions. Depression is the most common of these, affecting up to 40% of individuals following stroke. The most compelling reason to accurately identify and treat poststroke depression is the substantial impact it may have on quality of life, physical and intellectual recovery, and survival. The poststroke population represents a uniquely challenging group of individuals with a wide array of comorbid medical illnesses. For this reason, administration of antidepressant medication requires a thorough psychiatric and medical evaluation and careful clinical monitoring. The evidence strongly suggests, however, that the benefits of successful treatment of poststroke depression far outweigh the risks associated with the use of antidepressant medications. SSRIs in particular appear to hold the greatest promise for alleviating symptoms of depression without prohibitive side effects (Table 1).

There are several other psychiatric manifestations that may occur following stroke, and each affords the clinician with further challenges. For example, poststroke anxiety is frequently present in conjunction with depression and presents another host of symptoms to assess and treat. The relative benefits of SSRIs vs. tricyclics vs. benzodiazepines for this patient population have not been clearly elucidated and await further research. Other syndromes such as poststroke mania, bipolar disorder, apathy, and pathological lability also pose problems for the clinician and the demonstration of effective treatment regimens await controlled treatment studies. Additionally, lesion studies that provide insights into the anatomical and biochemical mechanisms of

TABLE 1 Clinical Syndromes Associated with Cerebrovascular Disease

Syndrome	Prevalence	Associated lesion location	Potential therapeutic agents
Major depression	20%	Left frontal lobe Left basal ganglia	SSRIs Tricyclics Novel agents ?
Minor depression	10%–40%	Right or left posterior parietal and occipital regions	As with major depressive disorder
Mania	Rare	Right basotemporal or right orbitofrontal lesions	Lithium, carbamazepine, valproic acid
Bipolar mood disorder	Rare	Right basal ganglia or right thalamic lesions	As with depression or mania, varies with clinical context
Anxiety disorder	27%	Left cortical lesions, usually dorsal lateral frontal lobe	SSRIs, tricyclics, benzodiazepines, busipirone
Apathy			May benefit from antidepressant treatment
without depression	22%	Posterior internal capsule	
with depression	11%		
Pathological laughing and crying	20%	Frequently bilateral hemispheric lesions May occur with almost any lesion location	May benefit from antidepressant treatment, possibly lithium or anticonvulsants

these disorders promise to aid in the development of specific pharmacological strategies.

ACKNOWLEDGMENTS

This work was supported in part by National Institute of Mental Health Grants Research Scientist Award MH00163 (to RGR), MH40355. The authors thank Thomas R. Price, John R. Lipsey, Rajesh Parikh, Carlos Castillo, Krishna Rao, Godfrey D. Pearlson, Lynn Book Starr, and Paula Andrezewski who participated in many of the studies described.

REFERENCES

1. Wolf PA, Kannel WB, Verter J. Cerebrovascular disease in the elderly: epidemiology. In: Albert ML, ed. Clinical Neurology of Aging. New York: Oxford University Press, 1984:458–477.

2. Starkstein SE, Fedoroff JP, Price TR, Leiguarda R, Robinson RG. Apathy following cerebrovascular lesions. Stroke 1993; 24:1625–1630.
3. Robinson RG, Starr LB, Kubos KL, Price TR. A two year longitudinal study of post-stroke mood disorders: findings during the initial evaluation. Stroke 1983; 14:736–744.
4. Parikh RM, Robinson RG, Lipsey JR, Starkstein SE, Fedoroff JP, Price TR. The impact of post-stroke depression on recovery in activities of daily living over two year follow-up. Arch Neurol 1990; 47:785–789.
5. Morris PLP, Robinson RG, Raphael B. Prevalence and course of depressive disorders in hospitalized stroke patients. Int J Psychiatry Med 1990; 20:349–364.
6. Robinson RG, Price TR. Post-stroke depressive disorders: A follow-up study of 103 outpatients. Stroke 1982; 13:635–641.
7. Burvill PW, Johnson GA, Jamrozik KD, Anderson CS, Stewart-Wynne EG, Chakera TMH. Prevalence of depression after stroke: The Perth Community Stroke Study. Br J Psychiatry 1995; 166:320–327.
8. House A. Depression after stroke. Br Med J 1987; 294:76–78.
9. Baldwin RC, Tomenson B. Depression in later life: A comparison of symptoms and risk factors in early and late onset cases. Br J Psychiatry 1995; 167:649–652.
10. American Psychiatric Association. Diagnostic and Statistical Manual of Mental Disorders, Third Edition (DSM-III). Washington, DC: American Psychiatric Press, Inc., 1980.
11. Spitzer RL, Endicott J, Robins E. Research diagnostic criteria: rationale and reliability. Arch Gen Psychiatry 1978; 35:773–782.
12. Eastwood MR, Rifat SL, Nobbs H, Ruderman J. Mood disorder following cerebrovascular accident. Br J Psychiatry 1989; 154:195–200.
13. American Psychiatric Association. Diagnostic and Statistical Manual of Mental Disorders—DSM-IV. Washington, DC: American Psychiatric Press, Inc., 1994.
14. Lipsey JR, Robinson RG, Pearlson GD, Rao K, Price TR. Nortriptyline treatment of post-stroke depression: a double-blind treatment trial. Lancet 1984; i:297–300.
15. Fedoroff JP, Lipsey JR, Starkstein SE. Phenomenological comparison of major depression following stroke, myocardial infarction or spinal cord lesion. J Affect Disord 1991; 22:83–89.
16. Lipsey JR, Spencer WC, Rabins PV, Robinson RG. Phenomenological comparison of functional and post-stroke depression. Am J Psychiatry 1986; 143:527–529.
17. Robinson RG, Benson DF. Depression in aphasic patients: frequency, severity and clinical-pathological correlations. Br Lang 1981; 14:282–291.
18. Starkstein SE, Robinson RG. Aphasia and depression. Aphasiology 1988; 2:1–20.
19. Benson DF. Psychiatric aspects of aphasia. Br J Psychiatry 1973; 123:555–566.
20. Herrmann M, Bartles C, Wallesch C-W. Depression in acute and chronic aphasia: symptoms, pathoanatomical-clinical correlations and functional implications. J Neurol Neurosurg Psychiatry 1993; 56:672–678.
21. Robinson RG, Bolduc P, Price TR. A two year longitudinal study of post-stroke depression: diagnosis and outcome at one and two year follow-up. Stroke 1987; 18: 837–843.
22. Astrom M, Adolfsson R, Asplund K. Major depression in stroke patients: a 3-year longitudinal study. Stroke 1993; 24:976–982.

23. Robinson RG, Szetela B. Mood change following left hemispheric brain injury. Ann Neurol 1981; 9:447–453.
24. Robinson RG, Kubos KL, Starr LB, Rao K, Price TR. Mood changes in stroke patients: relationship to lesion location. Compr Psychiatry 1983; 24:555–566.
25. Robinson RG, Kubos KL, Starr LB, Rao K, Price TR. Mood disorders in stroke patients: importance of location of lesion. Brain 1984; 107:81–93.
26. Morris PLP, Robinson RG, Raphael B. Lesion location and depression in hospitalized stroke patients: evidence supporting a specific relationship in the left hemisphere. Neuropsychiat Neuropsychol Behav Neurol 1992; 3:75–82.
27. House A, Dennis M, Mogridge L, Warlow C, Hawton K, Jones L. Mood disorders in the year after stroke. Br J Psychiatry 1991; 158:83–92.
28. Sinyor D, Jacques P, Kaloupek DG, Becker R, Goldenberg M, Coopersmith H. Post-stroke depression and lesion location: An attempted replication. Brain 1986; 109:539–546.
29. Starkstein SE, Robinson RG, Price TR. Comparison of cortical and subcortical lesions in the production of post-stroke mood disorders. Brain 1987; 110:1045–1059.
30. Starkstein SE, Robinson RG, Price TR. Comparison of patients with and without post-stroke major depression matched for size and location of lesion. Arch Gen Psychiatry 1988; 45:247–252.
31. Finset A. Depressed mood and reduced emotionality after right hemisphere brain damage. In: Kinsbourne M, ed. Cerebral Hemisphere Function in Depression. Washington, DC: American Psychiatric Press, Inc., 1988:49–64.
32. Morrison JH, Molliver ME, Grzanna R. Noradrenergic innervation of the cerebral cortex: widespread effects of local cortical lesions. Science 1979; 205:313–316.
33. Robinson RG. Differential behavioral and biochemical effects of right and left hemispheric cerebral infarction in the rat. Science 1979; 105:707–710.
34. Mayberg HS, Robinson RG, Wong DF, Parikh RM, Bolduc P, Starkstein SE, Price TR, Dannals RF, Links JM, Wilson AA, Ravert HT, Wagner HN Jr. PET imaging of cortical S_2-serotonin receptors after stroke: lateralized changes and relationship to depression. Am J Psychiatry 1988; 145:937–943.
35. Hamilton M. A rating scale for depression. J Neurol Neurosurg Psychiatry 1960; 23:56–62.
36. Balunov OA, O.G. S, Alemasova AY. Therapy of depression in post-stroke patients. Alaska Med 1990; 32:20–29.
37. Reding JJ, Orto LA, Winter SW, Fortuna IM, DiPonte P, McDowell FH. Antidepressant therapy after stroke: A double-blind trial. Arch Neurol 1986; 43:763–765.
38. Reding M, Orto L, Willensky P, Fortuna I, Day N, Steindler SF, Gehr L, McDowell F. The dexamethasone suppression test: An indicator of depression in stroke but not a predictor of rehabilitation outcome. Arch Neurol 1985; 42:209–212.
39. Grober S, Gordon W, Silwinski M, Hibbard M. Utility of the dexamethasone suppression test in the diagnosis of post-stroke depression. Arch Phys Med Rehabil 1991; 72:1076–1079.
40. Zis AP, Goodwin FK. Novel antidepressants and the biogenic amine hypothesis of depression. Arch Gen Psychiatry 1979; 36:1097–2011.

41. Dumbrille-Ross A, Tang SW, Seeman P. High-affinity binding of [3H]-mianserin to rat cerebral cortex. Eur J Pharmacol 1980; 114:119–122.
42. Lauritzen L, Bendsen BB, Vilmar T, Bendsen EB, Lunde M, Bech P. Post-stroke depression: combined treatment with imipramine or desipramine and mianserin: a controlled clinical study. Psychopharmacology 1994; 114:119–122.
43. Andersen G, Vestergaard K, Lauritzen L. Effective treatment of poststroke depression with the selective serotonin reuptake inhibitor citalopram. Stroke 1994; 25:1099–1104.
44. Greenblatt JD, Shader RI. Anticholinergics. N Engl J Med 1975; 288:1215–1219.
45. Ananth JV, Jain RC. Benzotropine psychosis. J Can Psychiatr Assoc 1973; 18:409–414.
46. Ettinger AB. Structural causes of epilepsy. Neurol Clin 1994; 12:41–56.
47. Giroud M, Gras P, Fayolle H. Early seizures after acute stroke: a study of 1640 cases. Epilepsia 1994; 35:959–964.
48. Lo YK, Yiu CH, Hu HH, Su MS, Laeuchli SC. Frequency and characteristics of early seizures in Chinese acute stroke. Acta Neurol Scand 1994; 90:83–85.
49. Lancman ME, Golimstok A, Norscini J, Granillo R. Risk factors for developing seizure after stroke. Epilepsia 1993; 34:141–143.
50. Johnston JA, Lineberry CG, Ascher JA. A 102-center prospective study of seizure in association with bupropion. J Clin Psychiatry 1991; 52:450–456.
51. Jick H, Dinan BJ, Hunter J. Tricyclic antidepressants and convulsions. J Clin Psychopharmacol 1983; 3:182–185.
52. Lingham VR. Methylphenidate in treating post-stroke depression. J Clin Psychiatry 1988; 49:151–153.
53. Lazarus LW, Winemiller DR, Lingam VR, Neyman I, Hartman C, Abassian M, Kartan U, Groves L, Fawcett J. Efficacy and side effects of methylphenidate for post-stroke depression. J Clin Psychiatry 1992; 53:447–449.
54. Johnson ML, Roberts MD, Ross AR, Witten CM. Methylphenidate in stroke patients with depression. Am J Phys Med Rehabil 1992; 71:239–241.
55. Murray GB, Shea V, Conn D. Electroconvulsive therapy for post-stroke depression. J Clin Psychiatry 1987; 47:458–460.
56. Currier MB, Murray GB, Welch CC. Electroconvulsive therapy for post-stroke depressed geriatric patients. J Neuropsychiatr Clin Neurosci 1992; 4:140–144.
57. Bolla-Wilson K, Robinson RG, Starkstein SE, Boston J, Price TR. Lateralization of dementia of depression in stroke patients. Am J Psychiatry 1989; 146: 627–634.
58. Robinson RG, Boston JD, Starkstein SE, Price TR. Comparison of mania with depression following brain injury: casual factors. Am J Psychiatry 1988; 145:172–178.
59. Gonzelez-Torrecillas JL, Mendelwicz J, Lobo A. Repercussion of early treatment of post-stroke depression on neuropsychological rehabilitation. Int Psychogeriatr, in press.
60. Starkstein SE, Fedoroff JP, Berthier MD, Robinson RG. Manic depressive and pure manic states after brain lesions. Biol Psychiatry 1991; 29:149–158.
61. Cummings JL, Mendez MF. Secondary mania with focal cerebrovascular lesions. Am J Psychiatry 1984; 141:1084–1087.

62. Evans DL, Byerly M, Greer R. Secondary mania: Diagnosis and treatment. J Clin Psychiatry 1995; 53(S3):31–37.
63. Bakchine S, Lacomblez L, Benoit N, Parisot F, Chain F, Lhermitte F. Manic-like state after orbitofrontal and right temporoparietal injury: efficacy of clonidine. Neurology 1989; 39:778–781.
64. Shukla S, Cook BL, Mukherjee S, Godwin C, Miller MG. Mania following head trauma. Am J Psychiatry 1987; 144:93–96.
65. Yassa R, Nastase C, Dupont D. Tardive dyskinesia in elderly psychiatric patients. Am J Psychiatry 1992; 149:1206–1211.
66. Stavrakaki C, Vargo B. The relationship of anxiety and depression: a review of the literature. Br J Psychiatry 1986; 149:7–16.
67. Starkstein SE, Cohen BS, Fedoroff P, Parikh RM, Price TR, Robinson RG. Relationship between anxiety disorders and depressive disorders in patients with cerebrovascular injury. Arch Gen Psychiatry 1990; 47:785–789.
68. Castillo CS, Starkstein SE, Fedoroff JP, Price TR, Robinson RG. Generalized anxiety disorder following stroke. J Nerv Ment Disord 1993; 181:100–106.
69. Castillo CS, Schultz SK, Robinson RG. Clinical correlates of early-onset and late-onset poststroke generalized anxiety. Am J Psychiatry 1995; 152:1174–1179.
70. Solomon K, Hart R. Pitfalls and prospects in clinical research on antianxiety drugs: Benzodiazepines and placebo: A review. J Clin Psychiatry 1978; 39:823–831.
71. Kahn RJ, McNair DM, Lipman RS, Covi L, Rickels K, Downing R, Fisher S, Frankenthaler LM. Imipramine and chlordiazepoxide in depressive and anxiety disorders. II. Efficacy in anxious outpatients. Arch Gen Psychiatry 1986; 43:79–85.
72. Adams RD, Victor M. Principles of Neurology. New York: McGraw-Hill, 1985.
73. Robinson RG, Parikh RM, Lipsey JR, Starkstein SE, Price TR. Pathological laughing and crying following stroke: Validation of measurement scale and double-blind treatment study. Am J Psychiatry 1993; 150:286–293.
74. Andersen G, Vestergaard K, Riis J. Citalopram for post-stroke pathological crying. Lancet 1993; 342(8875):837–839.

10
Depression and Cancer

Herbert Ward and Dwight L. Evans
University of Florida, Gainesville, Florida

I. INTRODUCTION

Diagnosis and treatment of depression in the elderly require an understanding of the biological and psychosocial substrates unique to this phase of life. When the aging brain and body is compromised by medical illness, the diagnostic and treatment challenge quickly escalates for the clinician. Of the physical threats to the elderly, cancer remains at the top of the list with 50% of all malignancies occurring in individuals 65 years and older (1,2). Currently, there is a paucity of formal investigation of depression in the elderly cancer patient. However, there has been considerable study of depression and cancer among mixed-age populations. A recent review of 18 studies involving 2100 cancer patients revealed a mean prevalence of depression of 24% (3). This chapter will examine the practical and theoretical concerns raised by these and other studies as they may apply to the elderly.

II. DIAGNOSIS

A. Psychosocial Context

An initial grief reaction to the loss of one's health and sense of independence is a normal response following a diagnosis of cancer. Comprehensive care of the cancer patient includes facilitation of this psychological adjustment and monitoring for pathological developments during normal bereavement. For the elderly, a diagnosis of cancer comes at a time in the life cycle when losses have already escalated. At any given point in time, the elderly cancer patient may be processing multiple losses, each at varying stages of resolution. Assessment of psychological symptoms of depression must therefore account for both the overlap between normal bereavement and depression, and the inevitable complexity of this stage of psychosocial development.

B. Medical Context

Many of the somatic symptoms of depression such as anorexia, weight loss, and fatigue overlap with symptoms of both cancer and the side effects of its treatment. Several studies have examined strategies for evaluating depressive symptoms in the medically ill patient. Cohen-Cole and colleagues have reviewed different approaches and summarized strengths and weaknesses of each (4). An "inclusive" approach counts all depressive symptoms toward the diagnosis of major depression, whether or not they may be secondary to a physical problem (5).

An "exclusive" approach eliminates anorexia and fatigue from the depression criteria (6). The clinical utility of the "inclusive" approach rests in its sensitivity, albeit at the expense of specificity. On the other hand, the specificity of the more "exclusive" criteria identifies a more homogeneous population that may be better suited for research purposes. Thus the inclusive approach, using clinical judgment on a case-by-case basis, is generally considered the best approach in clinical practice.

C. Medical Differential

Reversible or time-limited organic processes should be considered in the overall assessment of the elderly depressed cancer patient. A systematic approach to rule out treatable toxic, metabolic, structural, and infectious insults to the central nervous system (CNS) is essential in this population. For example, ectopic hormone production from lung cancer with secondary hyponatremia, hypercalcemia, hypomagnesemia, or Cushing's syndrome are not uncommon (7). In the elderly, it is often the additive effects of multiple "minor" metabolic or toxic derangements that result in cognitive or affective impairment. Early symptoms of delirium, which occur in one-third of all cancer patients, can be mistaken for depression (8). Metastases to the brain occur in approximately one-third of all patients with cancer (9). The direct effects of cancer on the CNS should always be considered.

Of the more common cancers in the elderly, breast, lung, and prostate cancer all have an increased propensity to metastasize to the brain (9). Dementia must be included in the differential for mental status changes in the elderly. However, as many as 12% of dementias are subsequently found to be "pseudodementia," or neurocognitive symptoms associated with depression which are responsive to antidepressant therapy (10). There is now considerable support for a relationship between cancer-related pain and depression. Spiegel and colleagues examined the prevalence of psychiatric diagnoses among patients with cancer who had low and high degrees of pain to better characterize this relationship. They found that 28% of the high-pain sample met the criteria for major depression, compared to 9% of the low-pain group (11). In a multicenter study of 215 cancer patients, Derogatis and colleagues found that 47% of the patients met Diagnostic and Statistical Manual (DSM-III) criteria for a psychiatric disorder. Most of these patients fell within a spectrum of depressive disorders, including adjustment disorder with depressed mood and major depression. Of this 47% with a psychiatric diagnosis, 39% reported severe pain, compared to 19% of patients without a psychiatric diagnosis (12). Ahles and colleagues compared cancer patients with and without pain and found that patients with pain obtained higher scores on measures of depression, hostility, somatization, and anxiety (13). These and other studies do not rule out a bidirectional relationship between cancer pain and psychiatric illness. However, there are sufficient data to support continual reappraisal of pain management in the cancer patient with depressive symptoms.

D. Biological Markers

There is a considerable body of literature characterizing the neuroendocrine changes seen in patients with major depression (14). In light of the difficulties in diagnosing depression in cancer patients, reliable biological markers could be of great clinical utility in this population. However, there are limited neuroendocrine data on patients with coexisting medical conditions (15) and, to date, only three studies examining biological markers specifically in depressed cancer patients. Joffe and colleagues evaluated 21 patients with pancreatic or gastric cancer. The mean age of their subjects was 54.8 years, with only two patients over 65 years of age. A subset of six pancreatic and six gastric cancer patients were administered the DST using a $\geq 5\ \mu g$ criteria.

Six of six pancreatic cancer patients (one of which was depressed) and five of six gastric cancer patients (none of which were depressed) failed to show suppression on the DST. They concluded that in this small group of patients that dexamethasone nonsuppression was a nonspecific finding (16). Evans and colleagues studied 83 women (aged 20–86 years; mean = 53 years) with cervical, endometrial, or vaginal cancer. Major depression was diagnosed in 23% of these women and adjustment disorder with depressed mood in an additional 24%. Forty percent of the women with major depression and 18% with adjustment disorder with depressed mood were nonsuppressors on the DST using a $\geq 7\ \mu g$ criteria. Sensitivity and specificity were 40% and 88%, respectively. Age was not significantly correlated with postdexamethasone serum cortisol levels.

However, they noted that 28% of patients screened were excluded because of the presence of medical factors known to influence the DST and that this high exclusion criteria may limit the clinical usefulness of the DST in this population (17).

In an ongoing study, Musselman and colleagues are examining the underlying pathophysiology of pancreatic cancer by measuring neuroendocrine changes in these patients. They report that many patients with cancer exhibit a dysregulation of the hypothalamic-pituitary-adrenocortical (HPA) axis that is similar to that in depressed patients without cancer (18). In the cancer patient, there are numerous potential limitations of the DST. Malignancies with ectopic ACTH production such as small cell bronchogenic carcinoma (19) and calorie or protein malnutrition (20) result in false-positive results on the DST. Several medications commonly used in cancer treatment interfere with the DST. Corticosteroids enhance dexamethasone suppression (21) and agents that increase hepatic metabolism, such as phenytoin (22), and barbiturates (23), prevent suppression. It should also be noted that the DST has not proven useful in differentiating dementia from major depression or "pseudodementia" in the elderly (24). However, Meyers and colleagues found 60% nonsuppression with the DST in healthy elderly depressed patients before treatment and 75% normalization after treatment (25).

Georgotas and colleagues found that 83% of a cohort of patients 60–85 years of age with major depression were nonsuppressors on the DST, and that the DST tended to normalize with clinical recovery (26). DST nonsuppression in elderly controls ranges from 0–11% (24). These studies seem to indicate that age per se does not take away from the clinical utility of the DST.

In the study by Evans and colleagues cited above, 27 of the 83 study patients also had evaluation of their hypothalamic-pituitary-thyroid axis. Two of seven patients with major depression (29%), three of seven with nonmajor depression (43%), and one of twelve with no psychiatric diagnosis (8%) had a blunted TSH response to TRH using a $<5\ \mu g/ml$ criterion. These percentages are consistent with studies of depressed psychiatric patients, with the exception of a higher percentage of blunted responses in the nonmajor depression group. The authors viewed these findings as preliminary in light of the small number of patients studied.

III. TREATMENT

Pharmacological treatment of depression in the elderly cancer patient occurs within a complex psychosocial framework and fragile biological system. It is not clear whether these or other factors are responsible for physicians setting diagnostic and treatment thresholds too high for these patients (27,28).

The optimal model for treatment in this setting would identify specific target symptoms known to respond to pharmacotherapy and clearly communicate these to the patient, family, and treatment team. These treatment goals may be occurring in parallel with bereavement, an accelerated realization of one's mortality, a necessary increased dependency on unfamiliar support systems, physical pain, and possibly preparation for death. A candid discussion of how antidepressant medication compliments the overall treatment efforts to restore health, relieve pain, improve quality of life, and facilitate emotional acceptance can be reassuring to the patient, family, and treatment team. Conceptualization of depression as a common medical complication of cancer will avoid inappropriate value judgments and provide a familiar theme for everyone involved. It is essential that these individuals see treatment for depression as fitting into their established cancer treatment priorities and not as evidence that there has been a change in priorities.

Two antidepressant treatment studies suggest that antidepressants relieve depression and improve quality of life in cancer patients with comorbid depression. Costa and colleagues studied 73 depressed women with cancer and found in a randomized placebo-controlled trial of mianserin vs. placebo that both depressive symptoms and quality of life improved (29). In a naturalistic pilot study, Evans and colleagues assessed the degree of depression and quality of life in 22 women (aged 26–74 years; mean = 45.7) with gynecological cancer after treatment with antidepressant medication (30). Twelve of these women received 150 mg of imipramine or its equivalent for at least 4 weeks. Ten women failed to complete a therapeutic trial secondary to noncompliance or intolerance to side effects and therefore emerged as a comparison group. Six of the twelve patients who received adequate treatment met criteria for DSM-III major depression. Five patients in the treatment group were diagnosed with adjustment disorder with depressed mood, and one patient had dysthymic disorder. Seven of the ten patients in the untreated group met DSM-III criteria for major depression. One patient met criteria for adjustment disorder with depressed mood, and two were diagnosed with dysthymic disorder. There was no significant difference in age or tumor load between treated and untreated groups. Depression was measured using the Hamilton Rating Scale (Ham-D) (31) and the Carroll Rating Scale (CRS) for depression (32). Quality of life was measured using the Psychosocial Adjustment to Illness Scale (PAIS) (33). Patients receiving an adequate trial of the antidepressant medication showed significant improvement in depression and better psychosocial adjustment to their cancer than patients who did not receive adequate antidepressant treatment. It should be noted that patients who did not meet full criteria for major depression (adjustment disorder and dysthymia) in the treatment group had similar levels of adaptation as measured by the PAIS to those in the treatment group with major depression. Although preliminary, these results suggest that cancer patients with both major depression and those who do not fully meet criteria for major depression have a significant reduction in their depressive symptoms and improved adaptation to their illness when adequately treated with antidepressant medication.

A. Mood Stabilizers

Patients receiving treatment for cancer, who are on lithium, require special monitoring and dosing considerations to avoid toxicity. General reviews of the use of lithium in the medically ill are available (34). However, Greenberg and colleagues use two case reports to generate a review of clinical management problems unique to patients maintained on lithium while receiving radiation and/or chemotherapy (35). Lithium-induced leukocytosis can be an advantage during cytotoxic chemotherapy since these granulocytes do possess full bactericidal function (36).

However, there is a concern that use of antineoplastic agents that preferentially target dividing cells may result in greater cell death while under the influence of lithium-induced lymphokines. For this reason, these authors conclude that lithium should be discontinued for 2 days prior to chemotherapy and restarted 1 day after treatment. Additionally, they discuss the theoretical concerns that lithium treatment in conjunction with repeated cytotoxic chemotherapy may hasten marrow depletion. Nausea, vomiting, diarrhea, and dehydration are common during chemotherapy. These side effects may obscure early signs of lithium toxicity, adding further support for suspension of lithium prior to chemotherapy.

Lithium therapy does not need to be withheld during radiation treatments, since the effects of radiation are not cell-cycle-specific. An exception to this would be during cranial radiation, when it would be difficult to distinguish between lithium neurotoxicity and the side effects of radiation. Lithium may need to be withheld during cranial radiation and reinstated judiciously to avoid neurotoxicity if treatment has resulted in cognitive impairment or white matter injury (37).

There is some evidence that lithium actually accelerates marrow repopulation (38). Hypercalcemia is the most common life-threatening metabolic disorder in cancer patients (39). Nausea, lethargy, confusion, and polyuria associated with hypercalcemia can mimic lithium toxicity. Although unusual, lithium itself can cause hypercalcemia through its effect on parathyroid hormone (40). Therefore, lithium may need to be discontinued in cancer patients with hypercalcemia. Since lithium is cleared primarily through renal excretion, direct involvement of the kidneys by tumor or the use of nephrotoxic agents such as cisplatin require more aggressive monitoring of serum lithium levels. The risk of hypothyroidism with lithium may be increased in cancer patients receiving radiation to the neck or antineoplastic agents known to also cause hypothyroidism, such as aminoglutathimide (41), interleukin-2, and other lymphokines (42). Other mood stabilizers such as divalproex may be useful in the elderly patient with cancer, given that divalproex is generally better tolerated than lithium in the elderly (43).

B. Cyclic Antidepressants

The side-effect profile of tertiary tricyclic antidepressants such as amitriptyline, imipramine, clomipramine, and doxepin can severely limit their use, and it is often not possible to achieve full antidepressant doses in the elderly cancer patient. The affinity for muscarinic, alpha-1, and histamine receptors results in constipation, cognitive impairment, orthostasis, and sedation. The secondary amines, such as desipramine and nortriptyline, generally have a more favorable side-effect profile, but are still prone to additive side effects when combined with agents routinely used in cancer therapy, such as antiemetics and analgesics. Additionally, therapeutic drug monitoring is critical to avoid cardiac and CNS toxicity (44). In the healthy patient, one steady-state blood level is sufficient to calculate final dosing (45). However, in the elderly cancer patient, blood levels must be rechecked if hepatic metabolism is changing over the course of their illness. In cases of progressive renal impairment due to direct involvement by tumor, or secondary to chemotherapy, hydroxymetabolites of the tricyclic antidepressants must also be monitored to avoid cardiac and CNS toxicity (46,47).

C. Selective Serotonin Reuptake Inhibitors

The relative selectivity of agents such as fluoxetine, sertraline, paroxetine, and fluvoxamine for the presynaptic reuptake site for serotonin have clearly given them a place in the treatment of depression in the medically ill (48,49). Although there are no controlled studies of the selective serotonin reuptake inhibitors (SSRIs) in elderly cancer patients, their side-effect profiles and use in healthy elderly patients would support their use in this population (50). Medication regimens for cancer patients can be complex, can involve multiple physicians, and can often change on a daily basis during high-acuity treatment periods. Thus, the potential for drug–drug interaction must be considered. All of the SSRIs approved for depression inhibit the hepatic cytochrome isoenzyme P450 2D6 and therefore can cause increased plasma levels of other agents that are metabolized through this system. Overall, the SSRIs are well tolerated; side effects with these agents in this population would include agitation, insomnia, nausea, diarrhea, and sexual dysfunction. Fluoxetine is available in a liquid form (20 mg/5 cc), which can be diluted to allow for unlimited dosing options and may be useful for patients dependent on tube feeding. However, it has active metabolites with a half-life of approximately 1 week.

D. Monoamine Oxidase Inhibitors

Because of dietary restrictions and incompatibility with narcotics and sympathomimetics, the monoamine oxidase inhibitors (MAOIs) such as phenelzine probably have no place in this patient population.

E. Bupropion

A potential advantage of this agent in the medically ill is its apparent lack of significant drug interactions. Its use, however, is associated with a higher risk of seizures than other agents and therefore would not be recommended in the patient with CNS tumor involvement, or nutritional or metabolic derangement which lower seizure threshold.

F. Venlafaxine

This agent appears to have a good drug–drug interaction profile. It has low protein binding, and there is no clear evidence that venlafaxine produces significant inhibition of cytochrome P450 isoenzymes. It has a similar side-effect profile to the SSRIs. Its inhibition of both norepinephrine and serotonin also make it a logical choice in elderly cancer patients with a history of depression responsive to tricyclics, but who are now too medically fragile to tolerate the tricyclic side effects. At higher doses (>300 mg/day), about 13% of patients will develop modest elevations in diastolic blood pressure. Although medically ill patients may respond well to lower doses, blood pressure should nonetheless be monitored.

G. Nefazodone

Like the SSRIs and venlafaxine, nefazodone has a relatively benign side effect profile. It is a potent inhibitor of cytochrome P450 3A4, which must be considered when coadministered with medications metabolized by this enzyme system. Use of this agent in this population may also be limited by its sedating effects and its mild orthostatic effects.

IV. SUMMARY

In the general population, depression can be described as common, often debilitating, and sometimes life threatening. This description also holds true for the depressed elderly cancer patient. The diagnostic overlap between depression, normal bereavement, and the physical symptoms of the patient's cancer should not impede diagnosis and treatment. The few studies evaluating efficacy of pharmacotherapy in mixed-age groups of cancer patients have confirmed clinical impressions that this population benefits from treatment for major depression. Additionally, there is some evidence that these patients may benefit even if their presentation does not fully meet criteria for major depression. The newer antidepressant medications have favorable side-effect profiles in the medically ill and low potential for toxicity. Couching pharmacological treatment for depression within established cancer treatment plans can optimize the chances for favorable acceptance by the patient, family, and treating clinicians.

Summary of Evaluation and Management Strategy for the Elderly Cancer Patient with Depression

- Optimize metabolic parameters
- Control pain
- Minimize use of anticholinergics and CNS depressants
- Rule out CNS metastatic involvement
- Use "inclusive" criteria to set threshold for diagnosis of depression
- Acknowledge the psychosocial and medical context of the depression
- Present treatment of depression as complementary to treatment of the cancer
- Choose low starting dose of an SSRI, bupropion, venlafaxine, or nefazodone
- Slowly titrate dose to minimize GI and CNS side effects
- Monitor for pharmacokinetic interactions

REFERENCES

1. Horrn JW, Asire AJ, Young JL, Pollack ES. SEER Program: Cancer incidence and mortality in the U.S., 1973–1981. Bethesda, MD: Department of Health and Human Services, NIH Publication No. 85-1837, 1984.
2. Young JL, Percy CL, Asire AJ. Incidence and mortality data: 1973–77. National Cancer Institute Monograph 57, DHHS No. (NIH) 81-2330. Washington, DC: U.S. Government Printing Office, 1981.
3. McDaniel JS, Musselman DL, Porter MR, Reed DA, Nemeroff CB. Depression in patients with cancer: diagnosis, biology, and treatment. Arch Gen Psychiatry 1995; 52:89–99.
4. Cohen-Cole SA, Brown FW, McDaniel SJ. Assessment of depression and grief reactions in the medically ill. IN: Stoudemire A, Fogel BS, eds. Psychiatric Care of the Medical Patient. New York/Oxford: Oxford University Press, 1993:53–69.

5. Rifkin A, Reardon G, Siris S, Karagji B, Kim YS, Hackstaff L, Endicott N. Trimipramine in physical illness with depression. J Clin Psychiatry 1985; 46:4–8.
6. Bukberg J, Penman D, Holland JC. Depression in hospitalized cancer patients. Psychosomat Med 1984; 46:199–212.
7. Odell WD. Ectopic hormones and humoral syndromes of cancer. In: Holland JF, Frei E, Bast RC, Kufe DW, Morton DL, Weichselbaum RR, eds. Cancer Medicine. Philadelphia and London: Lea and Febiger, 1993:896–904.
8. Farrell KR, Ganzini L. Misdiagnosing delirium as depression in medically ill elderly patients. Arch Intern Med 1995; 155(22):2459–2464.
9. Wright DC, Delaney TF. Treatment of metastatic cancer. In: De-vita VT, Hellman S, Rosenberg SA, eds. Cancer: Principles and Practice of Oncology, 3rd ed. Philadelphia: J. B. Lippincott, 1989:2245–2261.
10. O'Daniel R. Depressive pseudodementia. Psychiatr Ann 1981; 11:355–363.
11. Spiegel D, Sands S, Koopman C. Pain and depression in patients with cancer. Cancer 1994; 74(7):2079–2091.
12. Derogatis LR, Morrow GR, Fetting J, Penman D, Piasetsky S, Schmale AM, henrichs M, Carnicke CL. The prevalence of psychiatric disorders among cancer patients. J Am Med Assoc 1988; 249:751–757.
13. Achles TA, Blanchard EB, Ruckdeschel JC. Multidimensional nature of cancer-related pain. Pain 1983; 17:227–288.
14. Holsboer F. Neuroendocrinology of mood disorders. In: Bloom FE, Kupfer DJ, eds. Psychopharmacology: The Fourth Generation of Progress. New York: Raven Press, Ltd., 1995:957–969.
15. Perkins DO, Stern RA, Golden RN, Miller HL, Evans DL. Use of neuroendocrine tests in the psychiatric assessment of the medically ill patient. In: McCubbin JA, Kaufmann PG, Nemeroff CB, eds. Stress, Neuropeptides, and Systemic Disease. San Diego, CA: Academic Press, Inc., 1991:199–215.
16. Joffe RT, Rubinow DR, Denicoff KD, Maher M, Sindelar WF. Depression and carcinoma of the pancreas. Gen Hosp Psychiatry 1986; 8:241–245.
17. Evans DL, McCartney CF, Nemeroff CB, Raft D, Quade D, Golden RN, Haggerty JJ, Holmes V, Simon KS, Broba M, Mason GA, Fowler WC. Depression in women treated for gynecological cancer: clinical and neuroendocrine assessment. Am J Psychiatry 1986; 143:447–452.
18. Musselman DL, Nemeroff CB, McDaniel JS, Reed D, Wingard J, Seelig B, Porter MF, Landry JC. Cancer and depression: diagnostic considerations and biologic markers. 32nd Annual Meeting of the American College of Neuropsychopharmacology, Honolulu, Hawaii, Dec 14, 1993.
19. Martin JB, Reichlin S, Brown GM. Regulation of ACTH secretion and its disorders. In: Martin JB, Reichlin S, Brown GM, eds. Clinical Neuroendocrinology. Philadelphia: FA Davis Co., 1977:179–200.
20. Smith SR, Biedsoe T, Chetii MK. Cortisol metabolism and the pituitary-adrenal axis in adults with protein-calorie malnutrition. J Clin Endocrinol Metab 1975; 40:43–52.
21. Michael MI, Smith RE, Hermich EM. Adrenal suppression and intranasally applied steroids. Ann Allergy 1967; 25:569–574.

22. Jubiz W, Meikle AW, Levinson RA, Mizutani S, West CD, Tyler FH. Effect of diphenylhydantoin on the metabolism of dexamethasone: Mechanism of abnormal dexamethasone suppression in humans. N Engl J Med 1970; 283:11–14.
23. Brooks SM, Werk EE, Ackerman SJ, Sullivan I, Thrasher K. Adverse effects of phenobarbital on corticosteroid metabolism in patients with bronchial asthma. N Engl J Med 1972; 286:1125–1128.
24. Skare S, Pew B, Dysken M. The dexamethasone suppression test in dementia: a review of the literature. J Geriatr Psychiatry Neurol 1990; 3(3):124–138.
25. Meyers BS, Alpert S, Gabriele M, Kakuma T, Kalayam B, Alexopoulos GS. State specificity of DST abnormalities in geriatric depression. Biol Psychiatry 1993; 34 (1-2):108–114.
26. Georgotas A, Stokes PE, Krakowski M, Fanelli C, Cooper T. Hypothalamic-pituitary-adrenocortical function in geriatric depression: diagnostic and treatment implications. Biol Psychiatry 1984; 19(5):685–693.
27. Derogatis LR, Abeloff MD, McBeth CD. Cancer patients and their physicians in the perception of psychological symptoms. Psychosomatics 1976; 17:197–201.
28. Levine PM, Silverfarb PM, Lipowski ZJ. Mental disorders in cancer patients. Cancer 1978; 42:1385–1391.
29. Costa E, Mogos I, Toma T. Efficacy and safety of mianserin in the treatment of depression of women with cancer. Acta Psychiatr Scand 1985; 72:85–92.
30. Evans DL, McCartney CF, Haggerty JJ, Nemeroff CB, Golden RN, Simon JB, Quade D, Holmen V, Droba M, Mason GA, Fowler WC, Raft D. Treatment of depression in cancer patients is associated with better life adaptation: A pilot study. Psychosomatic Medicine 1988; 50:72–76.
31. Hamilton M. A rating scale for depression. J Neurol Neurosurg Psychiatry 1960; 23:56–62.
32. Carroll BJ, Feinberg M, Smouse PE, Rawson SG, Greden JF. The Carroll rating scale for depression. Br J Psychiatry 1981; 138:194–200.
33. Derogatis LR. The psychosocial adjustment to illness scale (PAIS). J Psychosomat Res 1986; 30(1):77–91.
34. Das Gupta K, Jefferson JW. The use of lihtium in the medically ill. Gen Hosp Psychiatry 1990; 12:83–97.
35. Greenberg DB, Younger J, Kaufman SD. Management of lithium in patients with cancer. Psychosomatics 1993; 34(5):388–393.
36. Boggs DR, Joyce RA. The hematopoietic effects of lithium. Semin Hematol 1983; 20:129–138.
37. Packer RJ, Simmerman RA, Belaniuk LT. Magnetic resonance imaging in evaluation of treatment-related CNS damage. Cancer 1986; 58:635–640.
38. Gallicchio VS, Chen MG, Watts TD. Ability of lithium to accelerate the recovery of granulopoiesis after subacute radiation injury. Acta Radiol Oncol 1984; 23:361–366.
39. List A. Malignant hypercalcemia. Arch Intern Med 1991; 151:437–438.
40. Shen FH, Sherrard DJ. Lithium-induced hyperparathyroidism: an alteration in the "set point." Ann Intern Med 1982; 96:63–65.
41. Dowsett M, Mehta A, Cantwell BM, Harris AL. Low-dose aminoglutethimide in postmenopausal breast cancer: effects on adrenal and thyroid hormone secretion. Eur J Cancer 1991; 27(7):846–849.

42. Atkins MB, Mier JW, Parkinson DR, Gould JA, Berkman EM, Kaplan MM. Hypothyroidism after treatment with Interleukin-2 and lymphokine activated killer cells. N Engl J Med 1988; 318:1557–1563.
43. Evans DL, Byerly MJ, Greer RA. Secondary mania: diagnosis and treatment. J Clin Psychiatry 1995; 56(suppl 3):31–37.
44. Pascualy M, Murburg MM, Veith RC. Cardiac risks of antidepressants in the elderly. In: Shamoian CA, ed. Psychopharmacological Treatment Complications in the Elderly. Washington, DC: American Psychiatric Press, 1992:17–44.
45. Preskorn SH, Fast GA. Therapeutic drug monitoring for antidepressants: efficacy, safety, and cost effectiveness. J Clin Psychiatry 1991; 52(suppl 6):23–33.
46. McCue RE. Plasma levels of nortriptyline and 10-hydroxynortriptyline and treatment-related electrocardiographic changes in the elderly depressed. J Psychiatry Res 1989; 23:73–79.
47. Nelson JC, Atillasoy E, Mazure C, Jatlow PI. Hydroxydesipramine in the elderly. J Clin Psychopharmacol 1988; 8:428–433.
48. Stoudemire A. Expanding psychopharmacologic treatment options for the depressed medical patient. Psychosomatics 1995; 36(2):S19–26.
49. Cunningham LA. Depression in the medically ill: choosing an antidepressant. J Clin Psychiatry 1994; 55(suppl A):90–97.
50. Preskorn SH. Recent pharmacologic advances in antidepressant therapy for the elderly. Am J Med 1993; 94(5A):2S–12S.

11
Depression and Parkinson's Disease

Norman Sussman
New York University, and Bellevue Hospital Center, New York, New York

I. INTRODUCTION

Idiopathic Parkinson's disease is a progressive, degenerative disorder associated with advancing age. Although the disease is characterized by such motor dysfunction signs as bradykinesia, gait disturbance, rigidity, and tremor, symptoms of depression are often part of the clinical picture. Indeed, it is generally held that depression is the most common psychiatric symptom of Parkinson's disease. In his original account of the disease, James Parkinson (1) characterized the typical patient as an "unhappy sufferer" who is prone to "melancholy." Subsequent research and clinical experience have confirmed a high prevalence of depression among patients with this disorder. Given the frequency of depression, and its adverse impact on the outcome of Parkinson's disease, it is important for clinicians to have empirically based guidelines for the management of these patients. Yet standard textbooks in neurology and general psychiatry offer little or no instruction on antidepressant drug selection and use for patients with parkinsonism. Clinical approaches vary markedly. Most neurologists delay initiating the pharmacotherapy of depression until dopaminergic medication is used to treat the motor symptoms. This strategy is based on the assumption that the depressive manifestations are a "normal" reaction to the physical symptoms or the result of the same alterations in monoamine functions that cause the movement disturbances. It is expected that mood will improve along with motor functions. Treatment with antidepressant drugs is usually begun when mood does not improve as expected, or when the depression is especially severe. An additional reason for the delay in starting antidepressant medications is the concern that they will complicate the treatment of motor symptoms and add to the side-effect burden of the patient.

II. CLINICAL RESEARCH LITERATURE

Ideally, clinicians should base their treatment decisions on the results of randomized, controlled studies. In the case of Parkinson's disease, most references to the pharmacology of depression are in the form of case reports, correspondence, or abstracts. The research literature is small and characterized by significant methodological limitations.

Klassen et al. (2) conducted an extensive literature search for controlled studies published between 1966 and 1993—in English, French, Dutch, or German—on the effect of antidepressant medications in depressed Parkinson's disease patients. To be included in the review, a study had to meet these conditions: it had to (1) be placebo-controlled; (2) involve a majority of patients with idiopathic parkinsonism; and (3) involve primary antidepressant drugs, as opposed to other drugs that might have mood effects [deprenyl, a monoamine oxidase inhibitor type B (MAO-B), was included because it was originally introduced as an antidepressant]. The authors found only 12 studies that met their inclusion criteria. Only six of the studies examined currently available antidepressants, and two of these studies involved deprenyl. None of the studies compared different antidepressants. In most of the studies, the dosage of antidepressant drug was subtherapeutic; one trial used a daily imipramine dose of 25 mg. In rating the quality of methodology used in the studies, the authors found other significant shortcomings and scored all the papers as "poor to moderate." Other investigators have also commented on the methodological limitations of the research literature regarding treatment of depression and anxiety in Parkinson's disease (3–5).

Selection bias is one weakness of studies investigating the effect of antidepressant medications in Parkinson's disease patients. Most studies are not population-based; they involve patients consecutively referred to academic centers or specialty units who are thus likely to have higher rates of psychiatric symptoms (5). In many studies, diagnosis is made by clinical impression alone. In the absence of validated diagnostic tools, it is impossible to know whether subjects represented cases of major depression or other mood disorder or if they were merely patients with subsyndromal mood symptoms.

The diagnosis of depression in parkinsonism is further complicated by the overlap of symptoms in Parkinson's disease, primary depression, and the physiological changes associated with normal aging (6). Signs and symptoms of Parkinson's disease, such as sleep difficulties, fatigue, apparent anhedonia (because of facial masking and bradykinesia), cognitive impairment, and stooped posture produce a clinical picture that appears consistent with depression, even in patients with a normal mood.

That several disorders share common clinical features with the idiopathic disorder and may not be recognized as separate conditions has also made diagnosis of Parkinson's disease depression difficult. These "Parkinson's plus syndromes" include progressive supranuclear palsy, corticobasal ganglionic degeneration, Alzheimer's disease, subcortical vascular disease, postencephalitic parkinsonism, and multisystem atrophy. Multiple system atrophy accounts for 4 to 22% of brains in parkinsonian brain banks (7). Any drug effects that manifest in one of these conditions will not have predictive value for the others, thus it is important to consider the accuracy of clinical diagnosis when interpreting the significance of studies or case reports.

Determination of both the motor and mood effects of medication in parkinsonism can be confounded by fluctuations in motor symptoms and associated mood alterations. The most perplexing variables in the assessment of mood effects in parkinsonism are the "on-off" and "end-of-dose" phenomena associated with levodopa treatment. During "off" periods, when the motor state is worse, patients experience increased depression and anxiety (8). Largely unpredictable, these periods may be very distressing, with crying and feelings of complete hopelessness.

III. NEUROCHEMICAL ASPECTS OF DEPRESSION IN PARKINSON'S DISEASE

It is often argued that the devastating nature of Parkinson's disease for most patients is sufficient reason to expect a "reactive" depression. However, studies consistently fail to demonstrate a correlation between the severity of motor symptoms, the degree of disability, and the presence of depressive symptoms (9). This suggests that mood disturbance in Parkinson's disease may have a biological basis. Several clinical findings support the hypothesis that depression in Parkinson's disease is a primary result of neurological changes (10). These include: a higher rate of depression among patients with right hemiparkinsonism (11); the abrupt onset of depressive episodes—in the absence of unusual psychosocial stressors—which occur during the presymptomatic phase of Parkinson's disease (i.e., before the manifestation of motor symptoms); the absence of any correlation between depression and specific measures of motor impairment; the alleviation of depression before amelioration of motor symptoms; and the persistence of depression in some patients, even after antiparkinsonian medication has significantly improved motor symptoms. Perhaps the strongest argument for the suggestion that biological factors are involved is based on the knowledge that the same neurotransmitter systems that have been shown to be disturbed in Parkinson's disease—dopamine and serotonin—are implicated in the pathophysiology of depression.

The dopamine system has been established as being critically involved in the pathophysiology of Parkinson's disease. Although other neurotransmitter functions are also disturbed in many parkinsonian patients, it is the loss of striatal dopamine neurons that produces motor symptoms. The high incidence of depression itself is suggestive evidence that dopamine hypofunction is etiologically involved in the mood symptoms, as is the fact that neuroleptics can produce depression as a side effect (12). The similarities between some of the symptoms of Parkinson's disease and those of depression also suggest that dopamine contributes to the pathophysiology of depression (13).

There is some indirect support for a relationship between nigrostriatal dysfunction and psychomotor slowing in major depression without Parkinson's disease (14). Several studies have suggested that L-tyrosine and levodopa, both precursors of dopamine, may have antidepressant efficacy in patients with psychomotor retardation or low pretreatment CSF homovanillic acid levels (15). Nomifensine, an antidepressant with predominantly dopaminergic effects, was briefly available in the 1980s and found to have robust antidepressant efficacy. Bupropion, a currently available agent with mainly noradrenergic and some dopaminergic activity, is also an effective antidepressant.

Growth-hormone response to apomorphine, which is thought to be a measure of central dopamine (D2) receptor sensitivity, has been used experimentally to explore the relationship between depression and parkinsonism. A finding that apomorphine-induced growth-hormone response is associated with measures of depression (16), particularly mild symptoms, suggests that dopaminergic mechanisms may account for the mood disturbance in some parkinsonian patients.

Even before the introduction of drugs that selectively inhibit reuptake of serotonin, there was evidence that the serotonin system modulates mood symptoms in Parkinson's disease. For example, reduced CSF levels of the serotonin metabolite 5-hydroxyindolacetic acid (5-HIAA) were found in depressed, but not in nondepressed, Parkinson's disease patients withdrawn from dopamine agonist therapy (17). Treatment with 5-hydroxytryptophan and L-tryptophan, both precursors of serotonin, have been reported to improve mood in depressed parkinsonian patients (18), although these compounds also cause motor symptom deterioration (19,20). In one case report (21), a patient with Parkinson's disease whose depression responded to fluvoxamine—a selective serotonin reuptake inhibitor (SSRI)—experienced an exacerbation of depression during tryptophan-depletion testing. The symptoms resolved following tryptophan repletion.

It has also been found that activity of tryptophan hydroxylase, the rate-limiting enzyme in serotonin synthesis, is reduced in the brains of Parkinson's disease patients (22). Tryptophan supplementation has been shown to moderate levodopa-induced motor fluctuations (23). An unknown factor in the use of dietary tryptophan as a treatment for parkinsonian patients, however, is possible tryptophan interference with the absorption of levodopa from the gastrointestinal tract and its transport into the CNS.

Fenfluramine, a drug that causes rapid release of serotonin, inhibits serotonin reuptake, and possibly has agonist properties at serotonin receptors (24), has been used in an acute challenge model to determine differences between depressed and nondepressed parkinsonian patients (25). Prolactin responses to fenfluramine were found to be significantly impaired in patients with Parkinson's disease when compared to controls, and the response was more blunted among the patients with major depression than those who were not depressed. The investigators interpreted these findings as evidence of diminished serotonergic responsivity in depression associated with Parkinson's disease (25).

Based on these biochemical findings and PET studies, Mayberg and Solomon (18) have attempted to describe the pathophysiological relationship between the serotonin and dopamine systems. These authors suggest that primary degeneration of dopamine neurons leads to the disruption of orbital frontal outflow to the dorsal raphe, hence, to secondary involvement of the serotonin system in some depressed parkinsonian patients. Postmortem studies have shown that marked variation in cell loss in subcortical structures may occur in Parkinson's disease. Cell loss in the serotonin-rich dorsal raphe ranged from 0–43% (26). Thus, although dysfunction of the dopamine system is the crucial factor in Parkinson's disease, serotonin and other systems are also involved, which adds to the unpredictability of successfully treating this disorder.

IV. MOOD EFFECTS OF DOPAMINERGIC AND ANTICHOLINERGIC MEDICATIONS

Most Parkinson's disease patients are taking dopaminergic or anticholinergic medications for their motor disturbances. These medications can themselves cause mood changes as well as interact with antidepressants, both on a pharmacodynamic and a pharmacokinetic level. Some studies have found that levodopa has no effect on depressed mood in Parkinson's disease (27), but others suggest levodopa is associated with treatment-emergent depression. Maricle et al. (8) have demonstrated that both depression and anxiety decrease following infusions of levodopa. It is impossible to determine from the available reports whether there is any cause-and-effect relationship between levodopa and depression (28). Beneficial mood effects are not frequent or pronounced.

Mania, hypomania, and euphoria have been reported as treatment-emergent effects of dopaminergic medications, including levodopa and those discussed below. The most common psychiatric side effect of dopaminergic drugs is psychosis. Bromocriptine, a D2/D3 agonist, has been documented in case reports as improving depression in patients who have not responded to conventional antidepressants (29). Recently, bromocriptine has been proven useful in reversing extrapyramidal side effects—loss of efficacy (tolerance) and fatigue—that are associated with SSRI treatment. Two double-blind trials published in 1981 found that bromocriptine was as effective as imipramine in patients with endogenous depression (30,31). Pramipexole, like bromocriptine, is a D2/D3 dopamine-receptor agonist and exerts its agonist activity at dopamine autoreceptors and postsynaptic dopamine receptors. Pramipexole has been found to have a more rapid onset of antihedonic effects in animal studies than conventional antidepressants (32).

Anticholinergic compounds, such as benztropine, trihexphenidyl, and biperiden, are generally not found to have antidepressant activity, and they may have a low potential for abuse, as drug abusers sometimes describe them as stimulating. In parkinsonian patients, however, anticholinergic compounds are more likely to produce confusion and cognitive difficulties. Delirium has been reported in nonparkinsonian patients treated with a combination of a neuroleptic, an SSRI, and benztropine (33). Although amantadine has exhibited antidepressant activity in animal models (34), and has the advantage of not being anticholinergic, it has not produced significant antidepressant effects in clinical practice, and can induce psychosis.

V. ANTIDEPRESSANT DRUGS: GENERAL CONSIDERATIONS

There are a number of special considerations regarding antidepressant drug use in Parkinson's disease patients. As for any special patient population, these considerations involve individualization of dosing and titration and close observation for potential side effects, drug–drug, and drug–disorder interactions.

The incidence of anxiety and panic symptoms among depressed patients with parkinsonism appears to be high (18,35–37). Parkinson's disease patients are more likely to experience anxiety early in the course of treatment, activated as a side effect of antidepressant medication, than are nonparkinsonism patients. It is not known whether this results from concurrent use of antidepressant medication with antiparkinsonian drugs. There is evidence that a predisposition to paniclike anxiety is a long-term complication of levodopa therapy (38), but other research suggests that anxiety results from the underlying neuropathology of Parkinson's disease (36,39).

Two studies have found that nearly half of Parkinson's disease patients have anxiety symptoms or mixed-anxiety–depression (37,39). It has been postulated that some "depressed" Parkinson's disease patients suffer from a distinct anxietylike syndrome. This could explain why some Parkinson's disease patients are susceptible to activation when treated with antidepressants, levodopa, or dopamine agonists. This amphetaminelike response is typical of the response observed in patients with panic disorder early in their course of antidepressant therapy. One study (40) found significant differences between Parkinson's disease patients and age- and sex-matched healthy controls with regard to complaints related to autonomic dysfunction (e.g., postural dizziness, frequency of micturition, urinary hesitancy, constipation, dry mouth, impotence, and loss of libido). The investigators also found a significant, positive correlation between autonomic complaints and measures of both depression and anxiety in the parkinsonism patients. The significance of the correlation persisted after the autonomic items were removed from the Hamilton scales. These findings suggest that some Parkinson's disease patients who are diagnosed as anxious or depressed may, in fact, be experiencing the subjective concomitants of autonomic failure. If there is such a subgroup, it might represent those who fail to respond or experience intolerable activating side effects from antidepressant therapy. For these patients, an antianxiety drug might prove beneficial. In some patients, panic is most pronounced during "off" periods, and is relieved by administration of levodopa. This has led to speculation that the induced panic may sometimes represent a form of levodopa abstinence syndrome (38).

Increased sensitivity to medication side effects in Parkinson's disease patients may also be related to alterations in drug metabolism. The poor debrisequine metabolizer phenotype significantly increased in Parkinson's disease patients (41). Thus, the cytochrome P450 system enzyme CYP 2D6 activity is reduced, which leads to impaired hepatic detoxification. The metabolism of various antidepressant drugs may thus be reduced, which could produce increased side effects and toxicity.

VI. ANTIDEPRESSANT SELECTION AND USE

In the absence of good double-blind studies and direct comparisons between drugs, it is not possible to characterize any drug or class of drugs as being "first-line" agents. Drug selection and use should be based on the benefit-risk profiles of each compound and published reports of its use in parkinsonian patients.

A. Tricyclic Antidepressants

The mainstay of antidepressant therapy since the mid-1950s, tricyclic antidepressants are the class of antidepressant drugs most used to manage depression in Parkinson's disease. Nevertheless, only five double-blind, placebo-controlled studies involving a depressed parkinsonian population treated with tricyclic antidepressants have been published (42–46). Tricyclics improved mood, did not worsen, and actually improved, some motor symptoms. These studies are limited in terms of their predictive value, however, not only by the already-noted methodological limitations, but also by their small total sample size of 143 subjects.

Tricyclic agents may improve motor abnormalities because of their anticholinergic activity, but these agents can also exacerbate confusion and psychosis and potentiate the anticholinergic effects of other medications. The typical tricyclic receptor interactions—anticholinergic, antihistaminic, and antiadrenergic—also interfere with compliance by adding to the distressing burden of side effects patients with Parkinson's disease already experience. For example, the hypotension associated with parkinsonism itself or caused by levodopa can be potentiated by α-adrenergic blockade. All tertiary tricyclics, and to a lesser extent secondary agents, have this troublesome effect.

Two tricyclics, trimipramine and clomipramine, have significant dopamine D2 blocking activity, but do not produce clinical extrapyramidal symptoms (as does amoxapine, a heterocyclic with comparable antidopaminergic activity) presumably because they are also anticholinergic. Clomipramine has been reported to cause tardive dyskinesia. In the absence of evidence that trimipramine and clomipramine have any advantages in the treatment of depression in patients with Parkinson's disease, there is little reason to use these drugs in this patient population.

B. Monoamine Oxidase Inhibitors

Three types of monoamine oxidase inhibitors (MAOIs) are available for clinical use. These are the nonselective, irreversible inhibitors; selective, irreversible inhibitors; and selective, reversible inhibitors. The nonselective inhibitors, phenelzine and tranylcypromine, have not been found in clinical practice to be particularly effective in depressed parkinsonian patients, although there are no studies documenting their use in this population. An overriding consideration regarding use of nonselective inhibitors, however, is their potential interaction with levodopa, which may result in severe side effects, including hypertension, increased involuntary movements, and delirium. In addition, these agents are associated with hypotension. The author has observed two cases in which patients experienced acute onset of severe depression, without apparent precipitating factors, before any manifestations of motor symptoms. The patients were successfully treated with MAOIs. When the MAOIs were discontinued, clinically significant Parkinson's disease manifested. It is not clear whether the MAOIs delayed the onset of motor symptoms or precipitated their expression through a drug withdrawal effect.

L-deprenyl is a relatively selective and irreversible inhibitor of MAO-B, which at the usual therapeutic dose of 5 to 10 mg per day has a significantly reduced risk of sympathomimetic crisis. It is indicated exclusively for use in the treatment of Parkinson's disease. This indication is based on studies that suggested deprenyl can slow the progression of Parkinson's disease and provide symptomatic improvement of existing motor symptoms. There is also evidence, although equivocal, that deprenyl might have antidepressant effects in some patients at a dose of 10 mg per day (47,48). Optimal antidepressant effects probably require daily doses in the range of 20 to 40 mg. With this dosage range, however, selectivity is lost and tyramine sensitivity occurs, abolishing the safety benefits of L-deprenyl. Severe toxicity among patients taking various SSRIs with L-deprenyl, even at doses of 10 mg per day, has been reported. Because of the potential for interactions, it is recommended that there be a 14-day lapse after discontinuing sertraline, fluvoxamine, and paroxetine before starting L-deprenyl therapy. A 5-week delay is recommended for fluoxetine because of its long half-life.

Moclobemide is a selective reversible inhibitor of MAO-A. This class of MAOIs, referred to as RIMAs, is available outside the United States for the treatment of depression. A major clinical advantage of moclobemide is that a hypertensive crisis ("tyramine effect") does not result from an interaction between it and dietary tyramine, pseudephedrine, meperidine, or other substances that must be avoided by patients taking such nonselective MAOIs as phenelzine or tranylcypromine. Although MAO-A accounts for only about 20% of the total MAO activity in the basal ganglia, it is as potent as MAO-B in deaminating dopamine. Thus, in theory, moclobemide should produce some positive effect on the motor symptoms of Parkinson's disease.

Moclobemide has been studied in nondepressed and depressed Parkinson's disease patients who were also treated with levodopa or dopaminergic agonists (49,50), and found to be effective and well tolerated as an antidepressant (49). When examined in a study that excluded depression or other psychiatric disorders, moclobemide produced "mild" symptomatic improvement for some experimental measures. In acute levodopa challenge, the latency of motor response was significantly shortened and its duration prolonged during moclobemide treatment. A slight reduction in "off" time after overnight withdrawal of dopaminergic medications also occurred. No adverse cognitive effects were observed. A dose of 150 mg three times per day was used in the study (50). Patients should not take moclobemide with deprenyl since the combination results in potentiation of the tyramine effect. If the two drugs must be used together, patients should follow an MAOI diet.

C. Selective Serotonin Reuptake Inhibitors

Because SSRIs selectively act on the serotonin reuptake transporter, the risk of their having any effect on parkinsonian movement disorders would appear to be slight. However, there have been anecdotal reports (51–53) of movement disorders caused by SSRIs in depressed nonparkinsonian patients. Included in these reports are cases of tardive dyskinesia (54). As of December, 1995, Eli Lilly and Company, the manufacturer of fluoxetine, had received reports of 76 cases of tardive dyskinesia associated with use of that drug (53).

SSRI-induced worsening of motor symptoms in parkinsonian patients has also been reported. Patients who are stable on levodopa for a long period of time have been observed to deteriorate after being treated with fluoxetine (55). In these patients, motor symptoms worsen after exposure to fluoxetine and improve when the drug is withdrawn. The reversibility of this deterioration when fluoxetine is stopped argues against the possibility that the worsening represents a natural progression of Parkinson's disease. Paroxetine has also been shown to exacerbate parkinsonian symptoms; motor symptoms improved after discontinuation (35). In addition, there are case reports of parkinsonian symptoms worsening after the addition of fluvoxamine to a stable regimen of antiparkinsonian medication (56).

Prompted by reports that SSRIs might induce or exacerbate parkinsonism, Caley and Friedman (57) retrospectively reviewed the medical records of 23 Parkinson's disease patients who were currently taking or had been treated with fluoxetine. Twenty of the 23 patients experiencing no worsening of motor symptoms while taking up to 40 mg per day of fluoxetine. Three patients worsened to a mild degree. Symptoms that increased included akinesia, tremor, rigidity, and gait. Motor symptoms improved in two patients. Iacono et al. (58) have reported on their clinical experience with sertraline (50 mg per day) and paroxetine (20 mg per day) in Parkinson's disease patients who were not selected on the basis of concurrent depression. The investigators found improvement in symptoms related to akinesia, postural instability, and gait problems. These improvements, especially those related to akinesia, were noted to make "important changes in [the patients'] activities of daily living." No significant side effects were reported. Adding support to the possibility that SSRIs can improve motor symptoms in Parkinson's disease, Meerwaldt (59) reported a marked reduction of hypokinesia following fluvoxamine therapy in a patient who had failed to respond to conventional antiparkinsonian medication. A prospective pilot study of 14 Parkinson's disease patients treated with fluoxetine for 1 month found no change in overall motor activity, but tremor was significantly reduced (60). It thus appears that although some individuals are susceptible to SSRI-induced worsening of Parkinson's disease, most patients experience either no change or some degree of improvement in their motor functions.

There are no restrictions on using SSRIs with antiparkinsonian medication, except caution when deprenyl is part of the regimen. There is, however, a single case report of a patient undergoing treatment with levodopa/carbidopa and fluoxetine who was given benztropine, an anticholinergic agent, to control motor symptoms. Even with fluoxetine therapy, the patient had residual depressive symptoms. Following the introduction of benztropine, the patient experienced improved motor symptoms, but he also developed mood instability, with mental status changes that ranged from delirium to mania, hypomania, and euthymia (61).

The reason why SSRIs appear to worsen motor symptoms in some patients, and have either no effect or cause some improvement in others, is not clear. Differences in medication response may reflect the known variability of involvement of different brain pathways in Parkinson's disease. The potential for SSRIs to influence motor activity emphasizes the close relationship between the serotonin and dopamine systems (62).

Considerable work has been done on the functional and anatomical aspects of depressed patients with Parkinson's disease. Both anatomical and neurochemical studies have revealed important serotonin inputs from the dorsal and median raphe nuclei to the substantia nigra and midbrain tegmentum. The nigrostriatal system, extrapyramidal, and limbic basal ganglia receive projections from the dorsal raphe (63). Research and clinical data suggest that serotonin may act by enhancing or decreasing striatal and frontal lobe dopamine release. Although the data are conflicting, there is evidence that SSRIs can decrease dopamine. It may be that acute SSRI administration increases dopamine turnover, whereas chronic administration may decrease turnover. The extent to which SSRIs produce extrapyramidal effects may relate to the status of the patient's monoamine neurotransmitter systems. Interestingly, some clinical experience shows that many of the side effects of SSRIs attributed to decreased dopamine activity can be reversed by adding such catecholamine agonists as dextroamphetamine or bromocriptine.

There are differences between SSRIs, even though they share the same primary mechanism of action. These differences include half-life, comparative monoamine reuptake selectivity and potency, and effects on nonserotonin receptors (64). For example, in vitro studies show that sertraline has the greatest dopamine reuptake blocking effect of any SSRI or other antidepressant currently available in the United States (64). This effect is quite small in magnitude when compared to sertraline's serotonin reuptake blocking effect, however, and its clinical relevance in the treatment of depression, with or without Parkinson's disease, remains unknown. Paroxetine has more anticholinergic activity than the other SSRIs, a property that might be of significance in some instances, although it has not been noted other than in side effects. Differences in reuptake potency, half-life, and protein binding also exist between the various SSRIs. Fluoxetine, paroxetine, and sertraline all utilize the CYP450 2D6 system, and may thus interact with other drugs. Perhaps more importantly, there is higher prevalence of poor metabolizers in Parkinson's disease patients.

This group may experience increased toxicity and side effects as the result of elevated plasma concentrations of the SSRI. SSRIs, particularly those with short half-lives (paroxeteine, sertraline, and fluvoxamine) are capable of causing discontinuation symptoms. It is not known to what extent, if any, this syndrome is associated with changes in the symptoms of parkinsonism, but it may produce a variety of symptoms that cause subjective distress.

Finally, an unexplored and potentially meaningful role for SSRIs in the management of Parkinson's disease is suggested by the high incidence of obsessive-compulsive symptoms in parkinsonian patients. Levin et al. (65) have reported that in a sample of "unequivocal" Parkinson's disease patients evaluated with the Layton Obsessional Inventory, 55% scored above the normative cutoff for the symptom score, and 73% scored above the normative cutoff for the trait score. In this latter group, use of SSRIs would be indicated.

D. Bupropion

Bupropion is unique among the currently available antidepressants in that it has no direct effect on serotonin reuptake or on any serotonin receptors. Although its precise mechanism of action is not known, bupropion, through one of its metabolites, appears to be primarily an inhibitor of norepinephrine reuptake. Bupropion also exerts a modest dopamine agonist effect by inhibiting dopamine reuptake. Only one study of bupropion use in Parkinson's disease has been published (66). Consistent with its known dopaminergic and cathecholaminergic properties, bupropion was found to produce some improvement in depressed mood and motor abnormalities. The incidence of side effects was low. Bupropion can cause psychosis as a side effect, however, and this effect may be greater in patients who are being treated with levodopa. Delirium and retropulsion have also been observed in nonparkinsonian patients taking bupropion for depression. In addition, a dose-related risk of seizures makes it important to follow the recommended dosing guidelines. Anxiety and insomnia are other side effects, which can be more pronounced in patients being treated concurrently with levodopa or bromocriptine. All this apart, bupropion is generally well tolerated.

It is tempting to speculate that drugs that act in part to block dopamine reuptake, such as nomifensine and bupropion, might be rendered less effective by the dopamine deficiency in parkinsonian brains. If there is less dopamine uptake to block, then there is less potential activity. However, not all dopamine neuron populations are equally involved in Parkinson's disease (67). Limbic and cortical dopamine neurons—those presumed to be most responsible for mood and cognitive dysfunctions in depression—may be much less affected by Parkinson's disease than nigrostriatal neurons. Thus, indirect-acting drugs that influence available dopamine systems should prove helpful.

E. Venlafaxine

Controlled studies involving venlafaxine have not been published. However, its profile as a mixed serotonin and norepinephrine reuptake inhibitor without anticholinergic activity suggests that it is well suited for the treatment of depression in Parkinson's disease. Initial clinical impressions are that it is both effective and well tolerated by Parkinson's disease patients. Its effects on motor abnormalities are not known. The most common side effects are nausea and headache.

F. Nefazodone

Nefazodone has not been studied in a parkinsonian population. The synaptic effects of nefazodone include reuptake blockade of serotonin at the presynaptic neurons and blockade of the serotonin 5HT-2A receptor at postsynaptic neurons. Nefazodone also induces a transient reuptake inhibition of norepinephrine. The most common side effects of nefazodone include nausea, headache, sedation, and dizziness. There is also a modest risk of orthostatic hypotension. Because of limited clinical experience and the absence of case reports, it is impossible to comment on the relative benefits and risks of using this drug in parkinsonian patients, with or without depression. A theoretical benefit of nefazodone may result from its 5HT-2A antagonist properties. Relatively pure 5HT-2A antagonists, such as ritanserin, have been shown to decrease drug-induced extrapyramidal symptoms and akathisia when added to haloperidol (68). It is possible that nefazodone may thus be beneficial for some patients because of the moderating effect of 5HT-2A antagonism on reduced dopaminergic states.

An unknown element regarding nefazodone use is the effect of *m*-chlorophenylpiperazine (*m*-CPP) on parkinsonism. *m*-CPP has been noted to exacerbate a number of psychiatric symptoms, including obsessive compulsiveness, panic, and psychosis. The effects of nefazodone, or *m*-CPP, on motor symptoms or interactions with levodopa are not known.

G. Trazodone

The major concern when using trazodone in Parkinson's disease patients is its α-adrenergic effect, which causes hypotension. Trazodone is also very sedating. Improved levodopa-induced dyskinesia in a depressed Parkinson's disease patient treated with trazodone has been reported (69).

H. Amoxapine

Amoxapine use in Parkinson's disease has not been studied, but there is a compelling argument against its use: amoxipine has clinically significant dopamine D2 antagonistic effects, which cause parkinsonian symptoms, and it has been reported to cause tardive dyskinesia. With many alternative agents available, there is little reason to consider amoxapine for treatment of Parkinson's disease patients. In theory, amoxapine might benefit a depressed patient with levodopa-induced psychosis, but this has not been described in the literature.

I. Maprotiline

Maprotiline is a relatively noradrenergic "tetracyclic" antidepressant that is generally well tolerated. The author has used it in Parkinson's disease patients without any unusual side effects. Maprotiline is associated with a dose-related risk of seizures, however.

VII. OTHER DRUGS USED IN THE TREATMENT OF DEPRESSION

There are a number of drugs with other indications that are used alone or as adjuncts in the treatment of depression.

A. Lithium

Lithium has inherent antidepressant activity when used alone and is used to augment response to primary antidepressant drugs. There is a textbook mention (70) of the successful use of lithium in the treatment of depression in Parkinson's disease, but there is no reference for the source of this observation. Tremor is a common side effect of lithium, so there may be parkinsonianlike side effects associated with its use. Cases of severe treatment-emergent parkinsonism involving lithium have been reported (71).

B. Clozapine

Clozapine has emerged as a clinically useful treatment for levodopa-induced psychosis (72). At low doses, clozapine does not appear to worsen, and can improve, the motor symptoms of Parkinson's disease. In addition, clozapine has been shown to possess mood-stabilizing properties (73), and may benefit patients who are depressed. The most common adverse effects of clozapine in Parkinson's disease patients are confusion, sedation, and orthostasis. Low doses—less than 100 mg per day—should be used. Because advanced age is a risk factor for clozapine-induced agranulocytosis, patients should be closely monitored.

C. Buspirone

Buspirone is a serotonin 5HT-1A agonist marketed as an anxiolytic, with typical daily doses of 15 to 30 mg prescribed. The drug has also been shown to have antidepressant activity when used alone (74), and is effective in the augmentation of antidepressant therapy (75–78). When buspirone is used as an antidepressant, doses above 30 mg per day are administered. Buspirone has a modest effect on the dopamine system; studies show that buspirone may either enhance or reduce dopamine synthesis (79). The compound has been observed to both cause and ameliorate drug-induced movement disorders. For example, buspirone has been noted to cause akathisia and dyskinesia and to suppress neuroleptic-induced akathisia and dyskinesia. Moss et al. (80) have reported that buspirone produced improvement in tardive dyskinesia when used at doses up to 160 mg per day. Bonifati (81) noted dramatic improvement in levodopa-associated dyskinesia at high doses. In both types of dyskinesia, patients with more severe symptoms showed the most benefit.

When used in Parkinson's disease patients at the anxiolytic dose, buspirone is unlikely to have any effect on motor symptoms (82,83). At doses above 60 mg per day, worsening of parkinsonian symptoms has been reported; the risk for exacerbation was higher in patients with more severe disease (82,83). High-dose buspirone should thus be avoided, unless it is used specifically to treat levodopa-induced dyskinesia.

D. Benzodiazepines

Antidepressants are usually effective in treating anxiety symptoms, whether or not they are part of a depressive disorder. However, many patients are extremely anxious and agitated, have significant insomnia, or are intolerant of antidepressants. In these cases, benzodiazepines are often used. There is no literature on the use of benzodiazepines in depressed parkinsonian patients, but in clinical practice, many patients do benefit from the symptomatic relief they provide. It is important to recognize that these drugs are associated with confusion, memory difficulties, and psychomotor impairment. Drugs with shorter half-lives, such as lorazepam, oxazepam, alprazolam, temazepam, triazolam, or clonazepam should be used in order to minimize risks of falls and sedation. Alprazolam probably has antidepressant properties, and might represent a reasonable choice. It is associated with a higher dependence liability than the other agents, however, and may require frequent dosing in order to minimize interdose rebound symptoms. Alprazolam has also been known to cause akathisia (Xanax, product information).

E. Psychostimulants

Amphetamine was used to treat muscular rigidity of parkinsonism before the introduction of specific dopamine agonists. One study involving intravenous methylphenidate (84) found that depressed parkinsonism patients had no euphoric response to the drug. Interestingly, nondepressed patients with Parkinson's disease, depressed patients without Parkinson's disease, and normal comparison subjects all experienced feelings of euphoria and well being, talkativeness, psychic activation, and greater locomotor activity. The authors speculated that the absence of a functional dopaminergic response prevented depressed Parkinson's disease patients from reacting to the methylphenidate challenge as the other subjects did.

VIII. OTHER BIOLOGICAL THERAPIES

Several other modalities have been reported to be beneficial or warrant consideration in the treatment of depression in Parkinson's disease.

A. Electroconvulsive Therapy (ECT)

ECT should be considered for depressed patients with Parkinson's disease who cannot tolerate medication for their symptoms. ECT has been shown to be helpful for both mood and motor symptoms in parkinsonian patients. Improvement of motor signs is not dependent on the improvement or even the existence of depression. For example, depression but not the parkinsonism may respond, and vice versa (85). ECT can markedly prolong the duration of the "on" phase of patients with "on–off" phenomena. Symptoms respond with 3 to 6 bilateral ECT treatments. Unilateral ECT is less effective in this population. Although some patients experience sustained neurological improvement lasting several months, symptoms more typically return within 4 to 6 weeks, so routine maintenance ECT is needed. Confusion and memory difficulties, which immediately follow treatment, are the most common and distressing side effects. The hypothesized mechanisms of ECT's antiparkinsonian effects include enhancement of dopaminergic transmission, and/or potentiation of response to dopamine agonists through increased permeability of the blood-brain barrier to those drugs (86).

B. Sleep Manipulation

Total sleep deprivation of one whole night has been widely demonstrated to possess antidepressant properties. Identical acute antidepressant effects have also been documented for partial sleep deprivation of the second half of the night. The response is transient, with relapse the following night after patients sleep again.

There are a number of references in the literature to the clinical effects of partial sleep restriction on both mood and motor symptoms in Parkinson's disease. Reist et al. (87) have reported that sleep deprivation significantly improved such motor symptoms as fluidity of gait and decreased rigidity. What is puzzling is that "sleep benefit"—in which motor symptoms improve after extended sleep—has also been reported. Moreover, Lauterbach (88) has pointed out that sleep deprivation can produce adverse mental status changes, including "on-"phase mania, agitation, confusion, and disorientation. Thus, sleep restriction may benefit some patients and worsen others.

It is interesting that animal studies have shown that sleep deprivation is associated with increased serotonin turnover in the brain as well as with increased dopamine and norepinephrine synthesis (89).

C. Light Therapy

Phototherapy, another established form of antidepressant therapy, is unexplored in the Parkinson's disease population. It merits consideration as a novel intervention, since there is evidence that the mechanism of action of light therapy involves the serotonin system (90), and SSRIs are effective antidepressants in parkinsonian patients. Reist et al. (87) have commented on changes in retinal sensitivity to light in Parkinson's disease patients (87). Attempts to treat seasonal affective disorder with levodopa therapy have produced negative results.

IX. CONCLUSIONS

The psychopharmacology of depression in Parkinson's disease patients is complex and is associated with many unanswered questions. The lack of any consensus on treatment strategies probably reflects a number of factors. First, depression and Parkinson's disease themselves are highly variable, both in clinical presentation and in their underlying neuropathology. The probability that the same neurochemical systems are involved in the pathophysiology of the mood and motor disturbances further complicates treatment since the treatment of one can destabilize the other. No single pharmacological intervention is universally effective in either disorder, and prediction of likely response to any single agent is not possible. Indeed, the need for individualized treatment characterizes depression and parkinsonism. There are also significant obstacles to conducting meaningful clinical drug studies. Diagnostic ambiguity, the inherent fluctuation of symptoms in parkinsonian patients, and the confounding effects of antiparkinsonian medications on ratings of antidepressant drug activity are some of these.

Nevertheless, a number of recommendations can be made. Most parkinsonian patients are elderly, have an increased sensitivity to side effects (especially activation), and are using one or more dopaminergic agents. Consequently, antidepressants should always be started at the lowest possible dose and titrated upward as tolerated. The treating physician should be well informed regarding the clinical profiles of all the drugs used by the patient in order to quickly recognize characteristic adverse events or synergistic effects. Because of the need for frequent adjustments of antiparkinsonian medications, it is best to avoid concurrent changes in antidepressant drugs or dose levels.

Neither research nor clinical experience has established a preferred individual drug or class of antidepressants for Parkinson's disease patients. The total number of patients studied is too small to permit any conclusions. Each drug carries its own risks and benefits. The effects of the SSRIs are of particular and immediate relevance because of their widespread clinical use. Available evidence and clinical experience suggest that these drugs are effective antidepressants in parkinsonian patients, and may even improve some motor functions. SSRIs can also abruptly and markedly worsen the movement disorder in some patients, however. This tends to underscore the element of unpredictability in treating depression in Parkinson's disease with any drug. Some patients benefit whereas others deteriorate from the same interventions. An unfortunate aspect of Parkinson's disease is that all therapies, for both depression and motor disturbances, are ultimately limited in their efficacy by the progressive and degenerative nature of the disorder, so they lose their effects over time.

Important questions remain unanswered. Should antidepressant medication be initiated concurrently with antiparkinsonian medication? Do antiparkinsonian medications have inherent antidepressant properties? Are certain drugs preferable to others in terms of efficacy and safety? Are there clinical, biochemical, or anatomical features that can be used to improve drug selection? Do available antidepressant therapies have any impact on the progression of the underlying disorder, and, if so, does early intervention alter the course of the disorder? Large-scale, well-designed studies are needed to resolve these issues.

REFERENCES

1. Parkinson J. An Essay on the Shaking Palsy. London: Sherwood, Neely and Jones, 1817.

2. Klassen T, Verhey FRJ, Sneijders GHJM, de Vet HCW, van Praag HM. Treatment of depression in Parkinson's disease: a meta-analysis. J Neuropsychiatry Clin Neurosci 1995; 7:281–286.
3. Dooneief G, Mirabello E, Bell K, Marder K, Stern Y, Mayeux R. An estimate of the incidence of depression in idiopathic Parkinson's disease. Arch Neurol 1992; 409:305–307.
4. Richard IH, Schiffer RB, Kurian R. Anxiety and Parkinson's disease. J. Neuropsychiatry and Clin Neurosciences 1996; 8:383–392.
5. Hantz P, Caradoc-Davis T, Weatherall M, Dixon G. Depression in Parkinson's disease. Am J Psychiatry 1994; 151:1010–1014.
6. Tandberg E, Larsen JP, Aarsland D, Laake K, Cummings JL. Risk factors for depression in Parkinson's disease. Arch Neurol 1997; 54:625–630.
7. Quinn C. Multiple System Atrophy. In: Marsden CD, Fahn S, eds. Movement Disorders 3. London: Butterworths, 1993.
8. Maricle RA, Nutt JG, Carter JH. Mood and anxiety fluctuation in Parkinson's disease associated with levodopa infusion: preliminary findings. Movement Disord 1995; 10:329–332.
9. Thiagarajan A, Anand KS. Parkinson's disease: incidence of depression, correlation of stages of depression to clinical staging and disability (abstract). Neurology 1994; 44(suppl 2):A254.
10. Chia LG, Cheng LJ, Chou LJ, Cheng FC, Cu JS. Studies of demential depression, electrophysiology and cerebrospinal fluid monoamine metabolites in patients with Parkinson's disease. J Neurol Sci 1995; 133:73–78.
11. Starkstein SE, Preziosi TJ, Bolduc PL, Robinson RG. Depression in Parkinson's disease. J Nerv Ment Disord 1990; 178:27–31.
12. Willner P. Sensitization of dopamine D2- or D3-type receptors as final common pathway in antidepressant drug action. Clin Neuropharmacol 1995; 18(suppl 1): S49–S56.
13. Brown AS, Gershon S. Dopamine and depression. J Neural Transm [GenSect] 1993; 91:75–109.
14. Flint AJ, Black SE, Campbell-Taylor I, Gailey GF, Levinton C. Abnormal speech articulation, psychomotor retardation, and subcortical dysfunction in major depression. J Psychiatric Res 1993; 27:309–319.
15. Mann JJ, Kapur S. A dopaminergic hypothesis of major depression. Clin Neuropharmacol 1995; 18:557–565.
16. Mellers JD, Quinn NP, Ron MA. Psychotic and depressive symptoms in Parkinson's disease: a study of the growth hormone response to apomorphine. Br J Psychiatry 1995; 167:522–526.
17. Mayeux R, Stern Y, Cote L, Williams JB. Altered serotonin metabolism in depressed patients with Parkinson's disease. Neurology 1984; 34:642–646.
18. Mayberg HS, Solomon DH. Depression in Parkinson's disease: a biochemical and organic viewpoint. Adv Neurol 1995; 65:49–60.
19. Chase TN. 5-hydroxytryptophan in Parkinsonism. Lancet 1970; 2:1029–1230.
20. Chase TN, Ng LKY, Watanabe AN. Parkinson's disease modification by 5-hydroxytryptophan. Neurology 1972; 22:479–484.

21. McCance-Katz EF, Marek KL, Price LH. Serotonergic dysfunction in depression associated with Parkinson's disease. Neurology 1992; 42:1813–1814.
22. Sawada M, Nagatsu T, Nagatsu I, Ito K, Iizuka R, Kondo T, Narabayashi H. Tryptophan hydroxylase activity in the brains of controls and parkinsonian patients. J Neural Transmission 1985; 62:107–115.
23. Sandyk R, Fisher H. L-tryptophan supplementation in Parkinson's disease. Int J Neurosci 1989; 45:215–219.
24. Murphy DL, Mueller EA, Garrick NA, Aulakh CS. Use of serotonergic agents in the clinical assessment of central serotonin function. J Clin Psychiatry 1986; 47:9–15.
25. Kostic VS, Lecic D, Doder M, Marinkovic J, Filipovic S. Prolactin and cortical responses to fenfluramine in Parkinson's disease. Biol Psychiatry 1996; 40:769–775.
26. Cummings JL. Depression in Parkinson's disease: a review. Am J Psychiatry 1992; 149:443–454.
27. Mayeux R, Stern Y, Sano M, et al. Depression in Parkinson's disease. Movement Disord 1988; 3:237–244.
28. Factor SA, Molho ES, Podskalny GD, Brown D. Parkinson's disease: drug-induced psychiatric states. Adv Neurol 1995; 65:115–138.
29. Inoue T, Tsuchiya K, Miura J, Sakakibara S, Denda K, Kashahara T, Koyama T. Bromocriptine treatment of tricyclic and heterocyclic antidepressant-resistant depression. Biol Psychiatry 1996; 40:151–153.
30. Theohar C, Fischer-Cornellson K, Akesson HO, et al. Bromocriptine as antidepressant: double-blind comparative study with imipramine in psychogenic and endogenous depression. Curr Ther Res 1981; 30:830–842.
31. Waehrens J, Gerlach J. Bromocriptine and imipramine in endogenous depression. A double-blind controlled trial in out-patients. J Affect Disorder 1981; 3:193–202.
32. Willner P, Lappas S, Cheeta S, Muscat R. Reversal of stress-induced anhedonia by the dopamine receptor agonist, pramipaxole. Psychopharmacology 1994; 115: 454–462.
33. Roth A, Akyol S, Nelson JC. Delirium associated with the combination of a neuroleptic, an SSRI, and benztropine. J Clin Psychiatry 1994; 55:492–495.
34. Moryl E, Danysz W, Quack G. Potential antidepressive properties of amantadine, memantine and bifemeline. Pharmacol Toxicol 1993; 72:394–397.
35. Jimenez-Jimenez FJ, Tejeiro J, Martinez-Junquerra G, Cabrera-Valdivia F, Alarcon J, Garcia-Albea E. Parkinsonism exacerbated by paroxetine. Neurology 1994; 44:2406.
36. Menza MA, Robertson-Hoffman DE, Bonapace AS. Parkinson's disease and anxiety: comorbidity with depression. Biol Psychiatry 1993; 34:465–470.
37. Stein MB, Heuser IJ, Juncos JL, et al. Anxiety disorders in patients with Parkinson's disease. Am J Psychiatry 1990; 147:217–220.
38. Vasquez A, Kumenez-Jimenez FJ, Garcia-Ruiz P, Garcia-Urra D. Panic attacks in Parkinson's disease: a long-term complication of levodopa therapy. Acta Neurol Scand 1993; 87:14–18.

39. Henderson R, Kurlan R, Kersun JM, Como P. Preliminary examination of the comorbidity of anxiety and depression in Parkinson's disease. J Neuropsychiatry Clin Neurosci 1992; 4:257–264.
40. Berrios GE, Campbell C, Politynska BE. Autonomic failure, depression and anxiety in Parkinson's disease. Br J Psychiatry 1995; 166:789–792.
41. Jolivalt C, Minn A, Vincent-Viry M, Galteau MM, Siest G. Dextromethorphan O-demethylase activity in rat brain microsomes. Neurosci Lett 1995; 187:65–68.
42. Indaco A, Carrieri PD. Amitryptiline in the treatment of headache in patients with Parkinson's disease. Neurology 1988; 38:1720–1722.
43. Boer BH, Erdman RAM, Onstenk HJVC, et al. Clomipramine, depresie en de ziekte van Parkinson. Tijdschr Psychiatrie 1976; 28:499–509.
44. Andersen J, Aabro E, Gulmann N, Hjelmisted A, Pedersen HE. Anti-depressive treatment in Parkinson's disease: a controlled trial of the effects of Nortriptyline in patients with PD treated with L-dopa. Acta Neurol Scand 1980; 62:210–219.
45. Laitinen L. Desipramine in the treatment of Parkinson's disease. Acta Neurol Scand 1969; 45:109–113.
46. Strang RR. Imipramine in the treatment of parkinsonism: a double-blind study. Br J Med 1965; 2:33–34.
47. Garcia-Monco JC, Padierna A, Gomez BM. Selegiline, fluoxetine, and depression in Parkinson's disease (letter). Movement Disord 1995; 10:352.
48. Allain H, Pollack P, Neukirch HC. Symptomatic effect of selegiline in de novo Parkinsonian patients. The French selegiline multicenter trial. Movement Disord 1993; 8(suppl 1):S36–S40.
49. Takats A, Tarczy N, Simo M, Szombathely E, Bodrogi A, Karpati R. Moclobemide/aurix treatment in Parkinson's disease with depression. New Trends Clin Neuropharmacol 1994; 8:260.
50. Sieradzan K, Channon S, Ramponi C, Stern GM, Lees A, Youdim MBH. The therapeutic potential of moclobemide, a reversible selective monoamine oxidase A inhibitor in Parkinson's disease. J Clin Psychopharmacol 1995; 15(suppl 2):51S–59S.
51. Brod TM. Fluoxetine extrapyramidal side effects (letter). Am J Psychiatry 1989; 146:1353.
52. Bouchard RH, Pourcher E, Vincent P. Fluoxetine and extrapyramidal side effects. Am J Psychiatry 1989; 146:1352–1355.
53. Leo RJ. Movement disorders associated with the serotonin reuptake inhibitors. J Clin Psychiatry 1996; 57:449–454.
54. Dubovsky SL, Thomas M. Tardive dyskinesia associated with fluoxetine. Psychiatr Serv 1996; 47:991–993.
55. Steur EN. Increase of Parkinson disability after fluoxetine medication. Neurology 1993; 43:211–213./
56. Vaucher M, Schulz P, Dick P. Potential interaction between fluvoxamine and treatment for Parkinson's disease. Encephale 1987; 13(suppl 4):266–267.
57. Caley CF, Friedman JH. Does fluoxetine exacerbate Parkinson's disease? J Clin Psychiatry 1992; 53:278–282.
58. Iocono RP, Toyama S, Meltzer C, Kumiyoshi S. Treatment of Parkinson's akinesia by selective serotonin reuptake inhibitors (abstract). Ann Neurol 1994; 36:296.

59. Meerwaldt JD. Treatment of hypokinetic rigid syndrome with fluvoxamine maleate. Lancet 1986; i:977–978.
60. Montastruc J-L, Fabre N, Blin O, Senard J-M, Rascol O, Rascol A. Does fluoxetine aggravate Parkinson's disease? A pilot prospective study (letter). Movement Disord 1995; 10:354–355.
61. Huszonek JJ. Anticholinergic effects in a depressed parkinsonian patient. J Geriatr Psychiatry Neurol 1995; 8:100–102.
62. Miyawaki E, Meah Y, Koller WC. Serotonin, dopamine and motor effects in Parkinson's disease. Clin Neuropharmacology 1997; 20:300–310.
63. Tsuiki K, Yamamoto L, Diksic M. Effect of acute fluoxetine treatment on the brain serotonin synthesis as measured by the a-methyl-L-tryptophan autoradiographic method. J Neurochem 1995; 65:250–256.
64. Tulloch IF, Johnson AM. The pharmacologic profile of paroxetine, a new selective serotonin reuptake inhibitor. J Clin Psychiatry 1992; 53(suppl):7–12.
65. Levin et al. 1994.
66. Goetz CG, Tanner CM, Klawans HL. Bupropion in Parkinson's disease. Neurology 1984; 34:1092–1094.
67. Goldstein, Menek. Personal communication.
68. Dubovsky SL, Thomas M. Serotonergic mechanisms and current and future psychiatric practice. J Clin Psychiatry 1995; 56(suppl 2):38–48.
69. el-Awar M, Freedman M, Seeman P, Goldenberg L, Little J, Solomon P. Response of tardive and L-dopa-induced dyskinesias to antidepressants. Can J Neurol Sci 1987; 14:629–631.
70. Wirshing WC. Neuropsychiatric aspects of movement disorders. In: Kaplan HI, Sadock BJ, eds. Comprehensive Textbook of Psychiatry. 6th ed. Baltimore: Williams & Wilkins, 1995:220–231.
71. Holyrod S, Smith D. Disabling parkinsonism due to lithium: a case report. J Geriatr Psychiatry Neurol 1995; 8:118–119.
72. Meltzer HY, Kennedy J, Dai J, Parsa M, Riley D. Plasma clozapine levels and treatment of L-DOPA-induced psychosis in Parkinson's disease. Neuropsychopharmacology 1995; 12:39–45.
73. Zarate CA Jr, Tohen M, Baldessarini RJ. Clozapine in severe mood disorders. J Clin Psychiatry 1995; 56:411–417.
74. Rickels K, Amsterdam JD, Clary C. Buspirone in major depression: a controlled study. J Clin Psychiatry 1991; 52:34–38.
75. Jacobsen FM. Possible augmentation of antidepressant response to buspirone. J Clin Psychiatry 1991; 52:217–220.
76. Bakish D. Fluoxetine potentiation by buspirone: three case histories. Can J Psychiatry 1991; 36:749–750.
77. Joffe RT, Schuller DR. An open study of buspirone augmentation of serotonin reuptake inhibitors in refractory depression. J Psychiatry 1993; 54:269–271.
78. Robillard M, Lieff S. Augmentation of antidepressant therapy by buspirone: three geriatric case histories. Can J Psychiatry 1995; 40:639–640.
79. Tunnicliff G, Brokaw JJ, Hausz JA, Matheson GK, White GW. Influence of repeated treatment with buspirone on central 5-hydroxy tryptamine and dopamine synthesis. Neuropharmacology 1992; 31:991–995.

80. Moss LE, Neppe VM, Drevets. J Clin Psychopharmacol 1993; 13:204–209.
81. Bonifati V, Fabrizio E, Cipriani R, Vanacore N, Meco G. Buspirone in levodopa-induced dyskinesias. Clin Neuropharmacol 1994; 17:73–82.
82. Ludwig CL, Weinberger DR, Bruno G, Gillespie M, Bakker K, LeWitt PA, Chase TN. Buspirone, Parkinson's disease, and the locus ceruleus. Clin Neuropharmacol 1986; 9:373–378.
83. Hammerstad JP, Carter J, Nutt JG, Casten GC, Shrotriya RC, Alms DR, Temple D. Buspirone in Parkinson's disease. Clin Neuropharmacol 1986; 9:556–560.
84. Cantello R, Aguggia M, Gilli M, et al. Major depression in Parkinson's disease and response to intravenous methylphenidate: possible role of the "hedonic" dopamine synapse. J Neurol Neurosurg Psychiatry 1989; 52:724–731.
85. Kellner CH, Beale MD, Poitchett JT, Bernstein HJ, Burns CM. Electroconvulsive therapy and Parkinson's disease: the case for further study. Psychopharmacol Bull 1994; 30:495–500.
86. Dubovsky S. Electroconvulsive therapy. In: Kaplan HI, Sadock BJ, eds. Comprehensive Textbook of Psychiatry, 6th ed. Baltimore: Williams & Wilkins, 1995: 2129–2140.
87. Reist C. Sokolski KN, Chen CC, Demet EM. The effect of sleep deprivation on motor impairment and retinal adaptation in Parkinson's disease. Prog Neuropsychopharmacol Biol Psychiatry 1995; 19:445–454.
88. Lauterbach EC. Sleep benefit and sleep deprivation in subgroups of depressed patients with Parkinson's disease. Am J Psychiatry 1994; 151:782–783.
89. Asikainen M, Deboer T, Porkka-Heiskanen T, Stenberg D, Tobler I. Sleep deprivation increases brain serotonin turnover in the Djungarian hamster. Neurosci Lett 1995; 198:21–24.
90. Lam RW, Zis AP, Grewal A, Delgado PL, Charney DS, Krystal JH. Effects of rapid tryptophan depletion in patients with seasonal affective disorder in remission after light therapy. Arch Gen Psychiatry 1996; 53:41–44.

12

The Assessment and Treatment of Depressed-Demented Patients

George S. Alexopoulos
Cornell University Medical College, White Plains, New York

I. INTRODUCTION

Depression and dementia often coexist. Studies of demented patients have shown a prevalence of comorbid depression ranging from 2 to 23% (1–5). Dementia was diagnosed in 14% of depressed patients (6). Identification and treatment of depression in demented patients can have important clinical implications. Appropriate treatment may reduce the suffering of depressed-demented patients and improve the qualify of life of their families. Improvement of depression can reduce "excess disability" in demented patients and allow them to remain in the community. Finally, antidepressant treatment can ameliorate the cognitive dysfunction contributed by depression and permit clinicians to determine the stage of dementia and advise patients and families about future treatment needs.

Despite the potential benefits of antidepressant treatment, many aspects of the diagnostic assessment and treatment of depressed-demented patients remain unclear. What follows is a review of findings and questions that need to be addressed.

II. ASSESSMENT OF DEPRESSION IN DEMENTED PATIENTS

The assessment of depressive symptomatology in demented patients is complicated by many factors. These include the overlap of depressive manifestations with symptomatology of dementia, the poor ability of demented patients to report their symptoms and the over-time fluctuation of the depressive syndrome in demented patients. Approaches that have been used to address these issues are summarized below.

A frequent clinical concern is the distinction of behavioral manifestations of depression from symptoms and signs of dementing disorders and medical illnesses. Somatic complaints are part of the depressive syndrome. Depression itself may enhance the symptoms of a medical illness. It has been reported that medically ill depressives have more somatic symptoms than medically ill nondepressed patients (7). Depression has been shown to add to disability caused by chronic medical illness (8).

Some of the symptoms and signs of frontal lobe syndromes are similar to the clinical symptomatology of depression. Lesions of the orbitofrontal circuit may lead to disinhibition, irritability, and diminished sensitivity to social cues (9). Impairment of the anterior cingulate may result in apathy and reduced initiative (9). Damage of the dorsolateral prefrontal circuit may result in cognitive impairment, including difficulties in set shifting, learning, and word list generation (9). These behavioral abnormalities resemble in part the depressive syndrome. If a frontal lobe syndrome is incorrectly diagnosed as depression, overtreatment with antidepressants may follow. However, depression itself may cause frontal lobe symptoms that can subside after antidepressant treatment. Finally, some patients with frontal lobe syndrome may develop depression. The most effective clinical approach to a patient with mixed depressive and frontal lobe symptomatology is to provide one or more antidepressant trials and attempt to distinguish the symptoms that respond from those that resist treatment. This strategy can reduce overtreatment of patients with a persistent frontal lobe syndrome.

The clinical complexity of depressed-demented patients led to the development of several assessment strategies (10). Rating instruments have used one or more of the following approaches: (1) Avoidance of items in areas where the symptoms and signs of depression overlap with those of medical illness (11) or of dementia (12–14); (2) exclusive rating of depressive signs since symptoms may be unreliably reported by demented-depressed patients (15); (3) reliance on informants' reports as well as patient evaluation (13,14); and (4) use of prolonged observation (13,14).

These approaches have made significant clinical and methodological contributions. However, several limitations remain. As a rule, informants are useful, but unreliable informants often complicate rather than help history taking. It has been observed, however, that caregivers are more sensitive than trained raters in identifying depressive symptoms and signs of demented patients (10). Restricting the definition of depression to areas that do not overlap with dementia or other neurological syndromes excludes disturbances in concentration and guilt, as well as somatic complaints, and may result in an insensitive identification of depression.

Recent studies began to evaluate the "all-inclusive" method in rating depressive symptoms and signs in depressed elderly patients. The "all-inclusive" approach accepts a broad range of depressive symptoms and signs regardless of whether they originate from the dementing disorder or depression. The Hamilton Depression Rating Scale (Ham-D) was found capable of discriminating demented patients with major depression from nondepressed demented patients (16). Moreover, there was no significant association between Ham-D scores and scores of cognitive impairment. However, specific studies need to be conducted in demented patients in order to ascertain the sensitivity and validity of scales that rate a broad range of depressive symptoms and signs.

Another method of assessing depression in demented patients may rely on a "diagnostic approach" that seeks to differentiate symptoms and signs of depression from manifestations of neurological disorders. The "diagnostic approach" can cover a broad range of depressive manifestations, but requires that clinicians accept symptoms and signs that in their view are part of the depressive syndrome and not part of dementia, frontal lobe syndrome, or other neurological or medical disorders. Although reliability and validity may be difficult to establish, it is possible that experienced clinicians are able to make these complex judgments reliably. However, the distinction of depressive from nondepressive manifestations of medical and neurological disorders introduces a "dualism" that can only be acceptable if the diagnostic approach is validated through a clinically useful method. A potential validation approach may demand that the diagnostic approach should be able to identify depressive syndromes with a response rate to antidepressant treatment comparable to that of nondemented patients. Even then, the diagnostic approach will be useful only if the all-inclusive approach is shown to identify patients with lower response rate to antidepressants. The assumption in this case will be that the all-inclusive approach incorrectly identifies as depressives patients who only have behavioral manifestations of dementia that do not respond to antidepressant treatment.

III. DEPRESSION WITH "REVERSIBLE DEMENTIA"

Approximately 18–57% of depressed patients present a syndrome of dementia that subsides after remission of depressive symptomatology (17). The clinical presentation of "reversible dementias" depends on the age of the patient, the underlying psychiatric disorder, and the setting in which the patient is treated (18–22). Early writers have suggested that patients with "reversible dementia" overdramatize their cognitive loss and often claim that they are unable to find the correct answers during a mental status examination (19). This presentation is perhaps relevant to middle-aged or "young-old" patients with personality, posttraumatic, or neurotic disorders. Geriatric studies did not observe excessive cognitive complaint responses in elderly depressives (17,23–25), and therefore this clinical presentation may not be relevant only to middle-aged populations with diagnoses other than depression. The depressive syndrome of elderly patients with "reversible dementia" usually is severe (26). These patients suffer from more intense motor retardation, hopelessness, helplessness, and anxiety than cognitively unimpaired elderly depressives and are more likely to demonstrate delusions (26–28). The dementia syndrome, on the other hand, tends to be of mild severity and consists principally of impairment in attention, free recall, motor speed, spontaneous elaboration of detail (26,29), word fluency, and syntactic complexity (17,21).

Biological investigations, including the dexamethasone suppression test (30), platelet monoamine oxidase activity (31), brain computerized tomography (32,33), electroencephalography (34), and sleep electroencephalographic studies (28,35), do not appear to help the differential diagnosis of reversible dementia. However, some of the electroencephalographic and neuroimaging studies have demonstrated group differences between depression with reversible dementia, irreversible dementia, or geriatric depression without dementia (28,32,33,35).

Clinical examination and laboratory tests often are unable to establish the diagnosis of depression with reversible dementia. Even in the most typical cases (e.g., an elderly patient who first develops mild dementia after a severe episode of late-onset depression characterized by retardation and depressive delusions), the clinician is unable to predict with certainty the outcome of dementia. Appropriate antidepressant treatment is necessary both in order to help depression and characterize the dementia syndrome as reversible or not. Dementia workup also needs to be pursued at this point in order to exclude treatable causes of dementia.

Studies on the course of geriatric depression with reversible dementia suggest that this syndrome is heterogeneous (36). Cognitive impairment frequently is part of the depressive syndrome, especially in the elderly. However, it is unclear why some elderly depressives develop severe cognitive dysfunction or even a transient dementia and others do not. One reason may be that at least some of these patients have an underlying dementing disorder. This is supported by the observation that many patients with reversible dementia do not achieve complete cognitive recovery even when their intellectual function improves following remission of depression (37). Moreover, recent studies (2, 38–40) observed development of irreversible dementia on follow-up at rates higher than those of nondemented geriatric depressives. The rates of development of dementia range from 11–23% per year, although lower percentages have been reported by others (2,38–40). A controlled study used survival analysis and observed that most depressed patients with an initial reversible dementia begin to develop irreversible dementia approximately 2 years after the initial recovery from depression and dementia (41); 43% of patients in this study became irreversibly demented after an average of 3 years.

A usual clinical evaluation and the Mini-Mental State Examination may not be sufficiently sensitive to identify elderly depressed, reversibly demented, patients who will later develop irreversible dementia. Cognitive dysfunction during depression may be an expression of decreased reserve cognitive capacity that becomes clinically evident only during a depressive episode. Therefore, some depressives with reversible dementia may already be suffering from a dementing disorder. Depression in some of these cases may be the first manifestation of a neurological brain disease that will later produce dementia. This is supported by the observation that the most frequent dementing disorders, such as Alzheimer's disease, multi-infarct dementia, and parkinsonism, have a high rate of comorbidity with depression, ranging from 17–50% (42–44). Approximately 30% of depressed Alzheimer's patients have a history of previous psychiatric illness (45), while 18% of all Alzheimer's patients were found to have a history of depression or paranoia (46). Furthermore, the percentage of demented patients in samples of elderly persons with major depression is approximately 10 times higher than that of the general elderly population (37, 42,44). Therefore, reversible dementia in the context of geriatric depression should be viewed as a risk factor for development of a progressive dementing disorder rather than as a benign entity.

Although a large percentage of elderly depressed patients develop reversible dementia on a background of subclinical dementing disorders, other cases do not progress into irreversible dementia. Various factors may contribute to the transient cognitive dysfunction of these patients. Geriatric depression with reversible dementia as a rule is a severe and often psychotic syndrome (41). The severity of depressive symptomatology may interfere with clinical examination. Some patients may be incorrectly identified as demented when in reality they are unable to cooperate with the cognitive function examination.

Cognitive dysfunction is often a part of severe geriatric depression. Cognitive dysfunction may be a primary sign in depression rather than an indirect consequence of depressed mood. Pharmacological probes may selectively affect cognitive function or mood symptoms. L-dopa and L-tryptophan may improve memory without significantly changing symptoms and signs related to mood (47). In contrast, lithium and imipramine were found to improve depressive manifestations disproportionately to memory improvement (47). These findings raise the question of whether cognitive and mood disturbances of depression are mediated by related, yet distinct, brain systems.

Nonprogressive brain lesions may predispose to cognitive dysfunction during depression without the eventual development of irreversible dementia. This view is supported by the observation that neurological symptoms and signs are exacerbated when patients become depressed (48). A positron emission tomography study showed that depressives with reversible dementia had a characteristic profile of regional cerebral blood flow abnormalities consisting of decreases in the left anterior prefrontal cortex and increases in the cerebellar vermis (49). These changes were distinct from those of Alzheimer's dementia. A speculation may be that some patients with depression and reversible dementia have a dysfunction of brain systems different from those of depression alone.

Finally, transient cognitive dysfunction in the elderly may be caused by a metabolic or drug-induced delirium or side effects of somatic treatments. The impact of these conditions may be heightened by the high sensitivity of the elderly population to metabolic, pharmacological, and environmental changes. One would expect that patients with delirium or drug-induced cognitive side effects should have a favorable long-term outcome, but specific studies are lacking.

IV. CLINICAL DIAGNOSIS IN DEPRESSED-DEMENTED PATIENTS

The above discussion focused on difficulties in differentiating depression from dementia in the elderly and in determining the long-term outcome of depressed-demented patients. It should be emphasized, however, that the syndromes of depression and dementia each occur in a high percentage of elderly patients. In some cases, depression and dementia may be relatively independent of each other and simply co-occur in the same patient. For example, a patient with a recurrent or chronic depression since early life who develops dementia in old age may have two independent disorders. However, even in such a case, the assumption that depression and dementia are independent of each other is not safe. The fact that a patient has had a recurrent early-onset depression does not preclude the current depressive syndrome from being a consequence of an underlying dementing disorder. In other cases, the syndromes of depression and dementia are caused by the same disorders. This may be the case in patients with vascular dementias, Parkinson's disease, Alzheimer's disease, hypothyroidism, and other disorders known to cause each of the two syndromes. Nonetheless, even in such cases, the clinician cannot establish that the two syndromes have common etiology.

In view of the complex relationships among depression and dementia syndromes in the elderly. Devanant and Nelson (50) have suggested that the best clinical approach is to consider each diagnosis independently rather than view the patient as having either depression or dementia. The diagnostic task may be facilitated by attention to the clinical presentation of various dementia syndromes. At least three dementia syndromes may be relevant to the evaluation of patients in whom depression and dementia are considered:

1. Subcortical dementia: The prominent symptoms of this syndrome are significant memory impairment and psychomotor retardation.
2. Cortical dementia: These patients have a broader spectrum of impairments, including memory impairment, apraxia resulting in disheveled appearance, language impairment leading to paraphasic errors, and construction problems (e.g., inability to draw a clock).
3. Frontal lobe dementia: The most prominent aspects of this syndrome are apathy, socially inappropriate behavior, and disinhibition that may be expressed as irritability. These symptoms may be prominent when the memory impairment is still mild.

The syndrome of depression shares several of the characteristics of the above dementia syndromes. Nonetheless, rather than seeking to identify the etiological origins of each symptom, it is clinically helpful to examine if the patient meets criteria for depression, dysthymia, or dementia independently. If criteria for one of the depressive syndromes are met or approximated, the clinician should consider an antidepressant treatment trial. The reasons for this recommendation are twofold. First, patients with depression should have the opportunity to receive a potentially effective treatment, regardless of whether they are demented or not. Second, improvement or recovery of the depressive syndrome can increase the clinician's ability to evaluate the severity of the dementing disorder and have a clearer idea of what the prognosis may be.

Prior to initiating antidepressant treatment, depressed-demented patients should be examined for inattention and fluctuating state of consciousness. Elderly patients often develop delirium in response to drug side effects and other toxic or metabolic factors.

Once the decision for an antidepressant treatment trial is made, attention needs to be given to the duration and intensity of antidepressant treatment. Research studies and controversies on the use of antidepressants in demented patients are summarized below. However, for clinical purposes, an antidepressant treatment trial is considered to be of adequate duration if it lasts 9–12 weeks (51). If tricyclics are to be used, nortriptyline or desipramine should be chosen because of their relatively favorable side-effect profile and the extensive research experience in the elderly (52). Similar plasma levels to those of younger adults should be attempted in the elderly (52). If serotonin reuptake inhibitors or other recently developed antidepressants are used, the dosage for geriatric depression should approximate that of younger adults.

Depressed-demented patients who fail to respond to one "adequate" antidepressant trial should be considered for a second antidepressant drug trial or electroconvulsant therapy (ECT). The determining factor in this decision should be the intensity of depressive symptomatology and not the presence or severity of the dementia syndrome. If a patient has a partial response to an "adequate" antidepressant trial, an augmentation technique should be considered, provided that the patient's medical health permits.

The multitude of conditions that may be present in patients with depression-dementia syndromes constitutes an indication for a thorough diagnostic workup seeking to identify treatable neurological disorders. Frequent follow-up is also necessary since dementing disorders may become clinically evident long after the initial recovery of the depression-dementia syndrome. Identification of an emerging dementia syndrome during the follow-up period may lead to the diagnosis of a treatable disorder or help early planning for appropriate living arrangements if the dementing disorder appears to be progressive.

V. TREATMENT OF DEPRESSED-DEMENTED PATIENTS

A. Treatment of Depression

Most experienced psychiatrists believe that depression of demented patients is a treatable condition. However, few controlled studies have specifically focused on the antidepressant treatment of demented patients. What follows summarizes the clinical research experience in the treatment of depression of demented patients, points out differences from the treatment of younger adults and nondemented patients, and outlines areas for new research.

In depression of Alzheimer's patients, open-label studies of tricyclics (53) and monoamine oxidase inhibitors (54) suggest a favorable treatment response. However, controlled treatment studies are sparse and difficult to interpret. An 8-week double-blind study compared imipramine (mean total plasma level: 119 ng/ml) with placebo in Alzheimer's patients who met Diagnostic and Statistical Manual (DSM-III) criteria and in nondepressed Alzheimer's patients (55). Ham-D scores improved in both groups. The efficacy of imipramine, however, was indistinguishable from that of placebo. The above study used a categorically defined population of Alzheimer's patients with major depression. Other studies focused on depressive symptomatology of Alzheimer's populations with a broad range of behavioral disturbances. In patients with Alzheimer's disease or vascular dementia, citalopram was more effective than placebo in reducing scores on the Ham-D and the Montgomery Asberg depression rating scales (56). Citalopram is a selective serotonin reuptake blocker with antidepressant and mood-stabilizing properties. Another study used depressed patients with mild-to-moderate dementia and noted that both low doses of trazodone (100 mg daily) and 5-methyltetrahydrofolic acid significantly reduced depressive symptomatology (57).

Pharmacological studies suggest that elderly depressives often require longer exposure to antidepressants than younger adults (51). The time to recovery of late-onset depressives was observed to be longer than that of early-onset geriatric depressives (58). Although specific studies are needed, one may speculate that late-onset depression may require longer antidepressant trials than early-onset depression. It is unclear, however, whether old age itself, late-onset, or coexisting dementing disorders, medical illnesses, and disability are responsible for the delay in treatment response.

Pharmacological studies of geriatric populations need to determine the role of cognitive impairment, medical burden, disability and even specific dementing disorders in prolonging the latency of response to antidepressant treatment.

There is some evidence that the antidepressant response of geriatric depression may be influenced by morphological brain characteristics, medical burden, disability, and blood chemistry parameters. Preliminary data suggest that large ventricular:brain ratio and third-ventricle-width:cranial width ratio predicted poor response to nortriptyline in geriatric patients with major depression (59). In a naturalistic treatment study of elderly depressives, growth curve analysis was used to observe the long-term course of depressive symptomatology up to the time of recovery. The strongest determinants of depressive symptomatology in this study were poor medical health, unfavorable living conditions, and high severity of depression at baseline (60). Finally, self-care deficits and low serum albumin were found to predict poor response to nortriptyline in a nursing home old-old population (61). Therefore, studies are needed to establish the role of cognitive impairment, appropriate neuroradiological parameters, medical burden, and disability in order to arrive at treatment guidelines for depressed-demented patients.

Most studies have shown that elderly patients with major depression require plasma levels of nortriptyline or desipramine comparable to those of younger depressives (52). However, there is evidence that cognitively impaired depressives and patients with ventriculomegaly may not have drug plasma concentration efficacy relations similar to those of younger adults. In a sample of elderly depressives treated with a fixed-dose nortriptyline regimen, a positive association was observed between nortriptyline plasma concentrations and improvement of depressive symptomatology in cognitively unimpaired patients. No such relationship could be identified in cognitively impaired depressives (62). The reasons for the lack of nortriptyline plasma concentration efficacy relationships in cognitively impaired depressives are unclear. However, cognitively impaired patients had a similar response rate to nortriptyline with the cognitively unimpaired depressives. Therefore, a possible explanation is that cognitive impairment influences the nortriptyline plasma concentration efficacy relationship through pharmacokinetic or pharmacodynamic mechanisms. In another sample, a positive association between plasma nortriptyline concentration and antidepressant response was observed in patients with small lateral brain ventricles. In contrast, there was no significant association between plasma levels and antidepressant efficacy in elderly depressives with large lateral ventricles (59). Poor response to nortriptyline may be the main reason for the lack of nortriptyline plasma concentration efficacy relationships in geriatric depressives with ventriculomegaly. However, one cannot exclude that pharmacokinetic and pharmacodynamic factors unique to patients with ventriculomegaly may influence the plasma concentration efficacy relationships of nortriptyline. These findings need to be followed by studies of the antidepressant concentration efficacy relationship in patients with specific dementing disorders in order to develop guidelines for adequate plasma levels in these populations.

Depressive syndromes are frequent in patients with vascular dementia or stroke. If left untreated, poststroke major depression may last approximately 1 year, while minor depression may last 2 years (63). Two placebo-controlled studies suggest that poststroke depression responds favorably to nortriptyline (35) and trazodone (65). A retrospective treatment study observed that poststroke depression responded favorably to a variety of antidepressants (63).

Some research experience exists on the course and treatment of depression in patients with Parkinson's disease. Despite the chronic course and the degenerative nature of the lesions of depressed Parkinsonian patients, preliminary evidence suggests that nortriptyline (66), desipramine (67), imipramine (68), and bupropion (32) may be effective in the treatment of these patients. ECT as a rule improves tremors, bradykinesia and rigidity early in treatment, while the antidepressant response occurs later (70). The encouraging results of the initial treatment studies should be followed by investigations that focus on specific clinical characteristics of depressed patients with Parkinson's disease, including areas of symptom overlap (motor retardation, cognitive abnormalities). Particular attention is needed on the relationship of antidepressant response to cognitive impairment and specifically to frontal lobe dysfunction since depressed patients with Parkinson's disease have more marked frontal lobe dysfunction compared to those without mood changes (70).

Knowledge about the probability of placebo response is important in the treatment of frail depressed-demented patients who are likely to be treated with ineffective dosages of antidepressants. In young adults, placebo response was found to be associated with early relapse (71). Geriatric studies of placebo responders and their long-term outcome are lacking. However, there is some evidence that placebo response may be frequent in some depressed-demented populations. Early clinical literature suggests that depressive symptomatology of demented patients is transient and recurrent (72). A controlled study observed that almost 50% of depressed Alzheimer's patients responded to placebo, a percentage comparable to imipramine response (55). Studies are needed to determine if cognitive impairment and perhaps presence of specific dementing disorder are associated with frequent response to placebo and a high relapse rate after an initial improvement to small dosages of antidepressants.

Tricyclic antidepressants have been reported to impair memory (73). Demented patients already have compromised memory. Prescribing tricyclics may add to the existing memory impairment of a demented patient. Therefore, follow-up assessment should determine whether the tricyclic-induced memory impairment is clinically significant or whether changes in antidepressant treatment are indicated.

Tricyclic antidepressants may cause delirium, mainly through central antimuscarinic action (52). Delirium is more likely to occur in patients with high tricyclic plasma levels (74). However, some patients have been reported to develop delirium while on therapeutic (75) or even subtherapeutic (76) levels of tricyclic antidepressants. Advanced age and female gender appear to increase vulnerability of delirium (77). Moreover, demented patients with a compromised central cholinergic system may be particularly prone to delirium. For these reasons, use of tricyclics in demented elderly should be monitored carefully. Changes in affective, psychotic, and cognitive symptoms have been observed to precede delirium by 15 days in a broad age-range population (77). These clinical changes should alert clinicians to the possibility of a pending delirium. It should be noted that a prospective naturalistic treatment study observed that depressed Alzheimer's patients did not develop delirium at greater frequency than other elderly patients even when treated with therapeutic concentrations of tricyclic antidepressants (78). Delirium appears to be infrequent in patients treated with serotonin reuptake inhibitors unless very high plasma levels are used (79). However, specific studies are lacking.

Stimulants may be of some help in depressed-demented patients. A review by Satel and Nelson (80) concluded that most of this literature has limitations. However, the existing controlled studies suggest that stimulants are rather ineffective in uncomplicated, primary depression (80). In contrast, controlled studies of stimulants in apathetic or depressed geriatric patients show partial efficacy (80). Moreover, favorable outcomes have been reported by uncontrolled studies of medically ill patients treated with stimulants (81,82). Stimulants are well tolerated and pose little risk for habituation and for drug-seeking behavior by the elderly. Despite the methodological limitations of studies on stimulants, these agents should be considered in depressed-demented patients who do not tolerate or fail to improve after treatment with antidepressants.

B. Treatment of Dementing Disorders

Pharmacological agents used in the treatment of dementing disorders may influence not only the course of dementia but also the course of depression in depressed-demented patients. The majority of depressed-demented patients have Alzheimer's disease, vascular dementia, or both disorders. While no definitive treatment for Alzheimer's disease is available, some drugs may reduce to some extent the cognitive and cognitive symptoms of Alzheimer's disease. Tetra-aminoacridine has been found to improve cognitive function in Alzheimer's patients with mild-to-moderate dementia (83). This drug may also help agitated Alzheimer's patients with advanced disease and is less toxic than neuroleptics. Ergotamine compounds (84) and the monoamine oxidase type B inhibitor 1-deprenyl (85) appear to reduce the noncognitive behavioral disturbances of Alzheimer's patients. It is clinically important to investigate whether these agents influence the acute treatment and whether they improve or worsen the relapse rate of depression in Alzheimer's patients.

Agents developed for the prevention of cerebrovascular disease may be relevant to the treatment of patients who develop depression in the context of vascular dementia or cerebrovascular disease that does not reach the level of dementia. Effective treatment of hypertension and hyperlipidemia can reduce cerebrovascular morbidity and mortality (86,87) and should be considered in depressed patients with hypertension or high cholesterol levels. Research is needed to examine whether specific antihypertensive or anticholesterinemia therapies improve the long-term outcome of depression as they reduce vascular events. Antiplatelet agents such as aspirin and ticlopidine have been found effective in reducing cerebrovascular episodes in large populations at risk for cerebrovascular disease (88). It remains to be investigated whether these agents can reduce the incidence or recurrence of depression in patients with risk factors for cerebrovascular disease.

Free radical scavengers may have a role in the prevention of new vascular events in patients with vascular dementia. Production of free radical appears to influence the pathophysiology of reperfusion of injury following transient ischemia. Tocopherol was found to decrease neuronal loss after ischemia and reduce cerebral ischemic edema if given prior to an ischemic event (89). Since antioxidants are well tolerated by elderly patients, studies need to investigate whether these antioxidants can prevent new episodes or recurrences of depression in patients with vascular dementia or vascular risk factors.

Agents that reduce damage after ischemic brain events may have relevance for the treatment of patients who develop depression in the context of vascular dementia or cerebrovascular disease. Nimodipine, a calcium channel blocker, was found to improve the outcome of ischemic stroke when administered in the first 12 h after the ischemic event (90). This action is thought to be mediated by reduction of calcium influx into the neuron, an event that follows excessive activation of postsynaptic glutamate NMDA receptors following ischemic injury (91). Gangliosides may limit postinfarction damage through their membrane-protective function and their neuroprotective action (92) and 21-aminosteroids may have a beneficial effect through their edema-reducing qualities (93). The role of these agents in depression of patients with cerebrovascular disease is unclear. However, research is needed to examine their efficacy as early interventions in patients with cerebrovascular disease who present a depressive recurrence or develop a new disability abruptly.

Drugs that alter monoamine neurotransmitter function appear to influence postischemic recovery. Amphetamine combined with physical therapy was reported to promote motor recovery (94) and bromocriptine appears to improve nonfluent aphasia (95). The effect of amphetamine on motor recovery is thought to be mediated by noradrenergic pathways. Support for this view comes from the fact that the α_2-antagonist yohimbine as well as the norepinephrine reuptake inhibitor desipramine facilitate motor recovery (96,97). In contrast, the α_1-receptor antagonists phenoxybenzamine and prazocin, as well as lesions of the locus ceruleus, reinstate functional deficits when administered during the recovery period after ischemic lesions (98,99). A mechanism by which noradrenergic agents facilitate recovery is thought to be their ability to reduce diaschisis and thus promote resolution of functional suppression in areas remote to the ischemic lesion (100). An alternative mechanism may be that enhancement of norepinephrine neurotransmission enables the locus ceruleus to switch control from the corticospinal tract to the rubrospinal tract during motor learning (101). The spinocortical pathway is active when new motor skills are learned and the rubrospinal pathway is active when already learned movements are performed (101,102). In lesions of the sensorimotor cortex, this switch can be beneficial to motor rehabilitation.

Dopamine agonists, cholinergic agents, GABAergic drugs, and some antidepressants may influence recovery from ischemic lesions. Bromocriptine (95) and apomorphine (103) were observed to reduce nonfluent aphasia and neglect in stroke victims while haloperidol may slow language recovery (104). Cholinergic agents may reduce functional deficits after ischemia by facilitating long-term potentiation and changing the synaptic efficacy that is thought to provide the physiological basis of information (105,106). Through this process, the intact part of the brain assumes the functions that had been performed by the areas damaged by the stroke. Benzodiazepines and phenytoin through a GABA-mediated action may suppress long-term potentiation and interfere with recovery (107,108). Several agents have been found effective in relieving depression of stroke patients, including trazodone (65), nortriptyline (64,109), amphetamine (110), and methylphenidate (111,112). However, animal experiments suggest that antidepressants have different effects on recovery after ischemic lesions. In rats, desipramine was noted to promote motor recovery while fluoxetine had no significant effect on recovery after ischemic damage (97). In contrast, trazodone and amitriptyline appeared to slow recovery or reinstate postischemia motor function deficits (97,113). These negative effects were thought to be mediated by antagonism of the α_1-noradrenergic receptor (114). Research is needed to examine if some antidepressants should be favored over others in depressed patients with cerebrovascular disease who are candidates for new ischemic lesions.

The stage of recovery may influence the choice and timing of interventions. After lesions of the bifurcating norepinephrine neurons of the locus ceruleus, "compensatory arborization" occurs and results in reactive sprouting of dendritic or axonal processes. Excessive sprouting beyond optimal levels has been proposed to account for the hypertonic state that some patients experience some time after the occurrence of cortical ischemic lesions (115). It has been suggested that drugs that reduce norepinephrine output, such as the α_2-agonist clonidine, may prevent hypertonicity (116) by reducing excessive sprouting. Pharmacological studies need to examine if interventions appropriately timed in relation to an ischemic event can be helpful in preventing postischemia depression.

VI. CONCLUSIONS

1. The diagnosis of depression in demented elderly patients is complicated by many factors. These include unreliable reports of symptoms, fluctuations of depressive symptomatology over time, and overlap of symptoms of depression with those of dementia. Prolonged observation and use of information from both patients and caregivers can improve the clinicians' ability to identify depression in demented patients. The most effective approach to diagnosis is to seek to identify various behavioral syndromes (e.g., depression, dementia, frontal lobe syndrome), rather than making the assumption that only one syndrome exists at a time. After all, dementing disorders do not confer immunity for depression. Instead, they increase the incidence of depression. If a depressive syndrome is identified, antidepressant treatment should be considered. Follow-up should then seek to ascertain whether the remaining symptoms are part of a residual depression or result from an underlying dementing disorder.
2. Most clinicians agree that antidepressants are effective in the treatment of depression of demented patients. However, several observations suggest that the guidelines for antidepressant treatment in these patients may be different than those of younger adults. "Placebo

response" may be frequent in demented patients who tend to have a spontaneously changing depressive symptomatology. Early improvement in depression of demented patients should not be interpreted as a pharmacological response. Such patients may have a worsening of their depression within a few days or hours. For this reason, they should be followed carefully.

3. The tricyclic plasma levels that are considered therapeutic in cognitively unimpaired elderly patients may not be relevant to depressed-demented patients. Emerging evidence suggests that cognitive impairment and ventriculomegaly influence the plasma level efficacy relationships. Studies of plasma levels of tricyclic antidepressants used in depressed-demented patients are needed.
4. Depression often develops in patients with cerebrovascular disease who have become demented or have cognitive impairment that has not reached the level of dementia. Assuming that vascular lesions can lead to a "vascular depression" syndrome, research needs to examine the impact of agents used in the prevention and treatment of cerebrovascular disease in changing the outcomes of late-onset depression. It is conceivable that effective prevention and treatment of vascular disease may reduce progression of cognitive impairment and even improve the depressive relapse rate in geriatric patients. Finally, animal studies suggest that some antidepressants promote neurological recovery after ischemic lesions while other antidepressants as well as haloperidol, phenytoin, and benzodiazepines inhibit recovery. Clinical studies are needed to establish treatment guidelines for depressed patients with clinical evidence of cerebrovascular disease.

REFERENCES

1. Reifler BV, Larson E, Hanley R. Coexistence of cognitive impairment and depression in geriatric outpatients. Am J Psychiatry 1982; 139:623–626.
2. Reding M, Haycox J, Blass J. Depression in patients referred to a dementia clinic. Arch Neurol 1985; 42:894–896.
3. Rovner BW, Broadhead J, Spencer M, Carson K, Folstein MF. Depression and Alzheimer's disease. Am J Psychiatry 1989; 146:1239.
4. Greenwald BS, Kramer-Ginsberg G, Martin DB, Laidman LB, Hermann CK, Mohs R, Davis KL. Dementia with coexistent major depression. Am J Psychiatry 1989; 146:1472–1478.
5. Weiner MF, Bruhn M, Svetlik D, Tintner R, Hom J. Experiences with depression in a dementia clinic. J Clin Psychiatry 1991; 52:234–238.
6. Nelson JC, Conwell Y, Kim K, Mazure CM. Concurrence of dementia in inpatients with affective disorder. Abstract of the Annual Meeting of the American Association of Geriatric Psychiatry, 1990.

7. Koenig HG, Cohen HJ, Blazer DG, Krishnan KR, Sibert TE. Profile of depressive symptoms in younger and older medical inpatients with major depression. J Am Geriatr Soc 1993; 41:1169–1176.
8. Wells KB, Stewart A, Hays RD, et al. The functioning and well being of depressed patients. Results from the Medical Outcomes Study. J Am Med Assoc 1989; 262: 914–919.
9. Benson DF, Stuss DT. Theories of frontal lobe function. Neurology and Psychiatry: A Meeting of the Minds. Mueller J, ed. Basel: Karger, 1989:266–283.
10. Alexopoulos GS, Abrams RC. Depression in Alzheimer's disease. Psychiatr Clin North Am 1991; 14:327–340.
11. Yesavage JA, Brink TL, Rose TL, et al. The geriatric rating scale: Comparison with other self-reports and psychiatric rating scales. In: Crook T, Gerris S, Bartus R, eds. Assessment in Geriatric Psychopharmacology. New Canaan, CT: Mark Powley Associates, 1983:153–165.
12. Sunderland T, Alterman IS, Yound D, Hill JL, et al. A new scale for the assessment of mood in demented patients. Am J Psychiatry 1988; 145:955–959.
13. Alexopoulos GS, Abrams RC, Young RC, Shamoian CA. Cornell scale for depression in dementia. Biol Psychiatry 1988; 23:271–284.
14. Alexopoulos GS, Abrams RC, Young RC, Shamoian CA. use of the Cornell scale on non-demented patients. J Am Geriatr Soc 1988; 36:230–236.
15. Katona CLE, Aldridge CR. The dexamethasone suppresion test and depressive signs in dementia. J Affect Disord 1985; 8:83–89.
16. Mulsant BH, Sweet R, Rifai AH, Pasternak RE, McEachran A, Zubenko GS. The use of the Hamilton rating scale for depression in elderly patients with cognitive impairment and physical illness. Am J Geriatric Psychiatry 1994; 2:220–229.
17. Emergy O. Pseudodementia: A Theoretical and Empirical Discussion: Interdisciplinary Monograph Series. Cleveland, Western Reserve Geriatric Education Center, Case Western Reserve University School of Medicine, 1988.
18. Kiloh L. Depressive illness masquerading as dementia in the elderly. Med J Aust 1981; 2:550–553.
19. Wells CE. Pseudodementia. Am J Psychiatry 1979; 136:895–900.
20. Alexopoulos GS, Young RC, Meyers BS, Abrams RC, Shamoian CA. Late-onset depression. Psychiatr Clin North Am 1988; 11:101–115.
21. Emery VO, Oxman TE. Update on the dementia spectrum of depression. Am J Psychiatry 1992; 149:305–317.
22. Rabins P, Merchant A, Nestadt G. Criteria for diagnosing reversible dementia caused by depression: validation by 2-year follow-up. Br J Psychiatry 1984; 144: 488–492.
23. Young RC, Manley M, Alexopoulos GS. "I don't know" responses in elderly depressives and in dementia. J Am Geriatr Soc 1985; 33:253–357.
24. Kahn RL, Zarit SH, Hilbert NM, Niederehe G. Memory complaint and impairment in the aged. Arch Gen Psychiatry 1975; 32:1569–1573.
25. Meyers BS. Adverse cognitive effects of tricyclic antidepressants in the treatment of geriatric depression: Fact or fiction? Edited by Shamoian CA. In Psychopharmacological Treatment Complications in the Elderly. Washington, DC, American Psychiatric Press, 1992:1–16.

26. Alexopoulos GS. Clinical and biological findings in late-onset depression. Tasman A, Goldfinger SM, Kaufmann CA, eds. American Psychiatric Press Review of Psychiatry 1990; 9:249–262.
27. Reynolds CF III, Hoch CC, Kupfer DJ, Buysse DJ, Houck PR, Stack JA, Campbell DW. Bedside differentiation of depressive pseudodementia from dementia. Am J Psychiatry 1988; 145:1099–1103.
28. Reynolds CF, Kupfer DJ, Houck PR, Hoch CC, Stack JA, Berman SR, Zimmer B. Reliable discrimination of elderly depressed and demented patients by electroencephalographic sleep data. Arch Gen Psychiatry 1988; 45:258–264.
29. Caine E. Pseudodementia: current concepts and future directions. Arch Gen Psychiatry 1981; 38:1359–1364.
30. Alexopoulos GS, Young RC, Haycox JA, Shamoian CA, Blass JP. Dexamethasone suppression test in depression with reversible dementia. Psychiatry Res 1985; 16: 277–285.
31. Alexopoulos GS, Young RC, Lieberman KW, Shamoian CA. Platelet MAO activity in geriatric patients with depression and dementia. Am J Psychiatry 1987; 144: 1480–1483.
32. Pearlson GD, Rabins PV, Kims WS, Speedie LJ, Moberg PJ, Burns A, Bascom MJ. Structural brain CT changes and cognitive deficits in elderly depressives with and without reversible dementia ("pseudodementia"). Psychol Med 1989; 19:573–584.
33. Pearlson GS, Rabins PR, Burns A. Centrum semiovale white matter CT changes associated with normal aging, Alzheimer's disease and late life depression with and without reversible dementia. Psychol Med 1991; 21:321–328.
34. Brenner R, Reynolds C, Ulrich R. EEG findings in depressive pseudodementia and dementia with secondary depression. Electroencephalogr Clin Neurophysiol 1989; 72:298–304.
35. Buysse D, Reynolds C, Kupfer D, Houck PR, Hock CC, Stack JA, Berman SR. Electroencephalographic sleep in depressive pseudodementia. Arch Gen Psychiatry 1988; 45:568–575.
36. Alexopoulos GS, Meyers BS, Young RC, Abrams RC, Shamoian CA. Brain changes in geriatric depression. Int J Geriatr Psychiatry 1988; 3:157–161.
37. Reifler BV, Larson E, Teri L, Poulsen M. Dementia of the Alzheimer's type and depression. J Am Geriatr Soc 1986; 34:855–859.
38. Kral V, Emery O. Long term follow-up of depressive pseudodementia. Can J Psychiatry 1989; 34:445–447.
39. Reynolds CF, Kupfer DJ, Hoch CC, Stack JA, Houck PR, Sewitch DE. Two-year follow-up of elderly patients with mixed depression and dementia. Clinical and electroencephalographic sleep findings. J Am Geriatr Soc 1986; 34:793–799.
40. Copeland JRM, Davidson IA, Dewey ME, Gilmore C, Larkin BA, McWilliam C, Saunders PA, Scott A, Sharma V, Sullivan C. Alzheimer's disease, other dementias, depression and pseudodementia: Prevalence, incidence and three year outcome in Liverpool. Br J Psychiatry 1992; 161:230–239.
41. Alexopoulos GS, Meyers BS, Young RC, Mattis S, Kakuma T. The course of geriatric depression with "reversible dementia": A controlled study. Am J Psychiatry 1993; 150:1693–1699.

42. Wragg RE, Jeste DV. Overview of depression and psychosis in Alzheimer's disease. Am J Psychiatry 1989; 146:577–589.
43. Alexopoulos GS. Heterogeneity and comorbidity in dementia-depression syndromes. Int J Geriatr Psychiatry 1991; 6:125–127.
44. Sano M, Stern Y, Williams J, Cote L, Rosenstein R, Mayeux R. Coexisting dementia and depression in Alzheimer's disease. Arch Neurol 1989; 46:1284–1286.
45. Rovner BW, Bradhead J, Spencer M, Carson K, Folstein MF. Depression and Alzheimer's disease. Am J Psychiatry 1989; 146:350–353.
46. Agbayewa MO. Earlier psychiatric morbidity in patients with Alzheimer's disease. J Am Geriatr Soc 1986; 34:561–564.
47. Henry GM, Weingartner H, Murphy DL. Influence on affective states and psychoactive drugs on verbal learning and memory. Am J Psychiatry 1973; 130:966–971.
48. Fogel B, Sparadeo FR. Focal cognitive deficits accentuated by depression. J Nerv Ment Disord 1985; 173:120–123.
49. Dolan RJ, Bench CJ, Brown RG, Scott LC, Friston KJ, Franckowiak RC. Regional cerebral blood flow abnormalities in depressed patients with cognitive impairment. J Neurol Neurosurg Psychiatry 1992; 55:768–773.
50. Devanant DP, Nelson JC. Concurrent depression and dementia: Implications for diagnosis and treatment. J Clin Psychiatry 1985; 46:389–392.
51. Georgotas A, McCue RE. The additional benefit of extending an antidepressant trial past seven weeks in the depressed elderly. Int J Geriatr Psychiatry 1989; 4:191–195.
52. Alexopoulos GS. Treatment of depression. In: Salzman C, ed. Clinical Geriatric Psychopharmacology, 2nd ed. Baltimore: Williams & Wilkins, 1992.
53. Reynolds CF, Perel JM, Kupfer DJ, Zimmer B, Stack J, Hoch CC. Open-trial response to antidepressant treatment in elderly patients with mixed depression and cognitive impairment. Psychiatry Res 1987; 21:111–122.
54. Ashford JW, Ford CV. Use of MAO inhibitors in elderly patients. Am J Psychiatry 1979; 136:1466–1467.
55. Reifler BV, Teri L, Raskind M, Veith R, Barnes R, White E, McLean P. Double-blind trial of imipramine in Alzheimer's disease patients with and without depression. Am J Psychiatry 1989; 146:45–49.
56. Gottfries C-G, Karlsson I, Nyth AL. Treatment of depression in elderly patients with and without dementia disorders. Int Clin Psychopharm 1992; 6(suppl 5):55–64.
57. Passeri M, Cucinotta D, Abate G, Senin U, Ventura A, Strama-Babiale M, Diana R, LaGreca P, LeGrazie C. Oral 5-methyltetrahydrofolic acid in senile organic mental disorders with depression: Results of a double-blind multicenter study. Aging Milano 1993; 5:63–71.
58. Alexopoulos GS, Meyers BS, Young RC, Kakuma T, Feder M, Einhorn A, Rosendahl E. Recovery in geriatric depression. Arch Gen Psychiatry 1996; 53: 305–312.
59. Young RC, Nambudiri D, Alexopoulos GS. Brain morphology and response to nortriptyline in elderly depressives. Abstract. Annual Meeting, American Association of Geriatric Psychiatry, 1990.

60. Alexopoulos GS. Predictors of recovery and disability in geriatric major depression. Unpublished data.
61. Katz IR, Simpson GM, Curlik SM, Parmelee P, Muhly C. Pharmacologic treatment of major depression for elderly patients in residential care settings. J Clin Psychiatry 1990; 51:41–47.
62. Young RC, Mattis S, Alexopoulos GS, Meyers BS, Shindledecker RD, Dhar AK. Verbal memory and plasma drug concentrations in elderly depressives treated with nortriptyline. Psychopharmacol Bull 1991; 27:291–294.
63. Federoff JP, Robinson RG. Tricyclic antidepressants in the treatment of post-stroke depression. J Clin Psychiatry 1989; 50:18–33.
64. Lipsey JR, Spencer WC, Rabins PV, et al. Phenomenological comparison of post-stroke depression and functional depression. Am J Psychiatry 1986; 143:527–529.
65. Reding MJ, Orto LA, Winter SW, et al. Antidepressant therapy after stroke. A double blind trial. Arch Neurol 1986; 43:763–765.
66. Andersen J, Aabro E, Gulmann N, Hjelmsted A, Pedersen HE. Antidepressant treatment in Parkinson's disease: A controlled trial of the effect of nortriptyline in patients with Parkinson's disease treated with L-dopa. Acta Neurol Scand 1980; 62:210–219.
67. Laitinen L. Despiramine in treatment of Parkinson's disease. Acta Neurol Scand 1969; 45:109–113.
68. Strang RR. Imipramine in treatment of Parkinsonism: A double-blind placebo study. Br Med J 1965; 2:33–34.
69. Goetz GG, Tanner CM, Klawans HL. Bupropion in Parkinson's disease. Neurology 1984; 34:1092–1094.
70. Cummings JL. Depression and Parkinson's disease: A review. Am J Psychiatry 1992; 149:443–454.
71. Quitkin FM, Stewart JN, McGrath PJ, Nunes E, Ocepek-Welikson K, Tricamo E, Rabkin JG, Ross J, Klein DF. Loss of drug effects during continuation therapy. Am J Psychiatry 1993; 150:563–565.
72. Roth M. The natural history of mental disorders in old age. J Ment Sci 1955; 01: 281–301.
73. Richardson JS, Keegan DL, Bowen RC, Blackshaw SL, Cebrian-Perez S, Dayal N, Saleh S, Shrikhande S. Verbal learning by major depressive disorder patients during treatment with fluoxetine or amitriptyline. Int Clin Psychopharmacol 1994; 9(1):35–40.
74. Livingston RL, Zucker DK, Isenberg K, Wetzel RD. Tricyclic antidepressants and delirium. J Clin Psychiatry 1983; 44(5):173–176.
75. Godwin CD. Case report of tricyclic-induced delirium at a therapeutic drug concentration. Am J Psychiatry 1983; 140(11):1517–1518.
76. Kutcher SP, Shulman KI. Desipramine-induced delirium at "subtherapeutic" concentrations: A case report. Can J Psychiatry 1985; 30(5):368–369.
77. Preskorn SH, Jerkovich GS. Central nervous system toxicity of tricyclic antidepressants: phenomenology, course, risk factors, and role of therapeutic drug monitoring. J Clin Psychopharmacol 1990; 10(2):88–95.
78. Meyers BS, Mei-Tal V. Psychiatric reactions during tricyclic treatment of the elderly reconsidered. J Clin Psychopharmacol 1983; 3(1):2–6.

79. Bangs ME, Petti TA, Janus MD. Fluoxetine-induced memory impairment in an adolescent. J Am Acad Child Adoles Psychiatry 1994; 33(9):1303–1306.
80. Satel SL, Nelson JC. Stimulants in the treatment of depression: A critical overview. J Clin Psychiatry 1989; 50:241–249.
81. Woods SW, Tesar GE, Murray GB, et al. Psychostimulant treatment of depressive disorders secondary to medical illness. J Clin Psychiatry 1986; 47:12–15.
82. Masand P, Pickett P, Murray GB. Psychostimulants for secondary depression in medical illness. Psychosomatics 1991; 32:203–208.
83. Farlow M, Croxcon SI, Hershey LA, Lewis KW, Soldowsky CH. A controlled trial of tacrine in Alzheimer's disease. J Am Med Assoc 1993; 269:2848–2850.
84. Schneider LS, Olin JT. Overview of clinical trials in hydergine in dementia. Arch Neurol 1994; 51:787–798.
85. Burke WJ, Rouaforte WH, Wengel SP, Bauer BL, Willcockson NK. L-deprenyl in the treatment of mild dementia of the Alzheimer type. J Am Geriatr Soc 1993; 41:1219–1225.
86. Insua JT, Sacks HS, Lau TS, Reitman D, Pagano D, Chalners TC. Drug treatment of hypertension in the elderly: a meta-analysis. Ann Intern Med 1994; 121:355–362.
87. Sirtori CR. The treatment of hypercholesterolemia in primary and secondary prevention. Ann Ital Med Int 1995; 10(suppl):48S–52S.
88. Raps EC, Galetta SL. Stroke prevention therapies and managing patient subgroups. Neurology 1995; 45 (2 Suppl 1):S19–S24.
89. Abe K, Yuki S, Kogure K. Strong attenuation of ischemic and postischemic brain edema in rats by a novel free radical scavenger. Stroke 1988; 19:480–485.
90. Mohr JP, Dilanni M, Muschett JL, Riccio RV, Bessalaar GH, et al. The Nimodipine Study Group. Nimodipine in acute ischemic stroke. Ann Neurol 1989; 26–124 (Abstract).
91. Fujisawa A, Matsumoto M, Matsuyama T, et al. The effect of the calcium antagonist nimodipine on the gerbil model of experimental cerebral ischemia. Stroke 1986; 17:748–752.
92. Karpiak SE, Li SU, Mahadik SP. Gangliosides (GM1 and AGF2) reduce mortality due to ischemia: protection of membrane function. Stroke 1987; 18:184–187.
93. Young W, Wojak JC, DeCrescito V. 21-Aminosteroid reduces ion shifts and edema in the rate middle cerebral artery occlusion model of regional ischemia. Stroke 1988; 19:1013–1019.
94. Crisostomo EA, Dunan PW, Propst MA, Dawson DB, Davis JN. Evidence that amphetamine with physical therapy promotes recovery of motor function in stroke patients. Ann Neurol 1988; 94–97.
95. Gupta SR, Michoch. Bromocriptine treatment of nonfluent aphasia. Arch Phys Med Rehabil 1992; 73:373–376.
96. Goldstein LB, Poe HV, Davis JN. An animal model of recovery of function after stroke: facilitation of recovery by an alpha2-adrenergic receptor antagonist. Ann Neurol 1989; 26:157 (abstract).
97. Boyerson MG, Harmon RL. Effects of trazodone and desipramine on motor recovery in brain-injured rats. Am J Phys Med Rehab 1993; 72:286–293.

98. Weaver MS, Farmer LJ, Feeney DM. Norepinephrine agonists and antagonists influence rate and maintenance of recovery of function after sensorimotor cortex contusion in the rat. Soc Neurosci Abstr 1987; 13:477 (Abstract).
99. Sutton RL, Feeney DM. Yohimbine accelerates recovery and clonidine and prazosin reinstate deficits after recovery in rats with sensorimotor cortex ablation. Soc Neurosci Abstr 1987; 13:913 (Abstract).
100. Feeney DM, Sutton RL. Pharmacotherapy for recovery of function after brain injury. CRC Crit Rev Neurobiol 1987; 3:135–197.
101. Kennedy PR. Corticospinal, rubrospinal and rubro-olivary projections: A unifying hypothesis. Trends Neurosci 1990; 12:474–479.
102. Massion J. Red nucleus: Past and future. Behav Brain Res 1988; 28:1–8.
103. Fleet W, Valenstein E, Watson RT, Heilman KM. Dopamine agonist therapy for neglect in humans. Neurology 1987; 37:1765–1770.
104. Porch B, Wyckes J, Feeney DM. Haloperidol, thiazides, and some antihypertensives slow recovery from aphasia. Soc Neurosci Abstr 1985; 11:52 (Abstract).
105. Feeney DM, Sutton RL. Pharmacotherapy for recovery of function after brain injury. CRC Crit Rev Neurobiol 1987; 3:135–197.
106. Tazaki Y, Sakai F, Otomo E. Treatment of acute cerebral infarction with a choline precursor in a multicenter double-blind placebo controlled study. Stroke 1988; 19:211–216.
107. Goldstein L. Pharmacologic modulation of recovery after stroke: Clinical data. J Neuro Rehab 1991; 5:129–140.
108. Brailowsky, Knight RT, Efron R. Phenytoin increases the severity of cortical hemiplegia in rats. Brain Res 1986; 376-71-77.
109. Lazarus LW, Moberg PJ, Langsley PR, Lingam V. Methylphenidate and nortriptyline in the treatment of post-stroke depression: A retrospective comparison. Arch Med Rehab 1994; 75:403–406.
110. Masand P, Murray GB, Pickett P. Psychostimulants in post-stroke depression. J Neuro Psychiatr Clin Neurosci 1991; 3:23–27.
111. Lingham VR, Lazarus LW, Groves L, Oh SH. Methylphenidate in treating post-stroke depression. J Clin Psychiatry 1988; 49:151–153.
112. Lazarus LW, Winemiller DR, Lingam VR, Robinson RG. Efficacy and side effects of methylphenidate for poststroke depression. J Clin Psychiatry 1992; 53: 447–449.
113. Boyerson MG, Harmon RL, Jones JL. Differential effects of fluoxetine, amitriptyline and serotonin S2 antagonist, markedly reduces infarct size following middle and cerebral artery occlusion in the rat. Neurology 1988; 38:1667–1673.
114. Boyerson MG, Jones JL, Harmon RL. Sparing of motor function after cortical injury. A new perspective on underlying mechanisms. Arch Neurol 1994; 51:405–414.
115. Crosby EC, Schneider RC, Jonge BR, Szonyl P. The alterations of tonus and movements through the interplay between the cerebral hemispheres and the cerebellum. J Comp Neurol 1966; 127–191.
116. Sanford PR, Sprengler SE, Sawasky KB. Clonidine in the treatment of brain stem spasticity: case report. Am J Phys Med Rehabil 1992; 71:301–303.

13
Use of Stimulants in Depressed Patients with Medical Illness

George B. Murray and Edwin Cassem
Massachusetts General Hospital, and Harvard Medical School, Boston, Massachusetts

I. HISTORY

SmithKline and French introduced the benzedrine inhaler for medicinal purposes over 50 years ago. For physicians, the ensuing decades brought first enthusiasm for the multiplicity of amphetamine uses, followed by disillusionment, when widespread abuse with its attendant morbidity was realized (1). Despite this, dextroamphetamine and methylphenidate have remained useful in the treatment of narcolepsy and attention deficit disorder with hyperactivity.

This chapter briefly reviews the history of amphetamines, their central mechanism of action, and focuses on the utility of psychostimulants in treating depression in patients with coexisting physical illness, especially the geriatric patient.

Racemic phenylisopropylamine, named amphetamine by the American Medical Association in 1932, was first synthesized in 1887 by the German pharmacologist, Edelean (2), although it was Barger and Dale in 1910 who first studied the effects of this and other "sympathomimetic amines." In addition to the peripheral alpha and beta actions common to the indirectly acting sympathomimetic drugs, amphetamine was noted to have potent CNS effects. Unlike epinephrine, however, it was effective after oral administration, with an effect lasting for several hours. In 1928, Alles reported that the dextro-isomer of amphetamine (i.e., dextroamphetamine) was three to four times more potent than the L-isomer in inducing euphoria, enhancing alertness, and diminishing fatigue (3).

Prompted by further reports from Alles of the efficacy of these drugs via the inhaled route, the benzedrine inhaler (D-L amphetamine) was introduced on the market in 1932, for use as a decongestant. The American Medical Association subsequently endorsed amphetamine in tablet form in 1937.

Physicians gave prompt and enthusiastic endorsement to these over-the-counter stimulants in the 1930s and soon the national media was publicizing the new "pep" and "superman" pills. Amphetamine was advocated widely for such conditions as narcolepsy, postencephalitic parkinsonism, nocturnal enuresis, barbiturate toxicity, depressive syndromes, and fatigue. The anorexogenic properties of amphetamines were reported in 1938, but the observation that tolerance developed quite consistently to this therapeutic effect was only realized later (4).

Before long, a steady stream of amphetamine congeners became available, including methamphetamine, synthesized in 1929, and later phenmetrazine, which was widely abused in Sweden in the 1960s. Methylphenidate (Ritalin), a stimulant of lesser potency than amphetamine, though possessing a greater CNS selectivity, was developed by Meier and others in 1954 (5).

Within 3 years after benzedrine's introduction in tablet form, U.S. sales rose to more than 50 million units. Attracted by its stimulant qualities, many began to abuse the amphetamines, particularly students, truck drivers, performers, and athletes.

The most striking psychiatric complication of stimulant abuse, the "amphetamine psychosis" was first reported in 1938 (1), and reviewed in detail by Connell 20 years later (6). The development of the psychosis usually was associated with a prolonged abuse pattern, with daily consumption in the range of 100–500 mg. A paranoid state with hallucinations was the characteristic presentation. It lacked the specific features of an organic delirium, namely, absence of a confusional state. Similar abuse of methylphenidate has led to an identical type of psychosis.

In the United States, a production of amphetamine tablets continued to rise after World War II. By 1969, an annual production of 8 billion tablets was estimated, with 50% of their total probably diverted into illegitimate channels. The 1960s also brought increasing popularity to high-dose, intravenous methamphetamine use, and the rise of a subculture of "speed freaks" with a unique set of experiences: euphoria ("the flash"), anorexia, insomnia, paranoia, violence, compulsivity, "over-amping," and death.

Compared to the 1960s, the current abuse of amphetamines has decreased substantially, due in part to the rise in popularity of cocaine. For the most part, after World War II and again in the 1960s and 1970s, the psychiatric community warned away from the psychostimulants, especially amphetamines (7).

II. PHARMACOKINETICS

Table 1 displays some pharmacokinetic elements of the two main psychostimulants used in inpatient use. We do not find great differences in their clinical use. Milligram for milligram, dextroamphetamine is just about twice as potent as methylphenidate, with an elimination half-life also about twice as long as that of methylphenidate.

We usually start a patient on 5 mg of dextroamphetamine or 10 mg methylphenidate, p.o. q.d., usually at about 0800 hours. We find that the duration of effect with dextroamphetamine is longer than the usually stated 6 h. Therefore, we tend not to use dextroamphetamine more than once a day. We often use b.i.d. dosage for methylphenidate, the second dose given before 1600 hours so as not to interfere with sleep.

Both agents have sustained-release preparations and are seldom used for medically ill inpatients. They are clinically relevant to patients who benefit from stimulants over a longer period of time. We almost never use them for inpatient consultations.

III. CLINICAL USE OF PSYCHOSTIMULANTS

The great bulk of our work was done on the Psychiatric Consultation Service at Massachusetts General Hospital (MGH). We were looking for a faster-acting antidepressant since most of the medical and surgical patients seen were not hospitalized for 2 or more weeks. Our anecdotal experience was that protriptylene, with a chemical structure somewhat similar to amphetamine, produced the fastest response. However, protriptylene was abandoned after about 2 years because of its strong anticholinergic effects, especially the production of tachycardia.

We then went directly to methylphenidate and dextroamphetamine. We did not use the psychostimulant pemoline (Cylert®) because of its long latency prior to a response.

TABLE 1 Pharmacokinetics

	Dextroamphetamine	Methylphenidate
Single-dose range	2.5–20 mg	5–20 mg
Daily-dose range	2.5–20 mg	5–40 mg
Usual start dose	2.5–5 mg q.d.	5–10 mg q.d.
Peak plasma level	3–4 h	1–3 h
Plasma elimination half-life	6–8 h	2–4 h
Onset of effect	1 h	1 h
Duration of effect	6–10 h	4–5 h

Academic studies on amphetamine and related substances were not clear in showing their greater efficacy relative to tricyclics and monoamine oxidase inhibitors (MAOIs) (8), but our clinical experience indicated that they were fast-acting and seemed to be antidepressant in effect. Wittenborn (9) reviewed the literature to understand why psychostimulants never attained unqualified acceptance. He mentions that most observers think depressive states in the geriatric population are clinically different from depressive states in young people. In 1958, Jacobsen (10) studied 54 geriatric patients split into two groups, those receiving psychotherapy alone and those receiving psychotherapy and methylphenidate. The second group had many fewer patients who had "no improvement." Katon and Raskind (11) describe three patients, all aged 72 years or older, who did well on 10 mg b.i.d. of methylphenidate. Wittenborn (9) concludes that although there was no real support for antidepressant efficacy of amphetamines and methylphenidate by controlled research, one of the obfuscating elements may well have been a difference between depression in the young and the old.

In reviewing all earlier papers about depression and psychostimulants, it must be borne in mind what "depression" meant to the various researchers. Only after Diagnostic and Statistical Manual (DSM-III) in 1980 was there a more or less homogeneous definition of depression. Chiarello and Cole (12) make this point to good effect.

The most up-to-date and concise critical view of psychostimulants in the treatment of depression is given by Satel and Nelson in 1989 (13). Their review found 10 outpatient placebo-controlled studies in primary depression; eight studies show no difference between placebo and stimulant. In four placebo-controlled studies on geriatric inpatients, two studies show no difference. Again, their conclusion is that controlled studies are not so convincing of the efficacy of psychostimulants; however, the case report literature is rather supportive of psychostimulant activity in depression.

Our first case study of clinical use of amphetamine was by Kaufman and Murray in 1982 (14). Of the three patients, only one (82 years old) was geriatric. All three were depressed and medically ill, and fulfilled DSM-III criteria for major depression. Further case histories showed good clinical response to dextroamphetamine or methylphenidate (15). In a study of five patients, three of whom were over 70 years of age and were put on methylphenidate with good results. Prior to this, one of them had had 12 sessions of unilateral electroconvulsive therapy (ECT) and, although it normalized his appetite, it still left him dysphoric, abulic, and uninterested in activities of daily living (ADL). A trial of methylphenidate 5 mg t.i.d. gave dramatic results: the patient performed full ADLs and had no dysphoria. The second patient, 71 years old, received methylphenidate 10 mg b.i.d.; within 24 h her depressive symptomology was greatly reduced. The third patient, a 71-year-old male, had had a stroke and was started on maprotiline 75 mg/day; after 2 weeks, he discontinued the medication due to too much sedation. In the hospital, he was started on methylphenidate 5 mg b.i.d. and in 12 h was in good spirits and highly motivated.

Close to 40% of the patients seen on the Psychiatric Consultation Service at MGH are 65 years or older. By far the great majority of patients given psychostimulants are in this geriatric age range.

Other papers of case reports were published in 1984 (16,17). A 4-year retrospective chart review of 3018 consecutive consultations showed 83, or 2.8% of these consultations, were prescribed psychostimulants (18). Only 66 of these patients were counted, however, because of lost charts or psychostimulant use for reasons other than depression. All of the patients met DSM-III criteria for depression and all but three of these qualified for secondary depression (19).

Of the 66 patients (34 women) studied (average age was 72 years; age range of 37–87 years), many had multiple system medical disease, all were seriously ill, some dangerously ill. Eight (12%) patients died during their index hospitalization, none of them while receiving a psychostimulant. Therapeutic trials numbered 71, of which 35 were dextroamphetamine (mean dose: 12 mg/day) and 36 were methylphenidate (mean dose: 13.5 mg/day). The Clinical Global Impressions (CGI) scale was used to rate improvement (20). Approximately 75% showed some improvement, in half of these improvement was marked or moderate. Of those improved, 93% reached peak response within the first 2 days. Side effects were notable for their relative absence (i.e., only five suffered side effects, all of which remitted on discontinuation of the drug).

In 1990, another retrospective review of 4740 consecutive psychiatric consultations was made from the years 1983 to 1988, which studied the geriatric medically ill with depression (21). There were 129 patients who received a psychostimulant. All depressive diagnoses fulfilled DSM-III criteria, all but two of whom met criteria for secondary depression (19). The average age was 74 years, with an age range of 65 to 88. Dextroamphetamine was prescribed for 104 patients (mean dose: 8.2 mg/day) and 25 patients were treated with methylphenidate (mean dose: 9 mg/day). A total of 105 patients (81%) experienced at least some improvement and 85 (66%) were rated as markedly or moderately improved. Within the first 2 days, 88 patients (68%) reached peak response. Seventeen patients (13%) experienced side effects (22).

IV. AMPHETAMINE VS. METHYLPHENIDATE

In these two larger studies (18,21) no significant difference was seen between amphetamine and methylphenidate. There was no follow-up on these patients after discharge; there was no report back to any of us by the patient's physician that there was any psychostimulant abuse after discharge. Decrease of appetite was not seen with any of our clinical studies; in fact, on low-dose amphetamine or methylphenidate appetite often increased (23). Olin and Masand (24) found in their studies that 12% of their patients had a marked improvement in appetite after they were given a psychostimulant; 17% were noted to have a moderate improvement; and 59% had minimal to no improvement in appetite.

There are several papers of a case report nature that affirm good overall response in the elderly with psychostimulants for depression and apathy (25–29). These studies varied in overall response rate from 54–87%.

There is now one double-blind, placebo-controlled study of psychostimulant use in patients with a mean age of 72 (30). Wallace and coworkers (30) randomized 16 patients to 4-day, double-blind treatment trials with either methylphenidate or placebo and then crossed them over without hiatus to the alternate treatment for an additional 4 days. Three patients, all taking placebo, dropped out. Among 13 patients completing treatment, depressive symptoms decreased dramatically in 7, moderately in 3, and minimally in 3 during treatment. They concluded that methylphenidate offers safe, well-tolerated antidepressant efficacy with the added benefit of relieving symptoms within 4 days.

In our clinical experience, we find dextroamphetamine to be slightly more effective than methylphenidate. We have gone over our data and although there is a mild trend that it is more effective, it is not significant. We have found no better tolerance, clinically, of the one or the other by younger patients or older patients. As to prescribing dextroamphetamine or methylphenidate, it can be said that older, more experienced clinicians tend to use dextroamphetamine; conversely, younger clinicians (e.g., residents, fellows) tend to use methylphenidate, presumably because of the unexamined belief in methylphenidate's greater safety. There is a pervasive avoidance by physicians of dextroamphetamine. The stigma caused by its abuse and as an anorexic lingers, decades later, as a significant mental block to its rational use. Not "politically correct," dextroamphetamine appears to be an irrationally feared agent.

V. SIDE EFFECTS AND SAFETY

We have used psychostimulants for patients with a whole host of medical and surgical illnesses. In one study of 129 patients (21), there were 306 medical diagnoses (see Table 2). Many patients had congestive heart failure, coronary artery disease, hypertension, cerebral vascular accident (31), renal failure, and diabetes mellitus. Of all of these, 13% (7) had side effects (listed in Table 3), and all resolved by lowering or discontinuing the dose.

TABLE 2 Medical Discharge Diagnoses

Category	Diagnosis	*n*
Cardiovascular	Arrhythmias	31
	Congestive heart failure	40
	Coronary artery bypass graft	3
	Coronary artery disease	31
	Hypertension	28
	Peripheral vascular disease	9
	Valvular disease	13
Pulmonary	Chronic obstructive lung disease	16
	Laryngeal/tracheal cancer	2
	Lung cancer	7
	Pneumonia	17
	Respiratory failure	9
Neurological	Cerebral vascular accident	14
	Normal pressure hydrocephalus	1
	Parkonsonism	2
	Seizures	4
Gastrointestinal	Liver disease	8
	Pancreatic disease	3
	Peptic ulcer disease	7
Endocrinological	Diabetes mellitus	25
	Thyroid disease	10
Urological	Prostate cancer	5
	Renal cancer	5
	Renal failure	19
Orthopedic	Degenerative joint disease	3
	Fractures	4
Total		306[a]

[a]Many patients had more than one diagnosis.

TABLE 3 Number of Patients with Side Effects

Side effect	Dextroamphetamine (n = 104)	Methylphenidate (n = 25)
Agitation	0	1
Anxiety	2	0
Atrial fibrillation	1	0
Confusion	3	1
Elevated blood pressure	1	1
Hypomania	2	0
Paranoid delusions	3	0
Sinus tachycardia	0	1
Spasticity	1	0
Total	13 (12.5%)	4 (16%)

We have reported three cases of hypomania on low-dose amphetamine (32). We also reported an exacerbation by 10 mg of dextroamphetamine of spasticity in a patient with motor neuron disease (33). The spasticity returned to baseline on discontinuing dextroamphetamine. All of these side effects are relatively minor as compared to side effects seen in intravenous amphetamine abusers.

Most of the touted side effects especially of amphetamine have been seen in street use of the drug at high doses. In 1981, Lundh and Trunving (34) reported four patients (three of them being I.V. users) who had a choreiform syndrome on several grams per day of amphetamine. One patient with the same syndrome used 300 mg orally t.i.d. Cerebral vasculitis from an oral overdose of amphetamine (i.e., at least 250 mg p.o.) has been reported (35). Intracerebral hemorrhage has been reported by Harrington et al. (36) in one patient who was a drug abuser of some years and whose daily dose of amphetamine was not known. However, after only 20 mg of dextroamphetamine orally, he had a headache and cerebral hemorrhage.

When one looks at the literature of serious side effects of psychostimulants, most of them resulted from intravenous use, large doses (usually >50 mg), or both. We have seen nothing like this in the oral doses (20 mg of amphetamine, most often less) that we use clinically.

VI. AMPHETAMINE MECHANISM

What us the mechanism of amphetamine? In the 1930s, it was thought to liberate norepinephrine more than dopamine. We now know that the major result of the introduction of amphetamine in the system is an increase of synaptic dopamine (37). However, it is known that low-dose dextroamphetamine suppresses norepinephrine functions (38), and has an effect on acetylcholine and serotonin (39). The exact mechanism of amphetamine in the clinical system is not known. It appears, however, that the low dose used clinically has its major effect on mesolimbic dopaminergic neurons, whereas the stereotopy produced by large doses (street abuse) is due to an activation of the nigrostriatal neurons (39).

Amphetamine's action is mediated by the catecholamine transporter (40). Amphetamine has three effects at the monoaminergic synapse: (1) inhibition of monoamine oxidase; (2) blockade of neurotransmitter uptake; and (3) promotion of its release into the synaptic cleft (41). Dopamine can be released through two mechanisms: exocytotic release, which is impulse-dependent, and transporter-mediated release, which is not impulse-dependent and appears to be the mechanism by which amphetamine releases catecholamines. Low doses of amphetamine (1–5 mg/kg) cause release of dopamine through exchange diffusion across the cell membrane (41).

VII. MOOD CHANGE WITH AMPHETAMINE

Psychostimulants have been viewed as containing a reward-enforcing element (42). There have been explorations of reward as the link to possible amphetamine addictions (43). Therefore, one suspects strongly that the nucleus accumbens is involved. The limbic striatum (nucleus accumbens) houses neuronal terminals whose cell bodies originate in the medial ventral tegmental region. It is thought that the nucleus accumbens is involved in the channeling of drive and affect (44). If dopaminergic transmission in the nucleus accumbens is selectively disrupted, the characteristic locomotor stimulation induced by low doses of amphetamine is reduced. Haloperidol and spiroperidol when microinjected into animal nucleus accumbens similarly block the locomotor effects of amphetamine (45). It is not known if or how inputs of corticolimbic origin play a role in the modulation of the accumbens function of locomotion and reward (46). However, it appears that low-dose amphetamine has its greatest effect on the nucleus accumbens, the limbic striatum, which we postulate energizes the clinically depressed geriatric patient.

It is possible that the depression relieved by psychostimulants in the medically/surgically ill geriatric patient may be, in effect, a different type of depression from that seen in the psychiatrist's office or on the psychiatric inpatient unit. First of all, our cases were all examples of "secondary" depression, which itself may differ from primary (psychiatric) depression. Prior to its inclusion in DSM-IV, this entity went unlisted except for the vague category of organic affective disorder. Second, secondary depression in the elderly may be a different illness from secondary depression in younger persons (47,48).

In all theories of mood disorder, neurotransmitters figure prominently. In normal aging, there is a decrease of norepinephrine, serotonin, and dopamine. At age 70–79, relative to ages >60, there are only about 67% of locus ceruleus neurons remaining in normals (49). Dopamine in the ventral tegmental area is also greatly diminished in the 65-year-old compared to the 25-year-old (50). Since epinephrine, serotonin, and dopamine are all decreased in normal aging, added stress of illness will decrease dopamine in the mesolimbic system (51), and perhaps cause depression more readily in the geriatric patient than the nongeriatric patient.

In a speculative mode, the dopamine theory of depression, first put forward by Randrup et al. (52) in 1975, seems worth considering here. Also of importance, it would appear, is an animal model of depression wherein chronic exposure to mild, unpredictable stress decreases rewarding properties of natural reinforcers (53). Dopamine agonists have been shown to be helpful in this animal model of depression (54).

Analogously, the depressive illness of the geriatric patient may result from chronic exposure to mild, unpredictable stress causing a deficiency of dopamine and thus a clinical depression (55). Psychostimulants, even intermittently as in animals, would act as the dopamine agonist in an antidepressantlike manner (54).

It is possible that secondary depression is less involved with the noradrenergic and serotonergic systems and more easily treated with dopamine agonists.

VIII. CONCLUSIONS

1. The history of psychostimulant abuse has cautioned psychiatrists against its use.
2. There is a paucity of controlled research on the effect of psychostimulants on depression in geriatric medical patients.
3. There appears to be no great clinical advantage in using methylphenidate over dextroamphetamine.
4. With use of a low-dose psychostimulant, no anorexia was observed; in fact, there was an improvement in appetite in about 25% of patients.
5. Most of the papers affirming good overall response to psychostimulants in the elderly are case reports.
6. There is one recent controlled study (30) using methylphenidate which demonstrated antidepressant efficacy.
7. Depression in medically/surgically ill geriatric patients can be treated effectively and quickly by psychostimulants.
8. Low doses of amphetamine affect mesolimbic dopaminergic neurons, whereas high doses tend to affect the nigrostriatal dopaminergic neurons.
9. Amphetamine has three effects at the monoaminergic synapse: (a) inhibition of monoamine oxidase; (b) blockade of dopamine uptake; and (c) promotion of release of dopamine into the synaptic cleft mainly by exchange diffusion across the cell membrane.
10. There are minimal data to suggest that amphetamine acts in elderly depression at the limbic system's nucleus accumbens.
11. It is probable that medically ill geriatric depression differs from primary psychiatric depression. (This suggests that nongeriatric patients may not get medically ill/secondary depression, and that geriatric patients may not get primary depression.)

ACKNOWLEDGMENT

The authors would like to thank Robert B. Shochet, M.D., Assistant Professor of Medicine, Johns Hopkins University, for his help with the historical part of the paper.

REFERENCES

1. Young D, Scoville WB. Paranoid psychoses in narcolepsy and possible danger of benzedrine treatment. Med Clin N Am 1938; 22:637–645.
2. Grinspoon L, Bakalar J. The amphetamines: medical uses and health hazards. Psychiatr Ann 1977; 7-8:381–390.
3. Monroe RR, Drell HJ. Oral use of stimulants obtained from inhalers. J Am Med Assoc 1947; 135:909–914.
4. Adlersberg D, Mayer ME. Results of prolonged medical treatment of obesity with diet alone, diet and thyroid preparations, and diet and amphetamines. J Clin Endocrinol Metab 1949; 9:275–284.
5. Meier R. Ritalin, eine neuartige synthetishe verbindung mit spezfischer zentralerregender wirkungss-komponete. Klin Wochenschr 1954; 32:445–450.
6. Connell PH. Amphetamine psychosis. Maudsley Monograph, No. 5, London: Chapman and Hall, 1958.
7. Edison GR. Amphetamines: a dangerous illusion. Ann Intern Med 1971; 74:605–610.
8. Overall JE, Hollister LE, Shelton J, Johnson M, Kimball I. Tranylcypromine compared with dextroamphetamine in hospitalized depressed patients. Dis Nerv Syst 1966; 27:653–659.
9. Wittenborn JR. Antidepressant use of amphetamines and other psychostimulants. Mod Probl Pharmacopsychiatry 1982; 18:178–195.
10. Jacobsen A. The use of Ritalin in psychotherapy of depressions of the aged. Psychiatr Q 1958; 32:474–483.
11. Katon W, Raskin M. Treatment of depression in the medically ill elderly with methylphenidate. Am J Psychiatry 1980; 137:963–965.
12. Chiarello RJ, Cole J. The use of pyschostimulants in general psychiatry. Arch Gen Psychiatry 1987; 44:286–295.
13. Satel SL, Nelson JC. Stimulants in the treatment of depression: a critical overview. J Clin Psychiatry 1989; 50:241–249.
14. Kaufmann MW, Murray GB. The use of d-amphetamine in medically ill depressed patients. J Clin Psychiatry 1982; 43:463–464.
15. Kaufmann MW, Murray GB, Cassem HN. Use of psychostimulants in medically ill depressed patients. Psychosomatics 1982; 23:817–819.
16. Kaufmann MW, Murray GB, Cassem NH, Jenike M. Use of psychostimulants in medically ill patients with neurological disease and major depression. Can J Psychaitry 1984; 29:46–49.
17. Kaufmann MW, Cassem NH, Murray GB, et al. The use of methylphenidate in depressed disorder after cardiac surgery. J Clin Psychiatry 1984; 45:82–84.
18. Woods SW, Tesar GE, Murray GB, Cassem NH. Psychostimulant treatment of depressive disorder secondary to medical illness. J Clin Psychiatry 1986; 47:12–15.
19. Feighner JP, Robins E, Guze SB, et al. Diagnostic criteria for use in psychiatric research. Arch Gen Psychiatry 1972; 26:57–63.
20. Guy W. ECDEU Assessment Manual for Psychopharmacology. USDHEW Publication No. 76-338, Washington, DC: US Government Printing Office, 1976.

21. Pickett P, Masand P, Murray GB. Psychostimulant treatment of geriatric depressive disorders secondary to medical illness. J Geriatr Psychiatry Neurol 1990; 3: 146–151.
22. Spier SA. Toxicity and abuse of prescribed stimulants. Int J Psychiatr Med 1995; 25:69–79.
23. Colle LM, Wise RA. Facilitory and inhibitory effects of nucleus accumbens amphetamine on feeding. Ann NY Acad Sci 1988; 537:491–492.
24. Olin J, Masand P. Psychostimulants for depression in hospitalized cancer patients. Psychosomatics 1996; 37:57–62.
25. Jacobsen A. The use of ritalin in psychotherapy of depressions of the aged. Psychiatr Q 1958; 32:474–483.
26. Landman ME, Preisig R, Perlmann M. A practical mood stimulant. J Med Soc NJ 1958; 55:55–58.
27. Kaplitz SE. Withdrawn, apathetic geriatric patients responsive to methylphenidate. J Am Geriatr Soc 1975; 2:271–276.
28. Clark ANG, Mankikar GD. d-Amphetamine in elderly patients refractory to rehabilitation procedures. J Am Geriatr Soc 1979; 27:174–177.
29. Askinazi C, Weintraub RJ, Karamouz N. Elderly depressed females as a possible subgroup of patients responsive to methylphenidate. J Clin Psychiatry 1986; 47: 467–469.
30. Wallace AE, Kofoed LL, West AN. Double-blind, placebo-controlled trial of methylphenidate in older, depressed, medically ill patients. Am J Psychiatry 1995; 152:929–931.
31. Masand P, Murray GB, Pickett P. Psychostimulants in post-stroke depression. N Neuropsychiatry 1991; 3:23–27.
32. Masand PS, Pickett P, Murray GB. Hypomania precipitated by psychostimulant use in depressed medically ill patients. Psychosomatics 1995; 36:145–147.
33. Rundell JR, Cassem EH, Murray GB. Exacerbation by dextroamphetamine of spasticity in a patient with motor neuron disease. J Clin Psychopharmacol 1988; 8:146.
34. Lundh H, Trunving K. An extrapyramidal choreiform syndrome caused by amphetamine addiction. J Neurol Neurosurg Psychiatry 1981; 44:728–730.
35. Matick H, Anderson D, Brumlik J. Cerebral vasculitis associated with oral amphetamine overdose. Arch Neurol 1983; 40:253–254.
36. Harrington H, Heller HA, Dawson D, Caplan L, Rumbaugh C. Intracerebral hemorrhage and oral amphetamine. Arch Neurol 1983; 40:503–507.
37. Kuczenski R. Biochemical actions of amphetamine and other stimulants. In: Creese I, ed. Stimulants: Neurochemical, Behavioral, and Clinical Perspectives. New York: Raven Press, 1983:31–61.
38. Huang YH, Maas JW. d-Amphetamine at low doses suppresses noradrenergic functions. Eur J Pharmacol 1981; 75:187–195.
39. Moore KE. The actions of amphetamines on neurotransmitters: a brief review. Biol Psychiatry 1977; 12:451–462.
40. Fischer JF, Cho AK. Chemical release from striatal homogenates: evidence for an exchange diffusion model. J Pharmacol Exp Ther 1979; 208:203–209.

41. Seiden LS, Sabol KE, Ricourte GA. Amphetamine effects on catecholamine systems and behavior. Ann Rev Pharmacol Toxicol 1993; 32:639–677.
42. Murray GB. Psychostimulants in general hospital psychiatry. Curr Affect Illness 1987; 6:5–10.
43. Wise RA, Bozarth MA. A psychomotor stimulant theory of addiction. Psychol Rev 1987; 94:469–492.
44. Mogenson GJ, Jones DL, Yim CY. From motivation to action: functional interface between the limbic system and the motor system. Prog Neurobiol 1980; 14:69–97.
45. Mogenson GJ, Yim CY. Electrophysiological and neuropharmacological behavioral studies of the nucleus accumbens: implications for its role as a limbic-motor interface. In: Chronister RB, DeFrance JF, eds. The Neurobiology of the Nucleus Accumbens. Haer Institute, 1981:210–229.
46. Pulvirenti L, Swerdlow NR, Hubner CB, Koob GF. The role of limbic-accumbens-pallidal circuitry in the activating and reinforcing properties of psychostimulant drugs. In: Wilner P, Scheel-Kruger J, eds. The Mesolimbic Dopamine System: From Motivation to Action. New York: John Wiley & Sons, Ltd., 1991:131–140.
47. Moffic HS, Paykel ES. Depression in medical inpatients. Br J Psychiatry 1995; 126:346–353.
48. Kathol RG, Petty F. Reaction of depression to medical illness. J Affect Disord 1981; 3:111–121.
49. Katzman R, Terry RD. Normal aging of the nervous system. In: Katzman R, Terry RD, eds. The Neurology of Aging. Philadelphia: F.A. Davis, 1983:15–50.
50. Van Domburg PHMF, ten Donkelaar HJ. The Human Substantia Nigra and Ventral Tegmental Area. New York: Springer-Verlag, 1991.
51. Willner P, Muscat R, Papp M, Sampson D. Dopamine, depression, and antidepressant drugs. In: Willner P, Scheel-Kruger J, eds. The Mesolimbic Dopamine System: From Motivation to Actions. New York: John Wiley & Sons, Ltd., 1991: 387–410.
52. Randrup A, Munkvad I, Fog R, et al. Mania, depression, and brain dopamine. In: Essnan WB, Valzelli L, eds. Current Developments in Psychopharmacology. New York: Spectrum Publications, 1975:207–229.
53. Zacharko RM, Arisman H. Stressor-provoked alterations of intracranial self-stimulation in the mesocorticolimbic system: an animal model of depression. In: Willner P, Scheel-Kruger J, eds. The Mesolimbic Dopamine System: From Motivation to Action. New York: John Wiley & Sons, Ltd., 1991:411–442.
54. Muscat R, Papp M, Willner P. Antidepressant-like effects of dopamine agonists in an animal model of depression. Biol Psychiatry 1992; 31:937–946.
55. Kapur S, Mann JJ. Role of dopaminergic system in depression. Biol Psychiatry 1992; 32:1–17.

14
Use of Lithium in Bipolar Disorder

Robert C. Young
The New York Hospital-Cornell Medical Center, White Plains, New York

I. INTRODUCTION

With continuing growth of the aged population, clinicians are faced increasingly often with geriatric patients having manic syndromes or bipolar disorders (1). Their treatment has been a relatively neglected area of investigation, however; few studies are available that address pharmacodynamic questions.

Somatic treatments that are effective for mania and for bipolar depression in younger patients can also be effective in the elderly. This chapter will focus on pharmacotherapy with lithium salts directed at acute suppression of symptoms, at continuation treatment to prevent immediate relapse, and at long-term maintenance.

In the management of geriatric manic or bipolar patients, exclusion of mood disorder due to medical conditions or substance-induced mood disorders is especially important, particularly in those with an older age of onset (1). Weighing the risks and benefits of treatments such as lithium is also important and may be more complicated in geriatric patients.

II. GENERAL ACUTE MANAGEMENT CONSIDERATIONS

A. Assessment

History

Documentation of the course of illness and its prior treatment are fundamental to psychiatric management. Sources of information will necessarily include family and other caregivers, and previous medical records. The differential diagnosis of geriatric patients with manic syndromes includes bipolar disorder, delusional disorder, schizoaffective disorder, mood disorder related to a medical condition or substance-induced mood disorder, dementia, and delirium. The differential diagnosis of bipolar depression in the elderly also includes major depression and dysthymia. Clarification of diagnosis rests on history.

In geriatric patients with affective syndromes, medical disorders and neurologic comorbidity are frequently noted (2–4). The chronology of such comorbidity and their treatments relative to the manic syndrome will identify potential etiological factors. In mixed-age patients, first onset of mania after age 40 is more often associated with medical and neurological illnesses and drug treatments (5). If present, these factors should be addressed. The medical history provides information relating to selection of lithium or other psychotropic agents, and highlights side effects of particular concern.

Selection of psychotropic treatment is based on knowledge of previous treatments and the associated response. Treatment history includes the drugs used, their dose, plasma levels achieved, and duration. This information permits judgments concerning the adequacy of previous therapeutic trials. Treatment history of bipolar family members may also suggest anticipated response in the patient.

Examination

A thorough physical, neurological, and mental status examination are essential in the geriatric patient for identification of potential etiological factors and comorbidity. Mental status examination prior to treatment includes assessment of psychotic features and cognitive status in addition to affective state. Pretreatment cognitive performance provides information regarding possible associated dementia, and an index for monitoring changes during treatment.

Laboratory Tests

Routine evaluation will include laboratory tests directed at differential diagnosis and assessment of comorbid conditions. Factors relevant to treatment with lithium and other agents are also assessed, as outlined below.

B. Treatment Setting

Manic states and bipolar depression can be treated in various settings, but hospitalization is often optimal. Judgment as to whether hospitalization is necessary is based on multiple factors including overall severity and duration, the patient's physical condition, the level of available supervision, and expected compliance in the existing setting. Hospitalization can provide an opportunity for rapid examination and laboratory assessment, staff expertise in use and evaluation of treatments, as well as restriction of socially damaging behavior in mania.

C. Other Aspects of Acute Management

Environmental control and behavioral interventions play a critical role in the acute management of manic patients. Flexible limitation of environmental and social stimulation through scheduled room restriction can be therapeutic. Interpersonal interactions should have a firm and directive style. Effective communication among staff avoids the "splitting" that can be common with manic patients. When agitation is severe, periods of monitored seclusion may be helpful. Physical restraint is used if necessary.

Effective use of such modalities will help to minimize the need for adjunctive medications, which will help to reduce the frequency of adverse reactions.

III. ACUTE LITHIUM PHARMACOTHERAPY

A. General Considerations

Selection of lithium, as described above, is directed by current assessment, prior treatment history, and consideration of comorbid medical conditions. In general, use of multiple drug classes simultaneously should be avoided in favor of monotherapy, if clinically feasible. Use of p.r.n. medications should be minimized in favor of frequent assessment of behavior and changes in standing orders. Multiple divided doses should be avoided when possible, as this is frequently not pharmacokinetically rational and is costly in terms of staff time.

B. Efficacy in Mania

Lithium salts have been and remain first-line agents for treatment of acute mania in the geriatric age group. The literature concerning their use in the elderly, while limited, is more extensive than that for other agents.

Response to lithium in acute mania has not been contrasted with placebo in geriatric patients; this reflects, in part, ethical concerns. Response to lithium has also not been contrasted in the elderly with response to other drugs such as neuroleptics.

Age effects have generally not been examined in treatment studies in mixed-age populations, which generally include few older patients (6–11). A prospective study of mixed-age patients receiving naturalistic treatment did suggest a weak negative age effect on response; however, only four patients were aged ≥60 years (12).

Reports focusing on older patients (Table 1) have been primarily retrospective analyses (3,13–15). Some have included demented patients (14).

C. Efficacy in Bipolar Depression

Pharmacological treatment of bipolar depression involves optimization of mood stabilizer dosage as a first strategy. In mixed-age patients, lithium is more effective than placebo (16). However, use of lithium salts in geriatric bipolar depression has received little study.

D. Guidelines for Practice

Pretreatment assessment includes a baseline electrocardiogram (ECG) to assess sinus node function, because use of lithium salts may be associated with sick sinus syndrome (17). This complication might be encountered particularly in older patients with coronary artery disease that has already compromised the sinus node.

Baseline evaluation also includes renal function tests. Serum creatinine is not a sensitive index of renal function, but collection of a 24-h urine sample to determine creatinine clearance is often difficult in an acute manic patient. Creatinine clearance can be approximated from age, body weight, and serum creatinine (18) in those patients with renal insufficiency who require careful monitoring and for whom collection of urine is not feasible.

TABLE 1 Therapeutic Response to Lithium in Elderly Manic Patients

Ref.	N	Diagnosis	Age (yrs)	Plasma levels (mEq/L)	Efficacy	Comments
52	81	Bipolar, manic	>55	Not reported	Good; delayed/poor in demented/ neurological	Retrospective
3	67	Bipolar, manic	≥60	Not reported	Good in 24 of 27 who received adequate trial	Retrospective
15	14	Bipolar, manic (DSM-III)	65–77	Range: 0.8–1.2	10 responded at range 0.5–0.8	No comparison group; no quantitative assessment
13	92	Bipolar manic (Feighner)	65–82	Not reported	Unchanged by cerebral organic impairment; not different than other treatment	Retrospective

Assessment of thyroid status, including thyroid-stimulating hormone (TSH), is especially important in the elderly. Diminished thyroid reserve accompanies aging (19), and lithium antagonizes thyroid gland function.

Dosing

Decreased proportion of body water with age influences the distribution of lithium, which is hydrophilic. Decreased volume of distribution is associated with higher plasma concentrations. Decreases in glomerular filtration rate and renal blood flow can occur with age. Because lithium is renally eliminated, reduction of renal function is associated with decreased lithium clearance and prolongation of its elimination half-life.

In addition, a number of age-associated medical disorders and drug and dietary regimens influence lithium distribution and elimination in this population. These pharmacokinetic issues are discussed in detail in Chapter 2.

Lower lithium doses, by 30–60%, may thus be required to achieve equivalent plasma lithium levels in elderly compared with younger patients. Changes in doses need to be made more slowly, as steady-state concentrations are reached more slowly (20). A conservative approach would be to start with 75–150 mg/day, usually in a single dose (21,22). Alternate day or less frequent dosing can also be used. Jensen et al. (23) have suggested that using a single nightly dose or 150% of the daily dose every other night reduces the side effects and improves compliance without decreasing effectiveness.

Lithium pharmacodynamics (i.e., the relationship between specific plasma concentrations and therapeutic or toxic responses) is not well understood in the elderly, despite clinical lore suggesting "increased sensitivity." Case reports (15) have suggested acute response in geriatric manics at lower levels (e.g., 0.4–0.8 mEq/L) than are optimal in mixed-age adults. However, a recent examination of naturalistic treatment suggested better response to higher lithium levels in a sample of both younger and geriatric patients (24).

The time course of response to lithium in geriatric mania has apparently not been investigated. Comparison with young manic patients treated equivalently is needed.

Manic patients may cycle into depression during treatment. In geriatric patients, Broadhead and Jacoby (25) noted that depressive episodes occurred more often during hospitalization for mania than in young patients.

E. Other Clinical Situations

Treatment of mania occurring in the context of dementia has received little investigation. Neurological status, including extrapyramidal syndromes and dementia, predicted delayed and/or poor response to lithium in a study of patients aged >55 years by Himmelhoch and associates (14); lithium levels were not specified.

Some studies have suggested that symptomatic or secondary manic states have poorer response to pharmacotherapy. Black and Winokur (26) reported that mixed-age patients with "complicated" manias (i.e., coexisting nonaffective psychiatric illness or serious medical illness) had poorer acute response to adequate lithium treatment compared to uncomplicated manics. Shukla and colleagues (27) also reported that mixed-age patients with secondary manias had a relatively poor acute lithium response. On the other hand, other experience in geriatric patients has not suggested a relationship between evidence of central nervous system disease and outcome of acute naturalistic pharmacotherapy (3,13).

F. Adjunctive Medication

Neuroleptics

Neuroleptic medications continue to have a role as adjuncts to lithium for initial management of acute mania. They have not been studied systematically in this context in the elderly. In this age group, concerns regarding toxicity include sedation, orthostatic hypotension, adverse cognitive effects, peripheral anticholinergic side effects, acute extrapyramidal reactions, and tardive dyskinesia. Low doses should be used if possible. Neuroleptics should be viewed as temporary measures; tapering of dosage and ultimate discontinuation should be attempted. Selection of low-dose, high-potency neuroleptics such as haloperidol will minimize anticholinergic and hypotensive effects, but extrapyramidal toxicity can be expected.

Recently, new neuroleptic agents have been introduced that may have differing toxicity profiles. Risperidone is an atypical agent with serotonergic as well as dopaminergic receptor antagonist properties that may have lower propensity for extrapyramidal side effects and anticholinergic effects than typical neuroleptics. There are apparently few data available concerning its use in the elderly. Clozapine also has a relatively low propensity for extrapyramidal side effects and can be useful in neuroleptic refractory patients (28–32). However, it has potent anticholinergic properties, and lethargy, sedation, respiratory distress, and leukopenia have been noted in the elderly despite low dosages. Agranulocytosis is also a risk. Thus, while risperidone and clozapine each have potential advantages, their efficacy, dosing requirements, and relative risks await systematic assessment.

Benzodiazepines

Benzodiazepines including lorazepam and clonazepam have both been reported to be useful in younger manic patients; nevertheless, high drop-out rates in recent studies of acute mania (11,33) suggest limited efficacy. They have not been studied systematically in elderly manic patients. In the elderly, the clinician must be vigilant for sedation, ataxia, cognitive toxicity, and paradoxical disinhibition. Use of long-acting agents with active metabolites should be avoided.

G. Adjunctive Antidepressant Pharmacotherapy

In one study in mixed-age bipolar depressed patients, imipramine was more effective than lithium or placebo (34). There is some evidence of increased resistance to tricyclic antidepressants in mixed-age bipolars compared to unipolar depressives (35) and of better response to tranylcypromine (14). These issues have not been addressed in the geriatric population. Presumably the need to minimize exposure to antidepressants in order to reduce the risk of mania and rapid cycling, which has been reported in younger patients, is also true in the geriatric population. Mania associated with antidepressant treatment has been reported in the geriatric population (36,37).

H. Lithium and ECT

Electroconvulsive therapy (ECT) has a clear role in treatment of mixed-age manic patients (38) in addition to bipolar depression. In mixed-age patients, concurrent lithium with ECT can increase severity of post-ECT confusion, memory loss, delirium, and prolong seizures (39–42). Abrams (42) has pointed out that lithium treatment concurrent with ECT can prolong muscular blockade of succinyl choline. The safety of continuing lithium during ECT in the elderly has not been established, and the risks may be significant.

IV. CONTINUATION AND MAINTENANCE PHARMACOTHERAPY

A. General Considerations

"Continuation" treatment means extension of treatment immediately following resolution of the acute episode to prevent relapse. "Maintenance" treatment refers to more prolonged efforts directed at prevention of recurrence. This distinction is not generally made, however, in the available literature concerning elderly manic patients. There is a great need for studies of continuation and maintenance treatment of mania in the elderly because of possible increasing vulnerability to relapse/recurrence in late-onset illness (43) and because of the potential complexity associated with comorbidity in the elderly.

B. Efficacy of Lithium Salts

A number of outpatient investigations of age effects have been available, but have design limitations confounding interpretation (Table 2). A report by Hewick et al. (44) is difficult to interpret due to lack of comparable plasma lithium levels in the geriatric and young patient groups. Abou-Saleh and Coppen (45) noted no difference in affective morbidity over an average of 5 years in elderly compared to younger patients maintained on similar, relatively high, lithium levels. Murray et al. (46) noted some increase in manic psychopathology, but not hospitalizations, in older compared with younger patients in a mixed-age sample that was followed prospectively at equivalent, moderate lithium levels.

Stone (4) found, retrospectively, no difference in hospital readmissions among those geriatric patients who had been treated with lithium and those who were not, but interpretation is limited by the naturalistic design.

C. Guidelines for Practice

Dosing

Optimum plasma concentrations for lithium continuation or maintenance treatment have not been defined through prospective investigations. Foster

TABLE 2 Therapeutic Response to Long-Term Lithium Treatment in the Elderly

Ref.	N	Diagnosis	Age (yrs)	Plasma levels (mEq/L)	Efficacy	Comments
46	82	Manic depression; recurrent unipolar depression	21–84	Range of means: 0.6–0.9	Trend for more morbidity at >50 yr	Retrospective; plasma levels lower in older group
55	148	Recurrent affective disorder	≥60	Range: 0.8–1.2	No difference in elderly (≥60 yr)	Prospective; unipolar and bipolar patients not distinguished
47	166	Bipolar and unipolar	21–78	Range: 0.4–0.8	Trend for increased prevalence and severity of mania with age	Prospective; equivalent plasma levels in elderly
4	92	Bipolar manic	≥65	Not stated	No effect in chronic inpatients; no difference in readmissions in those treated with lithium	Retrospective

and Rosenthal (47) recommended levels of 0.4–0.7 mEq/L for maintenance treatment based on their clinical experience. Shulman et al. (21) similarly recommended maintaining levels at approximately 0.5 mEq/L and using a single bedtime dose to reduce nephrotoxicity.

When a decision is made to discontinue lithium, the dose should probably be tapered gradually, as experience in mixed-age patients suggests that abrupt discontinuation may adversely affect outcome (48,49). Of course, there should be close subsequent clinical monitoring in the elderly patient.

D. Other Clinical Situations

The implications of comorbid dementia syndromes for continuation and maintenance treatment in elderly manic patients remains to be assessed.

E. Adjunctive Medication

A recent report in mixed-age adults highlights the frequent continuation of neuroleptic use after manic episodes (50). In geriatric patients the need to minimize long-term use of neuroleptics in order to reduce the risk of tardive dyskinesia is apparent. The long-term risks of benzodiazepine use, including tolerance and dependence, also argue strongly for tapering and discontinuation as soon as possible.

F. Adjunctive Nonsomatic Treatment Modalities

In the long-term management of geriatric patients with manic episode or bipolar disorder, individual or group psychotherapy can serve an important function that augments pharmacotherapy. Education about the nature of the disorder can be especially important in patients having their first episode in late life. Compliance with medication regimens can be enhanced by increasing the patient's understanding of the rationale for their use as well as their potential toxicity, by developing an alliance in terms of reporting symptoms and side effects, and by sharing decision making. Psychotherapeutic management can be provided by the psychiatrist and by other disciplines.

Daily rhythms are often irregular in bipolar patients (51). There is need for studies of the impact of regularizing daily routine on recurrence of psychopathology in geriatric patients as in younger adults.

Involvement of family and other caregivers in management is at least as important in geriatric as in younger patients. When there is concomitant cognitive impairment or dementia, their education concerning the nature of the disorder and its treatment becomes essential to compliance. Family and other caregivers are also sources of observational data used in assessing therapeutic effects and any toxicity.

ACKNOWLEDGMENTS

This work was supported by MH42522, MH01192, MH40726, and MH49762.

REFERENCES

1. Young RC, Klerman GL. Mania in late life: Focus on age at onset. Am J Psychiatry 1992; 149:867–876.
2. Alexopoulos GS. Psychiatric disorders in late life: Mood disorders. In: Kaplan HI, Sadock BJ, eds. Comprehensive Textbook of Psychiatry, 6th ed. Baltimore, MD: Williams & Wilkins, 1996.
3. Shulman K, Post F. Bipolar affective disorders in old age. Br J Psychiatry 1980; 136:26–32.
4. Stone K. Mania in the elderly. Br J Psychiatry 1989; 155:220–224.

   Strayhorn JM, Nash JL. Severe neurotoxicity despite "therapeutic" serum lithium levels. Disord Nerv Syst 1977; 38:107–111.
5. Krauthammer C, Klerman G. Secondary mania. Arch Gen Psychiatry 1978; 35(11): 1333–1339.
6. Shopsin B, Gerhson S, Thompson H, Collins P. Psychoactive drugs in mania. Arch Gen Psychiatry 1975; 32:34–42.
7. Stokes PE, Stoll PM, Shamoian CA, Patton MJ. Efficacy of lithium as acute treatment of manic-depressive illness. Lancet 1971; 1:1319–1325.
8. Taylor MA, Abrams R. Prediction of tretment response in mania. Arch Gen Psychiatry 1981; 38:800–803.
9. Secunda SK, Katz MM, Swann A, Koslow SH, Maas JW, Chuang S, Crougran J. Mania: Diagnosis, state measurement, prediction of treatment response. J Affect Disord 1985; 8:113–121.
10. Swann AC, Koslow SH, Katz MM, Maas JW, Javaid J, Secunda S, Robins E. Lithium carbonate treatment of mania. Arch Gen Psychiatry 1987; 44:345–354.
11. Bowden CL, Brugger AM, Swann AC, Calabrese JR, Janicak PG, Petty F, Dilsaver SC. Efficacy of Divalproex vs lithium and placebo in the treatment of mania. JAMA 1994; 271(12):918–923.
12. Young RC, Falk JR. Age, manic psychopathology and treatment response. Int J Geriatr Psychiatry 1980; 4:73–78.
13. Glasser M, Rabins P. Mania in the elderly. Age Aging 1984; 13:210–213.
14. Himmelhoch JF, Fuchs CZ, Symons BJ. A double-blind study of tranylcypromine treatment of major anergic depression. J Nerv Ment Disord 1982; 170:628–34.
15. Schaffer CB, Garvey MJ. Use of lithium in acutely manic elderly patients. Clin Gerontologist 1984; 3:58.

16. Goodwin FK. Jamison KR. Manic-Depressive Illness. New York: Oxford University Press, 1990:603–629.
17. Roose SP, Nurnberger J, Dunner D, et al. Cardiac sinus node dysfunction during lithium treatment. Am J Psychiatry 1979; 136:804–806.
18. Friedman JR, Norman DC, Yoshikawa TT. Correlation of estimated renal function parameters versus 24-hour creatinine clearance in ambulatory elderly. J Am Geriatr Soc 1989; 37:145–149.
19. Sawin CT, Castelli WP, Hershman JM, et al. The thyroid: thyroid deficiency in the Framingham study. Arch Intern Med 1985; 145:1386–1388.
20. Liptzin B. Treatment of mania. In: Salzman C, ed. Clinical Geriatric Psychopharmacology. New York: McGraw-Hill, 1984:116–131.
21. Shulman KI, Mackenzie S, Hardy B. The clinical use of lithium carbonate in old age: a review. Biol Psychiatry 1987; 11:159–164.
22. Jefferson JW, Griest JH, Ackerman DL, Carroll JA. Cardiovascular effects. In: Lithium Encyclopedia for Clinical Practice. Washington, D.C. APPI, 1979.
23. Jensen HV, Olaffson K, Bille A, Anderson J, Mellerup E, Plenge P. Lithium every second day: a new treatment regimen? Lithium 1990; 1:55–58.
24. Young RC, Kalayam B, Tsuboyama G, Stokes P, Mattis S, Alexopoulos GS. Mania: Response to lithium across the age spectrum. Abstract, Annual Meeting, Society for Neuroscience, 1992; 18(4):669.
25. Broadhead J, Jacoby R. Mania in old age: a first prospective study. Int J Geriatr Psychiatry 1990; 5:215–222.
26. Black DW, Winokur G, Bell S, Nasrallah A, Hulbert J. Complicated mania. Arch Gen Psychiatry 1988; 45(3):232–236.
27. Shukla S, Hoff A, Aaronson T, Cool BL, Jandorf L. Treatment outcome in organic mania. New Research Program, Annual Meeting, American Psychiatric Association, 1987:91, 134.
28. Bajulaiye R, Addonizio G. Clozapine in the treatment of psychosis in an 82 year old woman with tardive dyskinesia. J Clin Psychopharmacol 1992; 12(5): 364–365.
29. Ball CJ. The use of clozapine in older people. Int J Geriatr Psychiatry 1992; 7(9): 689–692.
30. Oberholzer AF, Hendricksen C, Monsch AU, et al. Safety and effectiveness of low-dose clozapine in psychogeriatric patients: a preliminary study. Int Psychogeriatr 1992; 4:187–195.
31. Salzman C, Vaccaro B, Lieff J, Weiner A. Clozapine in elderly patients with psychosis and behavioral disruption. Am J Ger Psychiatry 1995; 3:26–33.
32. Frankenberg FR, Kalunian D. Clozapine in the elderly. J Geriatr Psychiatry Neurology 1994; 7:129–132.
33. Pope HGJ, McElroy SL, Keck PE Jr, Hudson JI. Valproate in the treatment of acute mania: a placebo controlled study. Arch Gen Psychiatry 1991; 48:62–68.
34. Fieve RR, Platman SR, et al. The use of lithium in affective disorders I: Acute endogenous depression. Am J Psychiatry 1987; 144:35–40.
35. Thase ME, Kupfer DJ, et al. Characteristics of treatment-resistant depression. In: Zohar J, Belmaker RH, eds. Treating Resistant Depression. New York: PMA Pub, 1987:23–45.

36. Bittman B, Young RC. Mania in an elderly man treated with bupropion. Am J Psychiatry 1991; 148:541.
37. Jain H, Young RC. Antidepressants and late life mania. Abstracts, Annual Meeting, Society for Neuroscience, 1988; 505:15.
38. Mukherjee S, Sackeim HA, Schnur DB. Electroconvulsive therapy of acute manic episodes: A review of 50 years' experience. Am J Psychiatry 1994; 151(2): 169–176.
39. Alexopoulos GS, Young RC, Abrams RC. ECT in the high-risk geriatric patient. Convul Ther 1989; 5:75–87.
40. El-Mallabh RS. Complications of concurrent lithium and electroconvulsive therapy: A review of clinical material and theoretical considerations. Biol Psychiatry 1988; 23:595–601.
41. Penney JF, Dinwiddie SH, Zorumski CF, Wetzel RD. Concurrent and close temporal administration of lithium and ECT. Convulsive Therapy 1990; 6(2): 139–145.
42. Abou-Saleh MT, Coppen A. Prognosis of depression in old age: the case for lithium therapy. Br J Psychiatry 1983; 143:527–528.
43. Angst J, Baastrup P, Grof P, Hippius H, Poldinger W, Weis P. The course of monopolar and bipolar depression and bipolar psychosis. Psychiat Neurol Neurochir 1973; 76:489–500.
44. Hewick DS, Newburg P, Hopwood S, Naylor G, Moody J. Age as a factor affecting lithium therapy. Br J Clin Pharmacol 1977; 4:201–205.
45. Abou-Saleh MT, Coppen A. Prognosis of depression in old age: The case for lithium therapy. Br J Psychiatry 1983; 143:527–528.
46. Murray N, Hopwood S, Balfour DJK, Ogston S, Hewisk DS. Influence of age on lithium efficacy and side effects in outpatients. Psychol Med 1983; 13:53–60.
47. Foster JR, Rosenthal S. Lithium treatment of the elderly. In: Johnson FN, ed. Handbook of Lithium Therapy. Lancaster, England: MTP Press, 1980:414–420.
48. Suppes T, Baldessarini RJ, Faedda GL, Tohen M. Risk of recurrence following discontinuation of lithium treatment in bipolar disorder. Arch Gen Psychiatry 1991; 48:1082–1088.
49. Faedda GL, Tondo L, Baldessarini RJ, Suppes T, Tohen M. Outcome after rapid vs gradual discontinuation of lithium treatment in bipolar disorders. Arch Gen Psychiatry 1993; 50:448–455.
50. Sernyak MJ, Griffin RA, Johnson RM, Pearsall HR, Wexler BE, Woods SW. Neuroleptic exposure following inpatient treatment of acute mania with lithium and neuroleptic. Am J Psychiatry 1994; 151(1):133–135.
51. Halberg G. Physiologic considerations underlying rhythomometry with special reference to emotional illness. In: DeAjuriaguerra J, ed. Cycles Biologiques et Psychiatrie. Geneva: Masson et Cie, 1968.
52. Himmelhoch JM, Neil JF, May SJ, Fuchs S, Licata SM. Age, dementia, dyskinesias, and lithium response. Am J Psychiatry 1980; 137:941–945.

ADDITIONAL LITERATURE

Bushey M, Rotberg V, Bowers MB. Lithium treatment in a very elderly nursing home population. Compr Psychiatry 1963; 24:392–396.

Chacko RC, Marsh BJ, Marmion J, Dworkin RJ, Telschow R. Lithium side effects in elderly bipolar outpatients. Hillside J Clin Psychiatry 1987; 9(1):79–88.

Csernansky JG, Hillister LE. Using lithium in patients with cardiac and renal disease. Hospital Formulary 1985; 20:726–735.

de Paulo JR, Folstein MF, Correa EI. The course of delirium due to lithium intoxication. J Clin Psychiatry 1982; 43:447–449.

Foster JR, Silver M, Boksay IJ. Lithium in the elderly: A review with special focus on the use of intraerythrocyte (RBC) levels in detecting serious impending neurotoxicity. Int J Geriatr Psychiatry 1990; 5(1):1–7.

Gnam W, Flint AJ. New onset rapid cycling bipolar disorder in an 87 year old woman. Can J Psychiatry 1993; 38(5):324–326.

Hansen HE, Amdisen A. Lithium intoxication (report of 23 cases and review of 100 cases from the literature). Q J Med 1978; (N Ser XLVII) 186:123–144.

Jefferson JW. Lithium and affective disorder in the elderly. Compr Psychiatry 1983; 24:166–178.

Judd LL, Hubbard B, Janowsky DS, Huey LY, Takahashi K. The effect of lithium carbonate on the cognitive functions of normal subjects. Arch Gen Psychiatry 1977; 34:355–357.

Kelwala S, Pomara N, Stanley M, Sitarani N, Gershon S. Lithium-induced accentuation of extrapyramidal symptoms in individuals with Alzheimer's disease. J Clin Psychiatry 1984; 45:342–344.

Lazarus JH. Endocrine and Metabolic Effects of Lithium. New York: Plenum, 1986.

Makeeva VL, Gol'davskah IL, Pozdnyakova SL. Somatic changes and side effects from the use of lithium salts in the prevention of affective disorders. Sov Neurol Psychiatry 1975; 7:42–53.

Miller F, Menninger J, Whitchup SM. Lithium-neuroleptic neurotoxicity in the elderly bipolar patient. J Clin Psychopharmacol 1986; 6:176–178.

Mirchandani IC, Young RC. Management of mania in the elderly: An update. Ann Clin Psychiatry 1993; 5(1):67–71.

Nambudiri DE, Meyers BS, Young RC. Delayed recovery from lithium neurotoxicity. J Geriatr Psychiat Neurol 1991; 4:40–43.

Schou M. Lithium prophylaxis: Myths and realities. Am J Psychiatry 1989; 146(5): 573–576.

Shaw ED, Mann JJ, Stokes PE, Manevitz AZA. Neuropsychological effects of lithium. New Research Abstracts, Annual Meeting, American Psychiatric Association, 1985:76, 130.

Schou M. Long-lasting neurological sequelae after lithium intoxication. Acta Psychiatr Scand 1984; 70:594–602.

Smith RE, Helms PM. Adverse effects of lithium therapy in the acutely ill elderly patient. J Clin Psychiatry 1982; 43:3.

Vestergaard P. Clinically important side effects of long term lithium treatment: A review. Acta Psychiatr Scand 1983; 67(suppl):11–36.

Yassa R, Nair NPV, Iskandar H. Late onset bipolar disorder in psychosis and depression in the elderly. Psychiatr Clin North Am 1988; 11(1):117–131.

Young RC, Meyers BS. Psychopharmacology. In: Sadovoy J, Lazarus LW, Jarvik LF, eds. Comprehensive Review of Geriatric Psychiatry, 2nd ed. Washington, DC: American Psychiatric Press, 1996:752–817.

15
Lithium Toxicity in the Elderly

JAMES W. JEFFERSON
*DEAN FOUNDATION FOR HEALTH, RESEARCH AND EDUCATION,
MIDDLETON, WISCONSIN*

"The older we grow, the greater become the ordeals"
Goethe, *Maxims and Reflections*, early 19th century

One of the earliest reports of lithium toxicity in the elderly involved two cases recorded by Kolipinski in 1898 (1). An octogenarian had been prescribed one lithium citrate tablet daily, but apparently decided that five daily would be better. "He presented a state of general prostration, muscular weakness making locomotion impaired. The upper extremities, particularly the hands, presented a constant fine tremor of acute onset and so severe that he could no longer write his name, an act that he very readily could perform a few days previous." Stopping lithium was followed by full recovery within a few days. The other patient, a 60-year-old, also recovered fully after stopping his daily consumption of four or five lithium tablets. Symptoms included cold hands and feet, weakness, "marked tremor and unsteadiness when he puts on his shoes or his gloves, . . . a greater muscular effort to write his name" and, in general, "He feels himself suddenly very old, and is thereby much depressed in spirits."

In the late 1940s, a miniepidemic of lithium poisoning occurred in conjunction with the unregulated use of 25% lithium chloride as a salt substitute in patients with cardiovascular disease. Given the elderly's predilection toward cardiovascular disease, a predominance of the toxicity reports were in that age group. For example, Corcoran et al. (2) described a 70-year-old woman with severe arteriosclerotic disease who "was seized with giddiness and nausea, . . . showed mental confusion, apathy and gross tremor of the arms and legs."

Unaware of the role played by lithium, a neurologist commented, "I have never seen such striking muscular irritability in a cerebral lesion" and suggested strychnine poisoning, tetanus, and tetany as possible diagnoses. Since she received no lithium while hospitalized, her symptoms resolved over the next week, but following discharge she resumed use of the lithium-containing salt substitute. "Again tremor, confusion, and apathy developed; she passed into a coma and died on Aug. 27, 1948."

As an aside, the April 1949 issues of *Consumer Reports* took the FDA to task over the salt substitute poisonings, stating: "Whatever the reason, it is clear that the FDA had reason to challenge lithium chloride last year, had the power at least to bring charges after the salts were marketed, and failed to do so until tragedy forced its hand" (3).

These early misadventures may have delayed the acceptance of lithium in the United States as a treatment for bipolar and other psychiatric disorders, but over the years the drug established its well-deserved reputation as one of the marvels of psychopharmacology. While it has been used safely and effectively in the elderly, its narrow therapeutic index puts this age group at particularly high risk for toxicity. Consequently, clinicians must be especially aware of the varied manifestations of lithium intoxication, risk factors that increase the likelihood of misadventure, preventive measures that can abort disaster, and appropriate interventions to effectively treat the toxic patient.

I. MANIFESTATIONS OF LITHIUM TOXICITY

There are no pathognomonic features of lithium intoxication. Since the manifestations are primarily neurological, any alteration in CNS function in a patient taking lithium should be considered potentially lithium-induced. In instances of gradual intoxication, the onset may be subtle and consist of no more than the slow evolution of fatigue and weakness associated with mild but worsening tremor, slight slurring of speech, and mild difficulty with balance. Such findings may be easily overlooked in the elderly who often have coexisting neurological problems and medication side effects.

As intoxication worsens, the abnormalities become more obvious: the tremor generalizes, ataxia is more apparent, and speech becomes more difficult to understand. Neuromuscular irritability as manifested by muscle fasciculations and twitching is commonly seen. Extrapyramidal and cerebellar findings may appear. The level of consciousness is progressively depressed, coma may ensue, seizures may occur, and death may follow.

Nambudiri et al. described a 67-year-old who mistakenly increased his dose of lithium carbonate from 1200 mg to 4800 mg per day for 3 days (4). Symptoms associated with a lithium level of 1.83 mEq/L included impaired memory, dysarthria, tremor, and nystagmus. The syndrome was fully reversible with dosage reduction. A 63-year-old with more severe intoxication was minimally responsive to painful stimuli, had doll's eyes sign, hyperreflexia and myoclonus, and required mechanical intubation (5).

At times, choreoathetosis will be a prominent finding (6–9). A 73-year-old with a serum lithium level of 2.18 mEq/L had ". . . garbled speech, hyperreflexia, myoclonus, asterixis, perseveration, poor stereoagnosis, and graphesthesia." As the lithium level fell, the myoclonus and asterixis improved but he "developed marked choreoathetosis of his arms, ataxia, and jerky movements of his legs," which then resolved over the next few weeks (6). In 1949, a 57-year-old casualty of the lithium chloride salt substitute era developed similar (and reversible) findings: "Speech was slurred, at times explosive and unintelligible. The outstanding findings, however, were the profound generalized chorea-athetoid movements of the extremities accompanied by facial grimacing of bizarre nature, dystonic movements of the tongue, and smacking of the lips" (10).

Lithium has also been implicated in inducing a Creutzfeldt–Jakob-like syndrome either alone or when combined with other medications (11–16). For example, a 70-year-old taking lithium and levodopa developed "a precomatose state, mutism, rigidity, sporadic myoclonic jerks that were prominent in the lower limbs. . ." associated with EEG findings of slow-wave activity, triphasic waves, and diffuse sharp waves (13). Another patient with suspected Creutzfeldt–Jakob disease was scheduled for a diagnostic brain biopsy until the symptoms resolved following discontinuation of lithium and nortriptyline (11).

Lithium toxicity has also presented in the guise of mania (17–20). A 60-year-old was oriented, grandiose, and irritable with pressured speech and labile mood and met Diagnostic and Statistical Manual (DSM-III) criteria for an episode of mania, yet his serum lithium level was 2.19 mEq/L. With discontinuation of lithium and some p.r.n. chlorpromazine, his symptoms improved (17). A 73-year-old was initially thought to be "suffering from a manic exacerbation of her bipolar mood disorder that was possibly superimposed on a dementing illness." On admission, the serum lithium level was 1.2 mEq/L (compared to her usual level of 0.8 mEq/L). When vomiting and diarrhea developed on the eighth day of hospitalization, lithium was discontinued and improvement was rapid (20).

While lithium toxicity may be the sole cause of a manialike clinical presentation, it is also possible that overtreatment of a true manic episode with lithium could result in a similar picture. Also, a patient and/or a caregiver may misidentify early symptoms of toxicity as the onset of an affective episode and launch the patient on the road to severe toxicity with a well-intentioned increase in the lithium dose. Since many elderly patients have neurological symptoms due to other illnesses or medications, establishing the correct diagnosis may be difficult. This is especially true because serum lithium levels in the conventional therapeutic range may, nonetheless, cause toxicity (see below).

While neurotoxicity constitutes the core of lithium poisoning, other organ systems are commonly involved. Gastrointestinal manifestations include anorexia, nausea, vomiting, abdominal pain, and diarrhea. These, in turn, may further worsen the toxicity by causing dehydration, electrolyte imbalance, and further elevation of the lithium level. The same is true for nephrotoxic complications that can include both renal failure (21) and profound nephrogenic diabetes insipidus (22). Marked hypotonic volume depletion can, in turn, further elevate the lithium level and may also cause a hypernatremic encephalopathy. Cardiac arrhythmias have also been caused by lithium intoxication. They are usually associated with a global neurotoxicity but, at times, they may be a relatively isolated manifestation. For example, a 72-year-old developed sinus pauses and escape beats followed by sinus arrest, asystole, and cardiac arrest. He was successfully resuscitated, and as the lithium level fell from a high of 3.49 mmol/L, normal cardiac rhythm was reestablished (23). A similar occurrence was noted in a 75-year-old who collapsed suddenly because of a junctional bradycardia that was fully reversible when the lithium level of 2.13 mmol/L was successfully managed (24). While lithium-induced cardiotoxicity is not unique to the elderly, it is more likely to occur in that population (perhaps due to the progressive loss of sinus node pacemaker cells that occurs with aging). Sinus node dysfunction is a rare, but characteristic finding (at therapeutic or toxic lithium levels) that can present as arrhythmia, dizziness, syncope, or cardiac arrest (25). A bradyarrhythmia in an elderly patient on lithium should be considered lithium-induced until proven otherwise. If lithium is the culprit but cannot be safely discontinued, a cardiac pacemaker may be necessary; otherwise, another mood stabilizer should be considered.

Finally, fever and leukocytosis (sometimes exceeding 20,000 mm^3) often accompany lithium intoxication. A careful search for intercurrent infection is essential (an infection may have initiated the toxicity or evolved as a complication of it), but at times none will be found. In such cases, the fever may be due to the direct effect of lithium on brain stem thermoregulatory centers and the elevated white blood count due to a leukemoid reaction to stress.

Lithium intoxication is not an all or none phenomenon—either full recovery or death. Once the acute episode has resolved (and this may take weeks), patients may be left with irreversible neurological damage (23). Cerebellar abnormalities such as dysarthria, nystagmus, ataxia, and intention tremor are the most characteristic residua. For example, 1 year after being acutely toxic (serum lithium level 3.9 mEq/L), a patient was described as follows: "Her behavior was normal, and her intelligence . . . was also normal, with a full scale IQ of 131. She had ocular dysmetria and markedly slurred, monosyllabic, scanning speech. She was generally hyperreflexic . . . , and had markedly incoordinated limbs and intention tremor. She was very ataxic and unable to walk unassisted" (26).

It is important to realize that permanent lithium-induced neurotoxicity can affect areas other than the cerebellum. There have been reports of "choreoathetosis (basal ganglia), parkinsonism, corticospinal abnormalities, dementia, and peripheral neuropathy" (22).

II. RISK FACTORS

When episodes of lithium toxicity were assessed in a lithium clinic over an 18-month period, they had occurred in 12.9% of patients over the age of 60 (4/31) compared to only 1.2% (1/164) of younger patients (27). The normal process of aging brings with it a number of changes that increase the risk of lithium toxicity. For example, with regard to the kidney the following decrease with age: kidney size and volume; number of glomeruli; juxtamedullary nephron mass; glomerular filtration rate (GFR); ability to excrete a water load; and ability to maximally concentrate urine.

On average, creatinine clearance decreases about 1% per year beyond age 40 (28). In addition to a reduced ability to excrete lithium, the elderly are at increased risk for dehydration. Importantly, the ability to detect thirst decreases with aging (29). CNS angiotensin II production may be reduced in the elderly, thus reducing its thirst-stimulating effect. Finally, plasma renin activity and aldosterone secretion decrease with age as does vasopressin release (29,30).

Age-related cardiovascular changes may also contribute to the increased risk of lithium toxicity in the elderly. For example, only 10% of the number of sinus node pacemaker cells present at age 20 remain at age 75 (31). In addition, there are decreases in cardiac output, both at rest and with exercise, and a progressive reduction in the ability to increase heart rate in response to stress.

The above-mentioned decrements are so-called "normal" consequences of aging. Superimposed upon them are risk factors related to associated medical illnesses and the use of other medications. During a 1-month period, residents of an intermediate-care facility in Massachusetts received an average of 4.7 medications (32). Drugs commonly prescribed to the elderly that can cause increases in serum lithium level include thiazide diuretics, nonsteroidal anti-inflammatory drugs, and angiotensin-converting enzyme inhibitors. Finally, diets low in sodium will reduce renal lithium clearance and increase serum lithium levels.

Another factor that may contribute to lithium toxicity in the elderly is failure to adhere to treatment recommendations. One study of posthospitalization compliance found only 2 days after discharge that 64% of patients were taking at least one medication that was not ordered at discharge and 30% of the medications taken had not been ordered at discharge (33). Impaired cognition in the elderly (both patients and caregivers) may contribute to accidental overdosing. Misattributing symptoms of toxicity to other illnesses may result in failure to recognize toxicity in a timely fashion. Patients, significant others, and physicians have all been guilty of this error.

Finally, the elderly *may* be more sensitive to the toxic effects of lithium than younger individuals, as reflected in many reports of neurotoxicity occurring at "therapeutic" serum levels (20,34–36). It has not been firmly established, however, that old age alone is a risk factor since no controlled comparative research has been done and since such toxicity has also been described in younger individuals (37). Coexisting CNS pathology is more common in the elderly, and may be a predisposing factor. The bottom line is that a "therapeutic" lithium level does not exclude lithium as the cause of neurotoxic symptoms in any age group (although admittedly it does reduce the likelihood).

III. PREVENTION

> "The good doctor pays constant attention to keeping people well so that there will be no sickness."
>
> Huai-nan Tzu (d. 122 B.C.)

As previously stated, "The three keys to successful prevention of lithium intoxication are education (patients), education (physicians), and education (significant others)" (22). In view of the many risk factors likely to be present in the elderly, preventive measures must be carefully and consistently implemented. Office visits may need to be scheduled at closer intervals, serum lithium levels and other pertinent laboratory tests obtained more frequently, and significant others involved more often. There must be open and frequently used channels of communication linking together all involved in the care of the patient. Whenever there is clinical deterioration the questions must be asked, "Could lithium be responsible?" and "Has the risk for intoxication increased?" Whenever a new medication is taken or an old medication discontinued, the question must be asked, "Will this affect the lithium level?" Whenever the patient is exposed to a new intervention, such as a diet, a change in climate, or a surgical procedure, the possibility of altering the lithium level must be considered. All involved must recognize the early warning symptoms and signs of lithium intoxication so that corrective measures can be instituted promptly and progression to severe intoxication averted.

Written materials can do much to reinforce the messages conveyed during office visits. Booklets such as "Lithium and Manic-Depression: A Guide"

(38) and "Lithium Treatment of Manic-Depressive Illness: A Practical Guide" (39) are representative examples.

IV. TREATMENT

The treatment of lithium toxicity does not lend itself to controlled clinical trials, so it comes as no surprise that none have been done or are likely to be done in any age group. Even the widely accepted recommendation that lithium should be removed from the body as rapidly as possible in order to minimize the likelihood of death, disability, or prolonged recovery has been questioned. Schwartz and Jones suggest that rapid reduction of toxic lithium levels might actually increase the neurotoxicity. Consequently, they state: "dialysis for hyperlithemia after regular doses does not have self-evident justification, should be considered with caution, and according to the present data, may increase the risk of permanent neurologic sequelae" (40).

Nonetheless, clinical experience strongly suggests that the duration of exposure is a risk factor associated with poor outcome; therefore, unless proven otherwise, it seems reasonable to expect that the prompt and aggressive removal of lithium from the body should reduce this risk. As stated by Amdisen (41): "Because there is no antidote for lithium, the most important object of management is to shorten the duration of exposure to the toxic lithium load as efficiently as possible by removal of lithium from the effector sites which probably exist but have not yet been identified: i.e., to remove lithium from the body." In his review of 213 published case reports of acute lithium toxicity, El-Mallakh concluded: "Sequelae tended to occur in the more severe cases . . . , or in cases in which proper treatment was not undertaken or delayed . . ." (42).

The treatment of lithium intoxication has been summarized by many authors (5,22,41–46). There are no therapeutic interventions that are unique to the elderly. In general, all but the mildest intoxications usually require hospital observation and treatment. Obviously, lithium intake should be stopped and, in cases of acute overdose, gastric lavage is essential. Since delayed absorption occasionally occurs, repeated lavage or continuous gastric suction may be necessary. While activated charcoal is not particularly useful, there is growing evidence that an ion exchange resin, sodium polystyrene sulfonate, may effectively reduce lithium absorption and reabsorption (lithium is excreted via the bile and intestine) in both acute and chronic intoxications. Serum lithium levels *must* be monitored frequently to assess the rate of removal of lithium from the body. Blood levels alone, however, are insufficient guides to treatment; they must be coupled with careful clinical observation. It is well recognized that acute overdoses tend to be better tolerated than more gradual intoxications since tissue saturation is less complete. Despite case reports of remarkably high serum levels being well-tolerated and managed successfully with conservative treatment (I was recently contacted about a young adult who overdosed, remained asymptomatic, and recovered without sequelae despite a serum lithium level of 8.1 mEq/L and treatment with only intravenous hydration), there have also been reports of death following overdoses.

Hemodialysis is the most efficient way of removing lithium from the body and, consequently, it is the treatment of choice for severe intoxication. Under normal circumstances, renal lithium clearance is about 20 ml/min (probably lower in the elderly). This is often greatly reduced during intoxication because of the adverse effects of lithium on renal function and on fluid/electrolyte balance. Hemodialysis increases lithium clearance to well over 100 ml/min, which is a 5 to 10 times improvement over the ability of the kidneys to excrete lithium (47). Dialysis, however, is not risk-free (48) and deciding when to institute the procedure is not always easy. Jaeger et al. applied several sets of "when to dialyze" criteria to 14 of their lithium toxic patients (3 of 14 whom had been dialyzed). Had they acted on these various sets of criteria, they would have dialyzed 10, 8, 2, or 1 of these patients. They concluded that while hemodialysis is the preferred treatment for the lithium toxic patient, there are no universally applicable criteria. Rather, they state that the decision to dialyze should be based on the clinical condition of the patient, the serum lithium level, and the elimination kinetics of lithium (47). While they believe that the decision about dialysis can be made 8–12 h after admission, in some situations this could be viewed as an unnecessary delay. All too often, an obviously toxic patient is observed for days rather than hours before dialysis is considered, much to the detriment of the patient (21). The duration of dialysis and whether it is performed one or more times depends on the efficiency of the dialyzer being used, the postdialysis lithium level, and the extent of the postdialysis rebound in serum level.

Peritoneal dialysis is vastly inferior to hemodialysis as a way of removing lithium from the body, and it should be considered only if the latter is not available and if renal function is substantially compromised. If kidney function is normal, peritoneal dialysis will not improve upon the rate of renal lithium excretion.

Restoring or preserving normal fluid and electrolyte balance is an essential aspect of treating lithium intoxication, even if hemodialysis is not employed. Polyuria, which commonly exists either as a preexisting lithium side effect or as a complication of the toxicity, makes fluid restoration more difficult. In the presence of lithium-induced nephrogenic diabetes insipidus, hypertonicity is often a problem and hypernatremic encephalopathy may be an added complication. While volume expansion to restore normal renal function is important, the use of forced diuresis with isotonic saline is not generally advised (22,41, 43,47).

V. DELAYED RECOVERY

Regardless of how lithium is removed from the body, it is commonly observed that clinical recovery from the acute effects lags well behind the decrease in serum lithium level. This is especially true when the intoxication has been subacute or chronic and may reflect a slower decrease in intracellular lithium levels and/or a greater degree of cellular toxicity. It is not unusual to find that lithium is undetectable in the blood while the patient still displays some symptoms of toxicity. Whether delayed recovery is more common or more prolonged in the elderly has not been established with certainty, but clinical impression suggests that this is the case (4). In situations in which recovery is complete, restoration of baseline cognitive functioning may take days or weeks, and in cases in which there are permanent neurological residua, maximum improvement may not be realized for months.

VI. CONCLUSIONS

Lithium can be used in the elderly both safely and effectively. At the same time, a number of risk factors increase the danger of using the drug in this population. As in all of medicine, preventing toxicity is much preferred to treating it. Close clinical observation, frequent laboratory monitoring, collaboration across specialties, and patient and professional education will do much to minimize the likelihood of intoxication. When toxicity does occur, and occasionally it will, early recognition will greatly enhance the likelihood of full recovery. Treatment strategies for managing lithium poisoning have not evolved from controlled, prospective research trials. Nonetheless, they are based on extensive clinical observation, sound clinical judgment, and good common sense. At present, the greater fault in the management of such cases is not lack of knowledge, but rather failure to apply what is already known.

REFERENCES

1. Kolipinski L. Note on some toxic effects from the use of citrate of lithium tablets. Md Med J 1898-9; 40:4–5.
2. Corcoran AC, Taylor RD, Page IH. Lithium poisoning from the use of salt substitutes. J Am Med Assoc 1949; 139:685–688.
3. Aaron H. Dangerous drugs. Consum Rep 1949; 14:171–173.
4. Nambudiri DE, Meyers BS, Young RC. Delayed recovery from lithium neurotoxicity. J Geriatr Psychiatry Neurol 1991; 4:40–43.
5. Simard M, Gumbiner B, Lee A, et al. Lithium carbonate intoxication. Arch Intern Med 1989; 149:36–46.

6. Reed SM, Wise MG, Timmerman I. Choreoathetosis: a sign of lithium toxicity. J Neuropsychiatry 1989; 1:57–60.
7. Walevski A, Radwan M. Choreoathetosis as toxic effect of lithium treatment. Eur Neurol 1986; 25:412–415.
8. Matsis P, Fisher RA, Tasman-Jones C. Acute lithium toxicity—chorea, hypercalcemia and hyperamylasemia. Aust NZ J Med 1989; 19:718–720.
9. Zorumski CF, Bakris GL. Choreoathetosis associated with lithium: case report and literature review. Am J Psychiatry 1983; 140(2):1621–1622.
10. Peters HA. Lithium intoxication producing chorea athetosis with recovery. Wis Med J 1949; 48:1075–1076.
11. Finelli PF. Drug induced Creutzfeldt-Jakob like syndrome. J Psychiatr Neurosci 1992; 17(3):103–105.
12. Mazza S, Di Trapani G, Mennuni G, et al. Creutzfeldt-Jakob like syndrome induced by lithium treatment. A case report. Neurophysiol Clin 1990; 20(suppl):42S.
13. Broussolle E, Setiey A, Moene Y, et al. Reversible Creutzfeldt-Jakob like syndrome induced by lithium plus levodopa treatment. J Neurol Neurosurg Psychiatry 1989; 52(5):686–687.
14. Smith SJM, Kocen RS. A Creutzfeldt-Jakob like syndrome due to lithium toxicity. J Neurol Neurosurg Psychiatry 1988; 51:120–123.
15. Kemperman CJF, Notermans SLH. Creutzfeldt-Jakob like syndrome due to lithium toxicity. J Neurol Neurosurg Psychiatry 1989; 52:291.
16. Primavera A, Brusa G, Poeta MG. A Creutzfeldt-Jakob like syndrome due to lithium toxicity. J Neurol Neurosurg Psychiatry 1989; 52:423.
17. El-Mallakh RS, Kantesaria AN, Chaikovsky LI. Lithium toxicity presenting as mania. Drug Intell Clin Pharm 1987; 21:979–981.
18. Nurnberger JI. Diuretic-induced lithium toxicity presenting as mania. J Nerv Ment Disord 1985; 173:316–318.
19. Thiel A, Nau R, Lehmann, et al. Intoxication in manic patients following chaotic self-administration of lithium. Acta Psychiatr Scand 1993; 88:289–291.
20. Bassingthwaighte ME, Rummans TA. Lithium toxicity in an elderly woman. J Clin Psychiatry 1991; 52(4):181.
21. Rutherfoord Rose S, Klein-Schwartz W, Oderda GM, et al. Lithium intoxication with acute renal failure and death. Drug Intell Clin Pharm 1988; 22:691–694.
22. Jefferson JW. Lithium poisoning. Emerg Care Q 1991; 7(1):18–28.
23. Ong ACM, Handler CE. Sinus arrest and asystole due to severe lithium intoxication. Int J Cardiol 1991; 30:364–366.
24. Farag S, Watson RDS, Honeybourne D. Symptomatic junctional bradycardia due to lithium intoxication in patient with previously normal electrocardiogram. Lancet 1994; 343:1371.
25. Steckler TL. Lithium- and carbamazepine-associated sinus node dysfunction: nine-year experience in a psychiatric hospital. J Clin Psychopharmacol 1994; 14(5):336–339.
26. Donaldson IM, Cuningham J. Persisting neurologic sequelae of lithium carbonate therapy. Arch Neurol 1983; 40:747–751.
27. Roose SP, Bone S, Haidorfer C, et al. Lithium treatment in older patients. Am J Psychiatry 1979; 136:843–844.

28. Lubran MM. Renal function in the elderly. Ann Clin Lab Sci 1995; 25(2):122–133.
29. Silver AJ. Aging and risks for dehydration. Cleve Clin J Med 1990; 57:341–344.
30. Weinberg AD, Minaker KL. Dehydration: evaluation and management in older adults. J Am Med Assoc 1995; 274:1552–1556.
31. Wei JY. Age and the cardiovascular system. Mech Dis 1992; 327(24):1735–1739.
32. Beers M, Avorn J, Soumerai SB, et al. Psychoactive medication use in intermediate-care facility residents. J Am Med Assoc 1988; 260(20):3016–3018.
33. Beers MH, Sliwkowski, Brooks J. Compliance with medication orders among elderly after hospital discharge. Hosp Formul 1992; 27:720–724.
34. Brown AS, Rosen J. Lithium-induced delirium with therapeutic serum lithium levels: a case report. J Geriatr Psychiatry Neurol 1992; 5:53–55.
35. Kemperman CJF, Gerdes JH, De Rooij JAM, et al. Reversible lithium neurotoxicity at normal serum level may refer to intracranial pathology. J Neurol Neurosurg Psychiatry 1989; 52(5):679–680.
36. Bell AJ, Cole A, Eccleston D, et al. Lithium neurotoxicity at normal therapeutic levels. Br J Psychiatry 1993; 162:689–692.
37. Strayhorn JM, Nash JL. Severe neurotoxicity despite "therapeutic" serum lithium levels. Dis Nerv Syst 1977; 38:107–111.
38. Bohn J, Jefferson JW. Lithium & Manic Depression: A Guide, 8th rev ed. Madison, WI: Lithium Information Center, 1996.
39. Schou M. Lithium Treatment of Manic-Depressive Illness: A Practical Guide, 5th rev ed. Basel, Switzerland: S. Karger AG, 1993.
40. Swartz CM, Jones P. Hyperlithemia correction and persistent delirium. J Clin Pharmacol 1994; 34:865–870.
41. Amdisen A. Clinical features and management of lithium poisoning. Med Toxicol 1988; 3:18–32.
42. El-Mallakh RS. Acute lithium neurotoxicity. Psychiatr Dev 1986; 4:311–328.
43. Winchester JF. Lithium. In: Haddad LM, Winchester JF, eds. Clinical Management of Poisoning and Drug Overdose. Philadelphia: W.B. Saunders, 1990:656–665.
44. Karki SD, Holden JMC. Treatment of lithium intoxication. Psychiatr Ann 1988; 18(12):708–712.
45. Bellomo R, Boyce N. Current approaches to the treatment of severe lithium intoxication. Lithium 1992; 3:245–248.
46. Okusa MD, Crystal LJT. Clinical manifestations and management of acute lithium intoxication. Am J Med 1994; 97:383–389.
47. Jaeger A, Sauder P, Kopferschmitt J, et al. When should dialysis be performed in lithium poisoning? A kinetic study in 14 cases of lithium poisoning. Clin Toxicol 1993; 31(3):429–447.
48. Oliver DO. Chronic renal failure, dialyses, and transplantation. In: Weatheroll DJ, Ledingham JG, Warrell DA, eds. Oxford Textbook of Medicine. Oxford: Oxford University Press, 1983: 18,118-18,135.

16
Anticonvulsants in Bipolar Elderly

Charles L. Bowden
The University of Texas Health Science Center at San Antonio, San Antonio, Texas

I. CLINICAL CHARACTERISTICS OF BIPOLAR ELDERLY

Consider the characteristics that make lithium a difficult choice in elderly bipolar patients. Elderly patients are more likely to have secondary mania, which responds poorly to lithium (1,2). As reviewed in Chapter 15, several adverse effects characteristic of lithium tend to be more frequent and more severe in bipolar elderly. Cognitive impairment may occur even at low serum levels and can persist well beyond cessation of lithium use. A common variant of this is the patient with early-onset bipolar disease who has responded to and tolerated lithium well, only to gradually develop cognitive impairment, most often evident as short-term memory difficulties, during the fifth or sixth decade of life. Cardiovascular adverse effects of lithium most commonly occur in the elderly patient (3).

Changes in the course of the illness with older age for which valproate and other anticonvulsants may be particularly appealing may also warrant consideration of mood stabilizers. Patients who had frequently recurring major depression in early adulthood and/or middle age may shift to a course of illness that includes manic episodes in later life (4,5).

These characteristics of elderly bipolar patients are not strictly a function of age, since they differ from age-matched patients with major depressive disorder. These differences, summarized in Table 1, indicate more than a fourfold greater frequency of neurological disorders and more than double the mortality rate of major depressive disorder (6). Bipolar patients with neurological disorders are more likely to be subsequently hospitalized. Neurologically impaired patients are somewhat less likely than the entire manic sample

TABLE 1 Comparison of Elderly Manic and Major Depressed Patients

Variable	Manic $n = 50$	Major depressed $n = 50$	Adjusted odds ratio
Neurological disorder	36%	8%	8.0
Mortality rate	50%	20%	2.4

to have family history of affective disorder in first degree relatives (33 vs. 52%). Neurologically impaired patients are much more likely to have their illness commence with a manic episode than the non-neurologically impaired. To summarize, when compared with nonelderly bipolar patients, elderly patients with bipolar disorder are more likely to have manic and mixed presentations, comorbid neurological disorders, and other general medical disorders for which long-term use of lithium is often poorly tolerated (3).

II. CHARACTERISTICS OF IMPULSIVE AGGRESSION IN THE ELDERLY

A second focus in elderly patients with dementia is impulsive aggression. This has been even less extensively studied than bipolar disorder in nondemented elderly. A small number of promising reports of the effectiveness of carbamazepine and valproate have been published. The degree of linkage between impulsive aggression and bipolar disorder remains to be clarified. Dementia is present in the majority of nursing home patients. Behavioral aggression is the most common management problem in these patients, and was present in approximately one-half of all patients with a diagnosis of dementia in two independent studies (7,8).

Swearer et al. (9) have described the aggressive component of the disruptive behavior associated with dementia as encompassing angry outbursts with and without actual assaultive behavior. Lott et al. (10) suggest the descriptively useful definition of impulsive aggression as psychological distress or irritability coupled with inappropriate verbal behavior or physical combativeness. It is possible that impulsive aggression is independent of bipolar disorder, with only incidental overlap in the symptoms of hostility and mood lability. Alternatively, impulsive aggression can be at least phenomenologically analogous to secondary mania. The earlier illness history of these patients and associated family history, which should aid in clarification of primary diagnosis, have been little studied. Kahn et al.'s (11) three patients with episodic aggressive behavior who responded to divalproex were probably bipolar.

No medication is approved by the Food and Drug Administration (FDA) for treatment of impulsive aggression in the elderly. Numerous medications, including beta-blockers, benzodiazepines, neuroleptics, and lithium, have been utilized in impulsive aggression. Each of the above classes poses risks in such patients, in part due to the risk of further worsening of cognitive impairment from the drugs. Interest in valproate is influenced by evidence of antiaggressive properties of valproate in animals (12). Additionally, low, measured amounts of plasma (GABA) have been reported in dementia, and valproate is known to alter GABA activity by several mechanisms, including inhibition of GABA reuptake and interference with aldehyde reductase (13). A recent study indicated that higher pretreatment plasma levels of GABA were significantly correlated with greater improvement in manic symptoms among hospitalized manic patients treated with divalproex (14).

III. EFFICACY OF VALPROATE IN BIPOLAR ELDERLY

Compared to lithium, valproate is of further interest in bipolar elderly because of its superior effectiveness in patients with mixed manic episodes, which are more common in elderly patients (15,16). Open studies indicate that the high degree of effectiveness is maintained both with monotherapy and when combined with lithium for up to the 1-year period of study (17).

The evidence for the effectiveness of valproate comes from a small number of patients treated in open trials. McFarland et al. (18) treated seven patients with bipolar disorder, most of whom had mixed states. The patients ranged in age from 56 to 74 years, with a mean age of 66 years. All had failed to respond to other medications or electroconvulsive therapy (ECT). All had general medical problems. Following addition of divalproex to ongoing medication, increased to obtain serum levels between 50 and 150 μg/ml, the GAS improved from 28 to 57 over a 1-month trial. Risinger et al. (19) reported that divalproex given both as monotherapy and added to lithium was effective and well tolerated in four elderly bipolar patients.

Two larger series have recently been described. Kando and associates (20) retrospectively reviewed the response to valproate of 35 elderly patients, 24 of whom were manic. The mean age of the entire group was 71 (range: 63 to 85). Many received other psychotropic medications. Response for the 24 manic patients was not reported separately from the larger group. Twenty-nine patients appeared to receive an adequate trial. Among the 29 patients, valproate was mildly effective in 8 (28%), moderately effective in 17 (59%), and markedly effective in one patient (3%). Adverse events included reports of nausea in two patients, sedation in two patients, and confusion in one patient. Nausea led to drug discontinuation in one patient. In this study, the mean dose was 743 mg per day (range: 250 to 2000 mg per day). The mean valproate blood level was 53 μg/ml (range: 11 to 102 μg/ml). In a second series, Narayan and colleagues (21) described response of 20 elderly patients treated with divalproex at Yale New Haven Hospital. All 20 patients had the primary diagnosis of bipolar disorder, manic. The mean age of the patients was 71 years (range: 60 to 82). Five patients had dementia comorbid with bipolar disorder. In this retrospective study, the doses and blood levels were substantially higher than in the preceding study. The mean dose was 1362 mg per day (range: 500 to 3000 mg per day) and the mean valproate serum level was 82 μg/ml (range: 31 to 122 μg/ml). On a CGI scale, ten patients were rated as very much improved, eight patients were much improved, and two patients failed to respond. No patient was rated as worse or unchanged. The mean GAF score increased from 26.4 on admission to 50.3 at discharge. Two patients became sedated, but improved with a decrease in the valproate dose. No patient required discontinuation of treatment.

The association of neurological factors with bipolar elderly has been previously described. Stoll et al. (22) reviewed records of 115 patients who were hospitalized for bipolar or schizoaffective disorders and treated with valproate. Most of the patients had failed to respond to lithium. Patients with a history of seizure were more often improved substantially with valproate treatment than were patients without such history (70 vs. 35%). A history of head injury and abnormal EEG was also associated with a good response to valproate. Patients with any neurological abnormality had higher rates of good response than did neurologically normal patients (44 vs. 24%).

IV. EFFICACY OF CARBAMAZEPINE IN BIPOLAR ELDERLY

No studies of carbamazepine in elderly patients specifically have been published. Some evidence suggests that bipolar patients with associated organic disorders are more responsive to carbamazepine than to lithium (1). Some evidence supports the notion that patients with frequently recurrent severe major depression may be pathophysiologically bipolar. Mitchell and associates (23) reported on the effectiveness of carbamazepine in treatment of 16 depressed patients with a mean age of 64 years. Three had bipolar disorder and 13 had unipolar disorder. Fourteen had failed treatment with ECT, 11 with lithium. Four (44%) patients had moderate and three marked responses. Carbamazepine had to be discontinued in seven patients (44%). The reasons for discontinuation were rash (two patients), hyponatremia (two patients), and gastrointestinal upset or liver failure (three patients). Two patients who relapsed subsequently responded to valproate. Phrased differently, only 3 of 16 patients benefited long term from carbamazepine.

V. EFFICACY OF OTHER ANTIEPILEPTIC AGENTS

Several drugs recently approved for various forms of epilepsy have generated interest as possible mood-stabilizing drugs. These include lamotrigine, a drug that inhibits use-dependent sodium-channel activity in neurons. Lamotrigine has recently been reported to be effective in bipolar patients experiencing depressed, mixed, and manic episodes. In the open trial, lamotrigine was used both as monotherapy and added to stable drug regimens (24). A report of two previously treatment refractory bipolar patients who improved with lamotrigine has also been published (25). No controlled study data are available as yet.

Two antiepileptic drugs that enhance GABA activity, gabapentin and vigabatrin, have also generated recent interest because valproate is known to have effects on GABA. No studies in bipolar disorder have been published with either drug.

Each of the above drugs has a relatively benign adverse effect profile, thus enhancing its potential appeal in elderly patients if efficacy is shown in standard samples. It is premature to recommend these medications for any group of bipolar elderly.

VI. EFFICACY IN IMPULSIVE AGGRESSION IN THE ELDERLY

A. Valproate

Lott et al. (10) reported on ten patients between the ages of 71 and 94 with impulsive aggression and dementia, all of whom required nursing home care. Eight had no comorbid psychiatric condition. All had general medical disorders. Five were receiving no other medications. The patients were started on 125 mg of divalproex twice daily, with gradual increase in dosage until response was observed. One patient had complete remission of aggression, three had marked (>60%) reduction, and four moderate (>50%), one mild improvement, and one no improvement. Thus, in the aggregate, 80% had greater than 50% symptom reduction, which persisted for up to 1 year at last report. All patients tolerated the divalproex well. Plasma levels during improvement ranged from 13 to 52 μg/ml.

Two agitated patients, aged 63 and 68 years, were effectively treated with divalproex at standard serum levels (60–75 μg/ml). Clinical features suggestive of bipolar disorder were present in both patients (26). Mellow et al. (27) reported valproate markedly effective in two and transiently effective in one of four patients with dementia and associated behavioral disturbance.

Wilcox (28) reported on a diverse group of agitated patients in treatment at a state hospital, using time spent in seclusion as an objective measure of effectiveness of valproate. The mean pretreatment rate of 18 h per week in seclusion dropped to a mean value of 2 h per week after 2 weeks of valproate treatment. The best results were observed in patients who met criteria for mixed or atypical bipolar disorder.

Two retrospective medical record reviewers have also reported valproate effective in improving behavioral problems associated with dementia. Sival et al. (29) reported on 23 patients for whom disruptive behavior was completely eliminated in 26% and reduced in 52%. Narayan and Nelson reported on 23 patients between the ages of 62 and 86 years, 20 of whom had severe dementia (MMSE < 5) (30). Seven of the 14 patients who received divalproex alone were much improved, as were six of the nine patients for whom divalproex was added to previously ineffective neuroleptics, for an overall response rate of 57%. The mean serum valproate level was 63 μg/ml. Sedation was the only common adverse effect, occurring in seven patients, but diminishing with reduced divalproex dosage in six of the seven.

Kahn et al. (11) reported substantial improvement during divalproex treatment in three patients with aggression who had probable bipolar disorders. However, the ages of the patients ranged from 29 to 50 years. Also, Sovner (31) reported improvement in aggression with divalproex in five mentally retarded patients who also met some criteria for bipolar disorder. The patients were not elderly, ranging from 24 to 44 years of age.

Divalproex and carbamazepine have been compared directly in one retrospective study. Patients with impulsive aggression were assessed in terms of time spent in mechanical restraints during treatment with either divalproex or carbamazepine. Divalproex was reported as generally effective overall and much more effective than carbamazepine (32).

B. Carbamazepine

Smith and Perry (33) reviewed studies of carbamazepine in patients with aggression or agitation as the target behavioral problem. The review included studies on patients with dementia and organic mental disorders, but also younger patients with mental retardation and autism. The carbamazepine studies were considered inconclusive, in contrast to a more positive assessment of studies of beta-blockers. The authors recommended that carbamazepine be reserved for patients who had failed other regimens. The authors commented that most studies of carbamazepine had been poorly designed.

Patterson (34) reported on eight assaultive patients with organic mental disorders treated with carbamazepine, but did not say whether other drugs were used. The medication was generally effective, but two of the patients had to be discontinued because of diplopia and ataxia. A subsequent report by Patterson (35) of 13 patients also indicated a favorable response to carbamazepine. It is unclear whether these patients included the eight previously reported. Leibovici and Tariot (36) reported two demented patients who had improvement of agitation with carbamazepine treatment and tolerated the drug well. Lemke (37) studied 15 severely demented patients with aggression who had not responded to neuroleptic treatment for agitation and hostility. Carbamazepine was started at 100 mg daily and increased as needed. Carbamazepine serum levels at the end of the trial ranged from 2.4 to 5.2 ml. Haloperidol, which could also be added if clinically indicated, was used in ten patients, at an average dose of 3.4 mg/day. Activation and hostility factors from the BPRS improved significantly over the 4-week trial. Carbamazepine had to be discontinued in two subjects due to leukopenia and rash, respectively.

VII. DOSING AND TREATMENT MANAGEMENT GUIDELINES

The adverse effect profiles of valproate and carbamazepine have both been extensively studied (16,38). Relatively little data come from specifically elderly samples. However, certain features of both drugs may pose greater risks in elderly patients. Elderly patients tend to have lower levels of plasma proteins and thus have higher percentages of the free, active drug moiety. Rates of elimination of drugs by the liver are often reduced. Thus more cautious initial dosing, slower dosage escalation, and greater intervals between doses are likely to be useful in many, albeit not all, elderly bipolar or agitated patients.

A. Valproate

Bowden et al. (16) reported in a sample of 69 adult manic patients that serum valproate levels of 45 μg/ml or greater were associated with significantly greater likelihood of response than lower levels. Age was not significantly correlated with either the total or free serum level. Characteristic adverse effects were more common in patients who were between the ages of 18 and 65 years, and whose levels exceeded 125 ml (39). These results are similar to impressionistic reports of others (40).

In elderly patients with bipolar disorder, similar target values are indicated as a general guide to dosing until more explicit data become available. Valproate is highly bound to plasma proteins, and is readily displaceable by strongly lipophilic drugs such as salicylates. This results in an increase in the free, active fraction of valproate. Free levels are not routinely assayed, but generally constitute 5 to 20% of the total value (41).

Valproate should generally be initiated at a dose of 125 or 250 mg once or twice daily. If the patient is hospitalized or in another 24-h supervised facility, a more vigorous initial dosing can be considered, including use of a loading dose of 15–20 mg/kg body weight. If the patient's tolerance of initial dosage is good, the dosage may be rapidly increased until improvement occurs, intolerable adverse effects develop, or levels around 100 ml are reached. No systematic study of dosage and serum levels has been conducted in elderly patients, but individual patient experience indicates that some elderly patients respond to lower levels than the 45–125 μg/ml range, whereas others require the same levels as young patients (30). There are numerous anecdotal reports indicating that patients with other neurological disorders are less likely to tolerate standard doses, but may benefit at lower levels.

Pretreatment assessment in elderly patients is not different from that in younger adults, with baseline hematological and hepatic studies indicated. These parameters should initially be monitored somewhat more frequently given the likelihood of less reserve capacity of most organ systems with aging. However, the limited psychiatric and neurological literature do not suggest that frequency of any of the characteristic adverse effects of valproate is clinically significantly elevated in the elderly.

Cognitive Impairment

Studies indicate that valproate causes less cognitive impairment than phenytoin or carbamazepine (42,43). No direct comparisons with lithium have been published, but there is broad empirical support that valproate is much less likely to cause cognitive deficits than is lithium, as exemplified in the case report that follows. Nevertheless, some elderly patients have been observed to develop memory and attention problems at serum levels of valproate below 45 μg/ml. Therefore, alerting patients and nursing personnel to such possibilities is an important precaution. Valproate has no tendency to show delayed cognitive impairment; therefore, if a patient has not had memory difficulties by the time at which steady levels are attained, subsequent difficulties are unlikely.

Hair Loss

Hair loss occurs in around 3% of younger adults. Since it appears that this is associated with deficits of selenium and other trace metals such as zinc, which may be a consequence of gastrointestinal tract chelation with valproic acid, multiple vitamin supplementation with a selenium- and zinc-containing preparation is justified even prophylactically. Many less expensive multiple vitamins do not contain selenium or zinc. Formulations that have at least 150 mg of selenium and 10 mg of zinc include Centrum Plus and Glutofac.

Hematological Parameters

Thrombocytopenia is common with valproate treatment, but is not often clinically significant. Because hematopoietic activity may be diminished in the elderly, closer monitoring of both platelet count and clinical evidence of bruising or bleeding is warranted. The rate of blood dyscrasias is lower from valproate than from carbamazepine, and appear to be no higher than observed without drugs (38). Rarely, valproate can also reduce white blood count, possibly even to levels that require discontinuation of valproate.

Hepatic Function

Most hepatic abnormalities with valproate are associated with immature hepatic function, which is not at issue in the elderly. Preexisting liver disease may increase the risk of a hepatotoxic reaction to valproate, however. Therefore, enzymes should be monitored every month or so during the initial phase of treatment. Moderate elevation of liver enzyme activity (i.e., less than 3 times the baseline level) that does not continue to increase is not cause for action other than continued monitoring.

Tremor

Valproate may cause a fine or coarse intention tremor, which may be alleviated by reduced dosage, or lipophilic beta-blockers such as propranolol. Since elderly patients are increasingly likely to develop parkinsonism, careful baseline and continuing assessment for signs of extrapyramidal movements is indicated, lest the two relatively distinct syndromes of intention tremor with valproate and resting tremor with parkinsonism be confused.

Gastrointestinal Effects

Valproate is more prone to cause cramping, nausea, and diarrhea than is carbamazepine. These symptoms are less common and less severe with the divalproex preparation than with valproic acid (44). Gradual dosage escalation may allow some development of tolerance to these gastrointestinal effects. H_2-receptor blockers may also control such adverse effects. For patients taking relatively low daily dosages, use of the 125-mg sprinkle formulation will maintain a more even level with less peak level effects.

Drug Interactions

The principal interactions with valproate entail the displacement from plasma proteins by other lipophilic agents (salicylates, most psychotropic drugs, high-fat meals). This may be of such magnitude as to temporarily increase free levels to precipitate adverse effects. These effects may be minimized by separating dosing times of such drugs. A second group of interactions occur with oxidative and conjugating hepatic enzymes. In most patients treated with divalproex, the major metabolic pathway is by glucuronide conjugation. Relatively few drugs are so metabolized, but the potential for mutual increases for drugs with this primary route of metabolism is high. Concurrent use of lamotrigine, a recently introduced antiepileptic drug that is metabolized by conjugation, often results in a doubling of the levels for each drug over what would occur with monotherapy. The effects of oxidative inhibitors (paroxetine, fluoxetine) and inducers (carbamazepine) are usually modest. Nevertheless, because of the likely use by elderly patients of several medications, the best course is to assess initially the levels of any drugs of concern, including valproate, until a stable regimen has been maintained for several months. Subsequently, levels need to be monitored only if any regimen change occurs, adverse effects develop, or clinical state changes.

Valproate may be safely combined with other mood-stabilizing drugs. Pharmacokinetic interactions with carbamazepine and potential impact on hematological and hepatic function make the combination less advisable. Lithium and valproate are generally well tolerated, with empirical evidence that lower and thus better tolerated levels of lithium may be possible in combination with valproate. Nevertheless, the author's preference is to minimize complicated regimens in elderly patients, and to recommend efforts to discontinue lithium if valproate has been added to it.

Single Daily Dosing

Although the half-life of valproate is somewhat less than 24 h, many patients tolerate and maintain equivalent benefit from once-daily bedtime dosing schedules. This gives the benefit of improved adherence to medication schedule and may reduce transient adverse effects associated with increased levels shortly after dosing.

B. Carbamazepine

Pretreatment assessment prior to starting carbamazepine should include a complete blood count with differential and platelet count, hepatic function measures, serum sodium, thyroid function assessment, and an electrocardiogram. Serum levels should be determined for any drugs metabolized by the 3A4 isoenzyme for which therapeutic drug monitoring is indicated (e.g., bupropion). Because of the autoinduction by carbamazepine of its own metabolism, relatively frequent serum-level monitoring needs to be continued for the first 4 to 6 months.

Carbamazepine should be initiated as 200 mg per day, and slowly increased as tolerated. Even younger adults often develop neuromuscular adverse effects from carbamazepine (ataxia, diplopia, asthenia, sedation(. These complications may be more common in the elderly. Gleason reported that three of nine patients treated with 200 to 1000 mg per day of carbamazepine became ataxic (45). Similarly, Patterson reported diplopia and ataxia in two of eight patients (34) and Lemke reported that three of fifteen patients had to be discontinued for adverse effects over a 4-week period (37). These relatively high rates of discontinuance are consistent with reports in young subjects (46).

Plasma-level relationships of carbamazepine to response have not been found either in bipolar or epileptic patients. Dosing is therefore to the point of clinical response or tolerability. In younger adults, responses are generally observed between 6 and 12 μg/ml. It seems prudent to aim initially for levels in the lower end of that range, especially in patients with concurrent neurological disorders.

Several characteristic adverse effects of carbamazepine are either more frequent and or more problematic in the elderly. Hyponatremia, which occurs in young and old, is more likely to be clinically significant, causing weakness, in the elderly. Bradycardia and atrioventricular block occur principally in the elderly, with evidence of greater risk in women. A review of such complications in 26 patients found the average age of patients with these reported complications to be 65 years, with 81% female. Only 5 of the 26 cases occurred in patients less than 50 years of age. Seventy-three percent of the patients developed the various bradyarrhythmias at normal doses and levels. It is therefore important to obtain an electrocardiogram prior to starting treatment with carbamazepine in patients over 50 years of age, and to consider any existing degree of atrioventricular block as a relative contraindication (47).

Both leukopenia and thrombocytopenia are relatively common in elderly patients treated with carbamazepine (38). A somewhat more conservative threshold of concern seems warranted in the elderly because of their greater propensity to infections and bleeding problems. However, as with valproate, so long as white blood count does not fall below 3000/mm^3, only increased vigilance in monitoring is indicated.

Carbamazepine actively induces the 3A4 isoenzyme of the CYP450 family of oxidative liver enzymes. Since many psychotropic and general medical drugs are solely or largely metabolized through 3A4, combined use should be undertaken only if no other regimen is effective. A partial list of such drugs is shown in Table 2. If it is necessary to use carbamazepine with one of these drugs, when possible drug-level monitoring should be obtained to determine whether the levels are within the effective range.

VIII. CONCLUSIONS

The interest in use of drugs with antiepileptic properties to control manic episodes and mood cycling in elderly bipolar patients has been fueled by limitations in the tolerability of lithium, neuroleptics, and other sedative-type drugs

TABLE 2 Interactions of Carbamazepine with Drugs Metabolized by the 3A4 Oxidative Isozyme

Alprazolam	Terfenadine
Triazolam	Claritin
Bupropion	Ketoconazole
Nefazadone	Itraconazole
Birth control pills	Astemizole

in such patients. The relatively good tolerability of divalproex has been consistently reported in nearly all trials, both in elderly and nonelderly samples. Divalproex appears better tolerated than both lithium and carbamazepine (48). The difficulties in use of carbamazepine warrant concern about prescribing it in elderly patients unless other medications have failed.

The reported efficacy of divalproex in bipolar manic episodes and in impulsive aggression in the elderly has been consistently good. However, controlled, randomized, trial data are absent. Nevertheless, divalproex can be recommended for initial use in symptomatic bipolar elderly and agitated patients both because of its generally favorable safety profile and its ease of use. Additionally, no more compelling data are available for any other class of drug for these indications. The modest amount of available evidence should encourage systematic prospective studies to establish the effectiveness and predictors of response to valproate.

The efficacy of carbamazepine is less securely established than that of lithium or valproate. Although several reports indicate good outcomes, these often involved use of neuroleptics. This is consistent with studies of carbamazepine in nonelderly bipolar patients, wherein most received neuroleptic drugs (49). This suggests that carbamazepine may be more beneficial principally when combined with neuroleptics or possibly lithium or valproate.

Despite difficulties in diagnostic classification of behavioral agitation, it is clear that it is descriptively similar to many aspects of manic and mixed episodes (e.g., episodicity, impaired judgment, motor hyperactivity, irritability, and hostility). Even in the absence of studies to establish the degree of fitting within the spectrum of secondary mania, use of valproate, and secondarily, carbamazepine is warranted. Further systematic investigation of valproate in this serious medical problem area is indicated.

REFERENCES

1. Himmelhoch JM, Garfinkel ME. Sources of lithium resistance in mixed mania. Psychopharmacol Bull 1986; 22:613–620.

2. Prien RF, Himmelhoch JM, Kupfer DJ. Treatment of mixed mania. J Affect Disord 1988; 15:9–15.
3. Murray N, Hopwood S, Balfour DJK, Ogston S, Hewisk DS. The influence of age on lithium efficacy and side effects in out-patients. Psychol Med 1983; 13:53–60.
4. Shulman K, Post R. Bipolar affective disorder in old age. Br J Psychiatry 1980; 136:26–32.
5. Winokur G, Clayton P, Reich T. Manic-Depressive Illness. St. Louis: C.V. Mosby, 1969.
6. Tohen M, Shulman KI, Satlin A. First-episode mania in late life. Am J Psychiatry 1994; 151:130–132.
7. Rovner BW, Kafonek S, Filipp L, et al. Prevalence of mental illness in a community nursing home. Am J Psychiatry 1986; 143:1446–1449.
8. Chandler JD, Chandler FE. The prevalence of neuropsychiatric disorders in a nursing home population. J Geriatr Psychiatr Neurol 1993; 1:71–76.
9. Swearer JM, Drachman DA, O'Donnell BF, Mitchell AL. Troublesome and disruptive behaviors in dementia. Relationship to diagnosis and disease severity. J Am Geriatr Soc 1988; 36:784–790.
10. Lott AD, McElroy SL, Keys MA. Valproate in the treatment of behavioral agitation in elderly patients with dementia. J Neuropsychiatry Clin Neurosci 1995; 7: 314–319.
11. Kahn D, Stevenson E, Douglas CJ. Effect of sodium valproate in three patients with organic brain syndromes. Am J Psychiatry 1988; 145:101–111.
12. Simler S, Puglisi-Allegra S, Mandel P. Effects of N-dipropylacetate on aggressive behavior and brain GABA level in isolated mice. Pharmacol Biochem Behav 1983; 18:717–720.
13. Balfour JA, Bryson HM. Valproic acid: a review of its pharmacology and therapeutic potential in indications other than epilepsy. CNS Drugs 1994; 2:144–173.
14. Petty F, Rush AJ, Davis JM, Calabrese JR, Small JG, Swann AE, et al. Plasma GABA predicts response to divalproex in mania. Biol Psychiatry 1995; 37:593–683.
15. Freeman TW, Clothier JL, Pazzaglia P, Lesem MD, Swann AC. A double-blind comparison of valproate and lithium in the treatment of acute mania. Am J Psychiatry 1992; 149:108–111.
16. Bowden CL, Brugger AM, Swann AC, Calabrese JR, Janicak PG, Petty F, et al. Efficacy of divalproex vs lithium and placebo in the treatment of mania. J Am Med Assoc 1994; 271:918–924.
17. Calabrese JR, Delucchi GA. Spectrum of efficacy of valproate in 55 patients with rapid-cycling bipolar disorder. Am J Psychiatry 1990; 147:431–434.
18. McFarland BH, Miller MR, Straumfjord AA. Valproate use in the older manic patient. J Clin Psychiatry 1990; 51:479–481.
19. Risinger RC, Risby ED, Risch SC. Safety and efficacy of divalproex sodium in elderly bipolar patients. J Clin Psychiatry 1994; 55:215.
20. Kando JC, Tohen M, Castillo J, Zarate CA. The use of valproate in an elderly population with affective symptoms. J Clin Psychiatry 1996; 57:238–240.
21. Narayan M, Noaghiul S, Nelson JC. Divalproex treatment of mania in elderly patients. Presented at the American Society of Clinical Psychopharmacology Annual Meeting, Barbados, 1997.

22. Stoll AL, Banov M, Kolbrener M, Mayer PV, Tohen M, Strakowski SM, et al. Neurologic factors predict a favorable valproate response in bipolar and schizoaffective disorders. J Clin Psychopharmacol 1994; 14:311–313.
23. Mitchell P. Valproate for rapid-cycling unipolar affective disorder. J Nerv Ment Dis 1991; 179:503–504.
24. Anonymous editor. "Spectrum of efficacy" of lamotrigine in treatment-refractory manic depression 1995;
25. Weisler R, Risner ME, Ascher J, Houser T. Use of lamotrigine in the treatment of bipolar disorder. American Psychiatric Association Meeting, City, 1994 (Abstract).
26. Mazure CM, Druss BG, Cellar JS. Valproate treatment of older psychotic patients with organic mental syndromes and behavioral dyscontrol. J Am Geriatr Soc 1992; 40:914–916.
27. Mellow AM, Solano-Lopez C, Davis S. Sodium valproate in the treatment of behavioral disturbance in dementia. J Geriatr Psychiatr Neurol 1993; 6:205–209.
28. Wilcox J. Divalproex sodium in the treatment of aggressive behavior. J Clin Psychiatry 1994; 6:17–20.
29. Sival R, Haffmans P, vanGent P, et al. The effect of sodium valproate on disturbed behavior in dementia. J Am Geriatr Soc 1994; 42:906–907.
30. Narayan N, Nelson JC. Treatment of dementia with behavioral disturbance using divalproex or a combination of divalproex and a neuroleptic. Presented at the ASCP meeting, Montego Bay, Jamaica, 1996.
31. Sovner R. The use of valproate in the treatment of mentally retarded persons with typical and atypical bipolar disorders. J Clin Psychiatry 1989; 50:40–43.
32. Alam MY, Klass DB, Luchins DJ, et al. Divalproex sodium, valproic acid and carbamazepine in aggression. Presented at the annual meeting of the NCDEU, Orlando, FL, 1995.
33. Smith DA, Perry PJ. Nonneuroleptic treatment of disruptive behavior in organic mental syndromes. Ann Pharmacother 1992; 26:1400–1408.
34. Patterson JF. A preliminary study of carbamazepine in the treatment of assaultive patients with dementia. J Geriatr Psychiatr Neurol 1988; 1:21–23.
35. Patterson JF. Carbamazepine for assaultive patients with organic brain disorders. Psychosomatics 1987; 28:79–81.
36. Leibovici A, Tariot PN. Carbamazepine treatment of agitation associated with dementia. J Geriatr Psychiatr Neurol 1988; 1:110–112.
37. Lemke MR. Effects of carbamazepine on agitation in Alzheimer's inpatients refractory to neuroleptics. J Clin Psychiatry 1995; 56:354–357.
38. Tohen M, Castillo-Ruiz J, Baldessarini RJ, Kando KC, Zarate CA. Blood dyscrasias with carbamazepine and valproate: a pharmacoepidemiological study of 2,228 cases at risk. Am J Psychiatry 1995; 152:413–418.
39. Bowden CL, Swann A, Orsulak P, Davis J, Calabrese J, Morris D. Serum concentration-efficacy relationships of valproate in acute mania. Am Coll Neuropsychopharmacol 1994 (abstract).
40. Pope HG, Jr., McElroy SL, Keck PE, Jr., Hudson JI. Valproate in the treatment of acute mania: A placebo-controlled study. Arch Gen Psychiatry 1991; 48:62–68.

41. Gomez-Bellver MJ, Garcia-Sanchez MJ, Alonso-Gonzalez AC, Santos-Buelga D, Dominguez-Gil A. Plasma protein binding kinetics of valproic acid over a broad dosage range: therapeutic implications. J Clin Pharm Ther 1993; 18:191–197.
42. Trimble MR, Thompson PJ. Sodium valproate and cognitive function. Epilepsia 1994; 25(suppl 1):S60–S64.
43. Thompson PJ, Trimble MR. Sodium valproate and cognitive functioning in normal volunteers. Br J Clin Psychopharm 1981; 12:819–824.
44. Wilder BJ, Karas BJ, Penry JK, Asconape J. Gastrointestinal tolerance of divalproex sodium. Neurology 1983; 33:808–811.
45. Gleason RP, Schneider LS. Carbamazepine treatment of agitation in Alzheimer's outpatients refractory to neuroleptics. J Clin Psychiatry 1990; 51:115–118.
46. Denicoff KD, Smith-Jackson E, Disney E, Syed AO, Leverich GS, Post RM. Carbamazepone, lithium and the combination: a bipolar maintenance trial. Proceedings of the American Psychiatric Association, City, 1995.
47. Kasarskis EJ, Kuo CS, Berger R, Nelson KR. Carbamazepine-induced cardiac dysfunction. Arch Intern Med 1992; 152:186–191.
48. Citrome L. The use of lithium, carbamazepine, and valproic acid in a state operated psychiatric hospital. J Pharm Technol 1995; in press.
49. Okuma T, Yamashita I, Takahashi R, Itoh H, Otsuki S, Wantanabe S, et al. Comparison of the antimanic efficacy of carbamazepine and lithium carbonate by double-blind controlled study. Pharmacopsychiatry 1990; 23:143–150.

17
Treatment of Psychosis in Late Life

JOHN H. EASTHAM, JONATHAN P. LACRO, JAMES B. LOHR, AND DILIP V. JESTE
University of California, San Diego, La Jolla, and San Diego Veterans Affairs Medical Center, San Diego, California

I. INTRODUCTION

It has been estimated that more than 90% of nursing home residents have a major neuropsychiatric disability (1) and that nursing home patients receive antipsychotics for approximately 17 of every 100 patient days (2). As the most effective treatment of psychosis is the use of antipsychotic medications, neuroleptics are commonly prescribed to the elderly. In contrast to the large number of published studies of neuroleptics in young adult patients, there is relatively sparse literature regarding antipsychotics in older age. Treatment of late-life psychosis has generally involved extrapolating from studies of younger patients and gleaning information from small, uncontrolled studies that involved older patients. This chapter will discuss the evaluation and treatment of psychosis in late life. Evaluation consists of diagnostic workup, assessment of medical comorbidity and psychosocial factors, development of a treatment plan, and obtaining informed consent. Treatment considerations include the choice of antipsychotic medication, dosing guidelines, assessment of patient compliance, and neuroleptic maintenance strategies. To the extent possible, we will rely on the published literature despite its limitations and the fact that many of the published studies are uncontrolled.

II. PSYCHOSES

A. Early-Onset Schizophrenia

Schizophrenia patients who are first diagnosed in their adolescence or early adulthood may be termed as having early-onset schizophrenia (EOS). A majority of patients with EOS survive into old age. Although the course of schizophrenia has been poorly studied, it appears that most schizophrenia patients do not develop new positive symptoms as they get older. In about 60% of the patients, the illness remains relatively stable. Both positive and negative symptoms improve in about 20% of patients (3). The remaining 20% have a continued decline with the development of negative symptoms. A small proportion of patients improve sufficiently that neuroleptic medications are no longer required. Relapse and exacerbation may occur in elderly patients with chronic schizophrenia just as they do in younger patients.

B. Late-Onset Schizophrenia

Schizophrenia patients with an onset of symptoms after 45 years of age are considered to have late-onset schizophrenia (LOS) (4). Some studies have indicated that approximately 15% of schizophrenia patients have onset of symptoms after 45 years of age (5). LOS is similar to EOS in terms of clinical presentation of positive symptoms and the chronic nature of the disorder. LOS and EOS are also similar with respect to family history of schizophrenia and early childhood maladjustment (6). Nevertheless, some differences exist between LOS and EOS (5). LOS patients have fewer negative symptoms such as social withdrawal or emotional blunting than EOS patients. LOS is more common among women than men. Visual hallucinations are probably less common and cognitive impairment is less severe in LOS patients. We have found better organization of the semantic network (7) and larger thalamic volume on MRI in LOS as compared to EOS (8). Although treatment with typical antipsychotic medications elicits similar responses in both groups, LOS patients generally require up to one-third less dosage than do EOS patients of comparable age (6).

C. Delusional Disorder

Delusional disorder refers to persistent, nonbizarre delusions and may be misdiagnosed as schizophrenia. Delusions commonly involve erotomanic, grandiose, jealous, persecutory, and somatic themes. Delusional disorder generally presents in middle or late life. Delusional disorder can be differentiated from schizophrenia by the absence of prominent auditory or visual hallucinations and by the lack of functional deterioration outside the area of delusions in delusional disorder. Patients with delusional disorder also appear to have less neuropsychological impairment than do LOS patients (9).

D. Postpsychotic Depression

Depression secondary to psychotic symptoms may develop in up to 25% of schizophrenia patients during the course of their illness. This condition, termed postpsychotic depression (PPD), is characterized by a major depressive episode that occurs during the residual phase of schizophrenia (10). PPD patients experience a major depressive episode with mild or no psychotic symptoms, and they are more likely to have a psychotic relapse than schizophrenia patients without secondary depression. Depressive symptoms may be difficult to differentiate from the negative symptoms of schizophrenia, although this distinction is important for the differential diagnosis between PPD and schizophrenia. Like patients with major depressive episodes, patients with PPD may have suicidal ideation. Relatively little information is available on treating PPD; however, two reports of maintenance therapy with adjunctive imipramine have shown positive results in controlling depressive symptoms, although these studies of PPD have included mostly younger adults (11,12).

E. Other Psychoses

Other conditions of psychosis in elderly patients include dementia with delusions or hallucinations, mood disorder with psychotic features, psychosis NOS, Alzheimer's disease (13), Lewy-body dementia (14,15), levodopa-induced psychotic symptoms (16), Charles Bonnet syndrome-type visual hallucinations (complex visual hallucinations in the absence of a neuropsychiatric disorder) (17), and other organic psychiatric disorders.

III. GERONTOKINETICS/DYNAMICS

Pharmacokinetics can generally be considered to be the body's effect on the drug. Gerontokinetics refers to the numerous aged-related changes in physiology which affect pharmacokinetics. Changes may occur in the absorption, distribution, metabolism, and excretion of neuroleptics (18). In general, these changes may lead to higher blood levels of medications, prolonged pharmacological effects, and a greater risk for side effects (19). Changes in pharmacodynamics (the drug's effect on the body) are also likely to occur (gerontodynamics); however, these mechanisms are not well understood. The extent of *absorption* of neuroleptics in the elderly is probably comparable to that in younger adults. The aging process is also associated with decreased total body water, decreased muscle mass, and increased adipose tissue. As most neuroleptics are highly lipophilic, they are likely to have a larger volume of *distribution* in the elderly than they do in younger patients. This expanded volume of distribution seen in elderly patients may result in drug accumulation in fatty tissues. Some age-related comorbidity such as congestive heart failure may also result in an increased volume of distribution (19). The increased volume of distribution will prolong the elimination half-life of the drug but does not increase the plasma concentration.

Albumin and α_1-acid glycoprotein (AGP) are the principal binding proteins for acidic and basic drugs, respectively. *Protein binding* may be important because it is believed that only unbound neuroleptic drug (the free fraction) can exert a pharmacological effect. Decreases in protein levels may result in an increased free fraction of the drug that is bound to that protein. Correspondingly, increases in protein would result in a decreased free fraction. Rowell et al. (20) compared in vitro serum protein binding of fluphenazine in younger and older patients and reported a 29% higher fluphenazine free fraction in patients aged 72 to 88 than in those aged 25 to 29 years. Nevertheless, although decreased binding leads to an increased *free fraction*, the absolute value of the free concentration may be unchanged. The actual free concentration is dependent on the rate of clearance.

The liver undergoes changes in blood flow and volume with age. Phase I *metabolism* (e.g., oxidation, reduction, hydroxylation) may diminish with the aging process; however, there appear to be differences between isoenzyme pathways in terms of how they change with age. Phase II metabolism involves conjugation with an endogenous substrate (e.g., glucuronic acid, sulfate, acetate) and generally leads to inactive metabolites. Phase II metabolism does not decrease with age. Relatively few studies have examined changes in neuroleptic metabolism with aging (19).

A decline in renal function occurs as a natural consequence of aging. Renal blood flow, glomerular surface area, tubular function, and reabsorption mechanisms have all been shown to diminish with age. Diminished renal *excretion* may lead to a prolonged half-life of the drug, especially for those compounds more dependent on renal excretion. Neuroleptics and any pharmacologically active metabolites are likely to accumulate (19).

Dopamine and acetylcholine receptors have been shown to decrease with age, although it is unclear what happens to receptor subtypes, receptor density in specific brain regions, and second messenger systems. These changes are apparent in the side-effect profile of neuroleptics in the elderly population. For example, diminished central cholinergic function increases sensitivity to the anticholinergic effects of the neuroleptics. Diminished dopamine function may predispose to extrapyramidal symptoms (EPS).

One study which examined serum haloperidol levels in 32 patients aged 45–83 years reported a negative correlation of age and haloperidol dose ($r = -0.79$; $p < 0.001$) (21). Age was positively correlated ($r = 0.45$; $p < 0.05$) with the haloperidol level-to-dose ratio. At the same time, the haloperidol levels in this sample of older adults were much lower than those reported in younger adults. These findings suggest that there are age-related *pharmacokinetic* and *pharmacodynamic* changes in older patients.

IV. NEUROLEPTIC MEDICATIONS

Neuroleptic (antipsychotic) medications are generally divided into typical and atypical groups. Typical neuroleptics block dopaminergic D2 receptors and atypical antipsychotics antagonize both dopamine D2 and serotonin 5HT-2 receptors. Clozapine is unusual in that it antagonizes D4 receptors more than it does D2. Adrenergic and cholinergic antagonistic properties are present in both groups of antipsychotics.

A. Typical Antipsychotics

Typical neuroleptics may be subdivided into groups based upon either relative potency for blocking D2 receptors (low- versus high-potency) or chemical class (e.g., phenothiazines, butyrophenones). In spite of a large spectrum of typical neuroleptic agents, all the drugs are therapeutically equivalent with regard to the management of psychosis when given in therapeutic doses. Important differences exist only in side-effect profile and relative potency.

Low- and High-Potency Agents

At usual antipsychotic doses, low-potency neuroleptics generally have a high degree of sedative, anticholinergic, and adrenergic-blocking activity, and lower risk of EPS compared to high-potency drugs. Even at relatively low doses, the adrenergic-blocking activity of the low-potency agents may precipitate falls in elderly patients. Examples of low-potency neuroleptics include chlorpromazine and thioridazine. High-potency neuroleptics have relatively low sedative, anticholinergic, and orthostatic side effects but a high risk of EPS and possibly a higher risk of tardive dyskinesia (TD) (22). Haloperidol is the prototypical high-potency neuroleptic. Other examples include thiothixene and fluphenazine. Some drugs considered to have intermediate potency include perphenazine, mesoridazine, and loxapine.

Clinical Trials of Typical Neuroleptics

The therapeutic efficacy of typical neuroleptics has been documented in numerous controlled clinical trials. Only a few studies, however, have examined the effects of antipsychotics in elderly patients (23). A 24-week, double-blind study evaluated the efficacy of two phenothiazines in 308 men with schizophrenia (aged 54 to 74 years) (24). Acetophenazine and trifluoperazine were both more effective than placebo in treating psychosis, conceptual disorganization, and irritability and in improving personal neatness and social competence. Tsuang et al. (25) compared haloperidol and thioridazine in a 12-week, double-blind study of 50 patients aged 63 or older, most of whom had chronic schizophrenia. Patients had mean ages of 71 and 74 years for the haloperidol and thioridazine groups, respectively. Both medications were highly efficacious in reducing symptoms of anxiety, excitement, hostility, suspiciousness, and hallucinations. In a double-blind crossover study, Branchey et al. compared the effects of thioridazine and oral fluphenazine (26). All the patients had chronic schizophrenia and ranged in age from 60 to 81 years (mean 67 years). Both thioridazine and fluphenazine resulted in modest but significant improvement in psychopathology.

Several other studies have also been published on the efficacy of typical neuroleptics in the elderly (27–30). Although these studies were limited by lack of double-blind design, treatment with neuroleptics was generally reported to produce a clinically significant reduction in psychopathology (31).

B. Atypical Antipsychotics

Atypical antipsychotics have been defined in several ways, including decreased EPS and TD compared to typical neuroleptics, efficacy in treating negative symptoms, and pharmacological profile (dopamine and serotonin-blocking activity). Clozapine and risperidone were the first two atypical agents marketed in the United States, and both are combined dopamine and serotonin agonists. Other examples of atypical antipsychotics are sertindole, olanzapine, quetiapine, and ziprasidone (32–34). The data on the use of these medications in the elderly are very limited (35,36).

Clozapine

Clozapine has been shown to be effective in cases of treatment-resistant schizophrenia (35); however, its use in older patients is limited by the side effects of excessive sedation, anticholinergic toxicity, postural hypotension, and the necessity for weekly blood draws. As with other agents, the starting dose should be relatively low and the titration period should be longer relative to that used for younger patients (37,38). Salzman et al. reviewed the use of clozapine in 20 hospitalized psychotic patients aged 65 to 84 years (39). The mean daily dose required was 210 mg (ranging from 75 to 350 mg), well below the 300–600 mg/day range often used for younger adults. Although all the patients improved after clozapine was initiated, 12 of the patients reported sedation and lethargy, and serious respiratory complications (pneumonia, respiratory arrest) developed in four patients.

Oberholzer et al. (40) retrospectively reviewed the effects of clozapine in 18 patients aged 59 to 95 years (mean 81 years). Fourteen of the patients had Alzheimer's-type dementia and the remaining four had vascular dementia, normal pressure hydrocephalus, schizophrenia, and schizoaffective psychosis, respectively, and most were severely or moderately demented. The daily dose of clozapine ranged from 12.5 to 200 mg/day (mean 52 mg/day). One patient discontinued clozapine due to lack of clinical response. Three patients on doses of 25–75 mg/day discontinued clozapine due to adverse effects including an acute confusional state, somnolence, and increasing motor restlessness. In the remaining patients, clozapine appeared to be well-tolerated and safe. To evaluate the clinical effects of clozapine, the drug was abruptly discontinued in seven patients with severe Alzheimer's-type dementia and was then reinstituted if it was clinically necessary. Psychopathology assessments were made based on the Sandoz Clinical Assessment Geriatric scale (SCAG) (41) and the Nurses' Observation Scale for Inpatients (NOSIE) (42) immediately before clozapine discontinuation, at the end of the withdrawal phase, and 4 weeks after treatment resumption. Patients were receiving 12.5 to 75 mg/day (mean 41 mg/day) of clozapine. After 2 to 35 days (mean 12 days) of nontreatment, clozapine had to be reinstituted in all patients for agitation and aggressive behavior. In all seven patients, psychopathology worsened after clozapine was discontinued and improved after the drug was resumed. NOSIE factors worsened significantly in areas of irritability ($p = 0.0004$), social competence ($p = 0.023$), and social interest ($p = 0.008$) during the withdrawal period and returned to near previous levels after clozapine resumption. The SCAG factor for antisocial behavior worsened significantly ($p = 0.0071$) following clozapine withdrawal and returned to near its previous level after its resumption.

Clozapine use was also retrospectively examined by Changappa et al. in 12 female geriatric patients with psychosis who were aged 61 to 82 years (43). In six of these patients, a target dose of 300 mg/day was planned, but five did not reach the target dose or had to discontinue clozapine due to untoward side effects of the drug. Six other patients were titrated according to clinical response and side effects. Four of these patients remained on clozapine and received daily doses ranging from 25 to 300 mg/day (mean 150 mg/day). Clozapine improved psychotic symptoms markedly in two patients and moderately in five. Postural hypotension resulting in severe dizziness and ataxia was a relatively common adverse effect of clozapine and was experienced by seven of the 12 patients.

Frankenburg et al. retrospectively reviewed the use of clozapine in eight patients who ranged in age from 68 to 80 years (37). All of the patients were treatment-resistant and largely treatment intolerant; seven patients had developed severe Parkinsonian symptoms from typical agents and four had developed TD. Diagnoses varied: four had depression with psychotic features, three had schizophrenia, and one had organic delusional disorder. Clozapine was started at low doses and increased slowly, and the peak dose used ranged from 12.5 to 400 mg/day (mean 135 mg/day). Six patients showed at least moderate improvement of psychosis after clozapine was initiated, and all patients with parkinsonism or TD experienced a decrease in their symptoms. Clozapine was, however, poorly tolerated in this elderly group. Ataxia, falls, sialorrhea, and confusion required cessation of clozapine in one patient and another experienced urinary incontinence, confusion, and sedation which were attributed to clozapine. Marked orthostasis occurred in two patients. The authors commented that clozapine was useful for geriatric psychotic patients, but that doses should be started very low and adjusted with careful monitoring of mental status and blood pressure changes.

Several studies have indicated a beneficial effect of low-dose clozapine in treating psychosis in Parkinson's disease (44–47).

Risperidone

Risperidone is a useful antipsychotic agent in the elderly, but it should be used in considerably lower dosages than those commonly recommended for younger patients. As with other neuroleptics, side effects such as sedation and orthostasis can limit its use. Risperidone is much better tolerated in elderly patients, however, than clozapine.

We have studied risperidone use in middle-aged and frail elderly patients in open-label trials (48,49). In one trial, 10 patients (47 to 79 years of age) admitted to a tertiary-care county hospital were treated with risperidone. Seven of them had schizophrenia, two had organic delusional disorder, and one had bipolar disorder. The mean daily dose of risperidone was 3.9 mg and ranged from 0.5 to 8 mg/day. Seven of the patients improved markedly and two improved moderately, with their psychosis under control. Risperidone was generally well tolerated. One patient became lethargic and poorly responsive after risperidone was initiated but began improving 4 days after the drug was discontinued. Another patient receiving 1 mg/day experienced oversedation; however, the side effect resolved when the dose was reduced to 0.5 mg/day. In most of these middle-aged and elderly patients, the drug was very effective but the doses required varied widely.

In another trial, 15 stable middle-aged outpatients with schizophrenia, aged 45 to 64 years (mean 54 years), were titrated upward on risperidone over 3 days to a target dose of 6 mg/day, while their previous neuroleptic was being discontinued. While these were not geriatric patients, the findings are of relevance to geriatric psychopharmacology. Psychopathology and EPS were assessed at baseline (before initiation of risperidone) and every 2 weeks for 10 weeks with standardized rating scales. Nine of the 15 patients completed the 10-week study, and 11 completed at least 6 weeks of treatment. During the titration phase, four patients experienced sufficient lethargy, dizziness, and sedation to warrant withdrawal from the study. Three other patients reached the target dose of 6 mg/day, but required a dose reduction to 4 mg/day due to similar side effects. One patient experiencing continued psychosis had his daily dose increased to 8 mg/day. Psychopathology improved after risperidone was initiated. Positive symptoms decreased steadily from baseline to 10 weeks ($n = 8$; $p = 0.01$). The negative symptoms did not change appreciably during the first 6 weeks, but decreased from week 6 to week 10 ($p < 0.07$). Adverse effects to risperidone were experienced by several patients. Four patients discontinued the study during the titration phase and three others were unable to maintain the 6 mg/day target dose. Although this study was limited by open-label study design, the results indicated that risperidone may further reduce psychopathology over typical agents and that low doses of risperidone may be appropriate even in middle-aged patients.

We also examined risperidone use in frail elderly nursing home patients in a nonblind fashion. Risperidone was administered to fourteen nursing home patients with severe agitation or psychosis. Patients ranged in age from 54 to 100 years (mean 71 years), and were followed for 4 to 44 weeks (mean 13 weeks). The mean daily dose was 1.7 mg (range 0.25 to 6 mg). Six patients had marked improvement and six had moderate improvement after receiving risperidone. Two patients were considered therapeutic failures. Risperidone was well tolerated, and no serious side effects were observed. A dose analysis for the demented vs. nondemented patients (schizophrenia and other psychoses) revealed different risperidone dose requirements. Nondemented patients required a mean dose of 2.1 ± 2.3 mg/day, while demented patients required a mean dose of 1.0 ± 0.0 mg/day of risperidone. As these groups were similar in age (mean 69 and 71 years for nondementia and dementia groups, respectively), it appears that dementia patients require lower doses than schizophrenia patients do.

Risperidone's effects on cognition were assessed with the Mini Mental State Examination (MMSE) (50) in the last two of our studies. MMSE data sets of 19 patients from the two studies were combined for analysis. These patients were treated for 10.6 ± 7.0 weeks with risperidone. Their diagnoses were schizophrenia (13), dementia with psychosis features (3), delusional disorder (2), and psychosis NOS (1). Mean MMSE scores increased from 24.2 ± 5.5 at baseline to 28.2 ± 2.5 ($p < 0.005$) after risperidone treatment. Although these results indicating improved global cognition should be viewed with appropriate caution, they are similar to results from two other studies discussed below.

Borison et al. (51) treated patients with schizophrenia or Alzheimer's dementia with risperidone to assess safety and cognitive effects. Twenty-two patients (20 men and 2 women) aged 65 to 81 years (mean 69.8 years) were given risperidone for treatment of psychosis. All of the patients had previously been treated with antipsychotic agents and were experiencing significant psychotic symptoms at baseline. Risperidone was initiated at 2 mg/day and titrated to a target dose of 6 mg/day as the previous antipsychotic was discontinued. Seven days after the target dose was reached, risperidone was discontinued for 3 days (washout), reinstated at 6 mg/day, and then continued for 3 weeks. Side effects were assessed at each treatment period. Risperidone dosages of 6 mg/day were well tolerated by some, but not all, patients. Nine patients experienced side effects with risperidone. The most common adverse effects were hypotension, somnolence, and agitation, each of which occurred in a different patient. One episode of syncope led to cessation of the drug. Confusion, constipation, and tachycardia each occurred in two separate patients. The psychopathology and cognitive effects of risperidone were assessed at each treatment phase in a subset of patients. By the end of risperidone treatment, the mean global psychopathology decreased 14% ($p < 0.01$). Positive symptom scores also decreased significantly by 19% ($p < 0.05$), while negative symptom subscale scores decreased 12% (NS) from baseline to study completion. Cognition measures also improved. Mean MMSE scores increased from 19.7 ± 7.7 to 22.3 ± 8.4 ($n = 10$; $p < 0.05$), and the mean Digit Symbol score increased from 8.2 ± 12.3 to 40.5 ± 42.5 ($n = 8$; $p < 0.01$) from baseline to 6 weeks of risperidone treatment.

Berman et al. (52) conducted a double-blind study comparing the cognitive effects of risperidone and haloperidol in elderly patients. Twenty patients with stable schizophrenia, aged 57 to 77 years (mean 67.4 years), were given either risperidone or haloperidol. Doses of both medications were adjusted as clinically necessary; however, no patient required more than 6 mg of risperidone or 10 mg of haloperidol per day. Patients were administered the PANSS and cognitive tests including the MMSE, an abbreviated Boston Naming test, Digit Symbol, Digit Span, and Word Recall while receiving their previous antipsychotic medication and after at least 2 weeks of receiving a stable dose of the study medication. Significant improvements from baseline were seen on the Boston Naming test ($p = 0.05$) and MMSE ($p = 0.05$; $n = 8$) in the risperidone group but not in the haloperidol group. Changes in the other cognitive assessments from baseline were not significant in either study group. Patients in both groups remained psychiatrically stable. A trend for lower negative symptoms ($p = 0.07$) was seen in the risperidone group but not in the haloperidol group.

Encouraging results have also been reported on low-dose risperidone treatment of agitation and withdrawn behavior (53), and psychotic and behavioral symptoms in Lewy-body dementia (14), levodopa-induced hallucinations (16), and Charles Bonnet syndrome-type visual hallucinations (17).

V. SIDE EFFECTS

A. Sedation

Sedation is one of the most common side effects of neuroleptics that elderly patients experience. Low-potency neuroleptics are often employed for their sedative properties and may be useful in calming agitated patients or treating psychotic patients with insomnia. Sedation is likely to occur in the elderly at much lower doses than those prescribed for younger patients, and elderly patients are likely to experience daytime sedation from neuroleptics that were administered the previous night.

B. Hypotension

For elderly patients, hypotension is a serious side effect of neuroleptic medications, and both the phenothiazine and butyrophenone classes are associated with an increased risk of falls and femoral neck fractures in elderly patients (54). Because of decreased adrenergic tone and cardiac output, elderly patients may be more vulnerable to these orthostatic effects and may have severe orthostasis at relatively low doses. Orthostatic episodes are most likely to appear early in treatment, and during this period should be monitored closely. Patients and their caregivers should be instructed that the patient should rise slowly after being seated or supine and that extreme care should be taken if the patient wakes up during the night.

Patients should be assessed for orthostasis if they are suspected of, or are at risk for, an orthostatic episode. Assessments for orthostasis, however, are frequently improperly done. The patient should be supine for at least 20 min, and the standing blood pressure should be taken at 2 and 5 min after the patient has stood (55). Decreases in systolic blood pressure of 20 mm Hg or more on standing is orthostatic hypotension (56).

C. Anticholinergic Reactions

Elderly patients are much more sensitive to the anticholinergic side effects of medications than are younger adults. Addition of anticholinergic medications such as benztropine and trihexyphenedyl to treat EPS is very likely to result in anticholinergic side effects that may be especially troublesome for elderly patients in that they may aggravate previously existing comorbidity. Blockade of muscarinic receptors may increase intraocular pressure, worsen glaucoma, and decrease gastrointestinal motility, which may lead to constipation. Urinary retention due to benign prostatic hypertrophy may be exacerbated by anticholinergic toxicity.

The central effects of anticholinergics in the elderly are also important to consider as elderly patients are at risk for delirium and impaired cognition, attention, memory, and self-care capacity from muscarinic blockade (57–62). The higher risk of falls and hip fractures in the elderly associated with antipsychotics is due in part to the anticholinergic and sedative properties of these medications (63). In more severe cases, anticholinergic toxicity may be mistaken for an exacerbation of psychosis and the neuroleptic dose may be increased; this may result in patients becoming irritable and aggressive, and may even cause visual hallucinations.

Other medications also have anticholinergic activity. Nifedipine, theophylline, prednisolone, cimetidine, and digoxin have all been shown to have anticholinergic activity (60). The risk of toxicity increases with the concomitant use of these medications, neuroleptics with relatively high anticholinergic activity, and anticholinergic agents. Anticholinergic toxicity in elderly patients can be avoided by selecting a neuroleptic agent with minimal anticholinergic activity and judicious dosing of anticholinergic agents when these are required.

D. Cardiovascular

In addition to orthostatic hypotension, neuroleptics may also cause tachycardia and changes in electrocardiogram (ECG). Anticholinergic effects of the neuroleptics on the sinoatrial node may lead to tachycardia. Elderly patients receiving neuroleptics may have heart rates of 90 or more beats per minute. Neuroleptics, especially thioridazine, may induce nonspecific changes in T waves. The role of these T-wave abnormalities in predisposing a patient to more serious arrhythmias is uncertain.

E. Neuroleptic-Induced Movement Disorders

Extrapyramidal Symptoms

Extrapyramidal symptoms include akathisia, drug-induced parkinsonism, and dystonic reactions. The frequency of all EPS increases with the relative potency and dose of the typical neuroleptics. EPS can be very distressing to a patient and may contribute to medication noncompliance (64). Aspects of EPS prevalence and differential diagnosis that deserve special consideration in the elderly are listed in Table 1.

Akathisia

Akathisia is the most common EPS experienced by elderly patients, and it is believed to occur more frequently in the elderly than in younger patients. It is characterized by an inability to sit still, pacing, and restless movements especially in the lower extremities. Patients who are sitting may continually tap their feet, shift their body weight, or move in a rocking motion. Because a patient with akathisia appears to be restless, this may be mistaken for psychotic agitation. If this is the case and the neuroleptic dose is increased, the akathisia tends to worsen. As akathisia is poorly responsive to any treatment, the best course of treatment is to lower the neuroleptic dose. Akathisia may last for

TABLE 1 Special Considerations of Extrapyramidal Symptoms in the Elderly

Extrapyramidal symptom	Special consideration in the elderly
Akathisia	More common. DDx: Wandering: TD, restless leg
Drug-induced parkinsonism	More common. DDx: Idiopathic Parkinson's disease, Alzheimer's disease
Dystonia	Less common. DDx: Muscle cramps
Tardive dyskinesia (TD)	More common. DDx: Edentous dyskinesia, senile chorea, hyperthyroidism

DDx = Differential diagnosis.

several weeks, months, or even years. Because high-potency neuroleptics are more likely to cause akathisia, clinicians may wish to consider using a lower potency agent if the akathisia is severe.

Drug-Induced Parkinsonism

Drug-induced parkinsonism (DIP) is movement disorder characterized by bradykinesia, tremor, and rigidity which is often indistinguishable from idiopathic Parkinson's disease (65). Gait impairment may increase the risk of falls in the elderly (54). DIP develops insidiously after the offending agent is started, and most of the cases become apparent within 1 to 2 months. Because idiopathic Parkinson's disease is fairly common in older patients, DIP should be considered in the diagnostic workup if a patient presents with parkinsonism after recently starting a neuroleptic. The most effective treatment of DIP is removal of the offending agent. Because this can be extremely difficult in schizophrenia patients, attempts should be made at dose reduction or switching to a lower potency agent. Treatments with anticholinergic agents (amantadine, levodopa, and ritaserin) (66) have met with some success, although these agents have their own side effects and are best avoided in elderly patients. The anticholinergic drugs are particularly problematic in very elderly patients.

Dystonic Reactions

Dystonic reactions involve acute spasms of a muscle group and usually occur in the neck, face, or back. Dystonic reactions generally occur within 72 h after initiation of a neuroleptic and can occur after the first dose. They are usually extremely frightening for a patient and can often be very painful. Dystonic reaction is one of the few side effects that are less common in the elderly than in younger patients. Although dystonic reactions in younger patients appear to be dose-related, this is not necessarily the case with the elderly. Dystonic reactions are treated with anticholinergic agents. After the dystonia has resolved, subsequent lowering of the neuroleptic dose may also be indicated.

Tardive Dyskinesia

Tardive dyskinesia is a well-known side effect of neuroleptic agents, which occurs months or years after initiation of neuroleptic treatment (67). Essential features of TD include involuntary movements of the tongue, face, and jaw. Lip smacking, cheek puffing, and other facial movements may also be present. The orofacial region is the most common area of the body affected by TD. In more severe cases of TD, rhythmic purposeless movements of the arms and legs are present. Tongue movements are caused by contractions of the glossol muscles and may appear as fine contractions (vermicular or wormlike) or gross movements of the tongue. Movements of the jaw may cause repetitive chewing movements or clenching of teeth. Other common orofacial manifestations include lip smacking, puckering, sucking, and licking movements. Clinicians should be aware of the differential diagnosis of orofacial TD. In addition, lip smacking and tongue movements may be due to dry mouth induced by medications.

Nodding, lateral, or rotatory movements of the neck are examples of axial dyskinesias, which may present in more severe cases of TD. Truncal dyskinesias generally consist of rocking and oscillatory movements; however dyskinetic movements in the diaphragm, intercostal, and abdominal muscles are also possible. Possible lower extremity dyskinesias involving the leg include stamping or lateral movements, and repetitive weight shifting from one side of the body to the other. These may rarely lead to gait disturbance and falls.

The dyskinesia of TD may appear as choreiform (i.e., jerky and nonrepetitive), athetoid (continuous, slow, purposeless movements), or rhythmic (abnormal, involuntary) movements, generally limited to the face and distal extremities. Movements are reduced when the patient is relaxed and are exacerbated by emotional arousal. Tremors, myoclonus, and mannerisms are not considered a part of TD proper, although they may occur concomitantly with TD.

The predominant patient-related risk factor for developing TD is advanced age (68–70). Old age is also associated with increased incidence and prevalence, greater severity, and decreased remission of TD. We recently reported the results of a 3-year longitudinal study of 266 older outpatients (mean age 66 years) (22). The patients were early in the course of neuroleptic treatment, and the average neuroleptic dose was only 150 mg chlorpromazine equivalent daily over the course of the study. The cumulative annual incidence of TD was 26%, a rate which is five to six times that reported in younger adults (71). Significant risk factors for TD development were longer neuroleptic treatment duration, greater cumulative neuroleptic amounts (especially for high-potency agents), alcohol abuse or dependence, and subtle movement disorder at baseline. Although atypical antipsychotics are believed to have a lower risk of TD than are typical agents, there have been few long-term studies with these drugs in the elderly.

Time is the most important factor in the outcome of TD patients. TD generally remains relatively stable after 1 to 2 years, often with gradual improvement over the course of many years (67). One study showed that TD improved in 50% of patients whether or not antipsychotics were used (72). Nonetheless, it is advisable to consider tapering the neuroleptic or switching to atypical agents in patients with TD.

Although numerous medications have been studied for the treatment of TD, none has proved very effective. Current recommendations are to reduce the neuroleptic to the lowest dose possible or to change to an atypical neuroleptic such as clozapine, if not contraindicated. There is also some interest in treating TD with antioxidant compounds. Several studies of TD patients or patients receiving neuroleptics have reported elevated levels of lipid peroxidation and other oxidative stress measures (73–75). Transition metals, which are increased following the use of neuroleptics, may catalyze the formation of oxygen radicals. Several reports on the role of antioxidants in reducing the severity of TD have been reviewed by Lohr et al. (76). Although results have not been in complete agreement, the majority of studies have reported mild-to-moderate declines in the severity of TD, with some studies indicating that patients with TD for less than 5 years have a better response. Currently the effectiveness of vitamin E in TD is being studied in a multicenter Veterans Affairs cooperative study.

F. Other Side Effects

Neuroleptic Malignant Syndrome

Neuroleptic malignant syndrome (NMS) is a rare, but potentially fatal, drug reaction. Although most reported cases are in younger patients, the reaction can occur at any age. NMS is especially dangerous for elderly patients, as clinicians may fail to recognize it. The syndrome is characterized by rapid onset of autonomic dysfunction and EPS. The presentation of autonomic dysfunction may be highly variable; tachycardia, hypertension, hypotension, tachypnea, fever, diaphoresis, and urinary incontinence are all possible. A presumptive diagnosis can be confirmed if the patient has elevated creatine phosphokinase (CPK) levels, leukocytosis, and myoglobinuria. When NMS is suspected, the neuroleptic should be discontinued immediately. Treatment of NMS in older patients has been poorly studied. Clinicians are advised to treat NMS in elderly patients cautiously, with supportive therapy and, only if essential, bromocriptine or dantrolene given in low dosages.

Agranulocytosis

Agranulocytosis is a medication side effect most often associated with clozapine use. It is, however, possible (but much less common) with other neuroleptic agents as well. Agranulocytosis usually develops in the first 8 weeks after a neuroleptic has been initiated. With regard to the elderly population, women appear to be at a higher risk for agranulocytosis than men. The risk of clozapine-induced agranulocytosis increases slightly with age (77).

Weight Gain

Weight gain is frequently associated with neuroleptic use in both younger and elderly patients (78). The increase in weight may be of some concern for older patients as additional weight may compound other medical comorbidity such as cardiovascular disease, pulmonary disease, and diabetes. All of the neuroleptic agents are associated with weight gain except for molindone. However, few data are available regarding the atypical agents.

Miscellaneous Side Effects

Other side effects include sun sensitivity, allergic-type skin reactions, skin pigmentation, and retinal and corneal pigmentation. It is advisable to have annual slit-lamp evaluations in patients on high dosages of low-potency neuroleptics.

VI. EVALUATION PHASE

A. Psychiatric History and Evaluation

Psychiatric history may be obtained from multiple sources including the patients, caregivers, other relatives, physicians, and medical records. Medical records containing a psychiatric diagnosis from nonpsychiatric clinicians should be reviewed cautiously for justification and accuracy of diagnosis. Additionally, comments of "therapeutic failure" should be examined for adequacy of trial duration and dosing. A physical assessment is also an essential component of the evaluation phase and may reveal a nonpsychiatric etiology for the behavior disorder.

B. Diagnostic Workup

The possibility of a stroke, tumor, or metabolic encephalopathy should be examined in older patients who present with new onset of psychosis. Sudden onset of combativeness in an elderly patient may be a symptom of infection. In this case, a leukocyte count is probably warranted before prescribing drug treatment. Other laboratory tests that may be considered include thyroid function tests, toxicology screening, and serological tests for syphilis and HIV.

Drug-induced psychosis is frequently caused by levodopa, a common treatment of Parkinson's disease. Other medications are known to cause hallucinations, paranoia, and aggressiveness (79, 80). Elderly patients who present with disorientation and confusion should be examined for anticholinergic toxicity.

C. Medical Comorbidity

Medical comorbidity should be assessed before psychiatric treatment is begun. Thus, most neuroleptics, especially phenothiazines, should be used judiciously in patients with a seizure disorder as they are known to decrease seizure threshold. Patients with diminished pulmonary capacity are at a higher risk for bronchopneumonia when they are given neuroleptics. In addition, AIDS dementia patients should be administered antipsychotics judiciously as they appear to be more sensitive to EPS side effects (81,82). Similarly, low-potency neuroleptics with high anticholinergic properties should be avoided in patients with myocardial disease.

D. Psychosocial Assessment

Necessary psychosocial information can generally be obtained from a cooperative patient. Information on recent stressors, daily activities, and contact with friends or neighbors will aid in psychosocial assessment. For example, agitation may result from an elderly patient's moving to new and unfamiliar surroundings, and people who are close to the patient should be contacted regarding possible recent stresses the patient might have experienced. Psychosocial assessment also has potential implications for the management plan.

E. Management Plan

Development of a management plan should follow the diagnosis. The clinician should identify which of the patient's symptoms need to be treated (target symptoms). Review of prior treatment regimens may be useful for estimating the degree of symptom reduction obtainable with acute treatment. The plan should also include the selection of a neuroleptic medication and estimation of the likely trial duration. Possible side effects of the neuroleptic should be taken into consideration.

Psychosocial handicaps such as lower education, poor interpersonal skills, smaller network of friends, and societal stigmatization all have the potential of becoming amplified as the patient ages, and these handicaps may lead to a reduced utilization of health care and worsening of psychopathology. Clinicians should be aware of potential psychosocial handicaps and assist the patient in overcoming barriers to health care.

F. Informed Consent

The pertinent aspects of treatment, including its risk:benefit ratio, should be discussed with the patient (and, if appropriate, with the caregiver). Informed consent is important for clinical and medical/legal purposes. It should be documented that the decision maker understands the nature of the illness, nature of the medication, treatment risks and benefits, alternatives to the proposed treatment, and prognosis without treatment. This may be done by recording a summary of the discussion with the patient or caregiver about the neuroleptic consent or by obtaining a written informed consent.

Obtaining informed from patients with impaired decision-making capacity (i.e., demented or acutely psychotic patients) can be especially difficult. Laws governing medical treatment of impaired patients vary from state to state, and clinicians should be familiar with the laws and practice standards of their practice location.

VII. TREATMENT PHASE

A. Choice of Neuroleptic

The choice of one neuroleptic medication over another depends on what side effects the clinician would like to avoid in a given individual. High-potency agents should be avoided in patients with parkinsonism. Similarly, older individuals who are more sensitive to hypotensive and sedative side effects should probably not receive low-potency neuroleptics. Atypical agents are likely to decrease the overall risk of developing TD and help to diminish TD symptoms in those patients who have developed the disorder. Whether atypical antipsychotics will replace typical ones remains to be seen, but is possible.

B. Drug Interactions

Neuroleptics are associated with relatively few drug interactions. The most clinically significant interactions appear to be with carbamazepine, rifampin, and selective serotonin reuptake inhibitors (SSRIs).

Carbamazepine has been well documented to reduce the plasma levels of several neuroleptics (83–85). The effects of carbamazepine vary depending on the neuroleptic in question. Carbamazepine may decrease haloperidol and clozapine levels by up to 50–60% while its influence on thioridazine levels is essentially nil (85). Case reports of worsening pathology and exacerbation of psychosis have been attributed to this drug interaction (86).

Rifampin has been shown to significantly affect haloperidol concentrations (87). In a study involving 12 schizophrenia patients, haloperidol trough concentrations decreased to 30% of baseline 28 days following addition of rifampin. In another group of five patients, haloperidol levels increased to 329% of baseline levels 28 days after rifampin discontinuation. This drug interaction appears to be clinically significant as psychopathology increased slightly after rifampin was added. It is uncertain if the rise of haloperidol levels following rifampin discontinuation will result in an increased risk of EPS since the patients were receiving anticholinergic medications.

SSRIs, such as fluoxetine, sertraline, and paroxetine, inhibit metabolism of other medications that are metabolized by cytochrome P450 2D6. Most neuroleptics and some antidepressants (i.e., nortriptyline, desipramine, imipramine, and venlafaxine) are metabolized by this pathway (88). The combination of neuroleptics and SSRIs has been reported to result in dystonic reactions, EPS, and mental status changes (89–92).

Anticholinergics have been implicated in decreasing neuroleptic drug levels; however, this matter is controversial (93,94). Antacids containing aluminum, magnesium, or calcium may delay absorption of neuroleptics by altering gastric acidity or motility. Although the clinical significance of this interaction is probably minimal, it is prudent to avoid coadministering antacids with a stable regimen of neuroleptics.

Smoking is likely to enhance neuroleptic drug metabolism by stimulating the hepatic enzyme system (95). Unfortunately, monitoring of smoking habits is frequently neglected in the clinical assessment. Large changes in smoking habits are likely to have implications for drug clearance. If a patient dramatically changes smoking habits, the clinician should consider this in monitoring target symptoms.

C. Dosing Strategies

Elderly patients tend to be more sensitive to medications because of altered pharmacokinetic and pharmacodynamic factors (18). Hence, the principle of "start low and go slow" is critical to finding the lowest effective dose and to avoiding adverse effects. The starting dosage and titration rates for antipsychotic medications depend on the patient's characteristics such as physical comorbidity, body weight, past history of treatment response, etc. The starting dosage for elderly patients is often recommended to be one-third or one-fourth of the dose typically used for younger adult patients. Due to the high anticholinergic and antihistaminic properties of clozapine, very small initial dosages, as low as 6.25 mg, should be considered.

Depot forms of fluphenazine or haloperidol can be administered to patients with poor medication compliance. Intramuscular injections should generally be avoided in the thin and frail elderly, however, because of diminished muscle mass and the increased potential for erratic and unpredictable absorption.

D. Patient Compliance

A common reason for hospitalization of schizophrenia patients is poor medication compliance. Noncompliance is a persistent problem, and patients who have been compliant for years may still be at risk for stopping their medication. Continual surveillance of compliance and education are warranted for schizophrenia patients. Assessing medication noncompliance can be done with several methods including evaluations of appointment compliance, clinical outcome, and direct tracing methods such as electronic pill containers or pill counts. These methods, however, are imprecise or cumbersome. One instrument for assessing medication compliance in schizophrenia patients is the Rating of Medication Influences (ROMI) scale (96). There is obviously no substitute for a trusting patient-clinician relationship.

E. Maintenance Treatment

Once an effective total daily dose has been found, neuroleptic doses may be shifted to once-daily dosing at bedtime. Increased patient compliance, decreased need for hypnotic medications, and decreased cost are potential benefits of once-daily dosing. Because the peak blood levels occur while the patient is asleep, disturbances in the sleeping pattern and increased postural hypotension at night are possible.

The maintenance dose may be determined after target symptoms have been controlled and the patient is stable. By very slowly tapering the initial high dose downward, the clinician can find the lowest dose that is effective in controlling the target symptoms. In some cases, this may mean no drug. Relapses must be avoided by monitoring for the earliest symptoms of any exacerbation and by increasing the dose when these signs are seen (97,98).

ACKNOWLEDGMENTS

This work was supported, in part, by the National Institute of Mental Health grants MH43693, MH49671, MH45131, and by the Department of Veterans Affairs.

REFERENCES

1. Baldessarini RJ. Chemotherapy in Psychiatry, Principles and Practice. Cambridge: Harvard University Press, 1985.
2. Shorr RI, Fought RL, Ray WA. Changes in antipsychotic drug use in nursing homes during implementation of the OBRA-87 regulations. J Am Med Assoc 1994; 271: 358–362.
3. Belitsky R, McGlashan TH. At Issue: The manifestations of schizophrenia in late life: A dearth of data. Schizophr Bull 1993; 19:683–685.
4. American Psychiatric Association. Diagnostic and Statistical Manual of Mental Disorders, Third Edition-Revised. Washington, DC: American Psychiatric Press, 1987.
5. Harris MJ, Jeste DV. Late-onset schizophrenia: An overview. Schizophr Bull 1988; 14:39–55.
6. Jeste DV, Harris MJ, Krull A, Kuck J, McAdams LA, Heaton R. Clinical and neuropsychological characteristics of patients with late-onset schizophrenia. Am J Psychiatry 1995; 152:722–730.
7. Paulsen JS, Romero R, Chan A, Davis AV, Heaton RK, Jeste DV. Impairment of the semantic network in schizophrenia. Psychiatry Res 1996; 63(2–3):109–121.
8. Corey-Bloom J, Jernigan T, Archibald S, Harris MJ, Jeste DV. Quantitative magnetic resonance imaging in late-life schizophrenia. Am J Psychiatry 1995; 152:447–449.
9. Evans JD, Paulsen JS, Harris MJ, Heaton RK, Jeste DV. A clinical and neuropsychological comparison of delusional disorder and schizophrenia. J Neuropsychiatry Clin Neurosci 1996; 8(3):281–286.
10. American Psychiatric Association. Diagnostic Criteria from DSM-IV. Washington, DC: American Psychiatric Association, 1994.
11. Siris SG, Strahan A. Continuation and maintenance treatment trials of adjunctive impairments in post-psychotic depression. J Clin Psychiatry 1988; 49:439–440.
12. Siris SG, Bermanzohn PC, Mason SE, Shuwall MA. Maintenance imipramine therapy for secondary depression in schizophrenia. Arch Gen Psychiatry 1994; 51:109–115.
13. Jeanblanc W, Davis YB. Risperidone for treating dementia-associated aggression. Am J Psychiatry 1995; 152:1239.
14. Allen RL, Walker Z, D'Ath PJ, Katona CLE. Risperidone for psychotic and behavioral symptoms in Lewy body dementia. Lancet 1995; 346:185.
15. Lee H, Cooney JM, Lawlor BA. The use of risperidone, an atypical neuroleptic, in Lewy body disease. Int J Geriatr Psychiatry 1994; 9:415–417.

16. Meco G, Alessandria A, Bonifati V, Giustini P. Risperidone for hallucinations in levodopa-treated Parkinson's disease patients. Lancet 1994; 343:1370–1371.
17. Howard R, Meehan O, Powell R, Mellers J. Successful treatment of Charles Bonnet Syndrome type visual hallucinosis with low-dose risperidone. Int J Geriatr Psychiatry 1994; 9:677–678.
18. Pollock BG, Mulsant BH. Antipsychotics in older patients: A safety perspective. Drugs Aging 1995; 6:312–323.
19. Jeste DV, Klausner M, Brecher M, Clyde C, Jones R, the ARCS Study Group. A clinical evaluation of risperidone in the treatment of schizophrenia: A 10-week, open-label, multicenter trial. Psychopharmacology 1996; 131(3):239–247.
20. Rowell FJ, Hui SM, Fairbairn AF, Eccleston D. The effect of age and thioridazine on the in vitro binding of fluphenazine to normal human serum. Br J Clin Pharmacol 1980; 9:432–433.
21. Lacro JP, Kuczenski R, Roznoski M, Warren KA, Harris MJ, Jeste DV. Serum haloperidol levels in older psychotic patients. Am J Geriatr Psychiatry 1996; 4:229–236.
22. Jeste DV, Caligiuri MP, Paulsen JS, Heaton RK, Lacro JP, Harris MJ, et al. Risk of tardive dyskinesia in older patients: A prospective longitudinal study of 266 patients. Arch Gen Psychiatry 1995; 52:756–765.
23. Jeste DV, Lacro JP, Gilbert PL, Kline J, Kline N. Treatment of late-life schizophrenia with neuroleptics. Schizophr Bull 1993; 19(4):817–830.
24. Honigfeld G, Rosebaum MP, Blumenthal IJ, Lambert HL, Roberts AJ. Behavioral improvement in the older schizophrenic patient: Drug and social therapies. J Am Geriatr Soc 1965; 13:57–71.
25. Tsuang MM, Lu LM, Stotsky BA, Cole JO. Haloperidol versus thioridazine for hospitalized psychogeriatric patients: Double-blind study. J Am Geriatr Soc 1971; 19:593–600.
26. Branchey MH, Lee JH, Ramesh A. High- and low-potency neuroleptics in elderly psychiatric patients. J Am Med Assoc 1978; 239:1860–1862.
27. Kay DWK, Roth M. Environmental and hereditary factors in the schizophrenias of old age ("late paraphrenia") and their bearing on the general problem of causation in ssz. J Ment Sci 1961; 107:649–686.
28. Post F. Persistent Persecutory States of the Elderly. London: Pergamon Press, 1966.
29. Rabins P, Pauker S, Thomas J. Can schizophrenia begin after age 44? Comprehens Psychiatry 1984; 25:290–293.
30. Jeste DV, Harris MJ, Pearlson GD, Rabins P, Lesser I, Miller B, et al. Late-onset schizophrenia: Studying clinical validity. Psychiatr Clin North Am 1988; 11:1–14.
31. Tran-Johnson TK, Krull AJ, Jeste DV. Late life schizophrenia and its treatment: The pharmacologic issues in older schizophrenic patients. Clin Geriatr Med 1992; 8:401–410.
32. Ames D, Wirshing WC, Marder SR. Advances in antipsychotic pharmacotherapy: clozapine, risperidone, and beyond. Essential Psychopharmacol 1996; 1:5–26.
33. Jibson MD, Tandon R. A summary of research findings on the new antipsychotic drugs (review). Dir Psychiatry 1996; 16:i–vii.

34. Meltzer HY, Fibiger HC. Olanzapine: a new atypical antipsychotic drug. Neuropsychopharmacology 1996; 14:83–85.
35. Kane JM, Honigfeld G, Singer J, Meltzer H, Clozaril Collaborative Study Group. Clozapine for the treatment resistant schizophrenic: A double-blind comparison with chlorpromazine. Arch Gen Psychiatry 1988; 45:789–796.
36. Marder SR, Meibach RC. Risperidone in the treatment of schizophrenia. Am J Psychiatry 1994; 151:825–835.
37. Frankenburg FR, Kalunian D. Clozapine in the elderly. J Geriatr Psychiatry Neurol 1994; 7:129–132.
38. Pitner JK, Mintzer JE, Pennypacker LC, Jackson CW. Efficacy and adverse effects of clozapine in four elderly psychotic patients. J Clin Psychiatry 1995; 56:180–185.
39. Salzman C, Vacarro B, Lieff J, Weiner A. Clozapine in older patients with psychosis and behavioral disruption. Am J Geriatr Psychiatry 1995; 3:26–33.
40. Oberholzer AF, Hendriksen C, Monsch AU, Heierli B, Stahelin HB. Safety and effectiveness of low-dose clozapine in psychogeriatric patients: A preliminary study. Int Psychogeriatr 1992; 4:187–195.
41. Albus M, Maier W. Lack of gender differences in age at onset in familial schizophrenia. Schizophr Res 1995; 18:51–57.
42. Honigfeld G. NOSIE-30: History and current status of its use in pharmacopsychiatric research. In: Pichot P, ed. Modern Problems of Pharmacopsychiatry, 7: Psychological Measurements in Psychopharmacology. Basel: Karger, 1974:238–263.
43. Chengappa KNR, Baker RW, Kreinbrock SB, Adair D. Clozapine use in female geriatric patients with psychoses. J Geriatr Psychiatry Neurol 1995; 8:12–15.
44. Lew MF, Waters CA. Clozapine treatment of parkinsonism with psychosis. J Am Geriatr Soc 1993; 41:669–671.
45. Factor SA, Brown D, Molho ES, Podskalny GD. Clozapine: A 2-year open trial in Parkinson's disease patients with psychosis. Neurology 1994; 44:544–546.
46. Wolk SI, Douglas CJ. Clozapine treatment of psychosis in Parkinson's disease: A report of 5 consecutive cases. J Clin Psychiatry 1992; 53:373–376.
47. Wagner ML, Defilippi JL, Menza MA, Sage JI. Clozapine for the treatment of psychosis in Parkinson's disease: chart review of 49 patients. J Neuropsychiatr Clin Neurosci 1996; 8:276–280.
48. Jeste DV, Eastham JH, Gierz M, Field MG, Morgenstern M, Lacro JP. Use of risperidone in the elderly. The art of rational risperidone therapy. Baltimore: Ayd Medical Communications, 1997.
49. Jeste DV, Eastham JH, Lacro JP, Gierz M, Field MG, Harris MJ. Management of late-life psychosis. J Clin Psychiatry 1996; 57:39–45.
50. Folstein MF, Folstein SE, McHugh PR. Mini-Mental State: A practical method for grading the cognitive state of patients for the clinician. J Psychiatr Res 1975; 12:189–198.
51. Borison RL, Davidson M, Berman I. Risperidone treatment in elderly patients with schizophrenia or dementia (Poster). APA 46th Institute of Hospital and Community Psychiatry 1994; Abstract.
52. Berman I, Merson A, Allan E, Alexis C, Sison C, Losonczy M. Effect of risperidone on cognitive performance in elderly schizophrenic patients: a double-blind

comparison with haloperidol. NCDEU 35th Annual meeting 1995, Orlando, Florida; poster No. 93: Abstract.

53. Raheja RK, Bharwani I, Penetrante AE. Efficacy of risperidone for behavioral disorders in the elderly: A clinical observation. J Geriatr Psychiatry Neurol 1995; 8:159–161.
54. Campbell AJ. Drug treatment as a cause of falls in old age: A review of the offending agents. Drugs Aging 1991; 1:289–302.
55. Cassel CK, Walsh JR, Shepard M, et al. Clinical evaluation of the patient. In: Cassel CK, Riesenberg DE, Sorensen LB, et al., eds. Geriatric Medicine. New York: Springer-Verlag, 1990:102–110.
56. Johnson RH. Orthostatic hypotension in elderly people. In: Evans JG, Williams TF, eds. Oxford Textbook of Geriatric Medicine. Oxford: Oxford University Press, 1992:526–536.
57. Paulsen JS, Heaton RK, Sadek JR, Perry W, Delis DC, Kuck J, Zisook S, Braff D, Jeste DV. The nature of learning and memory impairments in schizophrenia. J Int Neuropsych Soc 1995; 1(1):88–99.
58. Thienhaus OJ, Allen A, Bennett JA, Chopra YM, Zemlan FP. Anticholinergic serum levels and cognitive performance. Eur Arch Psychiatry Clin Neurosci 1990; 240:28–33.
59. Tollefson GD, Montague-Clouse J, Lancaster SP. The relationship of serum anticholinergic activity to mental status performance in an elderly nursing home population. J Neuropsychiatr Clin Neurosci 1991; 3:314–319.
60. Tune L, Carr S, Hoag E, Cooper T. Anticholinergic effects of drugs commonly prescribed for the elderly: Potential means for assessing risk of delirium. Am J Psychiatry 1992; 149:10:1393–1394.
61. Tune LE, Strauss ME, Lew MF, Breitlinger E, Coyle JT. Serum levels of anticholinergic drugs and impaired recent memory in chronic schizophrenic patients. Am J Psychiatry 1982; 139:1460–1462.
62. Steinberg JL, Devous MD, Paulman RG, Gregory RR. Regional cerebral blood flow in first break and chronic schizophrenic patients and normal controls. Schizophr Res 1995; 17:229–240.
63. Ray WA, Griffin MR, Schaffner W, Baugh DK, Melton LJ. Psychotropic drug use and the risk of hip fracture. N Engl J Med 1987; 316:363–369.
64. Weiden PJ, Mann JJ, Dixon L, Haas G, DeChillo N, Frances AJ. Is neuroleptic dysphoria a healthy response? Comprehens Psychiatry 1989; 30:546–552.
65. Gershanik OS. Drug-induced Parkinsonism in the aged. Drugs Aging 1994; 5:127–132.
66. Bersani G, Grispini A, Marini S, Pasini A, Valducci M, Ciani N. 5-HT2 antagonist ritanserin in neuroleptic-induced parkinsonism: a double-blind comparison with orphenadrine and placebo. Clin Neuropharmacol 1990; 13:500–506.
67. Jeste DV, Caligiuri MP. Tardive dyskinesia. Schizophr Bull 1993; 19:303–315.
68. Kane JM, Jeste DV, Barnes TRE, Casey DE, Cole JO, Davis JM, et al. Tardive Dyskinesia: A Task Force Report of the American Psychiatric Association. Washington, DC: American Psychiatric Association, 1992.
69. American Psychiatric Association, Task Force on Late Neurological Effects of Antipsychotic Drugs. Tardive dyskinesia: Summary of a task force report of the American Psychiatric Association. Am J Psychiatry 1980; 137:1163–1172.

70. Jeste DV, Wyatt RJ. Understanding and Treating Tardive Dyskinesia. New York: Guilford Press, Inc., 1982.
71. Kane JM. Tardive dyskinesia: epidemiological and clinical presentation. In: Bloom FE, Kupfer DJ, eds. Pyschopharamcology: The Fourth Generation of Progress. New York: Raven Press, Ltd., 1995:1485–1495.
72. Casey DE, Gerlach J. Tardive Dyskinesia: What is the long-term outcome? In: Casey DE, Gardos G, eds. Tardive Dyskinesia and Neuroleptics: From Dogma to Reason. Washington, DC: American Psychiatric Press, 1986:75–97.
73. Lohr JB, Kuczenski R, Bracha HS, Moir M, Jeste DV. Increased indices of free radical activity in the cerebrospinal fluid of patients with tardive dyskinesia. Biol Psychiatry 1990; 28:535–539.
74. Sram RJ, Binkova B, Koclsova J, Topinka J, Fojtikova I, Hanel I, et al. Antioxidants effect on alcohol, drugs and aging. In: Mendelsohn ML, Albertini RJ, eds. Mutation and the Environment. New York: Wiley-Liss, 1990:237–337.
75. Tsai G, Goff D, Coyle JT. Oxidative stress and glutamatergic hypotheses of tardive dyskinesia. Neuroscience 1994; 20:671.8 Abstract.
76. Lohr LB, Browning JA. Free radical involvement in neuropsychiatry illnesses. Psychopharmacol Bull 1995; 31:159–165.
77. Alvir JMJ, Lieberman JA, Safferman AZ, Schwimmer JL, Schaaf JA. Clozapine-induced agranulocytosis. N Engl J Med 1993; 329(3):162–167.
78. Stanton JM. Weight gain associated with neuroleptic medication: a review. Schizophr Bull 1995; 21:463–472.
79. Eastham JH, Jeste DV. Differentiating behavioral disturbances of dementia from drug side effects. Int Psychogeriatrics 1996; 8(suppl 3):429–434.
80. Wood KA, Harris MJ, Morreale A, Rizos AL. Drug-induced pyschosis and depression in the elderly. Psych Clin Nor Am 1988; 11(1):167–193.
81. Sewell DD, Jeste DV, Atkinson JH, Heaton RK, Hesselink JR, Wiley C, et al. HIV-associated psychosis: A study of 20 cases. Am J Psychiatry 1994; 151(2):237–242.
82. Sewell D, Jeste DV, McAdams LA, Bailey A, Harris MJ, Atkinson JH, et al. Neuroleptic treatment of HIV-associated psychosis. Neuropsychopharmacology 1994; 11:284 Abstract.
83. Kidron R, Averbuch I, Klein E, Belmaker RH. Carbamazepine-induced reduction of blood levels of haloperidol in chronic schizophrenia. Biol Psychiatry 1985; 20: 219–222.
84. Jann MW, Ereshefsky L, Saklad SR, Seidel DR, Davis CM, Burch NR, et al. Effect of carbamazepine on plasma haloperidol levels. J Clin Psychopharmacol 1985; 5:106–109.
85. Tiihonen J, Vartiainen H, Hakola P. Carbamazepine-induced changes in plasma levels of neuroleptics. Pharmacopsychiatry 1995; 28:26–28.
86. Arana GW, Goff DC, Friedman H, Ornsteen M, Greenblatt DJ, Black B, et al. Does carbamazepine-induced reaction of plasma haloperidol levels worsen psychotic symptoms? Am J Psychiatry 1986; 143:650–651.
87. Kim YH, Cha IJ, Shim JC, Shin JG. Effect of rifampin on the plasma concentration and the clinical effect of haloperidol concomitantly administered to schizophrenic patients. J Clin Psychopharmacol 1996; 16:247–252.

88. Nemeroff CB, DeVane CL, Pollock BG. Newer antidepressants and the cytochrome P450 system. Am J Psychiatry 1996; 153:311–320.
89. Ketai R. Interaction between fluoxetine and neuroleptics. Am J Psychiatry 1993; 150:836–837.
90. Bouchard RH, Pourcher E, Vincent P. Fluoxetine and extrapyramidal side effects. Am J Psychiatry 1989; 146:1352–1353.
91. Tate JL. Extrapyramidal symptoms in a patient taking haloperidol and fluoxetine. Am J Psychiatry 1989; 146:399–400.
92. Hansen-Grant S, Silk KR, Guthrie S. Fluoxetine-pimozide interaction. Am J Psychiatry 1993; 150:1751–1752.
93. Goldstein G, Shemansky WJ. Influences on cognitive heterogeneity in schizophrenia. Schizophr Res 1995; 18:59–63.
94. Mukherjee P, Decina P, Scapicchio PL. Temporal course of cognitive impairment in elderly, chronic schizophrenic patients: A prospective longitudinal study. Schizophr Res 1993; 9:105.
95. Hansten PD. Smoking interactions with drugs. Drug Interact Newslett 1982; 2:13.
96. Weiden P, Rapkin B, Mott T, Zygmunt A, Goldman D, Horvitz-Lennon M, et al. Rating of medication influences (ROMI) scale in schizophrenia. Schizophr Bull 1994; 20:297–310.
97. Gilbert PL, Harris MJ, McAdams LA, Jeste DV. Neuroleptic withdrawal in schizophrenic patients. Arch Gen Psychiatry 1995; 52:173–188.
98. Jeste DV, Gilbert PL, McAdams LA, harris MJ. Considering neuroleptic maintenance and taper on a continuum: need for individual rather than dogmatic approach. Arch Gen Psychiatry 1995; 52:209–212.

18

Treatment of Psychosis in Parkinson's Disease

JONATHAN M. MEYER AND GEORGE M. SIMPSON
UNIVERSITY OF SOUTHERN CALIFORNIA, LOS ANGELES, CALIFORNIA

I. INTRODUCTION

Our current understanding of the pathophysiology and treatment of levodopa psychoses represents the culmination of a 30-year alliance between theoretical neuropharmacology and clinical observation. Levodopa-related mental status changes have long been a serious problem for the clinician who must balance the alleviation of motor symptoms with the psychological and social distress caused by the altered sensorium. Caught between the Scylla of dose reduction and the Charybdis of standard antipsychotic therapy with its exacting toll of dopaminergic antagonism, it is often the physician who evinced the more prominent tremor in the form of incessant hand-wringing over these unappealing alternatives. The magnitude of this dilemma is underscored by Goetz and Stebbins, who rated psychosis as the most frequent indicator for nursing home placement in their 1993 study (1). The advent of clozapine as a uniquely powerful treatment for psychosis in Parkinson's disease (PD) highlights the neuropharmacological complexity of central dopamine and serotonin systems in psychosis and parkinsonism, and the subtle differences in receptor specificity and distribution which permit this drug to act as an effective antipsychotic without distressing extrapyramidal side effects (EPS). The novel binding characteristics of clozapine have served as a focus for trials of newer agents that may possess its unique therapeutic properties without the concerns of agranulocytosis.

A. Historical Overview and Clinical Features of Psychosis in Parkinson's Disease

> Involuntary tremulous motion, with lessened muscular power; in parts not in action and even when supported; with a propensity to bend the trunk forward, and to pass from a walking to a running pace: the senses and intellects being uninjured (2).

Parkinson's original description of the "shaking palsy" delineates his impression that the natural history of this disorder was not marked by involvement of the cognitive processes or sensorium. A review of the literature from the prelevodopa era reveals the presence of psychotic symptoms in PD patients; however, these symptoms were largely confined to secondary forms of PD, especially postencephalitic PD (3–5). The physiological difference in central dopaminergic functioning between postencephalitic patients and those with idiopathic PD was borne out by the increased sensitivity noted in the former group to the psychiatric side effects of levodopa (6). Over the ensuing years, accumulated experience with levodopa and other antiparkinsonian agents has helped clarify the fact that all of these drugs can, to varying degrees, cause psychosis or delirium in the PD patient, with the population at greatest risk being those who have a concurrent diagnosis of dementia (7–9).

B. Psychosis, Delirium, and Confusional States: A Working Definition

It has been justifiably noted that the multiple uses and meanings attributed to the term psychotic have resulted in a "term [which] has lost its precision in current clinical and research practice" (10). Psychotic symptoms include delusions, hallucinations, and grossly disorganized thinking which contribute to functional impairment in social and work arenas. The presence of these symptoms implies severely impaired reality testing, with a concomitant lack of insight into their pathological nature (10); insight, however, is not an all-or-nothing phenomenon. Within the levodopa-induced psychoses in particular, the affected individual often recognizes the pathological nature of these symptoms (11). Psychotic symptoms are also features of many distinct illnesses including schizophrenia, severe forms of mania or depression, substance use, dementia, and delirium.

The disorganized psychotic patient may have difficulty in orientation items within the mental status examination; however, the presence of global cognitive impairment with diminished attention or clouding of consciousness necessitates the diagnosis of delirium. Fluctuation in arousal and difficulty attending to stimuli are the hallmarks of this condition, yet the presentation may include psychotic symptoms such as visual hallucinations, agitation, disorientation, sleep disturbance, and altered perceptions (13). Psychiatrists and neurologists differ on the use of this term, with the latter opting for the diagnosis of acute confusional state for those patients without significant signs of autonomic arousal (14). Implicit in the diagnosis of delirium is the presence of an offending agent, or underlying condition manifesting as generalized cortical dysfunction. The geriatric population is particularly sensitive to relatively minor metabolic derangements or infectious processes (13). An assiduous search for all etiologies must be undertaken in this age group due to the significant morbidity associated with untreated delirium.

C. Clinical Presentations of Psychosis and the Rule of Dementia

Extensive clinical experience with antiparkinsonian drugs over the past quarter century has clarified the clinical features of levodopa-induced psychosis and delirium; however, the increasing age of PD patients brings dementia into play as a complicating factor for the assessment and treatment of drug-induced mental status changes. The importance of this issue is underscored by Freidman, who estimates that up to 30% of PD patients have diagnosable dementia (14). The older PD patient is at risk for the development of secondary cerebral pathology, and, therefore, increased susceptibility to the CNS side effects of medications. In those who have PD and dementia, the prevalence of significant psychiatric side effects from antiparkinsonian medication ranges from 42–81%, compared to 5–17% in the nondemented patient (7,15,16). Although the etiology of dementia in the PD patient is an object of debate, over the past 30 years the mean age of PD patients has risen steadily, and with it an increased incidence in other forms of dementia. At the Boltzmann Institute (Vienna), the age of death for PD patients has risen from 65.8 [in 1950–1959 (n = 130)] to 78.2 [in 1980–1987 (n = 144)], with 40% of the current clinic population over the age of 80 (17). Danielczyk followed a cohort of 13 PD patients with psychometric testing to the time of death, and found that the specific visuospatial and other mild cognitive deficits measured early in the course of PD were not progressive in those individuals whose postmortem neuropathology revealed only changes consistent with PD (17). This finding, and those of other groups, point toward the dementia present in older PD patients being the result of secondary cerebral pathology, usually dementia of the Alzheimer type, and not the natural course of Parkinson's disease (18,19). Given the increased risk of dementia and medication sensitivity in the older PD patient, it is reasonable to perform a baseline mental status examination prior to the institution of antiparkinsonian medications, as this carries important prognostic significance for the development of delirium and psychosis. Reevaluation, with specific attention to sleep, memory, and visual perception, should precede significant changes in the drug regimen.

Rarely does the development of drug-induced psychosis and delirium arise de novo (20,21). More commonly, there is a "neuropsychiatric slippery slope" which begins as sleep disruption, and later progresses to psychosis or delirium in susceptible individuals (21). This initial sleep disturbance is characterized by sleep fragmentation and abnormal or vivid dreams that may lead the patient to awaken at night confused, behaving as if the dream was ongoing (14). Among the antiparkinsonian medications, the dopaminergic drugs are especially prone to induce abnormal dreams and sleep disruption (22). Sharf et al. (23) reported the incidence of three types of dream pathology associated with dopaminergic treatment in 88 PD patients: 27% complained of vivid dreams, 6.8% had night terrors, and 5.7% had nightmares. Night terrors, as opposed to nightmares or other dreams, occur in non-REM deep sleep, and are associated with thrashing or shouting for which the patient is amnestic in the morning. Patients may awaken after episodes of vivid dreaming believing the dream actually occurred; however, this is not a symptom of psychosis, and the proper intervention is to reassure the patient and the caregiver.

When visual hallucinations do present, they typically occur in the context of a clear sensorium, but may be accompanied by a mild delirium or confusional state in the older or demented patient (11). These hallucinations commonly present as nonthreatening, fully formed images of people, especially children, friends, or relatives, but may include animals or other objects (11). These objects or persons may appear in groups, and often are described as Lilliputian (24). Initially, these hallucinations tend to be nocturnal, but later are seen at other times and not influenced by changes in lighting (14). Patients may recognize the pathological nature of these hallucinations, yet talk or react to these images as though they possessed a reality "no more extraordinary than a visit from a neighbor" (11). Careful questioning will help distinguish visual hallucinations from benign hypnagogic hallucinations and *anwesenheit*, the illusion that someone or something is present just outside the range of vision (25). In about 28% of patients, these hallucinations are frightening, but the majority find these images tolerable, thereby permitting the preservation of motor function that would suffer from a decrease in medication dosage (21). The demented patient is much more likely to present with confusion, cognitive impairment, and limited insight into the pathological nature of these visions, resulting in behavior that is less manageable. Tactile and pure auditory hallucinations are rare, but an auditory component may accompany the visual hallucination in 26% of patients (21).

Delusions are defined by Diagnostic and Statistical Manual (DSM-IV) as false beliefs firmly held despite obvious proof to the contrary (26). The belief is one not ordinarily accepted within the culture or subculture (26). As with other psychotic symptoms, the degree of insight exists along a continuum, and may be ascertained by the resultant behavior. Klawans estimates the prevalence of delusions at 3% in individuals treated at least 2 years (20); nevertheless, delusions can create a significant management problem for the physician and caretaker. Typically, the delusions are paranoid in nature, involving family members, caretakers, and, at times, the physician (14). The patient may fear being poisoned or injured, or may accuse the family of stealing money, plotting to sell the house, or institutionalize the patient (27). There may be claims of spousal infidelity (jealous delusions), or that the family has been replaced by impostors (Capgras's syndrome) (28). The sensorium is typically clear, but delusions may present on a background of impaired cognition or memory as a mild delirium or confusional state.

The slow clinical progression in psychiatric side effects to antiparkinsonian medications has been the object of much scrutiny since the phenomenon was noted in the 1970s. Klawans invokes the role of dopaminergic-induced kindling to explain this inexorable progression from disruption of sleep with vivid dreams to a nonconfused psychosis, and in some, an organic confusional psychosis indistinguishable from delirium with psychotic features (20,21). The role of dopamine in psychosis, and the response of dopamine receptors to stimulation and blockade, is important to our understanding and treatment of the levodopa-induced psychoses.

II. DOPAMINE AND PSYCHOSIS

A. Dopamine Blockade

In 1963, dopaminergic blockade was postulated by Carlsson and Lindqvist as a mechanism of action common to the antipsychotics haloperidol and chlorpromazine (29). This finding, combined with the observation that dopaminergic agonists are capable of inducing states similar to schizophrenia led Randrup and Munkvad in 1965 to postulate a role for dopamine in schizophrenia (30). The further characterization of effective neuroleptics as dopamine (D_2) antagonists provided indirect confirmation of this hypothesis for the next 20 years and served as the backbone for most neuropsychopharmacological theories of psychosis (31); however, it became increasingly clear that this model was inadequate to explain the psychotomimetic activity of drugs such as lysergic acid diethylamide (LSD), a 5-hydroxytryptamine (5HT-2) agonist, or the substantial number of treatment failures on traditional antidopaminergic therapy (31). Conversely, the finding that EPS of neuroleptic treatment were indeed mediated by dopaminergic antagonism within the basal ganglia reinforced the understanding of Parkinson's disease as a state of nigrostriatal dopamine deficiency.

B. The Dopamine Receptor Family

Continued research on dopamine receptor physiology has led to the characterization of receptor subtypes with distinct profiles and distribution within the CNS. By 1979, two distinct classes of dopamine receptor were recognized, D_1 and D_2, differentiated by the coupling of D_1 receptor binding to the stimulation of adenylate cyclase via the stimulatory subunit (G_s), with inhibitory subunit (G_i) coupling postulated for D_2 (32). Currently, one speaks of the D_1 receptor family which encompasses the traditional D_1 receptor, now renamed D_{1A}, along with a newer receptor designated D_{1B} or D_5 (33). The D_{1A} receptor has a mesocortical, mesolimbic, and striatal distribution, unlike its newly recognized variant which possesses a mesocortical and mesolimbic distribution (33). Activation of D_{1A} receptors in addition to D_2 agonism is known to be important for the efficacy of dopaminergic agonists used to treat Parkinson's disease; however, the D_1 family is not a primary site of action for typical antipsychotic medications. The D_2 family consists of two functionally similar isoforms D_{2long} and D_{2short}, along with D_3 and D_4. D_2 shares a similar distribution to the D_{1A} receptor, while D_4 possesses a low-density localization to mesocortical and mesolimbic sites (33). Less is known about the clinical relevance for binding at D_3 sites compared to its cousins, although it shares a distribution in common with D_4. D_2 receptors were long postulated to be the sole sites for the antipsychotic activity of neuroleptics, with these drugs showing up to 100 times affinity for D_2 over D_4 receptors; however, clozapine is unique in possessing 15 times greater affinity for D_4 compared to D_2 (34). The *combination* of relative D_4 selectivity and antagonism of 5HT-2 receptors sets clozapine apart from typical neuroleptics both pharmacologically, and clinically, where it has demonstrated superior antipsychotic efficacy for chronic schizophrenia in the absence of extrapyramidal side effects (35).

Traditional neuroleptics have long been the bane of physicians attempting to treat levodopa psychosis in PD patients due to high affinity for D_2 receptors and the resultant exacerbation of parkinsonian symptoms. PET studies in normal volunteers given modest dosages of haloperidol (4–7.5 mg) reveal that near maximal (73–91%) occupancy of basal ganglia D_2 receptors occurs within several hours of the ingestion (36); moreover, continued high-level D_2 receptor occupancy (83–92%) persists for up to 30 h in those receiving a single 7.5-mg dose (36). By contrast, low doses (50 mg) of clozapine reveal essentially no binding (37), and moderate doses (125–200 mg daily) result in 20–33% occupancy of basal ganglia D_2 receptors (38). These binding characteristics are well below the 70–81% D_2 occupancy threshold associated with the development of akathisia or parkinsonism in schizophrenics (39). Interestingly, clozapine at 300–600-mg dosages also results in 35–52% occupancy of D_1 receptors, but the importance of this finding is still being explored (39).

C. Brief Comment on the Role of Serotonin

The significance for serotonin in psychosis has been present since early studies with hallucinogens such as mescaline (40); however, the recent recognition of clozapine's clinical efficacy and unique pharmacology has stimulated interest in the role of serotonin receptors in schizophrenia and other psychotic disorders. Clozapine is not unique in its antagonism of 5HT-2 receptors; however, it achieves approximately 85% cortical 5HT-2 receptor occupancy at dosages of 125–175 mg daily with only 20% basal ganglia D_2 occupancy (41). Clozapine also demonstrates a moderate affinity for the 5HT-3 receptor (42). Together, these findings propelled many investigators to examine the antipsychotic potential of compounds possessing 5HT-2 and 5HT-3 antagonism (43–45). That these trials had modest success in schizophrenia, but show more promise with the levodopa-induced psychoses, underscores the fact that schizophrenia is neuropharmacologically distinct from levodopa psychosis, with pervasive effects on multiple receptor subsystems. While clozapine has demonstrated significant efficacy in treating levodopa psychosis, only 30–50% of refractory schizophrenics show a therapeutic response to clozapine (46).

An incomplete understanding exists of the basic mechanisms underlying levodopa-induced psychosis, and the relative roles played by dopamine and serotonin receptors in the context of exogenously supplied dopamine. For many years, the concept of psychosis due to the overstimulation of supersensitive mesolimbic and mesocortical dopaminergic neurons was quite compelling (47); however, the finding of antipsychotic activity in pure serotonin antagonist drugs necessarily invokes a mechanism leading to stimulation of cortical serotonergic neurons (43–45). As an understanding of the neuropharmacology of psychosis slowly unravels, it becomes apparent that findings related to schizophrenia may not be applicable to psychosis in PD.

III. TREATMENT OF PSYCHOSIS IN PARKINSON'S DISEASE

A. Initial Approach

The PD patient who presents with psychotic symptoms must be carefully evaluated to determine the likelihood that etiologies other than antiparkinsonian medications are responsible. As with other geriatric patients, the presence of delirium raises the specter of underlying physical illness, particularly in the absence of recent medication changes (13). Distinguishing delirium with psychotic features from psychosis can be difficult, particularly in the demented patient, with the diagnosis resting on how "confused" the patient appears (14). Abrupt onset, agitation, alteration in the sleep cycle, difficulty in attending to interview, and failure to recognize individuals previously well known to the patient point toward a delirium, while preservation of baseline levels of alertness and orientation make delirium unlikely (13,14). When delirium is present, medical causes such as electrolyte disturbance, urinary tract or pulmonary infections should be investigated. If suspected, more extensive screening should be performed to rule out cerebrovascular incidents and structural lesions of the CNS. Although less common than drug-related psychosis, major depression with psychotic features is an instance when brief trials of standard (preferably low-potency) neuroleptics may be considered. The decrement in motor functioning is balanced by the rapid resolution of psychotic symptoms, ease of use, and low cost of these medications. The premorbid history should assist in the diagnosis, but psychiatric consultation should be obtained to assist in the management of these patients.

The decision to hospitalize primarily rests on the ability of caretakers to manage the patient without unnecessary risk to the patient or themselves. The patient who relates nonthreatening visual hallucinations or illusions with preservation of insight can often be managed by reassurance alone, with frequent office evaluation to assess the necessity of medication adjustment. When confusion and agitation are present, hospitalization is generally necessary, bearing in mind that this novel setting may exacerbate disorientation or paranoia, particularly in the demented patient. If an increase in medication has precipitated the event, the clinician must determine if the patient can tolerate a dose reduction. Adjunctive medications are reduced first (selegiline, anticholinergics), then dopaminergic agents (amantadine, bromocriptine), and last levodopa (14,24). Several days may be required for the resolution of psychotic symptoms (11). For those in whom symptoms persist, further reductions should be entertained, but weighed against the possibility of worsening motor symptoms.

B. Drug "Holiday"

The concept of a therapeutic drug holiday was studied during the prior decades in those patients whose psychiatric or motoric complications from drug therapy were significantly limiting (48). During hospitalization, medications were withdrawn over a 1- to 2-week period. Some investigators noted dramatic improvement in psychotic symptoms and increased responsiveness to levodopa immediately after the hiatus, but these benefits were often transitory (49). Moreover, attendant with this holiday was the cost of hospitalization, the need for extensive nursing care to prevent complications of immobility [decubitus ulcers, deep vein thrombosis, aspiration pneumonia (50,51)], and the frightening experience for the patient of becoming suddenly immobile, at times with impairment of swallowing. A potentially lethal condition similar to the neuroleptic malignant syndrome has also been described in those abruptly withdrawn from dopaminergic medications, in which the patient develops high fever, elevated creatine kinase and white blood cell counts, autonomic dysfunction, and lead-pipe rigidity (52,53). In the current era, this type of "holiday" is usually restricted to those psychotic PD patients who are unable to tolerate antiparkinsonian drug dose reduction or clozapine (52).

C. ECT

Long considered to be the gold standard of efficacy, particularly in the geriatric population with suicidal or psychotic depression, ECT is usually confined to those with refractory depression, despite its tendency to improve the motor symptoms in PD (54). Although generally well tolerated, the older PD patient is more likely to suffer from post-ECT confusion and memory impairment, especially when bilateral electrode placement is utilized. There is a report of complete remission in drug-induced psychotic symptoms with two nondemented PD patients treated by ECT (55), and another citing resolution of psychosis in a nondemented 74-year-old whose delusions failed to respond to 150 mg/day of clozapine (11). Nevertheless, the success of clozapine renders this modality useful mainly for refractory depression or psychosis.

D. Clozapine

The high level of D_2 blockade caused by standard neuroleptics has been a source of continued frustration in the treatment of psychotic PD patients. Even low-potency antipsychotics, such as thioridazine, itself strongly anticholinergic, were tolerated only briefly at low doses. The 1985 report by Scholz and Dichgans was the first of over a dozen studies in the next decade reporting the effectiveness of clozapine in treating the psychotic PD patient (56). Factor's 1995 review of 16 studies to date (all but one open label), revealed complete or partial resolution of psychotic symptoms in 82% (111/136) of patients (11). Among the remaining 18%, the majority withdrew due to intolerance of side effects, particularly among the demented PD population.

E. Pharmacology

Synthesized in 1958 in Bern, Switzerland, clozapine is a dibenzodiazepine compound structurally derived from tricyclic models (57). It lacks the classic neuroleptic ability to induce catalepsy in animals, or block amphetamine- or apomorphine-induced stereotypies in animals, properties which are dependent on a high level of D_2 blockade (57). Due to concerns over potentially fatal agranulocytosis, clozapine was not released in the United States until 1990. These concerns, along with a rigid monitoring system imposed by Sandoz on physicians and pharmacies, limited the utilization of clozapine despite data demonstrating superior efficacy in schizophrenia without extrapyramidal side effects. The 1993 publication by Alvir et al. of comprehensive data on 11,555 U.S. patients reporting the cumulative incidence of agranulocytosis at 0.91% over 18 months of treatment with only two deaths increased interest in this drug (58). These findings, combined with the development of protocols implementing the early use of granulocyte-macrophage colony stimulating factor (GM-CSF) for those few who do suffer agranulocytosis, have helped alleviate much of the anxiety over prescribing clozapine (59,60). Current recommendations for monitoring will be discussed below.

Clozapine is only available as an oral agent. It is well absorbed from the GI tract, with peak levels reached in 2 h, and possesses an elimination half-life of 12 h. Due to first-pass metabolism in the liver, the bioavailability ranges from 12–90%, with a mean between 50–60% (57). In addition to dopamine D_4 and serotonin 5HT-2 antagonism, clozapine is strongly anticholinergic (muscarinic), antihistaminic (H_1), and antiadrenergic (α_1 and α_2). Sedation is a significant problem due to histaminic and cholinergic blockade; moreover, the anticholinergic properties of clozapine may result in considerable confusion in the demented patient who can be intolerant of even very low (12.5 mg) doses (14). Typical anticholinergic side effects of tachycardia, urinary difficulties, and constipation have all been reported, but appear less frequent among PD patients compared with their schizophrenic counterparts (11). Interestingly, sialorrhea is a condition unique to clozapine. It develops early in treatment, and tends to persist. Patients mostly complain of drooling at night, waking in the morning with the pillow wet. Anticholinergics show little benefit, and should be avoided. The best solution is often a towel placed over the pillow at bedtime. Sugarless candies are often helpful in those few who complain of daytime drooling.

Hypotension related to adrenergic blockade may be a problem, especially in the older PD patient with poor vasomotor tone due to age or other medications. Rapid dose escalation, and initial doses over 75 mg are contraindicated in all patients (57). In the PD patient, the smallest starting dose, usually 6.25 mg, should be prescribed initially.

Lowering of seizure threshold is a dose-dependent phenomenon of significance at dosages approaching 300 mg per day, far in excess of those required for the PD patient with psychosis. In Factor's review of 136 cases, no seizures were reported (11). The risk for development of seizures is less than 1% at 300 mg/day, 2.7% between 300 and 600 mg/day, and 4.4% at dosages over 600 mg/day (61).

F. Treatment Strategy

Clozapine's usefulness is mitigated by its tendency toward side effects, especially in the cognitively impaired patient. The one double-blind placebo-controlled trial of clozapine performed by Wolters showed apparent worsening of parkinsonism with marked sedation and confusion in three of six patients studied (62). Unfortunately, the authors used a study design that maximized the propensity to side effects: high initial starting dosages, with rapid escalation to peak doses (75–250 mg/day) that are in excess of those currently recommended. One might speculate that the worsening parkinsonian signs observed may have been an effect of heavy sedation, given clozapine's lack of significant D_2 receptor blockade.

Once the clinician has exhausted other strategies and opted for a trial of clozapine, the patient should begin treatment utilizing 6.25 mg every other day. Two studies have documented the utility of a q.o.d. strategy in avoiding the more disabling side effects of sedation, confusion, and orthostasis (63,64). Unfortunately, as of this printing, the smallest available dosage is a 25-mg scored tablet. Due to the propensity for sleep disturbance in this group, Friedman advocates an h.s. schedule (14). Dosages should be titrated upward by either 6.25 mg daily, or 12.5 mg every other day, until symptoms start to remit or side effects become a problem. A temporary reduction in dosage will allow many patients to continue on clozapine who experience side effects during dose titration. Dosages above 62.5 mg daily are often not needed.

The issue of continued therapy has yet to be resolved. While those nondemented patients followed for up to 3 years continue to show benefit, the demented patient may become increasingly intolerant of the medication, necessitating a dose reduction or discontinuation (63,65–67). There has been one recent case report of a "therapeutic plunge" in a 62-year-old man with PD since age 37, titrated initially up to 75 mg per day of clozapine at age 57 for psychosis, who developed increasingly refractory psychotic symptoms over 10 months despite dosage reductions of both pergolide and carbidopa/levodopa, an increase of clozapine to 175 mg per day, and the addition of risperidone 1.5 mg (68). After a drug holiday, this patient was titrated up to 125 mg/day of clozapine, but could only tolerate lower doses of carbidopa/levodopa without psychosis. Should dose reduction become necessary, a gradual taper over many weeks is important to prevent cholinergic rebound, and to monitor for the return of psychotic symptoms.

The rationale for continued treatment once psychotic symptoms have resolved derives not only from the treatment flexibility that clozapine gives the physician, but from data showing improvement in certain areas of motor function. Several investigators have documented the ability of previously psychotic PD patients on clozapine to tolerate added medications, or levodopa dosage increases up to 68% over 2 years without psychotic symptoms (63,64,69). The additional benefits of improved motor function have been shown in several small studies. In one group of nine PD patients with prominent tremor, six of nine showed marked improvement, while the other three had moderate improvement using dosages ranging from 18–36 mg of clozapine daily (70). Similarly, Friedman treated five patients with tremor using 12.5–37.5 mg daily, with improvement in all five, one of which was deemed dramatic (71). Six patients given clozapine, 25 mg per day, were observed after an acute L-dopa test for on–off phenomena, and noted to have improved "off"-period scores, with higher ratings in all areas: rigidity, tremor, akinesia (72).

Agranulocytosis is a significant concern for patients and physicians, necessitating weekly monitoring of WBC counts. Alvir's U.S. data on agranulocytosis revealed a peak at 3 months (cumulative incidence 0.75%), with the risk dropping significantly after 6 months (58). Nevertheless, most physicians continue weekly monitoring for the duration of treatment. Any fever or sign of infection, especially during the first 18 weeks of treatment, demands a repeat WBC. Treatment should be interrupted if the total WBC falls below $3000/mm^3$, and the WBC monitored until counts are above this level. The use of clozapine must be permanently discontinued if the total WBC falls below $2000/mm^3$, or the absolute neutrophil count falls below $1000/mm^3$. This idiosyncratic response is immune-mediated, and rechallenge after recovery in patients who have experienced agranulocytosis results in the rapid return of agranulocytosis (73). Certain HLA types found among Ashkenazi Jews show a modest increased risk for agranulocytosis (HLA-BR8, -DR4, and -Dqw3) (74). Clozapine should not be administered concomitantly with other bone marrow suppressing agents, especially carbamazepine, and should be used with caution in those whose baseline WBC is below $3500/mm^3$. Although Sandoz had markedly relaxed the control over clozapine's dispensation, one must register as a physician, and subsequently register each patient entered into treatment. This can easily be done by telephoning Sandoz at (800) 448-5938. Clozapine remains expensive at $1.32 for 25-mg tables and $3.40 for 100-mg tablets, yet the cost is modest compared to full-time nursing care.

G. Newer Agents

Nearly every high-affinity binding site, including α_1 adrenergic receptors, have been implicated as the *deus ex machina* behind clozapine's unique clinical effectiveness. There is much evidence pointing to the importance of serotonergic antagonism (5HT-2 and 5HT-3), and a >10:1 affinity for D_4 over D_2 dopamine receptors, but the issue is far from settled. With this standard in mind, pharmaceutical compounds have been synthesized and tested attempting to harness these characteristics in a drug without the burden of weekly blood count monitoring. The finding that serotonergic blockade may be effective for levodopa-induced psychosis (75) raises questions regarding the dopamine-based model of psychosis as it applies to the PD population.

H. Risperidone

Risperidone is a benzisoxazole derivative with significant 5HT-2 antagonism, little affinity for muscarinic cholinergic receptors, and less D_2 binding than atypical neuroleptics. It has been shown to be an effective antipsychotic in clinical trials, but is not free from extrapyramidal side effects despite the lesser affinity for D_2 receptors (76). EPS are seen to occur in a dose-dependent fashion, especially at dosages over 8 mg per day, with PET studies of normal volunteers revealing 40–55% D_2 receptor occupancy in the basal ganglia after a single 1-mg dose (35). The absence of cholinergic antagonism, and a decreased propensity to EPS at lower dosages, has led to the trial of this agent in PD with psychosis. At least three reports have been published at the time of this writing, with a total of 18 patients. Meco's group in Rome found that low dosages (0.25–1.25 mg daily) were quite effective, and tolerated for up to 24 weeks without worsening of mental status or motor functioning (77). On the other hand, Ford reported worsening parkinsonian symptoms in all six patients treated with risperidone at a slightly higher average dose of 1.5 mg/day (78). Friedman treated four patients with idiopathic PD and two with presumed diffuse Lewy-body disease with risperidone for psychotic symptoms secondary to medication (PD patients) or disease progression (Lewy-body disease patients) (79). One PD patient was able to tolerate risperidone, 2 mg per day, for 3 months without worsening motor signs, but the other five patients were intolerant due to exacerbation of PD, or development of parkinsonism in the Lewy-body disease patients. Due to incomplete response at lower dosages, patients received an average of 2 mg per day (range 1–4 mg) prior to discontinuation. Of note is the fact that Friedman subsequently placed the five treatment failures on clozapine, with 100% resolution of psychosis and tolerance of the medication. Though the above data are somewhat conflicting, there appears to exist a small subset of PD patients who achieve relief of psychotic symptoms without significant worsening of motor functioning. Certain individuals may be considered for a judicious trial of risperidone, given its lower cost and absence of blood monitoring; however, failure to resolve psychotic symptoms at doses up to 1.0 mg, or exacerbation of parkinsonian symptoms should prompt discontinuation and a switch to clozapine.

Numerous other antipsychotic drugs possessing high affinity for 5HT-2 receptors, and decreased affinity for D_2 receptors compared to standard neuroleptics are in clinical trials: sertindole, seroquel, olanzapine, ocaperidone, zotepine, and ziprasidone (80). As the experience with risperidone has demonstrated, the measure of these drugs' usefulness for the psychotic PD patient lies heavily on D_2 binding characteristics, not simply antipsychotic efficacy.

I. Ondansetron

Several drugs have been synthesized and tested as antipsychotics which possess high affinity for 5HT-2 and 5HT-3 receptors. While exploiting a feature of clozapine postulated to play a role in its efficacy, these drugs would be free of the extrapyramidal side effects mediated by D_2 blockade. In a double-blind placebo-controlled study of 33 schizophrenics with prominent negative symptoms (apathy, avolition, withdrawal), ritanserin, a 5HT-2 antagonist, was used as an adjunctive treatment to standard neuroleptics with resulting significant improvement in negative symptoms and social functioning; moreover, there were no changes in measures of extrapyramidal symptoms (45). Another serotonergic antagonist, ondansetron, has been utilized in a trial with psychotic PD patients. Ondansetron is a 5HT-3 antagonist initially marketed as an antiemetic agent for chemotherapy patients. It showed promise in one trial with schizophrenic patients, with an absence of EPS, and has subsequently been given in open-label fashion to 16 patients with psychotic symptoms related to therapy for PD. Melamed et al. maintained patients on dosages of 12–24 mg per day for 4–8 weeks with no exacerbation of motor symptoms or dropouts due to side effects (81). Fifteen of 16 showed moderate or marked improvement in visual hallucinations, with one nonresponder. Confusion was decreased in 13 of 14, and paranoid delusions improved in 90% (9 of 10). Unfortunately, the authors did not comment on the need for hospitalization, or the time course of symptom resolution. Ondansetron is also quite expensive, costing $10 per 8-mg tablet; however, the limited success with drugs of this class is encouraging.

J. Partial Dopamine Agonists

A novel strategy for antipsychotic drug design utilizes the concept that certain drugs may act as D_2 antagonists under circumstances of high dopaminergic transmission, and agonists when dopamine activity is low (82). Unfortunately, the limited success using terguride to treat those aspects of schizophrenia—hallucinations and delusions—which most resemble the levodopa psychoses may not bode well for this group of agents as a possible treatment in PD psychoses (83).

K. Conclusions

Prior to publication of the Scholz and Dichgans study in 1985, the development of psychotic symptoms in the PD patient portended a bleak future for the affected individual. While clozapine has proved to be extremely effective at very low doses in relieving psychosis without exacerbation of parkinsonism, the demented PD population tolerate this medication less well, and continue to represent a challenge for the physician. New agents lacking clozapine's anticholinergic properties have been designed to exploit the high-affinity dopamine (D_4) and serotonin (5HT-2, 5HT-3) blockade believed central to clozapine's effectiveness, while sparing the D_2 antagonism which was the bane of standard neuroleptics. For the PD patient unable to tolerate clozapine, the addition of small doses of risperidone, olanzapine, or newer drugs may offer flexibility while preserving the options of ECT and drug holidays for this refractory group.

REFERENCES

1. Goetz GC, Stebbins GT. Risk factors for nursing home placement in Parkinson's disease. Ann Neurol 1992; 32:250.
2. Parkinson J. An essay on the shaking palsy. London: Whittingham and Rowland, for Sherwood, Neely, Jones, 1817.
3. Hoehn MM, Yahr MD. Parkinsonism: onset, progression and mortality. Neurology 1967; 17:427–442.
4. Jackson JA, Free GBM, Pike HV. The psychic manifestations in paralysis agitans. Arch Neurol Psychiatry 1923; 10:680–684.
5. Schwab RS, Fabing HD, Prichard JS. Psychiatric symptoms and syndromes in Parkinson's disease. Am J Psychiatry 1950; 107:901–907.
6. Calne DB, Stern GM, Laurence DR, Sharkey J, Armitage P. L-dopa in post-encephalitic parkinsonism. Lancet 1969; 1:744–746.
7. Damasio AR, Lobo-Antunes J, Macedo C. Psychiatric aspects in parkinsonism treated with L-dopa. J Neurol Neurosurg Psychiatry 1971; 34:502–507.
8. Celesia GG, Wanamaker WM. Psychiatric disturbances in Parkinson's disease. Dis Nerv Syst 1972; 33:577–583.
9. Goodwin FK. Psychiatric side effects of levodopa in man. J Am Med Assoc 1971; 218:1915–1920.
10. Kaplan HI, Sadock BJ, Grebb JA. Comprehensive Textbook of Psychiatry. Baltimore: Williams and Wilkins, 1995:681.
11. Factor SA, Molho ES, Podskalny GD, Brown D. Parkinson's disease. In: Weiner WJ, Lang AE, eds. Advances in Neurology, vol. 65. New York: Raven Press, 1995: 115–138.
12. American Psychiatric Association. Diagnostic and Statistical Manual of Mental Disorders. 4th ed. Washington, DC: American Psychiatric Association, 1994:129.
13. Kaplan HI, Sadock BJ, Grebb JA. Comprehensive Textbook of Psychiatry. Baltimore: Williams and Wilkins, 1995:729–732.
14. Friedman JH. Management of psychosis in Parkinson's disease. In: Koller WC, Paulson G, eds. Therapy of Parkinson's Disease. 2nd ed. New York: Marcel Dekker, 1995:521–532.
15. Sacks OW, Kohl MS, Messeloff CR, Schwartz WF. Effects of levodopa in parkinsonian patients with dementia. Neurology 1972; 22:516–519.

16. Girotti F, Soliveri P, Carella F, Piccolo I, Caffarra P, Musicco M, Caraceni T. Dementia and cognitive impairment in Parkinson's disease. J Neurol Neurosurg Psychiatry 1988; 51:1498–1502.
17. Danielczyk W. Mental disorders in Parkinson's disease. J Neural Transm 1992; 38(suppl):115–127.
18. McFadden L, Mohr E, Sampson M, Mendis T, Grimes JD. A profile analysis of demented and nondemented Parkinson's disease patients. In: Battistin L, Scarlato G, Caraceni T, Ruggieri S, eds. Advances in Neurology. vol. 69. Philadelphia: Lippincott-Raven, 1996:339–341.
19. Ross H, Hughes TA, Boyd JL, Biggins CA, Madeley P, Mindham RHS, Spokes EGS. The evolution and profile of dementia in Parkinson's disease. In: Battistin L, Scarlato G, Caraceni T, Ruggieri S, eds. Advances in Neurology. vol. 69. Philadelphia: Lippincott-Raven, 1996:343–347.
20. Klawans HL. Levodopa-induced psychosis. Psychiatr Ann 1978; 8:447–451.
21. Moskovitz C, Moses H, Klawans HL. Levodopa-induced psychosis: a kindling phenomenon. Am J Psychiatry 1978; 135:669–675.
22. Nausieda PA, Weiner WJ, Kaplan LR, Weber S, Klawans HL. Sleep disruption in the course of levodopa therapy: an early feature of the levodopa psychosis. Clin Neuropharmacol 1982; 5:183–194.
23. Sharf B, Moskovitz C, Lupton MD, Klawans HL. Dream phenomena induced by chronic levodopa therapy. J Neural Transm 1978; 43:143–151.
24. Steiger MJ, Quinn NP. Levodopa-based therapy. In: Koller WC, ed. Handbook of Parkinson's Disease. 2nd ed. New York: Marcel Dekker, 1992:391–410.
25. Thompson C. Anwesenehit: Psychopathology and clinical associations. Br J Psychiatry 1982; 141:628–630.
26. American Psychiatric Association. Diagnostic and Statistical Manual of Mental Disorders. 4th ed. Washington, DC: American Psychiatric Association, 1994:296–301.
27. Serby M, Angrist B, Lieberman A. Mental disturbances during bromocriptine and lergotile treatment of Parkinson's disease. Am J Psychiatry 1978; 135:1227–1229.
28. Lipper S. Psychosis in patients on bromocriptine and levodopa with carbidopa. Lancet 1976; 2:571–572.
29. Carlsson A, Lindqvist M. Effect of chlorpromazine and haloperidol on the formation of 3-methoxytyramine and normetanephrine in mouse brain. Acta Pharmacol Torticol 1963; 20:140–144.
30. Randrup A, Munkvad I. Special antagonism of amphetamine-induced abnormal behavior. Inhibition of stereotyped activity with increase of some normal activities. Psychopharmacologia 1965; 7:416–422.
31. Carlsson A. The dopamine theory revisited. In: Hirsch SR, Weinberger DR, eds. Schizophrenia. Cambridge, MA: Blackwell Science, 1995:379–400.
32. Kebabian JW, Calne D. Multiple receptors for dopamine. Nature 1979; 277:93–96.
33. Sibley DR, Monsma FJ. Molecular biology of dopamine receptors. Trends in Pharm Sci 1992; 13:61–69.
34. Van Tol HHM, Wu CM, Guan H-C, et al. Cloning of the gene for the human dopamine D_4 receptor with high affinity for the antipsychotic clozapine. Nature 1992; 350:610–614.

35. Waddington JL. The clinical psychopharmacology of antipsychotic drugs in schizophrenia. In: Hirsch SR, Weinberger DR, eds. Schizophrenia. Cambridge, MA: Blackwell Science, 1995:341–357.
36. Nordstrom AL, Farde L, Halldin C. Time course of D_2-dopamine receptor occupancy examined by PET after single oral doses of haloperidol. Psychopharmacology 1992; 106:433–438.
37. Brucke T, et al. Striatal dopamine D_2-receptor blockade by typical and atypical neuroleptics. Lancet 1992; 339:497.
38. Farde L, Nordstrom AL, Nyberg S, Halldin C, Sedvall G. D_1-, D_2-, and 5-HT-receptor occupancy in clozapine-treated patients. J Clin Psychiatry 1994; 55(9-suppl B):67–69.
39. Farde L, Nordstrom AL, Wiesel FA, Pauli S, Halldin C, Sedvall G. Positron emission tomographic analysis of central D_1 and D_2 dopamine receptor occupancy in patients treated with classical neuroleptics and clozapine. Arch Gen Psychiatry 1992; 49:538–544.
40. Meltzer HY, Fessler RG, Simonovic M, Fang VS. The effect of mescaline, 3,4-dimethoxyphenylethylamine and 2,5-dimethoxy-4-methylamphetamine on rat plasma prolactin: Evidence for serotonergic mediation. Life Sci 1978; 23(11):1185–1192.
41. Nordstrom AL, Farde L, Halldin C. High 5-HT_2 receptor occupany in clozapine-treated patients demonstrated by PET. Psychopharmacology 1993; 110:365–367.
42. Watling KJ, Beer MS, Stanton JA, Newberry NR. Interaction of the atypical neuroleptic clozapine with 5-HT_3 receptors in the cerebral cortex and superior cervical ganglion of the rat. Eur J Pharmacol 1990; 182:465–472.
43. White A, Corn TH, Feetham C, Faulconbridge C. Ondansetron in treatment of schizophrenia. Lancet 1991; 337:1173.
44. Wiesel FA, Nordstrom AL, Farde L, Eriksson B. An open clinical and biochemical study of ritanserin in acute patients with schizophrenia. Psychopharmacology 1994; 114(1):31–38.
45. Duinkerke SJ, Botter PA, Jansen AA, Van Dongen PA, Van Haaften AJ, Boom AJ, Van Laarhoven JH, Busard HL. Ritanserin, a selective 5-HT2/1C antagonist, and negative symptoms in schizophrenia. A placebo-controlled double-blind trial. Br J Psychiatry 1993; 163:451–455.
46. Baldessarini R, Frankenberg F. Clozapine: a novel antipsychotic agent. N Engl J Med 1991; 324:746–754.
47. Goetz CG, Tanner CM, Klawans HL. Pharmacology of hallucinations induced by long-term drug therapy. Am J Psychiatry 1982; 139:494–497.
48. Weiner WJ, Koller WC, Perlik S, Nausieda PA, Klawans HL. Drug holiday and management of Parkinson's disease. Neurology 1980; 30:1257–1261.
49. Sweet RD, Lee JE, Spiegel H, McDowell F. Enhanced response to low doses of levodopa after withdrawal from chronic treatment. Neurology 1972; 22:520–525.
50. Klawans HL, Goetz CG, Tanner CM, Nausieda PA, Weiner WJ. Levodopa-free periods ("drug holiday") in Parkinson's disease. In: Advances in Neurology. vol. 37. New York: Raven Press, 1983:33–43.
51. Direnfield L, Spero L, Marotta J, Seeman P. The L-dopa on-off effect in Parkinson's disease: treatment by transient drug withdrawal and dopamine receptor sensitization. Ann Neurol 1978; 4:473–475.

52. Friedman JH. "Drug holidays" in the treatment of Parkinson's disease: a brief review. Arch Intern Med 1985; 145:913–915.
53. Factor SA, Singer C. Neuroleptic malignant syndrome. In: Lang AE, Weiner WJ, eds. Drug-induced movement disorders. Mount Kisco, NY: Futura Press, 1992: 199–230.
54. Potter WZ, Rudorfer MV. Electroconvulsive therapy: A modern medical procedure. N Engl J Med 1993; 328:882.
55. Stern MB. Electroconvulsive therapy in untreated Parkinson's disease. Mov Disord 1991; 6:295.
56. Scholz E, Dichgans J. Treatment of drug-induced exogenous psychosis in parkinsonism with clozapine and fluperlapine. Eur Arch Psychiatr Neurol Sci 1985; 235: 60–64.
57. Kaplan HI, Sadock BJ, Grebb JA. Comprehensive Textbook of Psychiatry. Baltimore: Williams and Wilkins, 1995:1979–1987.
58. Alvir JM, Lieberman JA, Safferman AZ, et al. Clozapine-induced agranulocytosis: incidence and risk factors in the United States. N Engl J Med 1993; 329:162–167.
59. Lieschke G, Burgess AW. Granulocyte colony-stimulating factor and granulocyte-macrophage colony-stimulating factor. Drug Therapy 1992; 327:99–106.
60. Weide R, Kuppler H, Heymanns J, et al. Successful treatment of clozapine induced agranulocytosis with granulocyte colony-stimulating factor (G-CSF). Br J Haematol 1992; 80;557–559.
61. Devinsky O, Pacia SV. Seizures during clozapine therapy. J Clin Psychiatry 1994; 55(9-suppl B):153–156.
62. Wolters EC, Hurwitz TA, et al. Clozapine in the treatment of parkinsonian patients with dopaminomimetic psychosis. Neurology 1990; 40:832–834.
63. Lew MF, Walters CH. Clozapine treatment of parkinsonism with psychosis. J Am Geriatr Soc 1993; 41:669–671.
64. Factor SA, Brown D. Clozapine prevents recurrence of psychosis in Parkinson's disease. Mov Disord 1992; 7:125–131.
65. Friedman JH, Lannon MC. Clozapine in the treatment of psychosis in Parkinson's disease. Neurology 1989; 39:1219–1221.
66. Wolk SI, Douglas CJ. Clozapine treatment of psychosis in Parkinson's disease: a report of five consecutive cases. J Clin Psychaitr 1992; 53:373–376.
67. Pfeiffer RF, Kang J, Graber B, Hofman R, Wilson J. Clozapine for psychosis in Parkinson's disease. Mov Disord 1990; 239–242.
68. Greene P. Clozapine therapeutic plunge in patient with Parkinson's disease. Lancet 1995; 345:1172–1173.
69. Factor SA, Brown D, Molho ES, Podskalny GD. Clozapine: a two year open trial in Parkinson's disease patients with psychosis. Neurology 1994; 44:544–546.
70. Pakkenberg H, Pakkenberg B. Clozapine in the trreatment of tremor. Acta Neurol Scand 1986; 73:295–297.
71. Friedman JH, Lannon MC. Clozapine-responsive tremor in Parkinson's disease. Mov Disord 1990; 5:225–229.
72. Gomez-Arevalo GJ, Gershanik OS. Modulatory effect of clozapine on levodopa response in Parkinson's disease: a preliminary study. Mov Disord 1993; 8:349–354.

73. Frankenburg FR, Stormberg D, Gerson SL. Unsuccessful reexposure to clozapine. J Clin Psychopharm 1994; 14(6):428–429.
74. Yunis JJ, Corzo D, Salazar M, Lieberman JA, Howard A, Yunis EJ. HLA associations in clozapine-induced agranulocytosis. Blood 1995; 86(3):1177–1183.
75. Nausieda PA, Tanner CM, Klawans HL. Serotonergically active agents in levodopa-induced psychiatric toxic reactions. In: Fahn S, Calne DB, Shoulson I, eds. Advances in Neurology. vol 37. New York: Raven Press, 1983:23–32.
76. Janssen PAJ, Niemegeers CJE, Awouters F, Schellekens KHL, Megens AAHP, Meert TF. Pharmacology of risperidone (R 64 766), a new antipsychotic with serotonin-S_2 and dopamine-D_2 antagonistic properties. J Pharm Exp Therap 1988; 244:685–693.
77. Meco G, Alessandria A, Bonifati V, Giustini P. Risperidone for hallucinations in levodopa-treated Parkinson's disease patients. Lancet 1994; 343:1370–1371.
78. Ford B, Lynch T, Greene P. Risperidone in Parkinson's disease. Lancet 1994; 344: 681.
79. Rich SS, Friedman JH, Ott BR. Risperidone versus clozapine in the treatment of psychosis in six patients with Parkinson's disease and other akinetic-rigid syndromes. J Clin Psychiatry 1995; 56:556–559.
80. Kaplan HI, Sadock BJ, Grebb JA. Comprehensive Textbook of Psychiatry. Baltimore: Williams and Wilkins, 1995:2018–2019.
81. Zoldan J, Friedberg G, Weizman A, Melamed E. Ondansetron, a 5-HT_3 antagonist for visual hallucinations and paranoid delusional disorder associated with chronic L-dopa therapy in advanced Parkinson's disease. In: Battistin L, Scarlato G, Caraceni T, Ruggieri S, eds. Advances in Neurology. vol. 69. Philadelphia: Lippincott-Raven, 1996:541–544.
82. Coward D, Dixon K, Enz A, et al. Partial brain dopamine D_2 receptor agonists in the treatment of schizophrenia. Psychopharm Bull 1989; 25:393–397.
83. Olbrich R, Schanz H. An evaluation of the partial dopamine agonist terguride regarding positive symptoms reduction in schizophrenics. J Neural Transm (Gen Sec) 1991; 84:233–236.

19

Sedative-Hypnotics in the Elderly Population

Philip G. Janicak
The University of Illinois at Chicago, Chicago, Illinois

Frank J. Ayd, Jr.
Baltimore, Maryland

I. INTRODUCTION

The elderly are prescribed and utilize a disproportionate amount of medication, particularly sedative-hypnotics. For example, Monane and colleagues found that 65% (94/145) of elderly nursing home patients had sleep complaints. Over half had taken a sedative-hypnotic for at least 5 days in the past month, the majority on a daily basis (1). Most telling, there was no relationship between the use of these agents and the presence or absence of sleep complaints nor between sleep changes and increased or decreased drug use at 6 months follow-up.

In seeking guidance for the most appropriate use of such drugs in the elderly, the clinician often relies on data from younger patient groups. Age-related changes in pharmacokinetics and pharmacodynamics, however, make extrapolation of information from one age group to another an often harrowing task at best. In addition, expectable changes in organ systems, especially the liver and central nervous system, render the elderly patient much more sensitive to the effects of these agents. Complicating this reality is the frequent presence of comorbid medical and/or psychiatric conditions. These coexisting disorders will typically require medication management, setting the stage for a variety of potential adverse drug interactions when sedative-hypnotics are coprescribed.

Because of the risks of such unwanted adverse effects, sedative-hypnotics should be prescribed for the elderly with special caution. For example, with some benzodiazepines (BZDs), such as diazepam, an increase in the volume of distribution may result in lower plasma concentrations in older patients, but only after a single dose. Reactions such as oversedation persist longer and are more marked in the elderly, partly due to decreased rates of metabolism and to greater susceptibility to CNS depression (2). As a consequence, falls, fractures, and confusional states may be produced by small doses of some sedatives (3–6). Memory deficits such as forgetfulness and amnesia are also common in the elderly taking a BZD and should not automatically be attributed to an expected circumstance of aging (7,8). In this context, Salzman et al. found that cognitive function improved and sleep was no worse when bedtime BZDs were discontinued in an elderly nursing home population (9).

It is also imperative that prescribers be aware that pharmacodynamic changes with aging may result in an increased sensitivity to the effects of these agents for any given plasma concentration (10–14). As Rochon and Gurwitz (15) have emphasized: "While a physician can usually do little to alter the characteristics of individual older patients to affect the kinetics or the dynamics of drugs, the decision whether to prescribe anything at all, the choice of drug, and the manner in which it is used (e.g., dose and duration of therapy) are all factors that are under the control of the prescriber."

Lack of response to standard pharmacological treatment for anxiety and sleep disorders may be due to a number of causes, including inadequate medication trials; too low or too high a dose; too short a duration of treatment; an inadequate assessment; and the presence of comorbid psychiatric and/or medical disorders (16). Regarding this last issue, depression, substance abuse, and other anxiety disorders can cause symptoms that mimic various sleep problems. Comorbid axis II disorders (especially cluster A and B personality disorders) can also complicate the clinical picture. Furthermore, a number of medical conditions, as well as the medications required to manage them, can produce symptoms of anxiety and related sleep disturbances. Thus, elderly patients should be evaluated for hyperthyroidism, pulmonary conditions [e.g., chronic obstructive pulmonary disease (COPD)], and the physiological sequelae of alcohol and other drugs, including over-the-counter medications. Treatment-refractory symptoms warrant diagnostic reassessment and, when indicated, control of contributing comorbid disorders. When necessary, this should be followed by augmentation strategies targeted for specific symptom clusters. For the few patients who do not respond to these measures, alternative treatments should be considered (17).

II. NONPHARMACOLOGICAL THERAPIES FOR INSOMNIA

Appropriate nonpharmacological interventions should always be considered and, when possible, utilized in lieu of pharmacotherapy (18). When medication is necessary, nonpharmacological approaches may at least decrease the amount and duration of drug exposure (19). They include such techniques as: stimulus control; sleep restriction; relaxation techniques; paradoxical intention; and sleep hygiene education.

Stimulus control attempts to alter sleep-incompatible behaviors and to regulate the sleep–wake schedule. It incorporates instructions such as going to bed only when sleepy; using the bedroom only for sleep or sex; leaving the bedroom if unable to fall asleep within 15–20 min and returning again only when feeling sleepy; always arising at the same time each morning regardless of the amount of sleep; and never taking naps.

Sleep restriction attempts to decrease the amount of time spent in bed versus the actual amount of time spent sleeping, with a goal of achieving a window of sleep efficiency between 80–90%. If above or below this range, one would increase or decrease time in bed accordingly.

Relaxation techniques attempt to modify increased arousal, whether somatic, cognitive, or both. Somatic arousal is usually benefited by muscle relaxation and/or biofeedback, while increased cognitive arousal can be moderated by attention-focusing procedures such as imagery training or meditation.

Paradoxical intention focuses on staying awake as a means of diminishing performance anxiety.

Finally, *sleep hygiene* education emphasizes alterations in life style, such as improved *health practices* (e.g., diet, exercise, substance use); alteration of *environmental factors* (e.g., lighting, noise, temperature); and *basic information* about changes that occur in sleep patterns over the life cycle.

Regarding this last issue, it should be noted that the elderly tend to sleep less than younger individuals; their sleep architecture is altered; and there may be a phase advance in the sleep–wake cycle, culminating in an earlier bedtime and an earlier awakening the next morning.

Marin et al. recently reviewed this literature and performed a meta-analysis of the efficacy of various nondrug interventions (20). They included 59 treatment outcome studies involving over 2000 patients, and concluded that stimulus control and sleep restriction were the most effective single therapy procedures. Furthermore, clinical improvements were well maintained at an average follow-up of 6 months, documenting that nonpharmacological interventions produced reliable and durable positive changes in sleep latency and time awake after sleep onset in individuals with chronic insomnia.

III. PHARMACOTHERAPY OF SLEEP DISORDERS

To enable clinicians to rationally, safely, and effectively prescribe sedative-hypnotics, the following principles are recommended (18,21):

1. These agents should be prescribed only after the patient has been carefully evaluated for an underlying physical and/or psychiatric disorder.
2. These hypnotics should be prescribed only for the short-term management (7–14 nights) of insomnia (22). After 2 weeks, reassessment should be done before prescribing another course of medication.
3. If insomnia does not remit after 2 weeks of treatment, worsens, or new problems with thinking or behavior develop, an unrecognized psychiatric or physical disorder should again be considered.
4. These agents should be prescribed for patients with a history of alcohol or substance abuse or marked personality disorder only for short-term treatment and only under strict medical supervision.
5. Given that sleep disorders are often transient and intermittent, prolonged administration is generally neither necessary nor recommended.

Actual prescription of sedative-hypnotics should always include the following practices:

1. Do not prescribe more than a 1-month supply.
2. Before prescribing, fully inform the patient of the drug's risks and benefits, that treatment will be short term, and that refills will be limited. A patient information leaflet should be supplied and reviewed with the patient.
3. The patient should be fully cognizant of an agent's safe use.
4. Patients with a history of seizures should not abruptly stop therapy, even if taking concomitant anticonvulsant(s).

Regarding the elderly, the following issues should also be considered:

1. The risk of psychological and physical dependence should be minimized by prescribing the least amount of drug for the shortest period of time.
2. Do not prescribe in the presence of pain unless the insomnia persists after adequate analgesia.
3. Obtain a comprehensive history of prescription and over-the-counter drugs from the patient to avert any adverse drug–drug interaction(s).
4. Patients with pulmonary disease (e.g., COPD, sleep apnea) and dementia should receive sedative-hypnotics only when absolutely necessary and then with added vigilance for adverse effects.

A. Benzodiazepines

Sleep disorders are responsive to a wide variety of pharmacological and nonpharmacological treatments, but none has been shown to produce a cure.

Since these disorders are often chronic, long-term intermittent BZD treatment may be required to achieve optimal benefit. Even when long-term drug therapy is appropriate, periodic reassessment of its efficacy, safety, and necessity is good medical practice. Furthermore, as Griffiths has cogently observed: "While it is true that the majority of people who use benzodiazepines do so for relatively short periods of time (≤ 1 month), the majority of the drug dispensed is consumed by chronic long-term users under conditions in which efficacy has not been established and there are no generally accepted medical recommendations for use" (22). In support of his position, Griffiths cites a rigorous survey of the general population in the United States in 1990 that showed that 25% of past-year users of anxiolytics (primarily BZDs) reported daily use for 12 months or longer; for hypnotics, 23% of past-year users reported daily use for 4 months or longer (23). In this context, there are data indicating that: long-term users account for the bulk of anxiolytic and hypnotic BZDs sold in the United States (and probably worldwide); about 80% of hypnotics sold are consumed by individuals reporting daily use of 4 months or longer; and the number of long-term users of anxiolytics and hypnotic has increased in recent years, even though efficacy has not been established (22).

Finally, long-term BZD therapy for sleep or anxiety disorders has had various problems associated with it, especially in the elderly. These include excessive daytime drowsiness; cognitive impairment and confusion; psychomotor impairment, with an increased risk of falls; paradoxical reactions; depression; intoxication, even on therapeutic dosages; amnestic syndromes; respiratory problems; abuse and dependence; and breakthrough withdrawal reactions.

Biochemistry

There are three major BZD subgroups.

1. 1,4 BZDs, which contain nitrogen atoms at positions 1 and 4 in the diazepine ring and account for most therapeutically important agents. Bromazepam, chlordiazepoxide, clonazepam, clorazepate, diazepam, flunitrazepam, flurazepam, lorazepam, lormetazepam, midazolam, nitrazepam, oxazepam, prazepam, quazepam and temazepam are examples.
2. 1,5 BZDs, which contain nitrogen atoms at positions 1 and 5 in the diazepine ring. Clobazam is an example.
3. Tricyclic BZDs, which often consist of the 1,4 BZD nucleus plus a ring fused at positions 1 and 2. Alprazolam, adinazolam, loprazolam, midazolam and triazolam are examples (24).

In addition, another group features replacement of the fused benzene ring with heteroaromatic systems such as thieno or pyrazolo. Most compounds of this type are under investigation although brotizolam, a thienodiazepine, is currently available outside the U.S. Because pharmacological effects are comparable, both groups of diazepines are considered "BZDs" from a clinical standpoint.

Pharmacodynamics

In 1977, BZD receptors were identified and, along with a subpopulation of gamma aminobutyric acid type A ($GABA_A$) receptors, form the GABA-BZD-chloride ion channel complex. The high density of BZD receptors within the amygdala suggests this is an important site for these drugs' actions. BZDs act at this site to facilitate GABA-mediated transmission, thus serving as an indirect $GABA_A$ agonist. There are two BZD receptor subtypes in the brain, BZ_1 (type 1 or $omega_1$) and BZ_2 (type 2 or $omega_2$), and a third BZD receptor ($omega_3$) exists in peripheral tissues. There are also three types of ligands: agonists (e.g., diazepam), which are anxiolytic and anticonvulsant; antagonists (e.g., flumazenil), which are neutral; and inverse agonists (e.g., FG 7142), which are anxiogenic and proconvulsant.

Pharmacokinetics

Speed of onset and duration of action are two features of the BZD sedative-hypnotics that are independent and related to different aspects of pharmacokinetics. Thus, lipophilicity and absorption affect speed of onset, whereas duration of action and accumulation are determined by metabolism and elimination.

Lipophilicity. This physicochemical characteristic plays an important role in drug absorption. The more lipophilic a drug is the more readily it passes from the plasma through the blood/brain barrier to its sites of action. Diazepam, flurazepam, and quazepam are among the more lipophilic BZDs (25).

Absorption. BZDs differ in absorption speed (26,27). For example, the rate for triazolam is 1.3 h and for flurazepam 3.6 h. Among other effects, the rate of absorption determines the onset of action for a give hypnotic.

Protein Binding. BZDs also differ in their plasma protein binding capacity (26,27). For example, the percentage of unbound plasma protein binding for diazepam is 0–2% and for lorazepam 7–12%. Thus, physiological changes or drug interactions could substantially alter the availability of these agents' free fraction.

Metabolism. Based on metabolic profile, BZD hypnotics can be divided into three groups (26,27). The first is biotransformed by oxidative metabolism in the liver, primarily by *N*-demethylation or hydroxylation and often yields pharmacologically active metabolites that must undergo further metabolic steps prior to excretion. This group includes flunitrazepam and medazepam. The second are conjugated BZDs which do not have active metabolites and only the parent compounds account for clinical activity. This group includes lormetazepam and temazepam. The third group undergo a high first-pass effect prior to reaching the systemic circulation and may have short-lived but active metabolites. This group includes brotizolam, midazolam, and triazolam.

There are several important differences among these groups (26,27). First, metabolism of BZDs that require oxidation may be influenced by such factors as advanced age, liver disease, or coadministration of other drugs that may stimulate or impair hepatic oxidizing capacity. Second, BZDs that require oxidation (e.g., temazepam) tend to have longer elimination half-lives than agents that are conjugated directly. There are exceptions to this, notably the ultrashort-acting agents (e.g., triazolam), which have a high first-pass metabolism.

Elimination Half-Life. BZD hypnotics can also be classified by their elimination half-life: those that are long-acting because they are slowly eliminated; those that are intermediate-acting; and those that are short-acting due to rapid elimination (see Table 1) (26,27). It is important to note that patients receiving a short half-life BZD will react more quickly to dosage changes than those receiving long half-life agents. Long-acting BZD hypnotics usually have activity extending into the next day and not only help nocturnal awakenings

TABLE 1 Benzodiazepine Sedative-Hypnotics

Drug	Half-life (h)	Metabolites
Long-acting		
Flunitrazepam	20–30	None
Nitrazepam	15–38	None
Medazepam	65	*N*-desmethyldiazepam
Flurazepam	72–150	Several, including *N*-desalkylflurazepam
Quazepam	72–150	*N*-desalkylflurazepam
Intermediate-acting		
Estazolam	15–18	None
Lormetazepam	10–12	None
Temazepam	8–12	None
Short-acting		
Midazolam	1.5–3.5	None
Triazolam	1.5–5	None
Brotizolam	3–6	None

and late-onset insomnia (early morning awakening) but may also benefit a daytime anxiety component. These drugs accumulate on daily usage and include: flunitrazepam (20–30 h); nitrazepam (15–38 h); medazepam (65 h); flurazepam (72–150 h); and quazepam (72–150 h). The long half-lives of flurazepam and quazepam are due to their metabolism to desalkylfurazepam.

Intermediate-acting BZD hypnotics may have some residual effects the next day due to accumulation on daily ingestion and include: estazolam (15–18 h); lormetazepam (10–12 h); and temazepam (8–12 h).

Short-acting BZD hypnotics have a rapid fall in plasma level due either to a sustained distribution phase or to a rapid elimination. They are most useful in the treatment of early-onset insomnias (delayed sleep onset). The various drugs within this group have different rates of decline of plasma levels and therefore may sustain sleep to varying degrees. Generally, because of their short duration of action, rapidly eliminated BZD hypnotics do not have next-day residual effects, since they do not accumulate with daily usage. They include: midazolam (1.5–3.5 h); triazolam (1.5–5 h); and brotizolam (3–6 h). Midazolam and triazolam are ultrarapidly eliminated and their effect on sleep duration may be so short that patients may awaken earlier than they desire. Brotizolam, by contrast, has a half-life of about 5 h that places it in the middle of the range of activity of the rapidly eliminated hypnotics. Thus, brotizolam may not only induce sleep quickly but also sustain sleep without residual effects the next day and without accumulation on repeated ingestion.

The PDR aptly calls attention to the postulated relationship between the elimination rate and profile of common untoward effects (see Table 2). It points out that the type and the duration of effects and the profile of adverse effects during drug administration may be influenced by the biological half-life

TABLE 2 Differences Between Short- and Long-Acting Benzodiazepine Sedative-Hypnotics

Factor	Short-acting	Long-acting
mg potency	High	Low
Accumulation	Little or none	Common
Hypnotic hangover effects	None or mild	Mild to moderate
Rebound anxiety	Frequent	Infrequent
Dependency risk	++++	+–,++
Onset withdrawal symptoms	1–3 days	4–7 days
Duration withdrawal symptoms	2–5 days	8–15 days
Withdrawal severity	Severe	Mild to moderate
Paradoxical effects	Frequent	Infrequent
Anterograde amnesia	Frequent	Infrequent
Active metabolites	None or few	Many

of the parent compound and any active metabolites formed. When half-lives are long, drug or metabolites may accumulate during periods of nightly administration and be associated with impairment of cognitive and/or motor performance during waking hours, as well as enhancing the possibility of interactions with other psychoactive drugs or alcohol. By contrast, if half-lives (including half-lives of active metabolites) are short, drug and metabolites will be cleared before the next dose is ingested and carryover effects related to excessive sedation of CNS depression should be minimal or absent (28).

Some agents have a short half-life and no active metabolites. During nightly use for an extended period, pharmacodynamic tolerance or adaptation to some effects may develop. If the drug has a short elimination half-life, it is possible that a relative deficiency of the drug or its active metabolites (i.e., in relationship to the receptor site) may occur at some point in the interval between each night's use. This sequence of events may account for two reported clinical findings after several weeks on nightly, rapidly eliminated hypnotics, namely increased wakefulness during the last third of the night and increased signs of daytime anxiety.

Drug Interactions. BZD hypnotics, such as midazolam and triazolam, are primarily methylated via the P450 3A 3/4 microenzyme system. Other BZDs often utilized as hypnotics, such as diazepam, can also be metabolized by CYP 3A3/4 and CYP 2C19. Any drugs that act as inhibitors or inducers of these isoenzymes could increase or decrease BZD levels, respectively. Thus, ketoconazole and macrolide antibiotics, such as erythromycin, may decrease clearance and increase BZD levels to potentially toxic ranges. Selective serotonin reuptake inhibitors (SSRIs), such as paroxetine, sertraline, and fluoxetine, and, to a greater extent, fluvoxamine and nefazodone, also produce inhibition of CYP 3A3/4. But, at the present time, it is unclear how clinically meaningful these interactions are. Conversely, rifampin, carbamazepine, and dexamethasone may increase clearance and decrease BZD levels to potentially subtherapeutic ranges.

Specific Benzodiazepine Hypnotics

Estazolam (Prosom–Abbott). Estazolam is a 1,4 triazolobenzodiazepine hypnotic that depresses the CNS at limbic and subcortical sites. It potentiates the effect of gamma-aminobutyric acid on its receptor, which increases inhibition and blocks arousal. Estazolam is rapidly and completely absorbed through the gastrointestinal tract in 1 to 3 h; peak plasma levels occur within 2 h; it is highly lipid soluble; 93% is plasma protein bound; and it is extensively metabolized in the liver. Elimination half-life ranges from 15 to 18 h (29).

Estazolam is indicated for the short-term management of insomnia characterized by difficulty falling asleep, frequent nocturnal awakenings, and/or early morning awakenings. Because insomnia is often transient and intermittent, the prolonged administration of estazolam is generally neither necessary nor recommended (30). Caution should be exercised in prescribing this hypnotic for elderly or debilitated patients and those with impaired renal or hepatic function because these patients may be more sensitive to the sedative effects and/or have a reduced capacity to metabolize and eliminate this agent (31). The recommended initial dose is 1 mg, but some patients may need a 2-mg dose. For the elderly, a starting dose of 0.5 mg is usually appropriate and often sufficient.

Estazolam potentiates the CNS depressant effects of phenothiazines, narcotics, antihistamines, monoamine oxidase (MAO) inhibitors, barbiturates, alcohol, general anesthetics, and tricyclic antidepressants. Use with cimetidine, disulfiram, oral contraceptives, and isoniazid may diminish hepatic metabolism, resulting in increased estazolam plasma concentrations and enhanced CNS depressant effects. Heavy smoking (>20 cigarettes/day) and rifampin accelerate estazolam's clearance and decrease its half-life. Theophylline antagonizes estazolam's pharmacological effects.

Quazepam (Doral–Wallace). Quazepam is a 1,4 BZD hypnotic that acts on the limbic system and the thalamus by binding to BZD receptors responsible for sleep (32). It is well absorbed from the gastrointestinal tract, with peak plasma levels of about 15 ng/ml within 2 h. Steady-state plasma levels appear after 7 days of once-daily administration. The drug is more than 95% bound to plasma proteins. Mean elimination half-life of the parent drug and 2-oxoquazepam is 39 h; and 72 h for desalkylflurazepam (33). While the elimination half-life of the parent drug and 2-oxoquazepam are similar in younger and elderly patients, the elimination half-life of desalkylflurazepam in the elderly is twice that in young adults.

The indications, usage, and precautions for quazepam are similar to those for estazolam. Quazepam is available in unscored 7.5- and 15-mg strength tablets, with the latter dose initially used for healthy adults. In some patients, because of individual variations in responses, advanced age, or debilitation the starting dose should be 7.5 mg (34).

Use with alcohol, CNS depressants, antihistamines, opiate analgesics, and other BZDs increases CNS depression. Because of side effects secondary to accumulation, there is little, if any, use for long-acting BZDs such as flurazepam or quazepam in the elderly. An illustration is the occurrence of delirium, ataxia, and severe functional impairment caused by quazepam in a 76-year-old man. Within a week after its discontinuation, he was more alert, conversant, oriented, and his gait improved to the point that he was no longer wheelchair-bound (35).

Quazepam is a pregnancy risk category X drug and breastfeeding while taking it is not recommended.

Temazepam (Restoril–Sandoz). This BZD sedative-hypnotic depresses the CNS at limbic and subcortical levels. It potentiates the effect of GABA on its receptor, increasing inhibition and blocking cortical and limbic arousal. Temazepam is well absorbed through the gastrointestinal tract, with peak plasma levels occurring in 1–3 h and onset of action in 30–60 min. Temazepam is 98% protein bound with a half-life ranging from 8 to 12 h (36). Compared with other BZD hypnotics, temazepam is less lipid soluble and should be administered about 1 h before retiring. During this time patients should be advised to use nonpharmacological measures to induce relaxation.

Temazepam is rarely beneficial in patients with psychosis and may induce paradoxical reactions. It may exacerbate myasthenia gravis, Parkinson's disease, and chronic obstructive pulmonary disease (37). Temazepam may decrease plasma levels of haloperidol.

Abuse of temazepam in the United Kingdom has been increasing rapidly in recent years, with abusers melting the capsules and injecting the molten liquid (38). This process, called "hot-lining," has been the cause of local vascular damage and gangrene that may lead to amputation. The extent of abuse was so great in Britain that the U.K. Health Authorities removed the gelatin-filled capsules from the market. All other formulations of temazepam, however, are still available in the UK (39).

Triazolam (Halcion–Upjohn). Triazolam is a triazolobenzodiazepine sedative-hypnotic that depresses limbic and subcortical levels of the brain. It potentiates the effect of GABA on its receptor, which increases inhibition and blocks cortical and limbic arousal. It is well absorbed through the gastrointestinal tract, with peak levels reached in 1–2 h. Onset of action occurs in 15–30 min. Triazolam is 90% protein bound with an elimination half-life of 1.5 to 5 h.

Triazolam potentiates the CNS depressant effects of phenothiazines, narcotics, antihistamines, MAO inhibitors, barbiturates, alcohol, general anesthetics, and antidepressants. Nefazodone substantially decreases the clearance rate for triazolam, resulting in a 400% increase in this hypnotic's serum levels (40).

Erythromycin can also interfere with its metabolism, resulting in decreased clearance and possibly toxic plasma levels. Troleandomycin and other macrolide antibiotics, such as clarithromycin, flurithromycin, josamycin, midecamycin, or roxithromycin may also inhibit the metabolism of triazolam (41).

Triazolam can reach dangerous concentrations when administered to patients on systemic therapy with ketoconazole and may result in significant alterations in psychomotor test performance. In one study, volunteers were given low doses of triazolam (a single 0.25-mg dose) plus ketoconazole and peak plasma concentrations rose threefold, while the elimination half-life increased six- to sevenfold. Most volunteers experienced several hours of amnesia and felt tired and confused the next morning (42). Another study compared placebo to triazolam in healthy volunteers also on ketoconazole and produced comparable findings. In this second study, ketoconazole prolonged triazolam's half-life and reduced its clearance by about ninefold, while increasing impairment on neuropsychological performance (42). The coadministration of itraconazole and triazolam can also produce a marked elevation of the latter's plasma levels, associated with statistically significant impairment of psychomotor tests and a prolongation of adverse effects (e.g., amnesia, lethargy, and confusion) for hours after awakening (42). Cimetidine and disulfiram may also increase plasma concentrations of triazolam.

In high doses (≥ 1 mg), triazolam may cause a syndrome of severe anxiety, paranoia, hyperacusis, altered smell and taste, and paresthesia. With regular use, increased daytime anxiety typically occurs between doses, perhaps due to withdrawal effects because of its rapid elimination rate.

Other BZDs. If given in sufficient doses, any BZD may have sedative-hypnotic effects. For example, clorazepate and diazepam are often used when anxiety is a prominent symptom associated with insomnia. Clorazepate is a prodrug for *N*-desmethyldiazepam, a slowly eliminated metabolite, which makes clorazepate appropriate for this clinical indication. Desmethyldiazepam also has useful sedative-hypnotic activity and produces a steady anxiolytic effect through the next day. A single 15- or 22.5-mg bedtime dose is usually effective, but lower doses may be sufficient for older patients.

Diazepam and its active metabolite, desmethyldiazepam, are also slowly eliminated, tend to accumulate, and to have a daytime anxiolytic effect with repeated ingestion. Hence, like clorazepate, diazepam can be useful when anxiety is a prominent symptom associated with insomnia. A single 2.5-mg bedtime dose is usually sufficient for the elderly. Again, increased vigilance is required with these agents to anticipate and recognize adverse effects due to repeated dosing over time.

Adverse Effects

Residual sedation, anterograde amnesia, and rebound insomnia are common adverse effects of all BZD sedative-hypnotics. The rate of occurrence of these side effects varies from one drug to another, as well as with different doses of the same drug (43).

Physical Dependency vs. Addiction. Because of widespread lack of knowledge about the essential differences between physical dependency and addiction, dependency on BZDs is often erroneously labeled addiction by some physicians, as well as the media. Tables 3 and 4 review the definitions of these terms.

TABLE 3 Definitions of Drug Abuse, Addiction, and Dependence

Abuse	The use of a medication for *nonmedical or pleasurable purposes*. Abuse is present whenever drug use *results in adverse effects to self or others*, even though the user may be unwilling or unable to acknowledge this fact.
Dependence	Term with several meanings depending on context.
On therapeutic dose	Dependence on moderate therapeutic doses of a sedative/hypnotic drug with *no tendency to increase dosage*. It becomes apparent when withdrawal symptoms emerge following dosage reduction or drug discontinuation. Therapeutic dose dependence is difficult to terminate and may result in prolonged treatment.
Psychological	Condition in which a drug produces a *feeling of satisfaction and psychic drive* that requires periodic or continuous administration to produce pleasure or avoid discomfort (55). It is a subjective need for the drug independent of tolerance or withdrawal symptoms and is reflected by a fear of being without the medication.
Physical	An *adaptive state* characterized by intense physical disburbances (withdrawal or abstinence syndrome characteristic of the particular drug) when repeated drug administration is suspended (56).
Withdrawal	*Time-related reaction* experienced when the drug is stopped.

TABLE 4 Addiction vs. Dependence

- A complex behavioral disorder characterized by *loss of control over substance use*; continuous use *despite problems* caused by the substance overuse and *denial* both of the substance abuse and of the problems it causes.
- Addiction occurs *with* or *without physical dependence.*
- *Tolerance* more common in addiction.
- *Dose escalation* common and often marked.
- Addictive drugs are used for *nonmedical purposes* and usually harm users who typically *abuse multiple drugs*.
- May include abuse of *prescription medicines* as well as *illicit drugs*.
- Addictive drugs are often very *difficult to discontinue* and risk of *relapse is high* and common, even after prolonged abstinence. Addiction is a *life-long disease*.
- Occurs in *addiction-prone* individuals who have a family and/or personal history of chemical dependency (alcoholism, illicit drug use).

B. Nonbenzodiazepine Hypnotics

Zolpidem (Ambien–Searle)

Zolpidem is a non-BZD hypnotic of the imidazopyridine class that has no muscle-relaxant, anxiolytic, or anticonvulsant effects at sedative doses. It is rapidly absorbed after oral administration, reaching peak blood levels in about 2.2 h and is highly bound to plasma protein. Elimination half-life is 2.4 h in younger adults and 2.9 h in the elderly. Compared to earlier sedative-hypnotics, zolpidem has similar sleep-enhancing properties but is less likely to affect sleep architecture. Recommended starting dose for younger adults is 10 mg q.h.s. In older patients, however, doses as low as 2.5 mg may be more appropriate and sufficient.

Adverse Effects. Most drugs associated with sleepwalking and night terrors increase slow-wave sleep. Zolpidem increases delta sleep and this effect is dependent on the age of the subject (e.g., it is observed in young adults). For comparison, this agent affects sleep stages 3 and 4 to a greater extent than triazolam (44). Drug-induced sleepwalking, however, may require a combination of events including a past history of sleepwalking, a medication increasing delta sleep, and a precipitating external or internal (e.g., a full bladder) stimulus (45,46). A full comparison between zolpidem and triazolam is provided in Table 5.

Psychotic reactions to zolpidem have been reported, including two cases involving amnesia and hallucinations in an anorexic patient (47). In one case, zolpidem was prescribed for a 34-year-old woman with chronic insomnia. Twenty minutes after taking the recommended adult dose (10 mg) she experienced feelings of objects in her environment, then slept uneventfully,

TABLE 5 A Comparison of Zolpidem and Triazolam

Zolpidem	Triazolam
Rapidly absorbed, reaching maximum serum concentration in about 2 h	Rapidly absorbed, reaching maximum serum concentration in 1–2 h
Elimination half-life ranges from 2.4–2.9 h	Elimination half-life ranges from 1.5–5.5 h
Metabolites inactive	Metabolites inactive
Schedule IV drug	Schedule IV drug
Does not increase daytime sleepiness	May increase *daytime sleepiness*
No rebound insomnia	*Rebound insomnia*
Efficacy maintained up to 6 months	Efficacy diminished after 2 weeks
May impair cognitive function	May impair cognitive function
May produce *withdrawal symptoms*	Does produce *withdrawal symptoms*

recalling the unusual experience in the morning. Zolpidem has also been reported to cause transient cognitive and behavioral problems similar to those of benzodiazepines (48).

There is also the potential for abuse. For example, zolpidem (10 mg q.h.s.) was given to a 33-year-old male patient for insomnia associated with depression. The patient then increased the dose to 30 mg and noticed improvement of depressive symptoms. With continued dose escalation (up to 150–280 mg/day) tolerance developed. He occasionally noticed signs of intoxication with severe ataxia after doses of 80–100 mg, but never experienced the more common side effects of high-dose zolpidem (e.g., headaches, dizziness, drowsiness, nausea, diarrhea, or myalgia). Dose reduction caused depressive mood recurrence with apathy and drug craving, and a grand mal seizure occurred after ingesting 60–80 mg (49).

Zopiclone

Zopiclone (not presently available in the U.S.), a cyclopyrrolone derivative, is a nonbenzodiazepine hypnotic with high affinity for benzodiazepine receptors, competing directly for these receptor sites. It is chemically unrelated to other sedative-hypnotics currently in clinical use. Zopiclone has a half-life of 4–6 h and is rapidly absorbed after oral administration and extensively metabolized. *N*-desmethyl zopiclone and an *N*-oxide derivative are mostly inactive metabolites. The parent drug is effective in improving sleep onset latency, sleep quality, sleep duration, and frequency of nocturnal awakenings. The recommended dose is 7.5 mg, at which hangover effects are infrequent, becoming undetectable on the 3.75-mg dose. Since zopiclone has a short elimination half-life, its hypnotic effect may not be followed by performance impairment the next day, and it causes less daytime rebound anxiety than triazolam.

Its use should be restricted to short-term treatment, since most controlled clinical studied have involved short or intermediate-term administration. Compared to earlier compounds, zopiclone seems to have similar sleep-enhancing properties, but it is less likely to alter sleep architecture. It may, however, reduce both the quality and quantity of slow-wave sleep. Evidence is limited regarding tolerance and withdrawal.

Adverse Effects. Side effects include a metallic taste. It is claimed to be safe in overdose, which can be counteracted by flumazenil (50).

The combined use of this agent with alcohol produces immediate, enhanced impairment of the psychomotor effects without altering zopiclone's pharmacokinetics. The reaction is short-lived, usually lasting no more than 8 h (51). Co-administration also decreases rapid eye movement (REM) sleep duration during the first half of the night (52). Although coadministration of this agent with carbamazepine reduces plasma concentrations of each drug, it also produces clear additive impairment of psychomotor performance (51). Coadministration with metaclopromide also may decrease zopiclone plasma levels (53). In volunteers given simultaneous oral doses of trimipramine (50 mg) and zopiclone (7.5 mg), the pharmacokinetics of both drugs remained unchanged. Although a trend has been seen toward a decreased area under the curve which might lead to a lessened antidepressant effect of trimipramine, the clinical importance of this and other interactions remains undetermined (54).

Sedative Antidepressants

The use of low doses of sedating antidepressants (e.g., trazodone, doxepin) has been gaining popularity for a variety of short-term sleep disturbances. For example, doses of 25 to 50 mg of trazodone may be helpful while avoiding many of the undesirable effects of BZD sedative-hypnotic agents. Doxepin, however, possesses the same spectrum of effects as other tricyclics and must be used with caution in the elderly patient.

IV. CONCLUSION

Whenever considering drug treatment of dyssomnia in an elderly patient, several issues should be carefully considered. The first is whether a sleep disorder can be explained by another psychiatric or medical condition, which should be addressed (e.g., an antidepressant for sleep disruption secondary to a major depressive episode; analgesics in a patient with disabling pain secondary to arthritis). Next, consider if any prescribed or nonprescribed drugs could explain the disorder. Over-the-counter agents and excessive caffeine ingestion may go unappreciated unless inquired about. Nonpharmacological interventions often suffice. In particular, a detailed review of sleep hygiene issues combined with instruction about stimulus control and sleep restriction may be most useful.

If a medication is judged appropriate, we would suggest an initial trial with low-doses of zolpidem (e.g., 2.5–5 mg q.h.s.) or a short-to-intermediate acting BZD hypnotic (e.g., estazolam, 0.5 to 1 mg q.h.s.). When drug therapy is initiated, it is extremely important to monitor older patients for cumulative effects, given heightened organ system sensitivity (e.g., CNS) and decreased clearance rates (e.g., hepatic compromise). If sleep problems persist beyond 2 weeks, a careful reassessment of diagnosis should be undertaken before re-prescribing a sedative-hypnotic. Figure 1 summarizes the approach we would recommend.

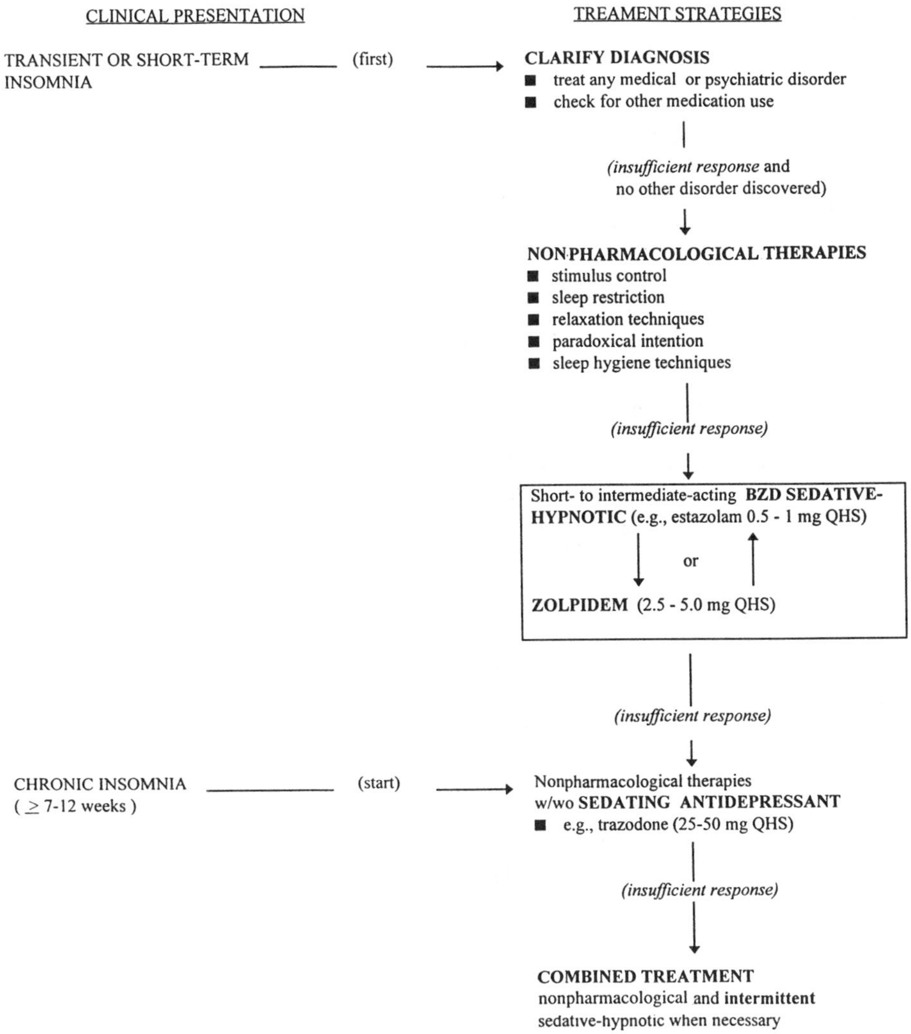

FIGURE 1 Strategy for the management of sleep disorders in the elderly. Adapted from Janicak PG, Davis JM, Preskorn SH, Ayd Jr FJ. *Principles and Practice of Psychopharmacotherapy*. 2nd Ed. Baltimore, MD: Williams & Wilkins, 1997.

REFERENCES

1. Monane M, Glynn RJ, Anarn J. The impact of sedative-hypnotic use on sleep symptoms in elderly nursing home residents. Clin Pharmacol Ther 1996; 59:83–92.
2. Ashton H. Toxicity and adverse consequences of benzodiazepine use. Psychiatr Ann 1995; 25:156–165.
3. Trewin VF, Lawrence CJ, Veitch GBA. An investigation of the association of benzodiazepines and other hypnotics with the incidences of falls in the elderly. J Clin Pharm Ther 1992; 17:129–133.
4. Ray WA, Griffin MR, Schaffner W, et al. Psychotropic drug use and the risk of hip fracture. N Engl J Med 1987; 316:363–369.
5. Sorock GS, Shiskin EE. Benzodiazepine sedatives and the risk of falling in a community-dwelling cohort. Arch Intern Med 1988; 148:2441–2444.
6. Ray WA. Psychotropic drugs and injuries among the elderly: a review. J Clin Psychopharmacol 1992; 12:386–396.
7. Gaind GS, Rosebuch PI, Mazurek MF. Lorazepam treatment of acute and chronic catatonia in two mentally retarded brothers. J Clin Psychiatry 1994; 55:20–23.
8. Rosebuch PI, MacQueen GM, Clarke JTR, et al. Late-onset Tay-Sachs disease presenting as catatonic schizophrenia: diagnostic and treatment issues. J Clin Psychiatry 1995; 56:347–351.
9. Salzman C, Fisher J, Nobel K, Glassman R, Wolfson A, Kelley M. Cognitive improvement following benzodiazepine discontinuation in elderly nursing home residents. Int J Geriatr Psychiatry 1992; 7:89–93.
10. Vogel G. Clinical uses and advantages of low doses of benzodiazepine hypnotics. J Clin Psychiatry 1992; 53(suppl 6):19–22.
11. Greenblatt DJ, Harmatz JS, Shader RI. Clinical pharmacokinetics of anxiolytics and hypnotics in the elderly: therapeutic considerations (part I). Clin Pharmacokinet 1991; 21:165–177.
12. Greenblatt DJ, Harmatz JS, Shader RI. Clinical pharmacokinetics of anxiolytics and hypnotics in the elderly: therapeutic consideration (part II). Clin Pharmacokinet 1991; 21:262–273.
13. Ayd FJ Jr. Prescribing anxiolytics and hypnotics for the elderly. Psychiatr Ann 1994; 24:91–97.
14. Salzman C. Practical consideration of the pharmacologic treatment of depression and anxiety in the elderly. J Clin Psychiatry 1990; 51(suppl):40–43.
15. Rochon PA, Gurwitz JH. Drug therapy. Lancet 1995; 346:32–36.
16. Monane M. Insomnia in the elderly. J Clin Psychiatry 1992; 53(suppl):23–28.
17. Hollander E, Cohen LJ. The assessment and treatment of refractory anxiety. J Clin Psychiatry 1994; 55(suppl 2):27–31.
18. Ayd FJ Jr, Janicak PG, Davis JM, Preskorn SH. Advances in the pharmacotherapy of anxiety and sleep disorders. In: Janicak PG, ed. Principles and Practice of Psychopharmacotherapy Update. Baltimore, MD: Williams & Wilkins, 1996.
19. Espie CA. Psychological Treatment of Insomnia. Chicester: Wylie, 1991.
20. Marin C, Culbert JP, Schwartz SM. Non-pharmacological intervention for insomnia. A meta-analysis of treatment efficacy. Am J Psychiatry 1994; 151:1172–1180.

21. Ayd FJ Jr. Principles of hypnotic prescribing. Int Drug Ther Newslet 1996 31:13–14.
22. Griffiths RR. Commentary on review by Woods and Winger. Benzodiazepines: long-term use among patients is a concern and abuse among polydrug abusers is not trivial. Psychopharmacology 1995; 118:116–117.
23. Balter MB, Uhlenhuth EH. New epidemiologic findings about insomnia and its treatment. J Clin Psychiatry 1992; 52(suppl 12):34–39.
24. Ayd FJ Jr. Lexicon of Psychiatry: Neurology, and the Neurosciences. Baltimore, MD: Williams & Wilkins, 1995:70.
25. Arnold J. Determinants of pharmacologic effects and toxicity of benzodiazepine hypnotics: role of lipophilicity and plasma elimination rates. J Clin Psychiatry 1991; 52(suppl):11–14.
26. Greenblatt DJ. Benzodiazepine hypnotics: sorting the pharmacokinetic facts. J Clin Psychiatry 1991; 52(suppl 9):4–10.
27. Greenblatt DJ. Pharmacology of benzodiazepine hypnotics. J Clin Psychiatry 1992; 53(suppl 6):7–13.
28. Greenblatt DJ, Miller LG, Shader RI. Neurochemical and pharmacokinetic correlates of the clinical action of benzodiazepine hypnotic drugs. Am J Med 1990; 88(suppl 3A):18S–24S.
29. Scharf MB, Roth PB, Dominquez RA, Ware JC. Estazolam and flurazepam: a multicenter, placebo-controlled comparative study in outpatients with insomnia. J Clin Pharmacol 1990; 30:461–467.
30. Pierce MW, Shu VS, Groves LJ. Efficacy of estazolam. The United States Clinical Experience. Am J Med 1990; 88(suppl 3A):6S–11S.
31. Kruse WH-H. Problems and pitfalls in the use of benzodiazepines in the elderly. Drug Safety 1990; 5:328–344.
32. Walmsley JK, Hunt ME. Relative affinity of quazepam for type-I benzodiazepine receptors. J Clin Psychiatry 1991; 52(suppl):15–20.
33. Hilbert JM, Battista D. Quazepam and flurazepam: differential pharmacokinetics and pharmacodynamic characteristics. J Clin Psychiatry 1991; 52(suppl 9):21–26.
34. Kales A. Quazepam: hypnotic efficacy and side effects. Pharmacotherapy 1990; 10:1–12.
35. Wengel SP, Burke WF, Ranno AE, et al. Use of benzodiazepines in the elderly. Psychiatr Ann 1993; 23:325–331.
36. Heel RC, Brogden RN, Speight TM, et al. Temazepam: a review of its pharmacological properties and therapeutic efficacy as a hypnotic. Drugs 1981; 21:321–340.
37. Mitler MM. Evaluation of temazepam as a hypnotic. Pharmacotherapy 1981; 1:3–13.
38. Carnwath T. Temazepam tablets as drugs of misuse. Br Med J 1993; 307:385–386.
39. Anon. Gelatin-filled temazepam capsules. Lancet 1995; 346:303.
40. Green DS, Dockens RC, Salazar DE, et al. Coadministration of nefazodone and benzodiazepines, I: pharmacokinetic assessment [abstract]. Clin Pharmacol Ther 1994; 55:141.
41. Varhe A, Olkkola KT, Neuvonen PJ. Oral triazolam is potentially hazardous to patients receiving systemic antimycotics ketoconazole or itraconazole. Clin Pharmacol Ther 1994; 56:601–607.

42. Greenblatt DJ, von Moltke LL, Harmatz JS, et al. Interaction of triazolam and ketoconazole. Lancet 1995; 345:191.
43. Roth T, Roehrs TA. Issues in the use of benzodiazepine therapy. J Clin Psychiatry 1992; 53(suppl 6):14–18.
44. Ayd FJ Jr. Lexicon of Psychiatry, Neurology, and the Neurosciences. Baltimore, MD: Williams & Wilkins, 1995:681–682.
45. Iruela LM. Zolpidem and sleepwalking. J Clin Psychopharmacology 1995; 15:223.
46. Mendelson WB. Sleepwalking associated with zolpidem (letter). J Clin Psychopharmacol 1994; 14:150.
47. Ansseau M, Pichot W, Hansenne M, et al. Psychotic reactions to zolpidem. Lancet 1992; 339:809.
48. Pies R. Dose-related sensory distortions with zolpidem. J Clin Psychiatry 1995; 56:35–36.
49. Gericke CA, Ludolph AC. Chronic abuse of zolpidem. J Am Med Assoc 1994; 272:1721–1722.
50. Ayd FJ Jr. Lexicon of Psychiatry, Neurology, and the Neurosciences. Baltimore, MD: Williams & Wilkins, 1995:682–683.
51. Kuitenen T, Mattila MJ, Seppala T. Actions and interactions of hypnotics on human performance: single doses of zopiclone, triazolam, and alcohol. Int Clin Psychopharmacol 1990; 5(suppl 2):115–130.
52. Misaki K, Kishi H, Koshino Y, et al. The influence on sleep by zopiclone or ethanol alone or in combination: a polysomnographic study. Jpn J Psychiatry Neurol 1991; 45:915–916.
53. O'Toole DP, Carlisle RJT, Howard PJ, Dunkee JW. Effects of altered gastric motility on the pharmacokinetics of orally administered zopiclone. Ir J Med Sci 1986; 155:136.
54. Callie G, DuSouich P, Spenard J, et al. Pharmacokinetics and clinical parameters of zopiclone and trimipramine when administered simultaneously to volunteers. Biopharm Drug Disp 1985; 5:117–125.
55. Eddy NB, Halbach H, Isbell H, Seevers MH. Drug dependence, its significance and characteristics. Bull WHO 1965; 32:721–723.
56. Ayd FJ Jr. Lexicon of Psychiatry, Neurology, and the Neuroscience. Baltimore, MD: Williams & Wilkins, 1995:194.

20

The Treatment of Generalized Anxiety Disorder, Panic Disorder, and Obsessive–Compulsive Disorder in the Elderly

MALCOLM LADER
UNIVERSITY OF LONDON, LONDON, ENGLAND

RAYMOND ANCILL
ST. VINCENT'S HOSPITAL, VANCOUVER, BRITISH COLUMBIA, CANADA

I. INTRODUCTION

Anxiety is a ubiquitous human emotion that can be experienced by anyone at any time and at any age. It is a normal response to threatening events in life and in turn mobilizes coping responses (cognitive, behavioral, and physiological) that enable readaptation to occur. Whether anxiety is more or less common in the elderly is unclear, although the nature of events that are perceived by the elderly as threatening will be somewhat different from those earlier in life. Thus, physical illness with secondary handicaps, financial worries and concerns about personal safety, with or without the perceptual disorders of dementia, become more prominent and may greatly dilute the quality of life in the elderly. The clinician must be empathetic in order to set such fears into their psychosocial context and to interpret these anxieties as normal or beyond normal limits. Concerns, anxieties, and fears that transcend normality, become excessive, and enter the realm of a clinical disorder, namely generalized anxiety disorder (GAD), major depression with anxiety, or organic anxiety disorder are the focus of this chapter.

Similar arguments can be advanced with respect to panic and obsessive–compulsive phenomena. Panic attacks can occur sometimes but do not become the clinical condition of panic disorder (PD) until they reach certain criteria of severity and frequency (see below). Obsessive–compulsive phenomena are also common and, again, criteria have been established with respect to the boundary between the trait of obsessionality and full-blown obsessive–compulsive disorder (OCD). However, the elderly as a group are especially prone to these disorders as syndromes secondary to neurodegenerative illnesses, such as Parkinson's disease, dementia of the Alzheimer type, dementia of the frontal type, and ischemic dementias.

Confusing the clinical picture further is the fact that with the cognitively impaired elderly, "typical" presentations are unusual and the usual presentation is one of dysfunctional behavior. These behaviors include agitation, aggression, yelling, and intrusiveness. A failure to appreciate this leads to an overevaluation of the behavior itself and the consequent misplaced clinical strategy of behavioral suppression, often with tranquilizers and usually with emergent toxicity. This spiral of toxicity is often the consequence of failing to make the proper diagnosis (1).

According to the Diagnostic and Statistical Manual (DSM-IV), criteria for GAD, PD, and OCD are listed in Table 1.

II. DIFFERENTIAL DIAGNOSIS

In the elderly, the exclusion of medical causes of anxiety is a prime consideration. Of course, the two can coexist with an anxiety disorder superimposed on a medical condition. The medical causes of anxiety are listed in Table 2. Of these, a few deserve special attention. Hyperthyroidism is commonly associated with symptoms of anxiety, particularly cardiovascular ones such as palpitations and flushing. A secondary hyperthyroidism, due to maintaining an elderly person on the same dose of levothyroxine that was appropriate to their physical state several years before, is a relatively common problem. Therefore, any elderly patient who presents with history of treated hypothyroidism should have a thyroid stimulating hormone (TSH) level. With modern radioimmune assay techniques, abnormally low levels of TSH, representing oversuppression by exogenous thyroxine, can be determined. Sometimes, an anxiety disorder ushers in frank hyperthyroidism with a delay of 1–2 years. Emphysema may give rise to symptoms akin to those of PD. Also nocturnal asthma can arouse the patient, with distressing symptoms that resemble those of PD. Acute anxiety secondary to paroxysmal nocturnal dyspnea may be the only sign of left ventricular failure. Treatments for these conditions may themselves be anxiogenic (e.g., digitalis or a sympathomimetic). Some elderly people have been

TABLE 1 Abbreviated Criteria for DSM-IV

Generalized Anxiety Disorder

- A. Excessive anxiety and worry (apprehensive expectation), occurring more days than not for at least 6 months, about a number of events or activities (such as work or school performance).
- B. The person finds it difficult to control the worry.
- C. The anxiety and worry are associated with three (or more) of the following six symptoms (with at least some symptoms present for more days than not for the past 6 months):
  1. Restlessness or feeling keyed up or on edge
  2. Being easily fatigued
  3. Difficulty concentrating or mind going blank
  4. Irritability
  5. Muscle tension
  6. Sleep disturbance (difficulty falling or staying asleep, or restless unsatisfying sleep).
- D. The focus of the anxiety and worry is not confined to features of an Axis I disorder.
- E. The anxiety, worry, or physical symptoms cause clinically significant distress or impairment in social, occupational, or other important areas of functioning.
- F. The disturbance is not due to the direct physiological effects of a substance or a general medical condition and does not occur exclusively during a mood disorder, a psychotic disorder, or a pervasive developmental disorder.

Panic Disorder

- A. Both (1) and (2):
  1. Recurrent unexpected panic attacks
  2. At least one of the attacks has been followed by 1 month (or more) of one (or more) of the following:
     - a. Persistent concern about having additional attacks
     - b. Worry about the implications of the attack or its consequences (e.g., losing control, having a heart attack, "going crazy")
     - c. A significant change in behavior related to the attacks.
- B. Absence of agoraphobia
- C. The panic attacks are not due to the direct physiological effects of a substance (e.g., a drug of abuse, a medication) or a general medical condition (e.g., hyperthyroidism).
- D. The panic attacks are not better accounted for by another mental disorder.

Obsessive-Compulsive Disorder

- A. Either obsessions or compulsions:

  Obsessions as defined by (1), (2), (3), and (4):
  1. Recurrent and persistent thoughts, impulses, or images that are experienced, at some time during the disturbance, as intrusive and inappropriate and that cause marked anxiety or distress
  2. The thoughts, impulses, or images are not simply excessive worries about real-life problems
  3. The person attempts to ignore or suppress such thoughts, impulses, or images, or to neutralize them with some other thought or action.

(continued)

TABLE 1 Continued

Obsessive-Compulsive Disorder (continued)

4. The person recognizes that the obsessional thoughts, impulses, or images are a product of his or her own mind (not imposed from without as in thought insertion).

Compulsions as defined by (1) and (2):

1. Repetitive behaviors (e.g., hand washing, ordering, checking) or mental acts (e.g., praying, counting, repeating words silently) that the person feels driven to perform in response to an obsession, or according to rules that must be applied rigidly
2. The behaviors or mental acts are aimed at preventing or reducing distress or preventing some dreaded event or situation; however, these behaviors or mental acts either are not connected in a realistic way with what they are designed to neutralize or prevent or are clearly excessive.

B. At some point during the course of the disorder, the person has recognized that the obsessions or compulsions are excessive or unreasonable.

C. The obsessions or compulsions cause marked distress, are time consuming, or significantly interfere with the person's normal routine, occupational functioning, or usual social activities or relationships.

D. If another Axis I disorder is present, the content of the obsessions or compulsions is not restricted to it.

E. The disturbance is not due to the direct physiological effects of a substance or a general medical condition.

on the same type of medication for many years and obsolescent drugs are often found in their medicine cabinets. The elderly often resort to over-the-counter remedies or rely on folk remedies from their childhood. Some of these substances, such as cough and cold remedies, may be taken regularly or even in excessive amounts. Careful questioning is essential to avoid overlooking these agents.

Alcohol-related problems may supervene or increase in the elderly. This can result in anxiety or panic attacks related to alcohol withdrawal—essentially subclinical delirium tremens. The patient complains of anxiety attacks typically in the morning after overindulgence the night before. Caffeine is another agent that can induce anxiety, and elderly people may become more sensitive to it as they do to other drugs. Insomnia with secondary anxiety (insomnophobia) is another consequence of caffeinism. Coffee or tea restricted to morning intake may still impact adversely on the following night's sleep. In such circumstances, strict adherence to decaffeinated beverages is required, especially if hypnotic medication is to be avoided.

Depression in the elderly is a major cause of the presentation of anxiety. Although there is some controversy as to the actual incidence and prevalence

TABLE 2 Organic Causes of Anxiety

Angina pectoris
Carcinoid syndrome
Cardiac arrhythmias
Cerebral arteriosclerosis
Cerebral neoplasm
Cushing's syndrome
Delirium of various types
Early dementia
Hyperventilation
Hypoglycemia; hyperinsulinism
Hypo- or hyperparathyroidism
Hypo- or hyperthyroidism
Hypoxic states
Mitral valve prolapse
Myocardial infarction
Partial complex seizures
Pheochromocytoma
Postconcussion disorders
Pulmonary embolism
Vestibular abnormalities

of major depression in the elderly, the generally accepted incidence of treatable depressive illness is around 10–15%. A confounding factor is copresentation with dementia. It is well recognized that depression is common in neurodegenerative diseases, with rates in Parkinson's disease being perhaps more than 50% (2) and about 30% in dementia of the Alzheimer's type and in multi-infarct dementia (3). Anxiety and agitation are common in this neuropsychiatric complex and may have several etiological components. Thus, agitation in a patient with parkinsonism (idiopathic or otherwise) may have poorly controlled dyskinesia, depression, drug toxicity, or any combination of these. The presence of appetite and sleep disturbance may predict an underlying depression, but in inadequately controlled Parkinson's disease, sleep may be disturbed because of rigidity or dystonias and appetite may appear affected if the patient avoids food because of a fear of choking. Thus DSM-IV criteria for any putative disorder must always be carefully assessed in the elderly with multiple pathologies.

III. EPIDEMIOLOGY OF ANXIETY DISORDERS IN OLD AGE

Earlier studies are difficult to interpret because diagnostic criteria for currently accepted nosological entities within the rubric of anxiety disorders had not yet been established; most were lumped together as the psychoneuroses. However, neither Leighton et al. (4) nor Pasamanic et al. (5) found any evidence of either an increase or a decrease in the prevalence of psychoneurotic disorders in old age. Two surveys in the U.K. found a prevalence of 10.2 and 11% of psychoneurosis in the elderly (6,7).

Another U.K. study surveyed over a thousand elderly people living in Liverpool using the Geriatric Mental State as a rating scale (8). The prevalence of anxiety disorder among females over the age of 65 was 1.5%, that in males 2.9%. Phobic Disorder was the next most common (1.2%), with hypochondriasis (0.5%) and OCD next (0.20%). Follow-up was continued for 3 years during which time the incidence was just under 0.5% per year (9). Some cases did remit over this time, but many suffered continued symptoms.

The most systematic data are available from the Epidemiologic Catchment Area survey (10). Over 18,000 subjects participated in the study based on institutional and community surveys of five sites in the U.S. At all age groups, GAD had fairly common (up to 5%) 1-year prevalence rates but tended to drop over the age of 65 (2.2%) (11). The age of onset of the condition tended to be in the twenties and virtually all cases in the over-65 age range were long standing. PD showed a marked fall off in 1-year prevalence with age, from around 4% in young adults to less than one-tenth of this in the elderly (12). The decline with OCD was less marked (2% to 0.9%) (13).

IV. PRINCIPLES OF TREATMENT

A. Pharmacokinetic

The general topic has been reviewed in an earlier chapter and elsewhere (14). By and large the elderly are more sensitive to most drugs because of changes in such pharmacokinetic parameters as volume of distribution, hepatic metabolism, and renal clearance rate. Sedatives, tranquilizers, and antidepressants are no exceptions to this rule. Furthermore, the elderly may become more sensitive because of changes in receptors and in receptor-effector coupling.

The practical implications are that the elderly may be more sensitive by a factor of 2, 3, or even more in the aged and multiply impaired (15). As drugs act longer, less frequent dosing may be feasible (16). It is usual to initiate drug treatment at half-dosage or even less, and to push the dose slowly: "Start low and go slow." Some elderly patients, however, may need full doses and appear to tolerate them; thus it is sometimes important not to stay "too low."

B. Available Treatments

Bromides were used extensively in the late nineteenth and early twentieth centuries. Their adverse effects were slow to become appreciated, toxic delirium being the most serious. This was a particular problem in the elderly because of their age-related decline in renal function, with subsequent cumulation in the body. Phenobarbital was also common, and other barbiturates were introduced for the treatment of anxiety: these included amobarbital and quinalbarbital. Unfortunately, the latter drugs were found to have a high likelihood of inducing dependence, toxicity in high doses, and danger in overdose, accidental or deliberate. All these compounds are now obsolete, but occasionally an elderly patient is encountered with life-long barbiturate usage.

The first compound in the search for a better anxiolytic was meprobamate. It enjoyed a brief popularity but was found to have most, if not all, of the drawbacks of the barbiturates. It was fairly rapidly superseded by the benzodiazepines, the first one of which (chloridiazepoxide) was introduced in 1959. Many others have followed. One in particular, alprazolam, is also indicated in the treatment of PD in the U.S.

Antidepressant drugs have also been evaluated as anxiolytics. The earliest example is the monoamine oxidase inhibitors (MAOIs), which were tried extensively in "atypical depression," often characterized by phobic anxiety and panics. More recently, imipramine and clomipramine, both tricyclic antidepressants (TCAs) have been evaluated in PD and the latter particularly in OCD. Efficacy has been established unequivocally, but these tricyclic drugs are often poorly tolerated in the elderly. Very recently, the selective serotonin reuptake inhibitor (SSRI) antidepressants have been tested in PD and OCD patients. All appear fairly effective in these conditions and one, paroxetine, has been licensed for those indications in the U.K. and Canada.

C. Available Medications

Detailed accounts of anxiolytic and antidepressant medications are available in standard textbooks. The following brief overview concentrates on their profile in the elderly.

Benzodiazepines

These compounds have been used for the past 3 decades or more as the main treatments for anxiety and related disorders. They act on the benzodiazepine (GABA) chloride ionophore receptor complex. These receptors are widespread throughout the brain, particularly in the cerebral and cerebellar cortex. They induce anxiolysis, sedation, sleep, muscle relaxation, and most have an anticonvulsive effect. They have little or no effect on autonomic function, but can produce profound impairments of psychomotor or cognitive function to the point of amnesia (see also Chapter 19).

Because many are metabolized slowly in the elderly, particular toxicity problems may arise. The most common subjective side effects are fatigue, tiredness, drowsiness, muscle weakness, dysarthria, ataxia, and tremor (17–19). At higher doses, confusion and depression can occur, with occasionally paradoxical anxiety, aggression, or mania (20).

Particular problems in the elderly to which attention has been drawn are the increased risk of falls and hip fractures (21,22) and the risk of road accidents (23).

Although benzodiazepines are generally fairly safe in the physically ill elderly, respiratory function can be further depressed in patients with chronic obstructive lung disease. The resulting anoxemia can induce a confusional state. As in younger patients, problems of habituation, dependence, and withdrawal syndromes can occur in the elderly. By simple chronology, the elderly are more likely to be long-term users of benzodiazepines than younger subjects.

Generally, the widespread use of benzodiazepines in the institutionalized elderly is a major cause of significant morbidity and probably mortality (24).

Buspirone

This anxiolytic was introduced several years ago. It acts on serotonin, not GABA, mechanisms. It is effective but has the drawback of a slow onset of action in contrast to the rather rapid effect of the benzodiazepines. Its side effects include nausea, dizziness, headache, and fatigue. Psychomotor and cognitive impairment is minimal, and dependence potential and abuse liability appear low (25). For all these reasons it may be of particular value in the elderly, particularly for those who cannot tolerate a benzodiazepine (26).

Antipsychotics

In some countries, low doses of antipsychotic medication are favored as antianxiety therapy (27). However, extrapyramidal effects such as akathisia may occur even at low dosage, and the elderly are more susceptible to these unwanted effects. In long-term treatment, tardive dyskinesia poses a risk. Neuroleptic malignant syndrome (NMS), or at least a transient variant of it, may be more common in the elderly than acknowledged. Acute confusion with rigidity, a high white cell count, rising creatinine kinase, and pyrexia are highly indicative of this potentially fatal syndrome. Early signs of NMS often include anxiety. The treatment is to stop the neuroleptic immediately and to reduce core temperature. Drugs such as dantroline or bromocriptine are usually unnecessary. Postural hypotension is another problem in the elderly, with the age-related impairment of maintaining blood pressure being exaggerated by the alpha-blocking effect of many neuroleptics. This may lead to falls and subsequent fractures.

Antihistamines

Hydroxyzine and diphenhydramine are sometimes prescribed for the anxious elderly. Antihistamines have concomitant anticholinergic effects such as dry mouth, blurred vision, confusion, and severe (sometimes obstructive) constipation to which the elderly are especially prone. Sedation is also quite marked and confusion and disorientation may occur. While it may be true that dependence does not develop, it is clear in the elderly that dose tolerance does. This will result in increasing toxicity over time.

Beta-blockers

These drugs are often used in patients with agoraphobia or social phobias. They reduce such symptoms as palpitations, tremor, and gastrointestinal upset. Some patients find them useful, others report only limited relief. The hypotensive effect of these drugs limits their use in the elderly.

Antidepressants

The various groups of antidepressants are being used increasingly in the management of anxiety disorders. Some are licensed for the indication of anxiety within the context of a depressive illness, others for mixed anxiety-depressive states. However, some antidepressants, clomipramine and SSRIs in particular, are effective in OCD. PD is another indication which is under increasing evaluation and SSRIs are proving quite effective. However, efficacy data in the elderly are lacking. Phobic anxiety has been traditionally a target for the MAOIs. For example, several studies attest to the efficacy of MAOIs in social phobia. Again, data in the elderly are not extant.

Among the antidepressants, the TCAs are often poorly tolerated in the elderly because of sedation and autonomic side effects, such as postural hypotension, dry mouth, and constipation. The traditional MAOIs are also poorly tolerated in the elderly, optimal dosage attainment being precluded by severe postural hypotension. The RIMA, meclobamide, is generally preferred as it is better tolerated despite some opinions that it is marginally less effective.

The SSRI compounds, fluoxetine, paroxetine, sertraline, citalopram, and fluvoxamine, appear to be effective in panic disorder and OCD, as well as in depression where their efficacy is more well established. Approval for use of each of these compounds in panic disorder and OCD varies with the compound and varies from country to country, but given the similar mechanism of action—blockade of serotonin uptake—it seems reasonable to assume that these drugs are more similar than they are different in terms of their efficacy in panic disorder and OCD.

Our knowledge of the use of these drugs in the elderly is limited. Their efficacy in panic disorder and OCD is demonstrated primarily in studies of younger patients, if at all. Our knowledge of the safety and tolerability of the SSRIs in elderly patients comes primarily from studies in depression and from our clinical experience. Paroxetine, initially at 10 mg, appears to be an effective choice for the treatment of depression in the elderly, especially those with anxiety. The long elimination time of norfluoxetine limits the value of fluoxetine in the elderly. Sertraline in the U.S. and citalopram in Europe are other alternatives. Sertraline displays less enzyme inhibition of the 2D6 hepatic isoenzyme than does paroxetine or fluoxetine. Fluvoxamine differs from the other SSRIs in that its clearance is dependent primarily on renal mechanisms rather than hepatic metabolism. This might be advantageous in some patients, but could be problematic in patients with renal disease.

Venlafaxine is a recently introduced antidepressant which blocks the uptake of both norepinephrine and serotonin and, perhaps, dopamine. It appears to be effective in cases of depression that have proven refractory to other agents (28), but its efficacy in panic and OCD is relatively untested.

Nefazodone is another new antidepressant. The principal action of nefazodone is 5HT-2 antagonism, but it also has modest serotonin reuptake blocking effects. In depressed patients, nefazodone appears to reduce anxiety more quickly than imipramine or placebo (29) and, unlike the SSRIs, it does not aggravate anxiety in the early stages of treatment. One brief report (30) suggested that it was more useful than imipramine for treatment of panic attacks occurring in the context of depression. Although the early clinical trial data suggest this drug may be particularly useful for the treatment of depression related to anxiety, it is not well studied in the elderly, and its efficacy in primary panic disorder and OCD is not established. Nefazodone is metabolized by the 3A4 isoenzyme (which appears to slow with advanced age), and blood levels following single initial doses are higher in the elderly than in younger patients. For this reason, if nefazodone is administered in the elderly, it is particularly important to start with lower doses (e.g., 50 mg b.i.d. or less). During steady dosing, blood levels in the elderly become more comparable to those in younger patients, and the doses ultimately required are relatively similar.

Electroconvulsive Therapy

Although electroconvulsive therapy (ECT) is not specifically indicated for anxiety, agitated elderly patients with depression may sometimes require this treatment. Often, these frail patients are not able to tolerate chemotherapy or have not responded to it. ECT is safe and effective. Furthermore, maintenance ECT, one to four treatments per month, as an outpatient may prevent relapse and subsequent readmission. For patients with Parkinson's disease and depression, ECT will benefit both the mood and motor symptoms and should be considered at an earlier stage than might otherwise be the case. The presence of a comorbid dementia is not a contraindication for ECT, and there continues to be no evidence that demonstrates that ECT causes further brain damage. To quote a leading authority in geriatric psychiatry: "There are no absolute contraindications to ECT apart from the absence of a head on which to place the electrodes" (31).

D. Practical Drug Management

Only broad guidelines can be given here and these reflect the personal preferences of the authors. First, the foundation of the treatment is explanation, reassurance, and discussion with the patient and caregivers. Second, the abnormal symptoms and behavior must be counteracted and brought back under the patient's control. This includes suppression of obsessive thoughts and compulsive rituals, lessening of panic attacks in terms of both frequency and severity, and amelioration of anticipatory and free-floating anxiety. Third, when these symptoms are maintained at a low and tolerable level, appropriate anxiety management and/or cognitive behavior therapy is instituted to alter behavior (e.g., agoraphobic avoidance) and to change cognitions. Finally, the drugs are slowly withdrawn.

Because the duration of this type of treatment strategy encompasses months rather than weeks, benzodiazepines are not suitable medication. This is especially so because dosages such as those of alprazolam will have to be high and, therefore, will be more likely to induce dependence. The only role for these drugs is as short-term (less than 2 weeks) therapy for the rapid relief of intolerable anxiety during an acute exacerbation.

In our opinion, SSRI antidepressants are the treatment of choice. In general, the doses needed to control OCD and suppress panic attacks are higher than the antidepressant doses. However, as SSRIs are *anxiogenic* during the first week or so of administration, half-doses should be given initially, and the patient must be warned of this side effect. Subsequently, the dosage can be titrated upward fairly slowly, as necessary. Although not licensed for this indication, it is our experience that the SSRIs are effective in GAD as well. The main side effects of the SSRIs in the elderly are headache, dizziness, and nausea, but these are usually markedly dose dependent and show tolerance. Sexual dysfunction is not a common complaint.

The subsequent psychological or behavioral treatment must be tailored to the individual needs of the patient. Such treatment must be expert: training in nonfocused techniques such as relaxation may not be helpful and some patients may become more panicky as they "relax." The patient must be prepared to invest time and energy (and in some countries, money) in cooperating with the treatment, which need not be prolonged. More traditional psychotherapies may be useful in some patients with complex and abnormal personal relationships.

V. CONCLUSIONS

Anxiety in the elderly, as it is in younger populations, is a nonspecific marker for distress as well as disease. However, neurodegenerative changes in the elderly further complicate this picture. Furthermore, the elderly often present with multiple illnesses requiring many different medications and, therefore, simply adding on the diagnosis of "anxiety," and prescribing a tranquilizer will invariably worsen the situation. Care must always be taken to obtain a detailed history with collateral informants, and to conduct a careful examination of both physical and mental states. The possibility of the anxiety or agitation being a presentation of drug toxicity should be considered early. Only when physical causes have been eliminated or, at least, stabilized, should psychiatric causes be explored.

Dementia and depression remain the most common causes of anxiety in the elderly. Clinical experience with tacrine, a cholinomimetic, has shown that "treating" the dementia may result in a reduction in anxiety. However, the treatment of dementia is in its infancy and symptomatic treatment is often indicated. As with antidepressants, anxiolytics should be chosen with care. Emergent toxicity should always be anticipated and the patient should be reviewed frequently. Supportive therapies may be helpful and realistic therapeutic goals need to be established.

While it is true that the world is a more threatening place for the elderly, it is equally true that the majority of old people are not frightened and cope extremely well. Prejudice and stereotyping must be avoided and each case must be assessed individually and thoroughly. This may take more time but the physician must avoid adding to the burden the patient has to bear.

REFERENCES

1. Ancill RJ, Carlyle WW, Liang RA, Holliday SG. Agitation in the demented elderly: a role for benzodiazepines? Int J Psychopharmacol 1991; 6:141–146.
2. Dooneief G, Mirabello E, Bell K, et al. An estimate of the incidence of depression in idiopathic Parkinson's disease. Arch Neurol 1992; 49:305–307.
3. Fischer P, Simamyi M, Danielczyk W. Depression in dementia of the Alzheimer type and in multi-infarct dementia. Am J Psychiatry 1990; 147:1484–1487.
4. Leighton DC, Harding DS, Macklin DB, et al. The Character of Danger. New York: Basic Books, 1963.

5. Pasamanic B, Roberts DW, Limkau PW, Krueger DB. A survey of mental disease in an urban population: prevalence by race and income. In: Pasamanic B, ed. Epidemiology of Mental Disorder. Washington, DC: American Association for the Advancement of Science, 1959:183–202.
6. Kay DW, Beamish P, Roth M. Old-age mental disorders in Newcastle-upon-Tyne. I. A study of prevalence. Br J Psychiatry 1964; 110:146–168.
7. Bergmann K. The neuroses of old age. In: Kay DW, Walk A, eds. Recent Developments in Psychogeriatrics. Ashford: Headley, 1971:39–50.
8. Copeland JRM, Dewey ME, Wood H, Searle R, Davidson RA, McWilliam C. Range of mental illness among elderly in the community: prevalence in Liverpool using GMS-AGECAT package. Br J Psychiatry 1987; 150:815–823.
9. Larkin BA, Copeland JRM, Dewey ME, et al. The natural history of neurotic disorders in an elderly urban population: findings from Liverpool longitudinal study of continuing health in the community. Br J Psychiatry 1992; 160:681–686.
10. Robins LN, Regier DA, eds. Psychiatric Disorders in America. New York: Free Press, 1990.
11. Blazer DG, Hughes D, George LK, Swartz M, Boyer R. Generalized anxiety disorder. In: Robins LN, Regier DA, eds. Psychiatric Disorders in America. New York: Free Press, 1990:180–203.
12. Eaton WW, Dryman A, Weissman MM. Panic and phobia. In: Robins LN, Regier DA, eds. Psychiatric Disorders in America. New York: Free Press, 1990:155–179.
13. Karno M, Golding JM. Obsessive-compulsive disorder. In: Robins LN, Regier DA, eds. Psychiatric Disorders in America. New York: Free Press, 1990:204–219.
14. Lader M. Neuropharmacology and pharmacokinetics of psychotropic drugs in old age. In: Copeland et al., eds. Principles and Practice of Geriatric Psychiatry, 1994: 79–82.
15. Salzman C, Shader RI, Harmatz JS. Response of the elderly to psychotropic drugs: predictable or idiosyncratic? Psychopharmacol Bull 1975; 4:48–50.
16. Cole JO, Stotsky BA. Improving psychiatric drug therapy. A matter of dosage and choice. Geriatrics 1974; 29:74–78.
17. Pomara N, Stanley B, Block R, et al. Adverse effects of single therapeutic doses of diazepam on performance in normal geriatric subjects: Relationships to plasma concentrations. Psychopharmacology 1984; 84:342–346.
18. Nikaido AM, Ellinwood EH Jr, Heatherley DG, Dubow D. Differential CNS effects of diazepam in elderly adults. Pharmacol Biochem Behav 1987; 27:273–281.
19. Larson EB, Kukull WA, Buchner D, et al. Adverse drug reactions associated with global cognitive impairment in elderly persons. Ann Intern Med 1987; 107:169–173.
20. Goodman WK, Charney DS. A case of alprazolam, but not lorazepam, inducing manic symptoms. J Clin Psychiatry 1987; 48:117–118.
21. Ray WA, Griffin MR, Schaffner W, et al. Psychotropic drug use and the risk of hip fracture. N Engl J Med 1987; 316:363–369.
22. Ray WA, Griffin MR, Downey W. Benzodiazepines of long and short elimination half-life and the risk of hip fracture. J Am Med Assoc 1989; 262:3303–3307.
23. Skegg DCG, Richards SM, Doll R, et al. Minor tranquillizers and road accidents. Br Med J 1979; i:917–919.

24. Ancill RJ, Embury GD, MacEwan GW, Kennedy JS. Lorazepam in the elderly—a retrospective study of the side-effects in 20 patients. J Psychopharmacol 1987; 2:126–127.
25. Lader M. Assessing the potential for buspirone dependence or abuse and effects of its withdrawal. Am J Med 1987; 82(suppl. 5a):20–26.
26. Singh AN, Beer M. A dose range finding study of buspirone in geriatric patients with symptoms of anxiety. J Clin Psychopharmacol 1988; 8:67–68.
27. Chou JCY, Sussman N. Neuroleptics in anxiety. Psychiatr Ann 1988; 18:172–175.
28. Nierenberg AA, Feighner JP, Rudolph R, Cole JO, Sullivan J. Venlafaxine for treatment-resistant unipolar depression. J Clin Psychopharmacol 1994; 14:419–423.
29. Fawcett J, Marcus RN, Anton SF, O'Brien K, Schwiderski U. Response of anxiety and agitation symptoms during nefazodone treatment of major depression. J Clin Psychiatry 1995; Suppl 6, 37–42.
30. Dassylva B, Fontaine R, Gammans D, Elie R. Efficacy of nefazodone in patients suffering from major depressive disorder and panic disorder. Biol Psychiatry 1992; 31:169A.
31. Katona C. The management of depression in old age. In: Katona C, ed. Depression in Old Age. Chichester: Wiley, 1993:105.

21

Use of Cognitive Enhancers in Dementing Disorders

STEVEN C. SAMUELS AND KENNETH L. DAVIS
MOUNT SINAI SCHOOL OF MEDICINE, AND MOUNT SINAI MEDICAL CENTER, NEW YORK, NEW YORK

I. INTRODUCTION

The primary goal of this chapter is to review the use of cognitive enhancing agents in dementia. Our emphasis is on Alzheimer's disease (AD). We include both clinical and preclinical data about compounds that are currently being used or are in active stages of development and expected to come to the marketplace or to clinical trials in the coming year. We also review future therapeutic approaches for AD. The compounds discussed are being used primarily to treat the cognitive deficits in dementia; for a review of the available treatments of the noncognitive syndromes in patients with dementia, the reader is directed to other chapters in this section of the book (1,2).

AD, affecting nearly 4 million persons and costing 80 billion per year in the U.S., is an age-related disease, exponentially increasing in prevalence from 0.3–3.0% at age 65 years (3,4) to 47.5% at age 85 years (3). After age 85 years, the prevalence rate levels off near 40% by age 95 years (5). Time from diagnosis until death averages 9 years, but there is individual variability (6).

Dementia is a disease affecting cognitive and noncognitive domains. Cognitive deficits occur in the areas of memory, language, motor function, sensory awareness and integration of new knowledge. Noncognitive deficits include the behavioral disturbances that may include physical or verbal agitation, wandering, sleep disturbance, inability to attend to activities of daily living (ADLs) and overall functional impairment.

II. CHOLINERGIC COMPOUNDS

In this section, we review the potential cholinergic approaches for treating AD, including precursors to acetylcholine, muscarinic agonists, and acetylcholinesterase inhibitors.

A. Cholinergic Function in AD

Cholinergic deficits in AD are consistently implicated. Evidence supporting the cholinergic hypothesis includes neurochemical studies in humans that correlate with dementia severity. Bierer and colleagues examined the relationship between neurochemical measures and dementia severity in a large AD sample after controlling for age (7). The dementia severity ratings were based on antemortem examination in about 47% and postmortem chart review in 53%. The activity of Choline acetyltransferase (ChAT), the enzyme responsible for the synthesis of acetylcholine, and clinical dementia ratings were highly correlated throughout the neocortex. Moreover, AD patients have preferential loss of cholinergic neurons in their brains (8). Anticholinergic drugs induce memory deficits in animals and humans. In some animal models of dementia, animals are treated with scopolamine to produce cognitive dysfunction. In the healthy elderly, anticholinergic agents are frequently associated with delirium or poor performance on structured neuropsychological tests. Animals and humans with drug-induced or structural deficits show improved attention and memory when cholinergic agents are administered. Further evidence implicating cholinergic depletion in AD comes from the controlled clinical trials with cholinergic agents.

B. Muscarinic Receptor Agonists

Muscarinic agonists have demonstrated some benefit in preclinical studies. A few compounds are now undergoing clinical trials. Continuous stimulation of receptors by cholinergic agonists does not mimic the pulsatile physiological stimulation and may result in receptor downregulation, possibly limiting the effectiveness of these compounds (9). However, tonic stimulation may be relevant to attention and arousal.

CI-979 (Milameline)

This compound is a nonselective partial agonist of muscarinic receptors that has demonstrated effectiveness in improving cognitive performance and increasing central cholinergic activity in rodents (10). CI-979 reverses scopolamine-induced memory deficits in rodents (11). In monkeys, CI-979 increases neocortical arousal as measured with EEG (10). The doses required for central cholinergic activity are below those required for peripheral cholinergic activity, allowing for good tolerability in healthy volunteers at doses up to 1 mg q 6 h (10). AD and healthy elderly patients tolerated a gradual increase in dose to 2–3 mg q 6 h. Dose-limiting side effects that occurred above 2 mg q 6 h were primarily gastrointestinal (GI) in nature (vomiting, nausea, and stomach pain). The duration of action is greater than 2 h in most tests. A multicenter clinical study of CI-979 for AD is currently in progress.

Xanomeline

This partial M-1 agonist has undergone safety trials in AD subjects. Initially developed in oral form, the most common adverse effects were GI distress and hypotension (12). The compound has biologically active metabolites (13) that may be partially responsible for the side effects. The oral form was discontinued from development and a phase II safety study with transdermal delivery of this compound is currently enrolling patients. Preliminary results suggested particular efficacy in noncognitive symptoms (14).

SB202026

This compound is a partial agonist with functional selectivity for the M-1 receptor (15). Phase III clinical trials with this agent are underway. Large phase II studies suggested efficacy at a dose as low as 0.25 mg (16).

Nicotine

Nicotine as a therapeutic agent for AD is based on a decreased number of nicotinic receptors in the postmortem Alzheimer's disease brains (17) and in living AD patients as measured with PET (18). Nicotine bitartrate administered to nonsmoking AD patients decreased the rate of intrusion errors (19). Nicotine use in AD patients, but not normal controls, was associated with adverse effects on mood (20). Prior studies have included intravenous infusion of nicotine; current studies are underway examining the transdermal nicotine delivery in AD patients. The therapeutic efficacy of nicotine may become reduced with AD progression as the cholinergic cells degenerate (21).

C. Acetylcholinesterase Inhibitors

To date, the acetylcholinesterase inhibitors have been the most successful of the cholinergic compounds in coming to the U.S. marketplace. Currently, two agents (tacrine and E2020) are approved. Other acetylcholinesterase inhibitors are expected to follow.

Physostigmine

Physostigmine, one of the earlier acetylcholinesterase inhibitors studied, enhances storage of long-term memory (22). The response to physostigmine appears related to cholinergic inhibition in the CSF (23) and in the plasma (24). The effects are dose-sensitive. Low dose improves long-term memory function in young adults, but higher doses worsen performance (25). Physostigmine has a 30-min half-life in plasma, which necessitates frequent dosing. Physostigmine significantly increased recognition memory at an individual's best dose (26). Physostigmine improved cognitive function transiently in a subgroup of AD patients, but significant cholinergic side effects, frequent dosing requirements, and rapid fluctuations in serum levels limit its use (27). Response to physostigmine was correlated with percentage increase in diurnal cortisol secretion (a marker of central cholinergic activity) (27). Physostigmine infusions were given to patients in a double-blind crossover study of L-Deprenyl or placebo. Subjects who received Physostigmine or L-Deprenyl alone or in combination did not demonstrate improvement in cognitive functioning as measured with digit span, verbal fluency, praxis, list learning, delayed recall, or delayed recognition. Both drugs were well tolerated (28). The short half-life of physostigmine makes it inconvenient to use and a longer acting form of physostigmine-salicylate is being developed for AD in an attempt to respond to some of the compound's current limitations for routine clinical use. Phase III trials with this agent have been completed, and showed efficacy (29).

Tacrine

Tacrine (9-Amino-1,2,3,4-tetrahydroacridine) was the first cholinesterase inhibitor approved in the U.S. for AD. The compound is a centrally acting noncompetitive reversible acetylcholinesterase and butyrylcholinesterase inhibitor (30). We have thoroughly reviewed Tacrine's role in the treatment of AD in another publication (31). Tacrine was shown to be effective in many clinical trials (31–42). The positive findings in both the Davis et al. 12-week study (41) and the Knapp et al. 30-week study (42) were pivotal for FDA approval of Tacrine. Prior studies with limited dosing and duration of Tacrine had precluded FDA sanction.

Limitations to Tacrine include q.i.d. dosing, serum monitoring for hepatic transaminase elevations, and gastrointestinal side effects. Tacrine doses of 80 mg/day to 160 mg/day are necessary for clinical response. At least 12 weeks of dose titration are required before a dose of 120 mg/day is realized. Often, gastrointestinal side effects or elevated hepatic transaminases increase the time required to titrate up to therapeutic doses. Transaminase elevations may result in discontinuation of tacrine. Patients may still be rechallenged with Tacrine, however, after the transaminase levels normalize. In one analysis,

88% of patients could tolerate Tacrine rechallenge and 72% of the patients tolerated higher Tacrine doses (43). The FDA allowed modification of the package insert reflecting less frequent transaminase monitoring and guidelines for rechallenge after clinical experience with the drug increased (44).

Tacrine and Brain Imaging. SPECT with AD patients on Tacrine demonstrate that technicium-99-labeled ethylene dicysteinate retention abnormalities (a measure of cerebral blood flow) are improved in mild-to-moderate AD patients who received 75 mg of Tacrine per day but not in those who received 25 mg q day (45). Utilizing Xe inhalation, rCBF was measured in probable AD patients before and after 14 months of Tacrine treatment. The group of patients that demonstrated cognitive improvement with Tacrine also revealed improvement or stabilization in rCBF compared with those patients who did not receive Tacrine. The trial was open-label with maximum dosage of Tacrine at 125 mg per day (46). Functional imaging studies of AD patients treated with acetylcholinesterase inhibitors should advance our understanding of how brain function correlates with clinical response to medication and further elucidate mechanisms of cholinergic dysfunction in AD.

Tacrine and the Cost of AD. In a pharmacoeconomic study, Lubeck et al. estimated that Tacrine could generate savings up to 17% of the current costs of AD or a total of 3.6 billion annually. Patients tolerating 80–160 mg/day showed an improvement of 1 point on the Mini-Mental State Exam (MMSE) and those able to tolerate 160 mg/day improved 2 points on the MMSE. The calculated savings were based upon 9.5 months to 12.1 months of reduced community and institutional costs, the amount of time that a 1–2-point improvement on the MMSE corresponds with (47). Industry-sponsored studies to further examine the cost of AD are underway. As more drugs are developed for AD, a drug's impact on the direct and indirect costs of the disease will become a standard for comparison and possibly will be used as a justification for choosing one agent over another.

Tacrine's Longer Term Effects on Quality of Life. Tacrine's effect on mortality and nursing home placement was studied in about 90% of the 663 patients in the Knapp 30-week study (42,48). These probable AD patients were followed openly for 2 years until they died or were placed in a nursing home. The patients who were receiving Tacrine doses greater than 80 mg/day were less likely to have died or have been admitted to a nursing home than patients on lower Tacrine doses (odds ratio >2.7). Limitations of this study include the lack of a control group and retrospective nature of the study. The dose-response nature of the findings suggest that the response is "real." The possibility that Tacrine may protect AD patients from mortality is intriguing and the findings of this report require replication.

E2020

In December, 1996, E2020 (donepezil hydrochloride) became the second acetylcholinesterase inhibitor approved for AD in the U.S. The drug blocks acetylcholinesterase in the brain. The inhibition is of mixed type (between competitive and uncompetitive inhibition). The inhibitor dissociation constant for E2020 is one or two orders of magnitude lower than Tacrine, indicating a stronger inhibitory effect of E2020 on acetylcholinesterase (49). The selective inhibition of E2020 is 1250 times greater for AchE than for butylcholinesterase (50). E2020 has also been shown to reverse scopolamine-induced deficits in rats (51).

E2020, marketed as Aricept (Pfizer and Eisai), has no evidence of hepatic toxicity, has convenient dosing (q h vs. q.i.d.), can be started at the target dosage (5 mg q h) and can be increased to 10 mg q h. The most common adverse effects include nausea and loose stool. In a 12-week double-blind placebo-controlled study, probable AD patients were treated with E2020 in doses of 1 mg, 3 mg, and 5 mg, or placebo. The E2020-treated AD patients demonstrated dose-related imposements in the ADAS cog and the MMSE. The 5 mg E2020 group demonstrated a statistically significant improvement in the ADAS cog compared with placebo. E2020 was not associated with hepatic toxicity and was well tolerated in this study (52). In a 6-month placebo-controlled study, patients receiving E2020 remained stable compared with the placebo patients who demonstrated decline on ADAS cog and ratings of clinical change made by clinicians and caregivers. The difference was statistically significant at the 5- and 10-mg dosage (53). It is expected that E2020 will become more widely used than Tacrine because of its ease of use, improved side-effect profile, and ability to immediately start at therapeutic doses. However, its reported efficacy on the ADAS, at its best, is not as large as has been reported for Tacrine, at its best, although direct comparative studies have not been done.

ENA-713

ENA-713 is a "pseudo-irreversible" carbamate acetylcholinesterase inhibitor that is brain-selective and demonstrates preferential selectivity for the hippocampus and cortex. The drug, neither metabolized nor eliminated by the liver, does not demonstrate hepatic toxicity. In one animal study utilizing the step-down avoidance paradigm, ENA 713 was shown to improve acquisition and retention memory in basal forebrain–lesioned rats (54). The phase I and II clinical trials of ENA 713 have been completed and the phase III trial program is ongoing. Efficacy of ENA 713 was demonstrated in two placebo-controlled studies involving 516 patients with probable AD. A dosage of 3 mg b.i.d. produced improvement in global symptoms and on cognitive function. Outcome measures included the Wechsler logic memory test, CIBIC-plus, Fuld-OME DSS, and CGIC. The drug was tolerated up to doses of 6 mg b.i.d. in the tolerability study (55). The phase III trial allows inclusion of patients with comorbid medical illness (56).

Galanthamine

Galanthamine is a tertiary amine of the phenthrene group and competitive inhibitor of acetylcholinesterase but not butyrylcholinesterase. The half-life is longer than physostigmine's and Galanthamine has shown promise in some studies (57) but not others (58). A multicenter clinical trial is currently underway in the U.S. and Europe for patients with AD. A large phase II trial reported statistically significant improvement in ADAS and a global measure, with a substantial subgroup of patients experiencing more than a 7-point improvement (59). The drug is already approved in Austria.

Eptastigmine

One randomized, double-blind placebo-controlled clinical trial of Eptastigmine was published at this writing (60). One-hundred-three patients with probable AD entered 4 weeks of double-blind placebo control followed by 1 week of washout then 8 weeks of open-label phase. Subjects had MMSE between 10 and 26. Dosing of Eptastigmine was based on weight after uniform dosing had resulted in nausea and vomiting in some patients. Outcome ratings included both physician and caregiver CGIC; test of logical memory, semantic word fluency, and trail making; and Index of Independence in Daily Living Scale (IADL). One hundred three patients entered the double blind phase (81 Eptastigmine, 22 placebo). After 4 weeks, 94 remained in the study (74 Eptastigmine, 20 placebo). Reasons for dropout included cholinergic side effects, uncooperation, protocol violation, and clinical worsening. At completion of the double-blind phase, the physician CGIC and IADL scales demonstrated significant difference between the groups favoring Eptastigmine. The memory scales, word fluency test, and trail making showed no difference between groups. Improvement occurred in 25–40% of the Eptastigmine group. Dose response was not linear but an inverted "U" shape. Six of 41 subjects who entered the open-label portion of the study dropped out for reasons unrelated to treatment. More clinical trial experience is needed with this cholinesterase inhibitor, particularly because in higher doses it produced agranulocytosis (61).

Metrifonate

This irreversible cholinesterase inhibitor is currently utilized to combat schistosomes (62). Metrifonate has greater inhibitory effects on butyrylcholinesterase than acetylcholinesterase (30), and is the prodrug of the long-acting organic cholinesterase inhibitor dichlorvos. The compound has demonstrated memory-enhancing effects in animals (63). Metrifonate has a short half-life, achieves long-acting and high levels of cholinesterase inhibition, and is well tolerated in AD patients and controls (64).

Metrifonate's mechanism of action as an antidementia agent may be attributable to characteristics other than cholinesterase inhibition. In one study using the Morris Water Escape Task in young rats, the relative effectiveness of metrifonate, dichlorvos, organophosphorous compounds diisopropylfluorophosphate and paraoxon, and structurally unrelated cholinesterase compounds, E2020, Tacrine and physostigmine were compared. Metrifonate, dichlorvos, diisopropylfluorophosphate, and, to a lesser degree, paraoxon enhanced the acquisition of the water escape task. Tacrine, E2020, and physostigmine did not affect learning and memory in the young-adult rat in the doses utilized (63). Metrifonate is currently under clinical investigation for AD.

Acetylcholinesterase Inhibitors and APP Processing

Abnormal processing of the amyloid protein precursor (APP) is involved in beta-amyloid production in AD. Normal processing results in release of the secretory components of APP. In a recent study using rat brain cortical slices, the effect of various acetylcholinesterase inhibitors on APP processing was examined (65). Physostigmine, heptylphysostigmine and 2,2-dichlorovinyldimethyl phosphate elevated release of APPs significantly above control levels. The authors suggested that acetylcholinesterase inhibitors may have a neuroprotective effect by activation of normal APP processing. Additional studies demonstrated Tacrine's reversible inhibition of APP secretion in cell cultures (66). A subcortically lesioned rat model of AD demonstrates many of the neurochemical and cognitive deficits of AD. The lesioned animals demonstrate altered APP mRNA processing. Transient functional denervation results in reversible changes in beta APP concentration and permanent lesions result in persistent induction (67).

III. ESTROGEN

Estrogen promotes the growth and survival of cholinergic neurons (68) and may decrease cerebral amyloid deposition (69). Estrogen appears to decrease the risk and delay the onset of developing AD. A longitudinal study of 1124 women in the New York City area who were initially free of AD revealed that 12.5% of the women took estrogen after menopause (70). Age at onset of AD was later in women who took estrogen compared with those who did not use estrogen. The relative risk of developing AD was 5.8% in estrogen users compared with 16.3% in nonusers, even after adjusting for education, Apolipoprotein E genotype, and ethnic origin.

In another study of female patients with AD, estrogen was shown to improve MMSE score over 3 and 6 weeks, increase the rCBF in the lower frontal region and primary motor area as measured with SPECT, and decrease the delta and theta band values on the EEG (71). In an analysis of patients who had AD diagnoses selected from a retirement community in southern California, the risk of having AD decreased significantly in women taking estrogen. The relationship was dependent on estrogen dosage and duration of use (72).

A multicenter study comparing two doses of estrogen by transdermal patch to placebo in AD patients is ongoing and preliminary reports presented at Society for Neuroscience on 10 AD women (five received 17-Beta estradiol and five received placebo for 5 weeks) reported beneficial effects on verbal memory and attention in those receiving estrogen compared with placebo (73). The results of this study in combination with the known literature will assist clinicians in making recommendations about estrogen replacement therapy to women at risk for AD and those who are already diagnosed with AD.

Combination treatments with estrogen and other antidementia treatments have not yet been systematically studied. However, in a retrospective analysis of women in the 30-week Tacrine trial (Ref. 42), those receiving estrogen replacement therapy responded better in measures of cognition and overall function than those not taking estrogen (74).

IV. GINGKO BILOBA

Gingko Biloba (EG6761), available in drug stores, health food stores, and mail order catalogues is commonly used by patients with memory impairment or frank dementia. The compound has been approved in Germany for the treatment of dementia (75). The clinical utility of this compound has not been well studied. In one study, 222 outpatients, aged over 55 years, with MID or Alzheimer's dementia of moderate severity received Gingko Biloba 120 mg b.i.d. or placebo prior to meals in the double-blind portion of the study (76). The design of the study was a single-blind 4-week placebo run-in followed by a 24-week active phase. Outcome measures were a clinician impression of change, a cognitive measure, and a behavioral rating. Response was defined as improvement in at least two of the three outcome measures. Six of the 222 subjects dropped out during the 4-week single-blind run in phase. Two-hundred-five of 216 completed the 24-week active phase; 21 dropped out; and 28 had protocol violations leaving 156 who were analyzed (77 Gingko and 77 placebo). Using intent-to-treat analysis, 23% responded to Gingko and 10% responded to placebo. Headache was the only notable adverse effect. Although the results of this study are intriguing, well-designed clinical trials with Alzheimer's disease patients with different stages of disease are needed before this drug can be endorsed as useful for patients with AD.

V. NOOTROPICS

In many countries the standards for drug approval are less stringent than those required for FDA approval in the United States. As a result, many compounds known as nootropics were developed and are available for indications ranging from "loss of memory" to "circulatory problems." These agents have not demonstrated benefit under the scrutiny necessary to recommend clinical use and will not be reviewed in this chapter.

VI. FUTURE APPROACHES TO SLOW THE COURSE OF ALZHEIMER'S DISEASE

In addition to the aforementioned cognitive enhancers, there are a number of compounds that may slow the progression of the disease and are at various stages of clinical development. The rationale for pursuing treatment with these agents is discussed in this section.

A. Anti-Inflammatory Agents

The anti-inflammatory basis of therapeutics in AD is based upon the presence of the following inflammatory factors at the sites of neurodegeneration (77): (1) increased amounts of IL-1 and IL-6; (2) acute phase reactants are found in senile plaques; (3) Clq, an early complement cascade component; and (4) activated microglial cells.

Causation is implied by the following: (1) IL-6 overproduction in a transgenic mouse model leads to increased neurodegeneration (78); (2) IL-1 increases APP production in cell culture (79); (3) Clq interacts with Abeta, resulting in an increase in aggregation and increased Abeta toxicity (80); (4) IL-1 augments Abeta1-42 toxicity in rat pheochromocytoma cell lines (81); (5) neurotoxin release from mononuclear inflammatory cells (82).

Anti-inflammatory and anti-immune agents that are currently being investigated in AD include prednisone, colchicine, and hydroxychoroquine. Epidemiological studies have revealed other agents that may be candidates for further investigation including methotrexate, sulfasalazine and beta-interferon. There is strong fundamental basic science work supporting the use of anti-inflammatory agents in the treatment of AD. Clinical research is required with many of these agents.

B. Glutaminergic Compounds

Excitatory amino acids (EAA) such as glutamate or aspartate, are found throughout the brain, but are in especially high concentrations in the hippocampus, corticocortical projections and corticostriatal connections. EAA have three ionotropic receptor subtypes: NMDA, AMPA (formerly called quisqualate) and kainate receptors that are associated to cationic channels. Glutaminergic compounds are the focus of investigation because stimulation with glutamate results in long-term potentiation of neurons, a correlate of memory production. Overstimulation may result in neurotoxicity. The NMDA receptor, a glutamate receptor subtype, has an agonist binding site that can bind glutamate, aspartate, and NMDA, and is involved in memory and learning (83). The NMDA receptor also has a glycine site and polyamine site that mediate allosteric regulation and modulate glutamate's effects. There is also a site located within the channel for activity-dependent antagonists. The channel is calcium permeable and blocked by magnesium in a voltage-dependent manner. Antagonists of NMDA receptors and AMPA receptors may have a neuroprotective role.

Milacemide

Milacemide gets converted to glycine and glycinamide after it crosses the blood-brain barrier. One multicenter study of 228 patients with AD did not demonstrate any efficacy of milacemide (84). Another study of 48 healthy adults did not support the effectiveness of milacemide as a cognitive enhancer (85). It is not clear whether this agent will undergo further development.

Aniracetam

Aniracetam, a pyrrolidinone derivative, may positively modulate the metabotropic glutamate receptors and AMPA-sensitive glutamate receptors. It may also facilitate cholinergic transmission (86). Aniracetam has demonstrated memory-enhancing effects in animals and reduces memory deficits in animals induced by cholinergic antagonists, cerebral ischemia, and electroconsulsive shock. In healthy human volunteers, the compound reduced EEG changes induced by hypoxia and reduced scopolamine-induced cognitive impairment (86).

Clinical trials with Aniracetam have demonstrated the cognitive-enhancing effects of this agent. Aniracetam 1500 mg/day demonstrated increased effectiveness compared with placebo at 4 and 6 months in one study of 109 probable AD patients with mild-to-moderate severity utilizing the Sandoz Clinical Assessment Geriatric (SCAG). Aniracetam-treated patients improved 12–35% compared with placebo receivers who demonstrated 9–19% deterioration. The 6-month extension phase of this study continued to demonstrate superiority of Aniracetam to placebo (87). In a 3-month study with lower doses of Aniracetam (1000 mg/day) and including some severely affected Alzheimer's disease patients, there was no difference between the treatment and placebo group (88). In a nonplacebo-controlled study of Aniracetam (1500 mg/day) and piracetam (2400 mg/day), the Aniracetam was more effective in 8 of 18 variables of the SCAG in patients with mild-to-moderate AD. Aniracetam-treated patients improved 17–29% compared with piracetam-treated patients, who improved 9–20% (89).

The most common adverse effects of Aniracetam include unrest, anxiety, uneasiness, and insomnia. Other mild adverse effects included headache, somnolence, vertigo, mild epigastric pain, nausea, diarrhea, and rash. No increases in liver enzymes were noted and the adverse effects did not necessitate drug discontinuation (86). Aniracetam appears to be effective, well tolerated, and safe in preliminary trials of AD patients. Further evaluation is warranted with well-designed clinical trials.

C. Ampakines

In AD, decreased AMPA receptor subunits may influence neuronal vulnerability through alterations in calcium homeostasis (90). Ampakines enhance the activity of AMPA receptors and may facilitate memory by enhancing long-term potentiation (91).

D. Nerve Growth Factor

Nerve growth factor (NGF) is essential for neuronal function, regeneration, and survival. Nerve growth factor acts selectively on cholinergic neurons and it is taken up by neurons in a retrograde fashion. NGF is primarily located in the hippocampus, basal forebrain, and cortex. Basal forebrain cholinergic neurons possess the NGF receptors and produce increased choline acetyltransferase in response to NGF (92). NGF administration attenuates degenerative changes in neurons experimentally lesioned and elevates levels of acetylcholine production (93). NGF restored spatial memory in animals with strategically placed lesions (94).

One case study reports improvement in verbal memory, increased nicotine binding, and increased cerebral blood flow in a patient treated for 1 month with NGF (95). An NIA work group made recommendations regarding the study of NGF in AD (96). Clinical trials of this agent will require alternate means of drug delivery as NGF must currently be given via the intracerebral ventricular route of administration as the compound does not cross the blood-brain barrier (97). The intracerebral ventricular route of administration is inconvenient and has a high complication rate. Alternatively, drugs that potentiate NGF and can cross the blood-brain barrier may be worthy of further study (98,99).

E. Antioxidants

Antioxidants and free radical scavengers have a theoretical basis in the treatment of AD. Free radicals may be mediators of A-beta peptide-induced toxicity. Agents that minimize free radical damage to neurons are being evaluated in preclinical and clinical studies.

Vitamin E and Selegiline

Vitamin E and Selegiline, a monoamine oxidase-B (MAO-B) inhibitor, both have antioxidant properties. A double-blind, placebo-controlled clinical trial of Selegiline and vitamin E, alone and in combination, compared with placebo was recently completed. Outcome measures compared over 2 years were: change from CDR of 1 or 2 to CDR of 3; death; nursing home placement; or complete loss of two or three ADLs on the Blessed. The results of this study were not available at the time of this writing.

Idebenone

This benzoquinone derivative is structurally related to ubiquinone, an intermediate in the ATP generating oxidative phosphorylation pathway. Idebenone has been available in Japan since 1986 and is one of the most commonly prescribed drugs there. Over 8 million persons have been prescribed the drug in Japan and it is also available in Europe, Asia, and South America.

Idebenone has been demonstrated to be effective for patients with probable AD in double-blind placebo-controlled trials (100–102). In one study (102), 450 patients were randomized to receive either placebo or Idebenone at 30 mg t.i.d., 60 mg t.i.d., or 90 mg t.i.d. The ADAS sum score at 6 months compared with baseline significantly favored Idebenone. The ADAS cog, CGI, and an ADL scale also favored Idebenone in a dose-dependent manner. The results at 12 months demonstrated even greater differences between placebo and Idebenone. Favorable results with Idebenone were also reported in other double-blind, placebo-controlled studies using lower doses of Idebenone (100,101).

The adverse effects of Idebenone most commonly reported in AD patients included an influenzalike syndrome, bronchitis, and lumbar pain. The adverse events most commonly attributable to Idebenone include dizziness, agitation, sleep disorder, insomnia, nausea, and abdominal pain. The incidence for placebo was similar. A multisite double-blind, placebo-controlled clinical trial with three doses of Idebenone and placebo is currently underway in the U.S.

F. Agents Affecting Calcium

Calcium's role as a chemical messenger has been well substantiated. Neuron destruction may be attributable to alterations in calcium homeostasis. Attempts to restore calcium balance have led to trials of calcium antagonists in Alzheimer's disease.

Nimodipine

Nimodipine is an example of a calcium antagonist that has been investigated. Nimodipine administration to rabbits improved memory and learning (103). In a randomized, double-blind, placebo-controlled, multicenter trial, 227 patients with AD received either placebo or Nimodipine 90 mg or 180 mg per day (104). Subjects receiving Nimodipine 90 mg, but not Nimodipine 180 mg, had improved performance on a word list memory test. This selective dose response may reflect neuron functional sensitivity to calcium levels. Other studies supported Nimodipine's positive effect on cognition in AD patients (105,106).

G. Agents That Affect Amyloid Beta Processing and Deposition

Abnormal processing of the amyloid protein precursor (APP) may lead to overproduction of beta-amyloid (A-beta). A-beta is found in senile plaques in brains of persons with AD. A recent paper reviewed the potential pharmaceutical interventions that may be utilized with regard to A-beta in AD processing. The author suggested that the following interventions be considered: (1) activation of serine and/or cysteine proteases which are involved in APP processing; (2) suppression of binding between apoE and amyloidogenic proteins; (3) prevention of aggregation of A-beta molecules; (4) inhibition of the proteases that result in A-beta overproduction; (5) modulation of the lysosomal proteases to affect APP fragment production; (6) degradation of already formed and deposited A-beta; (7) protecting membrane stability, improvement of brain circulation, antioxidants that will assist in the prevention of denaturation of proteolytic systems (107). Clearly, this is an active avenue of research still in the preclinical stages of development.

H. Alteration in Tau Processing

In addition to senile plaques, neurofibrillary tangles are one of the histopathological hallmarks of AD. Abnormal phosphorylation of tau may be involved in tangle formation. Agents that modify the processing of tau may have beneficial effects on the microtubule stability. These agents may protect neurons from the destruction that may be related to tangle formation.

I. Adrenergic Agents

Idazoxan

The neurochemistry of AD is complex and cholinergic activity may be potentiated by other neurotransmitter systems. The alpha-2 antagonists may presynaptically affect cholinergic transmission. Idazoxan, an alpha-2 antagonist, acts presynaptically to increase synaptic concentration of norepinephrine. The compound is selective for noradrenaline and has a low affinity for dopamine and 5HT. The rationale for studying the effects of an alpha-2 antagonist follow from clonidine (alpha-2 agonist)-induced deficiencies in frontal lobe function tests.

One study with rats utilized the passive avoidance learning paradigm, inhibition of acetylcholinesterase enhanced learning. A subthreshold dose of acetylcholinesterase inhibitor with Idazoxan increased learning. The authors concluded that noradrenergic activation through presynaptic alpha-2 adrenoreceptor blockade may potentiate cholinergic activity in the formation of long-term memories (108). Another study in three patients with frontal lobe dementia reported improvement in frontal lobe function after treatment with Idazoxan. The compound did not improve deficits in spatial or working memory (109). Further research with these compounds is needed.

VII. CLINICAL USE OF THE CURRENTLY AVAILABLE COGNITIVE ENHANCERS

Based on tolerability of the currently available cognitive enhancers, we recommend that patients with probable AD be started on Donepezil rather than Tacrine. If they fail Donepezil, a trial of Tacrine may be reasonable. The patient should also be given the option of volunteering for a clinical trial of a cognitive enhancer that is not yet FDA approved. Patients with more severe Alzheimer's disease have decreased quantity and quality of cholinergic neurons. Therefore, patients with more advanced disease may have decreased response to cholinesterase inhibitors. However, patients with moderate disease should not be deprived of a trial with Donepezil or Tacrine. Based on the clinical trial data, the treatment failure with Donepezil may be considered if there is no improvement in function per the treating physician or caregiver by 24 weeks. If either the physician or caregiver notes improvement in function, the treatment should be continued. Patients with severe behavioral disturbances were not included in the clinical trials of Tacrine or Donepezil. These patients may be receiving a number of concurrent psychotropic medications to manage the behavioral change. Our current practice recommendations do not preclude patients with behavioral disturbances from receiving Donepezil or Tacrine. However, we recommend that any patients with dementia and behavioral disturbances have a thorough evaluation to search for general medical conditions (e.g., urinary tract infection, constipation, pain) or medications that may be contributing to the behavioral change. We have found some patients whose behavioral disturbances have worsened while on cholinesterase inhibitors, others whose behaviors appeared to improve, and still others who had no change. Further studies of cholinesterase inhibitors on behavioral disturbances in AD patients need to be performed. This will generate the data to better guide clinical practice with respect to drug interactions and predictors of behavioral change from the cholinesterase inhibitors.

VIII. CONCLUSIONS

The cause of AD is not yet fully understood. Clues from basic science have led to the development of cholinergic drugs, some of which are now available for patients to use. Continued preclinical and clinical research will advance our understanding of disease pathogenesis and ultimately change clinical practice. In the near future, research with antioxidants, agents that affect calcium, neurotrophic agents, membrane stabilizers, hormonal therapies, agents that modify beta-amyloid and tau processing, excitotoxins, and yet unidentified compounds will hopefully result in the increased availability of well-tolerated therapeutic agents that are effective not only in slowing down disease progression, but ultimately in reversing or preventing the devastating effects of Alzheimer's disease and other dementias.

REFERENCES

1. Devanand DP. Neuroleptics for behavioral complications of dementia. In: Nelson JC, ed. Geriatric Psychopharmacology. New York: Marcel Dekker, 1998:405–426.
2. Tariot PN, Schneider LS. Nonneuroleptic treatment of complications of dementia: applying clinical research to practice. In: Nelson JC, ed. Geriatric Psychopharmacology. New York: Marcel Dekker, 1998:427–454.

3. Evans DA, Funkenstein HH, Albert MS, et al. Prevalence of Alzheimer's disease in a community population of older persons. J Am Med Assoc 1989; 262:2551–2556.
4. Rocca WA, Hofman A, Brayne C, Breteler MM, Clarke M, Copeland JR, Dartigues JF, Engedal K, Hagnell O, Heeren TJ, et al. Frequency and distribution of Alzheimer's disease in Europe: a collaborative study of 1980-1990 prevalence findings. The EURODEM Prevalence Research Group. Ann Neurol 1991; 30:381–90.
5. Ritchie K, Kildea D. Is senile dementia "age-related" or "aging related"?—evidence from meta-analysis of dementia prevalence in the oldest old. Lancet 1995; 346:931–4.
6. Walsh JS, Welch HG, Larson EB. Survival of outpatients with Alzheimer-type dementia. Ann Intern Med 1990; 113:429–434.
7. Bierer LM, Haroutunian V, Gabriel S, et al. Neurochemical correlates of dementia severity in Alzheimer's disease: Relative importance of the cholinergic deficits. J Neurochem 1995; 64:749–760.
8. Marin DB, Davis KL. Experimental Therapeutics. In: Bloom FE, Kupfer DJ, eds. Psychopharmacology: The Fourth Generation of Progress. New York: Raven Press, 1995:1417–1426.
9. Flynn DD, Weinstein A, Mash DC. Loss of high-affinity agonist binding to M1 receptors in Alzheimer's disease: Implications for the failure of the cholinergic replacement therapies. Ann Neurol 1991; 29:256–262.
10. Sedman AJ, Bockbrader H, Schwarz RD. Preclinical and Phase 1 Clinical characterization of CI-979/RU35926, a novel muscarinic agonist for the treatment of Alzheimer's disease. Life Sci 1995; 56:877–882.
11. M'Harzi M, Palou AM, Oberlander C, Barzaghi F. Antagonism of scopolamine-induced memory impairments in rats by the muscarinic agonist RU 35,926 (CI-979). Pharmacol Biochem Behav 1995; 51:119–24.
12. Sramek JJ, Hurley DJ, Wardle TS, et al. The safety and tolerance of xanomeline tartrate in patients with Alzheimer's disease. J Clin Pharmacol 1995; 35:800–806.
13. Kasper SC, Bonate PL, DeLong AF. High-performance liquid chromatographic assay for xanomeline, a specific M-1 agonist, and its metabolite in human plasma. J Chromatogr B Biomed Appl 1995; 669:397–403.
14. Altsteil L. Cholinomimetic Therapy in Alzheimer's Disease: Experience with the Muscarinic Agonist Xanomeline. Second Annual Conference on the Therapeutics of Alzheimer's Disease, 1996, Garden City, New York.
15. Kumar R. Efficacy and Safety of SB 202026 as a Symptomatic Treatment for Alzheimer's Disease. Ann Neurol 1996; 40:504.
16. McCafferty J. SB2020226 Muscarinic Partial Agonist. Second Annual Conference on the Therapeutics of Alzheimer's Disease, 1996, Garden City, New York.
17. Nordberg A, Winblad B. Reduced number of [3H]nicotine and [3H]acetylcholine binding sites in the frontal cortex of Alzheimer brains. Neurosci Lett 1986; 72:115–119.
18. Nordberg A. Neuroreceptor changes in Alzheimer's disease. Cerebrovasc Brain Metab Rev 1992; 4:303–382.
19. Newhouse PA, Sunderland T, Tariot PN, et al. Intravenous nitocine in Alzheimer's disease: a pilot study. Psychopharmacology (Berl) 1988; 95:171–175.

20. Sunderland T, Tariot PN, Newhouse PA. Differential responsivity of mood, behavior and cognition to cholinergic agents in elderly neuropsychiatric populations. Brain Res 1988; 472:371–389.
21. Riekkinen P, Riekkinen M. Effects of tetrahydroaminoacridine and nicotine in nucleus basalis and serotonin-lesioned rats. Eur J Pharmacol 1995; 279:65–73.
22. Davis KL, Mohs RC, Tinkleberg JR, Pfefferbaum A, Hollister LE, Kopell BS. Physostigmine: improvement in long term memory processes in humans. Science 1978; 201:272–274.
23. Thal LJ, Fuld PA, Masur DM, Sharpless NS. Oral physostigmine and lecithin improve memory in Alzheimer disease. Ann Neurol 1983; 13:491–496.
24. Asthana S, Grieg NH, Hegedus L, Holloway HH, Raffaele KC, Schapiro MB, Soncrant TT. Clinical pharmacokinetics of physostigmine in patients with Alzheimer's disease. Clin Pharmacol Ther 1995; 58:299–309.
25. Davis KL, Hollister LE, Overall J, Johnson A, Train K. Physostigmine: effects on cognition and affect in normal subjects. Psychopharmacology 1976; 51:23–27.
26. Davis KL, Mohs RC. Enhancement of memory processing in Alzheimer's disease with multiple dose intravenous physostigmine. Am J Psychiatry 1982; 139:1421–1424.
27. Mohs RC, Davis BM, Johns CA, et al. Oral physostigmine treatment of patients with Alzheimer's disease. Am J Psychiatry 1985; 142:28–33.
28. Marin DB, Bierer LM, Lawlor BA, Ryan TM, Jacobson R, Schmeidler J, Mohs RC, Davis KL. L-Deprenyl and physostigmine for the treatment of Alzheimer's disease. Psychiatry Research 1995; 58:181–189.
29. Schwartz G. Results of extended release physostigmine in the treatment of Alzheimer's disease. ACNP, 1996 San Juan, Puerto Rico.
30. Pacheco G, Palacios Esquivel R, Moss DE. Cholinesterase inhibitors proposed for treating dementia in Alzheimer's disease: selectivity toward human brain acetylcholinesterase compared with butyrylcholinesterase. J Pharmacol Exp Ther 1995; 274(2):767–770.
31. Samuels SC, Davis KL. A risk benefit assessment of Tacrine for the treatment of Alzheimer's disease. Drug Safety 1996; 16(1):66–77.
32. Summers WK, Viesselman JO, Marsh GM, et al. Use of THA in treatment of Alzheimer-like dementia: pilot study in twelve patients. Biol Psychiatry 1981; 16: 145–153.
33. Summers WK, Majovski V, Marsh GM, et al. Oral tetrahydroacridine in long-term treatment of senile dementia, Alzheimer type. N Engl J Med 1986; 315:1241–1245.
34. Chatellier G, Lacomblez L. Tacrine (tetrahydroaminoacridine; THA) and lecithin in senile dementia of the Alzheimer type: a multicentre trial. Br Med J 1990; 300: 495–99.
35. Gauthier S, Bouchard R, Lamontagne A, et al. Tetrahydroaminoacridine-Lecithin combination treatment in patients with intermediate-stage Alzheimer's disease. N Engl J Med 1990; 322:1272–1276.
36. Wilcock GK, Surmon DJ, Scott M, et al. An evaluation of the efficacy and safety of tetrahydroacridine (THA) without Lecithin in the treatment of Alzheimer's disease. Age Aging 1993; 22:316–324.
37. Eagger SA, Levy R, Sahakian BJ. Tacrine in Alzheimer's disease. Lancet 1991; 337:989–992.

38. Eagger SA, Morant NJ, Levy R. Parallel group analysis of the effects of Tacrine versus placebo in Alzheimer's disease. Dementia 1991; 2:207–211.
39. Farlow M, Gracon SI, Hershey LA, et al. A controlled trial of Tacrine in Alzheimer's disease. J Am Med Assoc 1992; 268:2523–2529.
40. Maltby N, Broe GA, Ceasey H, et al. Efficacy of Tacrine and Lecithin in mild to moderate Alzheimer's disease: a double blind trial. Br Med J 1994; 308:879–883.
41. Davis KL, Thal LJ, Gamzu ER, et al. A double-blind, placebo controlled multicenter study of Tacrine for Alzheimer's disease. N Engl J Med 1992; 327:1253–1259.
42. Knapp MJ, Knopman DS, Soloman PR, et al. A 30-week randomized controlled tiral of high dose Tacrine in patients with Alzheimer's disease. J Am Med Assoc 1994; 271:985–991.
43. Watkins PB, Zimmerman HJ, Knapp MJ, et al. Hepatotoxic effects of tacrine administration in patients with Alzheimer's disease. J Am Med Assoc 1994; 271:992–998.
44. Tacrine Prescribing Information from US package insert. Warner-Lambert Company, Parke-Davis Division, 1995.
45. Riekkinen P, Kuikka J, Soininen H, Helkela E-L, Hallikainen M, Riekkinen P. Tetra hydroxyamoniacridine modulates technitium-99m labeled ethylene dicysteinate retention in Alzheimer's disease measured with single photon emossion computed tomography imaging. Neurosci Lett 1995; 195:53–56.
46. Minthon L, Nilsson K, Edvinsson L, Wendt PE, Gustafson L. Long-term effects of Tacrine on regional cerebral blood flow changes in Alzheimer's disease. Dementia 1995; 6:245–251.
47. Lubeck DP, Mazonson PD, Bowe T. Potential Effects of Tacrine on Expenditures for Alzheimer's Disease. Med Interface 1994; xx:130–138.
48. Knopman D, Schneider L, Davis K, et al. Long-term tacrine (Cognex) treatment: effects on nursing home placement and mortality. Neurology 1996; 47:166–177.
49. Nochi S, Asakawa N, Sato T. Kinetic study on the inhibition of acetylcholinesterase by 1-benzyl-4-[(5,6-dimethoxy-1-indanon)-2-yl]methylpiperidine hydrochloride (E2020). Biol Pharm Bull 1995; 18(8):1145–1147.
50. Sugimoto H, Iimura Y, Yamanishi Y, Yamutsu K. Synthesis and structure relationships of acetylcholinesterase inhibitors: 1-benzyl-4-[(5,6-dimethoxy-1-oxoindan-2-yl)methyl]piperidine hydrochloride and related compounds. J Med Chem 1995; 38:4821–4829.
51. Dawson GR, Iversen SD. The effects of novel cholinesterase inhibitors and selective muscarinic receptor agonists in tests of reference and working memory. Behav Brain Res 1993; 57:143–153.
52. Rogers SL, Friedfoff LT. The efficacy and safety of donepezil in patients with Alzheimer's disease: Reuslts of a US multicentre, randomized, double-blind, placebo controlled trial. Dementia 1996; x:293–303.
53. Friedhoff LT, Farlow MR, Mohs RC, Rogers SL. Donepezil (E2020) demonstrates significant improvement in cognitive and global function in patients in mild-to-moderately severe Alzheimer's disease. ACNP, 1996, San Juan, Puerto Rico.
54. Niigawa H, Tanimukai S, Hariguchi S, Nishimura T. Effects of SDZ ENA 713, a novel acetyl cholinesterase inhibitor, on learning of rats with basal forebrain lesions. Prog Neuropsychopharmacol Biol Psychiatry 1995; 19:171–186.

55. Anand R, Garabawi G, Enz A. Efficacy and safety results of the early phase studies with Exelon (TM) (ENA-713) in Alzheimer's disease: An overview. Journal Drug Devel Clin Prac 1996; 8:109–116.
56. Anand R, Gharabawi G. Clinical development of Exelon (TM) (ENA-713): The ADENA (R) programme. J Drug Devel Clin Pract 1996; 8:117–122.
57. Thomsen T, Bickel U, Fischer JP, et al. Galanthamine hydrobromide is a long-term treatment of Alzheimer's disease: selectivity toward human brain acetylcholinesterase compared with butyrylcholinesterase. J Pharmacol Exp Ther 1995; 274(2): 767–770.
58. Dal-Bianco P, Maly J, Wober C, et al. Galanthamine treatment in Alzheimer's disease. J Neural Transm 1991; xx(suppl):59–63.
59. Wilcox G, Wilkinson D. Galanthamine Hydrobromide-Interim results of a group of Galanthamine-Hydrobromide-Interim result of a group. Fifth International Conference on Alzheimer's Disease and Related Disorders, 1996, Osaka, Japan.
60. Canal N, Imbimbo BP, Bassi S, et al. Relationship between pharmacodynamic activity and cognitive effects of eptastigmine in patients with Alzheimer's disease. Clin Pharmacol Ther 1996; 60:218–228.
61. Troetel WM, Imbimbo BP. Overview of the Development of Eptastigmine, a long acting cholinesterase inhibitor. Fifth International Conference on Alzheimer's Disease and Related Disorders, 1996, Osaka, Japan.
62. Cioli D, Pica-Mattoccia L, Archer S. Antischistosomal drugs: past, present ... and future? Pharmacol Ther 1995; 68:35–85.
63. van der Staay FJ, Hinz VC, Schmidt BH. Effects of Metrifonate, its transformation product, dichlorvos, and other organophosphorus and reference cholinesterase inhibitors on Morris water escape behavior in young-adult rats. J Pharmacol Exp Ther 1996; 278:697–708.
64. Unni LK, Womack C, Hannant ME, Becker RE. Pharmacokinetics and pharmacodynamics of metrifonate in humans. Meth Fund Exp Clin Pharmacol 1994; 16:285–289.
65. Mori F, Lai CC, Fusi F, Giacobini E. Cholinesterase inhibitors increase secretion of APPs in rat brain cortex. Neuroreport 1995; 6:633–636.
66. Lahiri DK. Reversibility of the effect of tacrine on the secretion of the beta-amyloid precursor protein in cultured cells. Neurosci Lett 1994; 181(1-2):149–152.
67. Wallace W, Haroutunian V. Using the subcortically lesioned rat cortex to understand the physiological role of amyloid precursor protein. Behav Brain Res 1993; 57:199–206.
68. Honhjo H, Tamura T, Matsumoto Y, Kawata M, Ogino Y, Tanaka K, Yamamoto T, Ueda S, Okada H. Estrogen as a growth factor to central nervous cells. Extrogen treatment promotes development of acetylcholine-positive basal forebrain neurons transplanted in the anterior eye chamber. J Steroid Biochem Mol Biol 1992; 41:633–635.
69. Jaffe AB, Toran Allerand CD, Greengard P, Gandy SE. Estrogen regulates metabolism of Alzheimer amyloid beta precursor protein. J Biol Chem 1994; 269: 13065–13068.
70. Tang MX, Jacobs D, Stern Y, Marder K, Schofied P, Gurland B, Andrews H, Mayeux R. Effect of oestrogen during menopause on risk and age at onset of Alzheimer's disease. Lancet 1996; 348:429–432.

71. Ohkura T, Isse K, Akazawa K, Hamamoto M, Yaoi Y, Hagino N. Evaluation of estrogen treatment in female patients with dementia of the Alzheimer type. Endocr J 1994; 41:361–371.
72. Paganini-Hill A, Henderson VW. Estrogen deficiency and the risk of Alzheimer's disease in women. Am J Epidemiol 1994; 140:256–261.
73. Asthana S, Craft S, Baker LD, Raskind MA, Avery E, Lofgreen C, Wilkinson CW, Falgraf S, Veith RC, Plymate SR. Transdermal estrogen improves memory in women with Alzheimer's disease [Abstract]. Society for Neuroscience Abstracts, Vol 22, Pt 1:200. 26th Annual Meeting, 1996, Washington, DC.
74. Schneider LS, Farlow MR, Henderson VW, Pogoda JM. Effects of estrogen replacement therapy on response to tacrine in patients with Alzheimer's disease. Neurology 1996; 46:1580–1584.
75. Itil T, Martorano D. Natural substances in psychiatry (Gingko Biloba in Dementia). Psychopharm Bull 1995; 31:147–158.
76. Kanowski S, Herrmann WM, Stephen K, et al. Proof of efficacy of the gingko biloba special extract Egb 761 in outpatients suffering from mild to moderate primary degenerative dementia of the Alzheimer type or multi-infarct dementia. Pharmacopsychaitry 1996; 29:47–56.
77. Aisen PS, Davis KL. Inflammatory mechanisms in Alzheimer's disease: implications for therapy. Am J Psychiatry 1994; 151:1105–1113.
78. Campbell IL, Abraham CR, Masliah E, et al. Neurologic disease induced in transgenic mice by cerebral overexpression of interleukin 6. Proc Natl Acad Sci USA 1993; 90:10061–10065.
79. Buxbaum JD, Oishi M, Chen HI, et al. Cholinergic agonists and interleukin 1 regulate processing and secretion of the Alzheimer beta-A4 amyloid protein precursor. Proc Natl Acad Sci USA 1992; 89:10075–8.
80. Webster S, O'Barr S, Rogers J. Enhanced aggregation and beta structure of amyloid beta peptide after coincubation with Clq. J Neurosci Res 1994; 39:448–456.
81. Fagarasan MO, Aisen PS. Il-1 and anti-inflammatory drugs modulate A-beta cytotoxicity in PC12 cells. Brain Res 1996; 723:231–234.
82. Guilian D, Li J, Li X, et al. The impact of microglia-derived cytokines upon gliosis in the CNS. Dev Neurosci 1994; 16:128–136.
83. Ito I, Tanabe S, Kohda A, Sugiyama H. Allosteric potentiation of quisqualate receptors by a nootropic drug aniracetam. J Physiol 1990; 424:533–543.
84. Dysken MW, Mendels J, LeWitt P, et al. Milacemide: A placebo-controlled study in senile dementia of the Alzheimer's type. J Am Geriatr Soc 1992; 40:503–506.
85. Camp-Bruno JA, herting RL. Cognitive effects of milacemide and methylphenidate in healthy young adults. Psychopharmacology (Berl) 1994; 115:46–52.
86. Lee Cr, Benfield P. Aniracetam, an overview of its pharmacodynamic and pharmacokinetic properties, and a review of its therapeutic potential in senile cognitive disorders. Drugs Aging 1994; 4(3):257–273.
87. Senin U, Abeate G, Fieschi C, Gori G, Guala A, et al. Aniracetam (Ro13-5057) in the treatment of senile dementia of the Alzheimer type (SDAT): results of a placebo controlled multicentre clinical trial. Eur Neuropsychopharmacol 1991; 1:511–517.

88. Sorander LB, Portin R, Molsa P, Lahdes A, Rinne UK. Senile dementia of the Alzheimer's type treated with aniracetam: a new nootropic agent. Psychopharmacology 1987; 91:90–95.
89. Parnetti L, Bartorelli L, Bainiouto S, Cucinotta D, Cuzzopoli M, et al. Aniracetam (Ro 13-5057) for the treatment of senile dementia of the Alzheimer's type: results of a multicentre clinical study. Dementia 1991; 2:262–267.
90. Armstrong DM, Ikonomovic MD, Sheffield R, Wenthold RJ. Glutamate receptor subtype immunoreactivity in the entorhinal cortex of non-demented elderly and patients with Alzheimer's disease. Brain Res 1994; 639:207–216.
91. Searching for Drugs that Combat Alzheimer's [News]. Science 1996; 273:50–53.
92. Dreyfus CF. Effects of nerve growth factor on cholinergic brain neurons. Trends Pharmacol Sci 1989; 10:145–149.
93. Koliatsos VE, Clatterbuck RE, Nauta JHW, et al. Human nerve growth factor prevents degeneration of basal forebrain cholinergic neurons in primates. Ann Neurol 1991; 30:831–840.
94. Hefti F, hartikka J, Knusel B. Function of neurotrophic factors in the adult and aging brain and their possible use in the treatment of neurodegenerative diseases. Neurobiol Aging 1989; 10:515–533.
95. Olson L, Nordberg A, von Holst H, et al. Nerve growth factor affects C-nicotine binding, bloow flow, EEG, and verbal episodic memory in an Alzheimer's disease patient. J Neural Transm 1992; 4:79–95.
96. Phelps CH, Gage FH, Growden JH, et al. Potential use of nerve growth factor to treat Alzheimer's disease. Neurobiol Aging 1989; 10:205–207.
97. Parnetti L. Clinical pharmacokinetics of drugs for Alzheimer's disease. Clin Pharmacokinet 1995; 29:110–129.
98. Knuesel B, Kaplan DR, Winslow JW, et al. K-252b selectively potentiates cellular actions and trk tyrosine phosphorylation mediated by neurotrophin-3. J Neurochem 1992; 59:715–722.
99. Furukawa S, Furukawa Y. Nerve growth factor synthesis and its regulatory mechanisms: an approach to therapeutic induction of nerve growth factor synthesis. Cerebrovasc Brain Metab Rev 1990; 1:328–344.
100. Senin U, Parnetti L, Barbagallo-Sangiorgi G, Bartorelli L, Bocola V, Capurso A, Cuzzupoli M, Denario M, Marigliano V, Tammaro AE, Fioravanti M. Idebenone in senile dementia of the Alzheimer's type: a multicentre study. Arch Gerontol Geriatr 1992; 15:249–260.
101. Bergamasco B, Scarzella L, La Commare P. Idebenone, a new drug for the treatment of cognitive impairments in patients with dementia of the Alzheimer's type. Funct Neurol 1994; 9:161–168.
102. Weyer G, Erzigkeit H, Hadler D, Kubicki S. Efficacy and safety of Idebenone in the long-term treatment of Alzheimer's disease: a double-blind, placebo controlled multicentre study. Hum Psychopharmacol 1996; 11:53–65.
103. Deyo RA, Staube KT, Disterhoft JF. Nimodipine facilitates associative learning in aging rabbits. Science 1989; 243:809–811.
104. Tollefson GD. Short term effects of the calcium channel blocker nimodipine (Bay-e-9736) in the management of primary degenerative dementia. Biol Psychiatry 1990; 27:1133–1142.

105. Ban TA, Morey L, Aguglia E, et al. Nimodipine in the treatment of old age dementias. Prog Neuro Psychopharmacol Biol Psychiatry 1990; 14:525–551.
106. Parnetti L, Senin U, Carosi M, et al. Mental deterioration in old age: results of two multicenter, clinical trials with nimodipine. Clin Ther 1993; 15:394–406.
107. Li K. The role of B-amyloid in the development of Alzheimer's disease. Drugs Aging 1995; 7(2):97–109.
108. Camacho F, Smith CP, Vargas HM, Winslow JT. -2-Adrenoreceptor antagonists potentiate acetylcholinesterase inhibitor effects on passive avoidance learning in the rat. Psychopharmacology 1996; 124:347–354.
109. Coull JT, Middleton HC, Robbins TW, Sahakian BJ. Clonidine and diazepam have differential effects on tests of attention and learning. Psychopharmacology (Berl) 1995; 120:311–321.

22

Neuroleptics for Behavioral Complications of Dementia

D. P. Devanand
New York State Psychiatric Institute, and Columbia University, New York, New York

Patients with dementia often develop behavioral disturbances (e.g., agitation and aggression) or psychotic features (e.g., delusions and hallucinations) (1). The term "behavioral complications" will be used here to include both behavioral disturbances and psychotic features. Behavioral complications occur in most forms of dementia. The most common type of dementia in the elderly is Alzheimer's disease (AD), where brain autopsy characteristically demonstrates amyloid plaques and neurofibrillary tangles (2). This chapter will focus on behavioral complications and their treatment with neuroleptics in AD, with reference to other causes of dementia (e.g., multi-infarct dementia or frontal lobe dementia), as appropriate.

The evaluation of behavioral complications in dementia is intrinsically limited by several factors. First, memory loss and other intellectual impairments make it difficult for many demented patients to accurately report symptoms. Therefore, in addition to direct evaluation of the patient's mental status, informants need to be interviewed to gather relevant information. These informants are commonly family members for outpatients and ward staff for inpatients and nursing home patients. This strategy is unavoidable for practical reasons, but the inability of patients to directly report on the symptoms that they experience (e.g., hallucinations may not be reported by the patient who manifests hallucinatory behavior) introduces a potential confound that must be taken into account. Also, it is difficult to separate formal thought disorder from aphasia, since some degree of aphasia invariably develops with disease progression. Many types of delusions (e.g., "someone is stealing my things") can be considered a type of confabulation to fill in the gaps resulting from memory impairment (3). Therefore, the use of precise operational definitions is important in the evaluation of delusions and hallucinations in AD (4).

First, the extant literature on behavioral complications in dementia will be reviewed. Of note, most studies have been based on samples in outpatient clinics where patients often present because behavioral complications have occurred. Therefore, the reported prevalence of specific behavioral symptoms is likely to be higher than in patients residing in the community. Second, the current state of knowledge on the use of neuroleptics to treat these behavioral complications will be reviewed.

I. BEHAVIORAL COMPLICATIONS OF DEMENTIA

A. Behavioral Disturbance

Behavioral disturbances are usually outward manifestations that are observable by others, and the patient may not complain or even recognize the changes (5). In AD, behavioral complications are both common and heterogeneous in their presentation (3,6,7). Personality changes may be the earliest manifestation of dementia. These personality changes are initially subtle, and include apathy, anhedonia, irritability, inability to pay attention, and loss of emotional connection with significant others (8). In later stages, varying degrees of agitation may occur in up to half of AD patients in outpatient clinics (9,10) and nursing homes (11), with aggressive behavior being less common (10,12). Within the broad framework of disinhibited behaviors, demented patients can manifest a wide range of symptoms. These include pacing, wandering, verbal and physical aggression, repetitive calling out and screaming, and rarely self-mutilating behaviors. Catastrophic reactions, including bursts of anger and even violent behavior, can occur when patients are required to perform tasks beyond their cognitive capacities (9). Stubbornness, or refusal to complete essential activities of daily life, can be particularly frustrating for caregivers.

Most studies of behavioral disturbance have been cross-sectional (9, 12–15) and only recently have data from longitudinal studies become available (7,10,16). These follow-up studies suggest that behavioral disturbance of both the apathetic and disinhibited type increase with severity of dementia. Recently, we completed a study of the course of psychopathology in patients with mild-to-moderate AD (10). Two-hundred-thirty-five patients with early, probable AD were recruited at three sites and followed at 6-month intervals for up to 5 years. Trained research technicians administered the Columbia University Scale for Psychopathology in Alzheimer's Disease (CUSPAD) to informants. Using dichotomous ratings (present or absent) for each symptom category,

Markov analyses were used to predict the probability of developing or maintaining the specific symptom at the next visit. The transition probability for the development of a new symptom was 0.31 for agitation (i.e., 31% of patients without agitation at one visit manifested agitation at the next visit; 6-month interval). The transition probability for the persistence of agitation was 0.74, indicating that 74% of patients with agitation at one visit again manifested agitation at the next visit (6-month interval). Wandering or agitation occurred at ≥ three of four consecutive visits (2 years) in the majority of patients. Overall, behavioral disturbance was the most frequent and highly persistent category, with wandering/agitation mainly accounting for this effect. The high prevalence and persistence of behavioral symptoms, particularly agitation, highlights the importance of treatment for these symptoms.

B. Psychosis

The prevalence of delusions has been reported to range from 0% to 50% in AD in different studies (6,17,18). Isolated symptoms may be two to three times as common as diagnosable psychotic disorders (19). Paranoid delusions of theft and suspicion are among the most common types of delusions (6,19). However, these symptoms often do not meet strict definitional criteria for delusions, and patients may intermittently acknowledge that their suspicions are not realistic. These fluctuating features make delusional symptoms hard to classify according to traditional psychiatric nomenclature (4). Misidentifications are also common, particularly in intermediate to late stages of illness. Symptoms are typically misidentifying people (including Capgras syndrome), misidentification of the patient's own mirror image or characters on television, and the conviction that the house is not one's home. The latter can be particularly problematic for family members, because patients sometimes insist that they immediately leave the house for their "real" home. It remains unclear as to how misidentifications should be classified (i.e., are they delusions, perceptual disorders, or a direct manifestation of cognitive impairment?). Perhaps misidentifications in dementia merit their own independent category. In contrast to paranoid ideation and misidentification, systematized complex delusions and grandiose delusions are relatively rare in AD and other dementias (5,6). This finding indirectly supports the view that relatively intact cognition is necessary for the formation of systematized complex delusions.

Hallucinations are more commonly visual than auditory. In mild-to-moderate AD, they occur in only 5–10% of patients (6,10) with a slightly higher frequency in severely demented samples (19). In AD, one common type of hallucination is the idea that someone else is in the house (i.e., phantom boarder syndrome) (5). Illusions also occur in demented patients, and these often have a component of misidentification (e.g., a coat on its hanger is mistaken for an individual dressed in a coat).

In our recent study of 235 AD patients with mild-to-moderate AD who were followed prospectively for up to 5 years, approximately half the patients with paranoid delusions or hallucinations were likely to manifest the same symptom 6 months later (10). The moderately high rate of persistence emphasizes the importance of developing appropriate treatment strategies for these psychotic features. However, paranoid delusions or hallucinations occurred at ≥ three of four consecutive visits (2 years) in only 10–15% of patients. The fact that these psychotic symptoms may not persist for prolonged periods raises the question of how long patients need to be continued on psychotropic medications after treatment response.

We previously reported that symptoms of both psychosis and behavioral disturbance were present in eight of nine patients who participated in a pilot study of haloperidol treatment of behavioral complications in AD (20). Similarly, 48 of 66 AD outpatients participating in an ongoing haloperidol dose-comparison study have met criteria for psychosis, and all 66 patients have met criteria for behavioral disturbance. The "pure" psychotic AD patient without associated behavioral disturbance appears to be rare in clinical practice (21).

From a theoretical perspective, behavioral changes may be a direct expression of underlying brain pathology, and should not be assumed to be solely secondary to cognitive deficits (22). However, brain-behavior correlations for psychopathology in AD have not been established. There is limited evidence that patients with multi-infarct dementia are more likely to exhibit mood lability and affective syndromes than patients with AD (13,23,24), and that patients with frontal lobe dementia are more likely to exhibit disinhibited behaviors (25). Patients with subcortical dementia (multisystem atrophy, progressive supranuclear palsy, progressive subcortical gliosis) may be more likely to manifest lack of energy and psychomotor retardation (25). In dementing disorders due to relatively uncommon causes, data about the nature and course of psychopathology are lacking.

In summary, the extant studies indicate that behavioral complications are frequent in AD (1,5,10), are heterogeneous in their presentation (19), and may be associated with a worse prognosis (26–28). Untreated behavioral symptoms are distressing to patients and caregivers (29,30), and may lead to institutionalization (31,32). Concomitant medical illness can induce or exacerbate these symptoms, and adequate medical management is important. In other cases, nonpharmacological interventions may be effective: change in room, reduction in noise level, brief periodic nursing contacts, behavior modification, or family education (33). Nonetheless, a large proportion of demented patients with behavioral complications require psychopharmacological intervention.

II. NEUROLEPTICS FOR BEHAVIORAL COMPLICATIONS

A. Prevalence of Neuroleptic Use

Early studies indicated that nearly half the inpatients with dementia in VA hospitals (34) and other settings (35) received psychotropic medications, primarily neuroleptics and benzodiazepines (36–39). Despite subsequent federally mandated restrictions on the use of such medications in long-term care facilities, these agents are still widely used (40–42). This indirectly suggests that clinicians still find neuroleptics to be valuable therapeutic agents.

B. Efficacy of Neuroleptics

Neuroleptics have been studied more widely than any other class of medications to treat the behavioral complications of dementia (43,44). Most studies have involved patient samples with dementia or organic brain syndrome from a variety of causes. With the exception of AD, neuroleptic trials in specific diagnostic subtypes of dementia (e.g., frontal lobe dementia) have not been conducted. Trials of neuroleptics in dementia, both uncontrolled and controlled, generally have been of relatively short duration (3 to 8 weeks on average).

Uncontrolled Studies

Several early uncontrolled trials evaluated the efficacy and side effects of neuroleptics in geriatric inpatients or in nursing homes. Patients were diagnostically heterogeneous in most of these studies, and some samples even included patients with schizophrenia or major affective disorder (45–52). Studies of predominantly demented patient samples also tended to be diagnostically heterogenous (51,53,54), but recent studies have restricted the inclusion criteria to AD only (55–57). Overall, these uncontrolled reports suggest that anywhere from 25–75% of a broad spectrum of demented patients with behavioral complications respond to neuroleptics.

Controlled Studies

Most controlled studies of neuroleptics in dementia have suffered from major methodological limitations, and these have been discussed in a number of reviews (3,43,58,59). In these studies, diagnostic heterogeneity was a common feature, methods of assessment were often global and inadequate, the effects of neuroleptics on core psychotic features versus other forms of behavioral disturbances were not assessed, and samples comprised mainly severely demented inpatients. Only a few of the published studies utilized a randomized, double-blind, placebo-controlled design (Table 1) (60–67).

TABLE 1 Randomized Double-Blind Placebo-Controlled Studies of Neuroleptics in Samples of Mainly Demented Patients

Report	Year	*n*	Diagnosis	Length (weeks)	Meds mg/day	Outcome measures	Results
Abse et al.	1960	32	OBS + senile psychosis	8	Chlorpromazine 75	Global Target symptoms	Improvement on both drug and placebo
Hamilton and Bennett	1962	27	OBS with psychosis 78%	8	Trifluperazine 4-8	Behavior and Nursing scales	Worse on medication compared to placebo
Hamilton and Bennett	1962	19	OBS with psychosis	3-8	Acetophenazine 40	Behavior and Nursing scales	Worse on medication compared to placebo
Sugarman et al.	1964	18	OBS	6	Haloperidol 0.5-4.5 Benzotropine p.r.n.	Psychotic reaction profile scale	Agitation, hostility improved
Rada and Kellner	1976	42	Nonpsychotic OBS 57% Psychotic OBS 43%	4	Thiothixene 6-15	BPRS NOSIE	Lack of efficacy but safe
Barnes et al.	1982	53	PDD 55% MID 38% Other 7%	8	Thioridazine 62.5 Loxapine 10.5	BPRS SCAG CGI NOSIE	All groups improved on BPRS
Petrie et al.	1982	61	PDD 49% MID 43% Other 8%	8	Haloperidol 4.6 Loxapine 21.9	BPRS SCAG CGI	Response rates: 35% Hal 32% Lox 9% Plac
Finkel et al.	1995	33	PDD	11	Thiothixene 0.25-18	CMAI	Thiothixene superior to placebo

OBS = organic brain syndrome; MID = multi-infarct dementia; PDD = primary degenerative dementia; BPRS = Brief Psychiatric Rating Scale; SCAG = Sandoz Clinical Assessment-Geriatric; CMAI = Cohen-Mansfield Agitation Inventory; CGI = Clinical Global Improvement; NOSIE = Nurses Observation Scale for Inpatient Evaluation.

Early studies comparing chlorpromazine to placebo in samples restricted to organic mental disorders failed to demonstrate significantly superior efficacy for chlorpromazine (36,61). Other controlled studies found evidence of moderate efficacy for neuroleptics in the treatment of behavioral complications (60,64). During the last two decades, results from only four random assignment, double blind, placebo-controlled trials of neuroleptics in dementia have been published (Table 1). All four studies were conducted in inpatients or in nursing homes. In a 4-week trial, thiothixene ($\leq$ 15 mg/day) demonstrated marginal superiority over placebo in the treatment of 42 patients with organic brain syndrome (18 psychotic and 24 nonpsychotic patients) (65). Lack of information about diagnosis, nonstratified assignment of psychotic patients to the treatment groups, short trial duration, and a high placebo response rate (55%) were problematic. In another study of 61 patients with dementia (30 AD and 26 multi-infarct), global clinical improvement was significantly greater with haloperidol (35% improvement, mean daily dose 4.6 mg) or loxapine (32%, mean daily dose 21.9 mg) compared to placebo (9%). Besides the large proportion of patients with multi-infarct dementia (42.6%), the use of antiparkinsonian agents and chloral hydrate were major limitations (60). In another study of 53 patients, loxapine and thioridazine showed a small advantage over placebo but led to more side effects (66). Diagnostic heterogeneity (55% AD, 38% multi-infarct dementia), the use of concomitant sedative (chloral hydrate) and anticholinergic (trihexiphenidyl) medications, and the high placebo response rate limited these findings. In a recent study of 33 demented patients in a nursing home, thiothixene (variable dose, 0.25–18 mg daily) was superior to placebo in the treatment of agitation (67).

Schneider et al. (43) conducted a meta-analysis of the available literature on placebo-controlled trials of neuroleptic treatment of behavioral complications in patients with any form of organic brain syndrome. Clinical worsening, dropout and side effects were not accounted for in this meta-analysis. The problems of diagnostic heterogeneity in sample selection and permitted use of other psychotropics were among the methodological limitations that characterized these studies, compromising the utility of the meta-analytic approach. In this meta-analysis, neuroleptics were found to be moderately more efficacious than placebo (one-tailed $p = .004$), with effect size reduced by the high placebo response rate in some studies (65,66). These high placebo response rates raise the concern that the inclusion of patients with very mild symptoms (to enhance sample size) increased type II error (i.e., finding no difference when in fact a "true" difference existed). Of note, these were inpatient studies, and it is unclear if similar findings will be obtained in outpatients where few controlled data have been published.

From these limited data, one can conclude that neuroleptics are efficacious in the treatment of behavioral complications in some demented patients.

In Alzheimer's disease, classical psychotic symptoms such as delusions and hallucinations are less common than behavioral problems such as agitation and catastrophic reactions (10,68). Thus, the presentation of these nonpsychotic behavioral symptoms, particularly agitation, more commonly leads to treatment with neuroleptics. The notion that agitation and other behavioral symptoms may be less responsive to neuroleptics than classical psychotic features remains to be confirmed by empirical research (43,69). Raskind and Risse (69) suggested that neuroleptics may be effective in the treatment of bizarre and disturbing behaviors in AD that cannot be understood in terms of impaired memory or aphasia. However, making this distinction can be difficult, particularly in severely demented patients with poor communication abilities (3). Conversely, it remains unclear if some delusions that are clearly secondary to cognitive impairment (e.g., the belief that deceased parents are alive) are less likely to respond to neuroleptics.

Comparisons Between Neuroleptics

There is little evidence to indicate superior efficacy for a specific neuroleptic, or class of neuroleptics, in the treatment of behavioral complications in dementia (44,58). The few studies that compared a low potency neuroleptic (thioridazine) to a high potency neuroleptic (haloperidol) did not demonstrate any consistent differences in efficacy (70–73). These studies were limited by the lack of a placebo control, and the fact that the patient samples were diagnostically heterogeneous. Similarly, comparisons between loxapine and haloperidol (60,74) and between loxapine and thioridazine (66) failed to demonstrate a significant advantage for any one medication.

A more relevant question is whether the use of a specific neuroleptic would result in a particularly advantageous side-effect profile in demented patients. At comparable doses, low-potency neuroleptics like thioridazine and thorazine are less likely to cause extrapyramidal signs (EPS) than high-potency neuroleptics like haloperidol. However, these low-potency neuroleptics are more likely to cause orthostatic hypotension, which increases the risk of falls and fractures (38). In addition, low-potency neuroleptics have a greater propensity for anticholinergic side effects that may worsen the cognitive deficit in demented patients. Unfortunately, little work has been done on the effects of neuroleptics on cognition and activities of daily life in AD (20), and it remains unclear if the anticholinergic effects of low-potency neuroleptics like thioridazine have more deleterious effects on cognitive function than high-potency neuroleptics like haloperidol. Nonetheless, the choice of neuroleptic should be based on side-effect profiles rather than expectations of differential efficacy (e.g., thioridazine should be preferred to haloperidol in a patient with preexisting EPS, and haloperidol should be preferred to thioridazine in a patient with preexisting orthostatic hypotension).

Clozapine and Risperidone

Traditional neuroleptics can induce short-term (sedation, EPS) and long-term (tardive dyskinesia; TD) side effects. The newer neuroleptics have a lower propensity to cause EPS. Clozapine may be more efficacious than other neuroleptics in schizophrenia, and the risk of developing TD is very low (75). However, the use of clozapine can lead to orthostatic hypotension, which increases the risk of falls and fractures (76). Critically, there is a need for intensive monitoring for blood dyscrasias (75). These safety issues are of major importance for elderly AD patients with behavioral complications, particularly for outpatients where close monitoring is not possible and caregivers often find it difficult to bring the patient for frequent visits. Probably for these reasons, there have been no published controlled trials using clozapine to treat behavioral complications in AD patients.

Risperidone also has a decreased propensity for EPS. In a multicenter study of young adults with schizophrenia that compared 2, 6, 12, and 16 mg daily of risperidone to 20 mg daily of haloperidol, 6 mg risperidone daily led to the best therapeutic profile (77). However, the optimal risperidone dose range is likely to be far lower in elderly AD patients (78). Comparing doses between traditional neuroleptics and risperidone is complicated by the differential effects of risperidone and haloperidol in varied animal models (79,80), and by risperidone being both a D_2 antagonist and 5HT-2 antagonist unlike the predominantly D_2 antagonist haloperidol (81). Open trials in demented patients have used risperidone in doses from 0.25 to 5 mg daily, with some evidence of positive results (82,83). A few patients had to discontinue the medication because of orthostatic hypotension, raising concerns that even low-dose risperidone may lead to falls with the risk of fractures in the demented elderly (82). Ongoing industry-sponsored trials are likely to provide important information on the risk–benefit ratio of using risperidone in demented patients with behavioral complications.

Dose-Finding Studies

Although neuroleptics were introduced and began to be widely used in the 1950s, it took many decades before it became clearly established that relatively low doses are adequate for both acute and maintenance treatment in most patients with schizophrenia (84,85). Given this historical lesson, it is clearly important to avoid the problem of using excessive neuroleptic doses in elderly demented patients who are particularly prone to side effects (e.g., EPS). On the other hand, using too low a dose may result in lack of efficacy. Studies comparing different doses of the same neuroleptic are necessary to clarify the issue of optimal dosage, including the possibility that there is a "therapeutic window" that results in an optimal trade-off between efficacy and side effects.

However, there are no published controlled studies comparing different doses of the same neuroleptic medication.

In a pilot study that employed a single-blind ABA (A=4 weeks placebo, B=8 weeks haloperidol) design, we found that haloperidol in doses of 1 to 5 mg daily was efficacious in the treatment of nine AD outpatients with behavioral complications. However, some patients could not tolerate the higher doses (> 4 mg daily), primarily due to EPS. Haloperidol treatment was associated with a small, but significant, decline in cognitive function, assessed by the modified Mini Mental State Exam (MMSE) (20). These findings suggested that even lower doses may be necessary (i.e., very low, homeopathic, doses might retain the efficacy seen at higher doses, while avoiding side effects). To address this issue, we are in the process of completing a random assignment, parallel group, double-blind, placebo-controlled study in which standard-dose haloperidol (2–3 mg daily), low-dose haloperidol (0.5–0.75 mg daily), and placebo are compared in a 6-week trial with a subsequent crossover phase. A total of 66 patients (56 completers) have participated in this trial. The results will not be published until this double-blind study is completed. The results from this sample of AD outpatients with behavioral complications should help provide information on the optimal dose range in the treatment of these patients.

Neuroleptics vs. Other Medications

The few studies that compared neuroleptics to benzodiazepines suffered from methodological flaws, particularly with respect to sample selection and study design (50,86–88). One report claimed superiority for oxazepam over several neuroleptics in a diagnostically heterogeneous sample of geriatric patients (50). However, other studies demonstrated superiority for thioridazine over benzodiazepines in the treatment of anxiety and agitation in nursing homes and similar facilities (86–88). In 21 demented inpatients with behavioral complications on a psychogeriatric unit, both haloperidol (0.5–3 mg daily) and oxazepam (10–30 mg daily) led to moderate improvement in target behaviors (89). These limited data do not indicate superiority for benzodiazepines over neuroleptics in the treatment of behavioral complications in demented patients.

The known pharmacological profile of benzodiazepines suggests that these medications may be effective in the treatment of insomnia and agitation but not classical psychotic symptoms (i.e., delusions and hallucinations). However, this remains to be established in demented patients with behavioral complications. Given the known heterogeneity in the manifestation of behavioral complications in dementia, studies with large patient samples will be required to evaluate treatment responsivity of individual symptoms or groups of symptoms to specific medications.

Benzodiazepines can lead to tolerance and dependence, and worsening of cognition is a concern (90). Despite the known deleterious effects of benzodiazepines on learning and memory in normal subjects (91–93), particularly among the elderly (94), side-effect comparisons of neuroleptics and benzodiazepines in demented patients have not been reported.

As reviewed in Chapter 23, several other medications have been reported to be efficacious in demented patients with behavioral complications. These include trazodone (95,96), selective serotonin reuptake inhibitors (SSRIs) (97,98), lithium (99), carbamazepine (100,101), valproate (102), and propranolol (103). However, published systematic, controlled studies comparing these agents to neuroleptics are lacking (90).

Optimal Duration of Neuroleptic Treatment

In clinical practice, it is often possible to taper or withdraw neuroleptics over time, presumably because some demented patients experience a remission of behavioral complications due to changes in specific brain regions that accompany disease progression. There is only limited indirect evidence to support this view. In a nursing home sample of 91 patients of whom half had dementia, Lantz et al. (41) found that more than half the patients received a psychotropic medication during their 5 years of residence, but less than one-quarter were continuously medicated during this period.

In our recent multicenter study of 235 patients, the highly persistent nature of agitation indirectly suggested that treatment of this target behavior may need to be relatively prolonged (10). Paranoid delusions and hallucinations were somewhat less persistent, suggesting that not all patients need long-term neuroleptic treatment for these symptoms. However, these data were confounded by the use of psychotropic medications that were based on doctor's choice. To date, there have been no controlled studies that have examined the likelihood of relapse following neuroleptic discontinuation in patients whose behavioral complications have improved with neuroleptic treatment. The need for continuation of neuroleptic treatment in dementia, and the optimal duration of such treatment, remain to be evaluated in empirical research. Also, potential predictors of both response and relapse remain to be identified.

C. Neuroleptic Side Effects

In elderly patients, there is an increased propensity to both short-term (anticholinergic, EPS) and long-term (TD) side effects (104–107). As a result, elderly schizophrenics tend to be maintained on neuroleptic doses that are one-third to one-half that used in young adults (104,108). Even lower doses should be used in demented patients, because not only are there physiological changes due to aging, but progressive neuronal degeneration may alter behavioral symptoms and increase vulnerability to side effects (22). However, there is little information on the risk of TD with chronic use of neuroleptics in AD (109).

In their placebo-controlled trial that compared haloperidol and loxapine in 61 demented patients with behavioral complications, Petrie et al. reported that EPS (38%) and sedation (38%) were common side effects (60). The doses used (mean haloperidol 4.6 mg daily and loxapine 21.9 mg daily) were somewhat higher than those currently recommended for use in AD (44,57). In our single-blind pilot study of nine AD patients with behavioral complications, side effects, particularly EPS, suggested that haloperidol doses above 4 mg daily are generally not advisable. In another pilot study of ten AD patients, depot neuroleptic treatment with low-dose fluphenazine decanoate (1.25–3.75 mg intramuscularly bimonthly) was efficacious, with few side effects observed during a 16-week trial (56). In an open trial of 30 AD patients with behavioral problems who received low-dose haloperidol (0.5–3 mg daily) or thioridazine (12.5–75 mg daily), Tune et al. (57) found that only three patients completed the study without experiencing significant side effects. During a 3-month stabilization follow-up phase, late emergent side effects developed in 7 of 18 patients. It remains unclear if these late emergent side effects are purely a function of neuroleptic usage or the progression of AD brain pathology. Short-term and longer term side effects are frequent limiting factors during neuroleptic usage in AD, even when low doses are used.

Other complications include neuroleptic malignant syndrome and cardiac side effects, including orthostatic hypotension with low-potency neuroleptics (110). Less common side effects include hepatotoxicity (chlorpromazine), retinopathy (thioridazine), agranulocytosis (clozapine), dermatological reactions, arrhythmias, and, rarely, sudden death. In the elderly, the increased risk of cardiovascular side effects and the anticholinergic symptoms of confusion, urinary retention, and constipation may lead to the use of haloperidol as the medically safer choice. These factors need to be weighed against the greatly increased sensitivity to EPS with high-potency agents like haloperidol (20, 57). The use of multiple medications is of concern in the elderly, and significant drug interactions also need to be taken into account (58).

Effects on Cognition and Activities of Daily Life

Few studies have evaluated the effects of neuroleptics on cognition or activities of daily life in dementia (20,55). One concern is that the anticholinergic activity of neuroleptics may further compromise the already damaged central cholinergic projections in AD (111,112). The level of cognitive impairment may be increased by the use of neuroleptics with strong anticholinergic properties (e.g., thioridazine) or by the addition of anticholinergic agents to treat drug-induced EPS. At another level, the sedation produced by neuroleptics may enhance the degree of disorientation and cognitive impairment in AD. These theoretical concerns remain to be validated by systematic research.

D. Pharmacodynamics and Pharmacokinetics

As indicated in Chapter 1, dopamine neurons degenerate with aging, particularly after age 70. Also, there is a decrease in cholinergic neurons in AD (111, 112). These pharmacodynamic changes may reduce the tolerance of the elderly to neuroleptics, and increase the likelihood of side effects.

From a pharmacokinetic perspective, drugs have slightly longer half-lives in the elderly compared to the rest of the adult population (113,114). Tolerance decreases and the therapeutic index narrows (115). Age-related decreases in gut motility and the anticholinergic effects of neuroleptics may decrease absorption rates. Therefore, drugs take longer to reach therapeutic blood levels and also take longer to leave the system, thereby prolonging side effects. The concomitant use of antacids may lower neuroleptic blood levels (116,117). Neuroleptic drugs undergo biotransformation primarily in the liver, with the gastrointestinal tract, lungs, and kidneys being secondary sites.

There has been little work examining the utility of monitoring neuroleptic blood levels in demented patients. In our ongoing study that compares haloperidol (2–3 mg daily, 0.5–0.75 mg daily) and placebo, plasma haloperidol levels were detectable in all patients on 2–3 mg daily. In 18 patients who received 0.5–0.75 mg daily, haloperidol levels were below the limit of detection by the RIA assay in seven patients. In these cases, the lower limit of assay detection was used as the value for the haloperidol level. Despite the consequent restriction of range in plasma levels, correlations between oral dose (0.5, 0.75, 2, or 3 mg daily) and blood levels were moderately strong ($r = 0.72$; $p < .001$). Of note, only three patients had ever received neuroleptics prior to entering the study. The neuroleptic naivete of these AD patients may have precluded the alterations in drug absorption and metabolism that occur with chronic neuroleptic treatment in schizophrenia with resultant distortion of the relations between oral dose and blood level (4).

In patients with schizophrenia, there is a postulated (controversial) therapeutic window for haloperidol of ~5–15 ng/ml (118–120). Interestingly, we observed therapeutic effect in our series of AD patients at blood levels that were invariably below this postulated therapeutic window. In fact, in our ongoing study, the highest blood level recorded was 3.8 ng/ml for one patient who received 3 mg haloperidol daily. Also, EPS developed in some patients at these low blood levels, which indicates that the increased sensitivity to neuroleptics in dementia is not likely to be due to pharmacokinetic changes. A pharmacodynamic explanation (e.g., degeneration of dopaminergic neurons leading to greater sensitivity to even low oral doses of neuroleptic medication) is more likely. Of note, the pharmacokinetics of nortriptyline in the elderly do not appear to differ from what has been previously reported in young adult patients (121).

We previously reported in a small sample that compared to oral dose, blood levels show stronger associations with improvement in symptoms and severity of EPS in AD patients with behavioral complications (122). While intriguing, these preliminary findings on the utility of monitoring neuroleptic blood levels require further extension and independent replication in demented patients, where only limited data are available (123).

III. RECOMMENDATIONS FOR CLINICAL PRACTICE

There are a paucity of rigorous controlled studies to guide clinical practice. The following recommendations are based on the current state of knowledge in the field, and are likely to change based on the results obtained from ongoing and future research.

Neuroleptics are difficult to use in the demented elderly, and careful evaluation of the trade-off between efficacy and side effects is necessary. The choice of medication depends more on likely side effects than differential efficacy (e.g., low-potency agents like thioridazine for patients with preexisting EPS, high-potency agents like haloperidol for patients with preexisting orthostatic hypotension or prostatic enlargement). The equivalent of haloperidol 1–2 mg daily is suggested as a starting dose, but this often needs to be titrated individually to achieve an optimal trade-off between efficacy and side effects. There are few data on blood-level monitoring, which at this stage cannot be recommended for routine clinical practice. Anticholinergic agents to treat EPS should be avoided, particularly in AD, with lowering of neuroleptic dose being the preferred strategy. The concomitant use of a hypnotic (e.g., chloral hydrate at low dose) may be required in some patients. A trial of 6–12 weeks in duration is usually sufficient to determine the outcome of neuroleptic treatment. If the optimal neuroleptic dose is reached quickly, clinical response may occur within the first week or two. On the other hand, the need to adjust dosage due to side effects may require a relatively prolonged trial period. Nonresponse or intolerable side effects should lead to consideration of another class of neuroleptic or an alternative type of medication (e.g., valproate).

The heterogeneous nature of behavioral complications suggests that specific target symptoms should be identified before initiating neuroleptic treatment, and these target symptoms should be monitored serially during the course of treatment. In addition to neurological and other common neuroleptic side effects, cognition and activities of daily living need to be monitored, preferably with brief instruments like the MMSE. In patients maintained for extended periods on neuroleptics, assessment for TD should be conducted at regular intervals. Periodic attempts should be made to taper or discontinue the neuroleptic, although the optimal period of continuation neuroleptic treatment remains to be established.

REFERENCES

1. Reisberg B, Borenstein J, Salob SP, et al. Behavioral symptoms in Alzheimer's disease: phenomenology and treatment. J Clin Psychiatry 1987; 48:9–15.
2. McKhann G, Drachman D, Folstein M. Clinical diagnosis of Alzheimer's disease: Report of the NINCDS-ADRDA Work Group under the auspices of Department of Health and Human Services Task Force on Alzheimer's Disease. Neurology 1984; 34:939–944.
3. Devanand DP, Sackeim HA, Mayeux R. Psychosis, behavioral disturbance, and the use of neuroleptics in dementia. Compr Psychiatry 1988; 29:387–401.
4. Devanand DP, Miller L, Richards M, et al. The Columbia University Scale for Psychopathology in Alzheimer's disease. Arch Neurol 1992; 49:371–376.
5. Burns, 1992. Psychiatric phenomena in dementia of the Alzheimer type. Int Psychogeriatr 1992; 4 (suppl 1):43–54.
6. Reisberg B, Franssen E, Sclan SG, Kluger A, Ferris SH. Stage specific incidence of potentially remediable behavioral symptoms in aging and Alzheimer's disease. A study of 120 patients using the BEHAVE-AD. Bull Clin Neurosci 1989; 54:95–112.
7. Rubin E, Morris J, Berg L. The progression of personality changes in senile dementia of the Alzheimer's type. J Am Geriatr Soc 1987; 721–725.
8. Rubin EH, Kinscherf DA. Psychopathology of very mild dementia of the Alzheimer type. Am J Psychiatry 1989; 146:1017–1021.
9. Devanand DP, Brockington CD, Moody BJ, et al. Behavioral syndromes in Alzheimer's disease. Int Psychogeriatr 1992; 4:161–184.
10. Devanand DP, Jacobs DM, Tang M-X, Castillo-Castaneda CD, Sano M, Marder K, Bell K, Bylsma FW, Brandt J, Albert M, Stern Y. The course of psychopathology in mild to moderate Alzheimer's disease. Arch Gen Psychiatry 1997; 54:257–263.
11. Cohen-Mansfield J, Marx MS, Rosenthal AS. A description of agitation in a nursing home. Gerontology 1989; 3:M77–M84.
12. Swearer JM, Drachman DA, O'Donnell BF, Mitchell AL. Troublesome and disruptive behaviors in dementia. J Am Geriatr Soc 1988; 36:784–790.
13. Cummings JL, Miller B, Hill MJ, Neshkes R. Neuropsychiatric aspects of multi-infarct dementia and dementia of the Alzheimer type. Arch Neurol 1987; 44:389–393.
14. Teri L, Larson EB, Reifler BV. Behavioral disturbance in dementia of the Alzheimer's type. J Am Geriatr Soc 1988; 36:1–6.
15. Jeste DV, Wragg RE, Salmon DP, et al. Cognitive deficits of patients with Alzheimer's disease with and without delusions. Am J Psychiatry 1992; 149:184–189.
16. Wagner AW, Teri L, Orr-Rainey N. Behavior problems among dementia residents in special care units: changes over time. J Am Geriatr Soc 1995; 43:784–787.

17. Bucht G, Adolfsson R. The comprehensive psychopathological rating scale in patients with dementia of Alzheimer type and multi-infarct dementia. Acta Psychiatr Scand 1983; 68:263–270.
18. Mayeux R, Stern Y, Spantaon S. Heterogeneity in dementia of the Alzheimer type: evidence of subgroups. Neurology 1985; 35:453–461.
19. Wragg RE, Jeste DV. Overview of depression and psychosis in Alzheimer's disease. Am J Psychiatry 1989; 146:577–587.
20. Devanand D, Sackeim H, Brown R, Mayeux R. A pilot study of haloperidol treatment of psychosis and behavioral disturbance in Alzheimer's disease. Arch Neurol 1989; 46:854–857.
21. Mulsant BH, Gershon S. Neuroleptics in the treatment of psychosis in late life: a rational approach. Int J Geriatr Psychiatry 1993; 3:979–992.
22. Fairburn CG, Hope RA. Changes in behaviour in dementia: A neglected research area. Br J Psychiatry 1988; 152:406–407.
23. Rosen WG, Terry RD, Fuld PA, et al. Pathological verification of ischemia score in differentiation of dementias. Ann Neurol 1980; 7:486–488.
24. Bucht G, Adolfson R, Winbald B. Dementia of the Alzheimer type and multi-infarct dementia: A clinical description and diagnostic problems. J Am Geriatr Soc 1984; 32:491–497.
25. Gonzalez MP, Lopez OL, Sudilovsky A, et al. Differences in neuropsychiatric profile in Alzheimer's disease and non-Alzheimer's disease dementias. American Psychiatric Association meeting, Miami, FL, 1995 (NR31).
26. Stern Y, Mayeux R, Sano M, et al. Predictors of disease course in patients with probable Alzheimer's disease. Neurology 1987; 37:1649–1653.
27. Drevets WC, Rubin EH. Psychotic symptoms and the longitudinal course of dementia of the Alzheimer type. Biol Psychiatry 1989; 25:39–48.
28. Rosen J, Zubenko GS. Emergence of psychosis and depression in the longitudinal evaluation of Alzheimer's disease. Biol Psychiatry 1991; 29:224–232.
29. Grad J, Sainsbury P. The effect that patients have on their families in a community care and a control psychiatric service - a 2 year followup. Br J Psychiatry 1968; 114:265.
30. Small GW, Jarvik LF. The dementia syndrome. Lancet 1982; 11:1443–1445.
31. Rabins PV, Mace NL, Lucas MJ. The impact of dementia on the family. J Am Med Assoc 1982; 248:333–335.
32. Haller E, Binder RL, McNeil DE. Violence in geriatric patients with dementia. Bull Am Acad Psychiatry Law 1989; 17:183–188.
33. Leibovici A, Tariot PN. Agitation associated with dementia: a systematic approach to treatment. Psychopharmacol Bull 1988; 24:39–42.
34. Prien Y, Haber PA, Caffey EMJ. The use of psychoactive drugs in elderly patients with psychiatric disorders: survey conducted in twelve Veterans Administration hospitals. J Am Geriatr Soc 1975; 23:104–112.
35. Michel K, Kolakowska T. A survey of prescribing psychotropic drugs in two psychiatric hospitals. Br J Psychiatry 1981; 138:217–221.
36. Barton R, Hurst L. Unnecessary use of tranquilizers in elderly patients. Br J Psychiatry 1966; 112:989–990.
37. Gilleard CJ, Morgan K, Wade BE. Patterns of neuroleptic use among the institutionalized elderly. Acta Psychiatr Scand 1983; 68:419–425.

38. Ray WA, Federspiel CF, Schaffner W. A study of antipsychotic drug use in nursing homes: epidemiologic evidence suggesting misuse. Am J Public Health 1980; 70: 485–491.
39. Reynolds MD. Institutional prescribing for the elderly: patterns of prescribing in a municipal hospital and a municipal nursing home. J Am Geriatr Soc 1984; 32: 640–645.
40. Beardsley RS, Larson DB, Burns BJ, et al. Prescribing of psychotropics in elderly nursing home patients. J Am Geriatr Soc 1989; 37:327–330.
41. Lantz MS, Louis A, Lowenstein G, Kennedy GJ. A longitudinal study of psychotropic prescriptions in a teaching nursing home. Am J Psychiatry 1990; 147:1637–1639.
42. Avorn J, Soumerai SB, Everitt DE, et al. A randomized trial of a program to reduce the use of psychoactive drugs in nursing homes. New Engl J Med 1992; 327:168–173.
43. Schneider LS, Pollock VE, Lyness SA. A meta-analysis of controlled trials of neuroleptic treatment in dementia. J Am Geriatr Soc 1990; 38:553–563.
44. Devanand DP. Role of neuroleptics in treatment of behavioral complications. In: Lawlor BA, ed. Behavioral Complications in Alzheimer's Disease. Washington, DC: American Psychiatric Press, Inc., 1995:131–151.
45. Lehmann E, Ban A. Comparative pharmacotherapy of the aging psychotic patient. Laval Med 1967; 38:588–595.
46. Jackson EB. Mellaril in the treatment of the geriatric patient. Am J Psychiatry 1961; 118:543–544.
47. Cavero CV. Evaluation of thioridazine in the aged. J Am Geriatr Soc 1966; 14:617–622.
48. Kral VA. The use of thioridazine (Mellaril) in aged people. Can Med Assoc J 1961; 84:152–154.
49. Robinson DB. Evaluation of certain drugs in geriatric patients. Arch Gen Psychiatry 1959; 1:41–47.
50. Tewfik GI, Jain VK, Harcup M, Magowan S. Effectiveness of various tranquilizers in the management of senile restlessness. Gerontol Clin 1970; 12:351–359.
51. Tobin JM, Brousseau ER, Lorenz AA. Clinical evaluation of haloperidol in geriatric patients. Geriatrics 1970; 25:119–122.
52. Branchey MH, Lee JH, Amin R, Simpson GM. High- and low-potency neuroleptics in elderly psychiatric patients. J Am Med Assoc 1978; 239:1860–1862.
53. Terman L. Treatment of senile agitation with chlorpromazine. Geriatrics 1955; 10:520–522.
54. Raskind M, Risse S, Lampe T. Dementia and antipsychotic drugs. J Clin Psychiatry 1987; 48:16–18.
55. Steele C, Lucas M, Tune L. Haloperidol vs. thioridazine in the treatment of behavioral symptoms in senile dementia of the Alzheimer's type: preliminary findings. J Clin Psychiatry 1986; 47:310–312.
56. Gottlieb GL, McAllister TW, Gur RC. Depot neuroleptics in the treatment of behavioral disorders in patients with Alzheimer's disease. J Am Geriatr Soc 1988; 36:642–644.
57. Tune LE, Steele C, Cooper T. Neuroleptic drugs in the management of behavioral symptoms of Alzheimer's disease. Psychiatr Clin North Am 1991; 14:353–373.

58. Salzman C. Treatment of agitation in the elderly. In: Meltzer HY, ed. Psychopharmacology: The Third Generation of Progress. New York: Raven Press, 1987:1167–1176.
59. Sunderland T, Silver M. Neuroleptics in the treatment of dementia. Int J Geriatr Psychiatry 1988; 3:79–88.
60. Petrie WM, Ban TA, Berney S, et al. Loxapine in psychogeriatrics: a placebo- and standard-controlled investigation. J Clin Psychopharmacol 1982; 2:122–126.
61. Abse DW, Dahlstrom WG, Hill C. The value of chemotherapy in senile mental disturbance. J Am Med Assoc 1960; 174:2036–2042.
62. Hamilton LD, Bennett JL. Acetophenazine for hyperactive geriatric patients. Geriatrics 1962; 17:596–601.
63. Hamilton LD, Bennett JL. The use of trifluperazine in geriatric patients with chronic organic brain syndrome. J Am Geriatr Soc 1962; 10:140–147.
64. Sugarman AA, Williams H, Adlerstein AM. Haloperidol in the psychiatric disorders of old age. Am J Psychiatry 1964; 120:1190–1192.
65. Rada RT, Kellner R. Thiothixene in the treatment of geriatric patients with chronic organic brain syndrome. J Am Geriatr Soc 1976; 24:105–107.
66. Barnes R, Veith R, Okimoto J, et al. Efficacy of antipsychotic medications in behaviorally disturbed dementia patients. Am J Psychiatry 1982; 139:1170–1174.
67. Finkel SI, Lyons JS, Anderson RL, Sherrell K, Davis J, Cohen-Mansfield J, Schwartz A, Gandy J, Schneider L. A randomized, placebo-controlled trial of thiothixene in agitated, demented nursing home patients. Int J Geriatr Psychiatry 1995; 10:129–136.
68. Tariot PN, Mack JL, Patterson MB, et al. The CERAD behavior rating scale for dementia (BRSD). Am J Psychiatry 1995; 152:1349–1357.
69. Raskind MA, Risse SC. Antipsychotic drugs and the elderly. J Clin Psychiatry 1986; 47:17–22.
70. Smith GR, Taylor CW, Linkous P. Haloperidol versus thioridazine for the treatment of psychogeriatric patients: A double-blind clinical trial. Psychosomatics 1974; 15:134–138.
71. Cowley LM, Glen RS. Double-blind study of thioridazine and haloperidol in geriatric patients with a psychosis associated with organic brain syndrome. J Clin Psychiatry 1979; 40:411–419.
72. Tsuang M, Lu LM, Stotsky BA, Cole JO. Haloperidol versus thioridazine for hospitalized psychogeriatric patients: double-blind study. J Am Geriatr Soc 1971; 19: 593–600.
73. Rosen JH. Double-blind comparison of haloperidol and thioridazine in geriatric outpatients. J Clin Psychiatry 1979; 40:17–20.
74. Carlyle W, Ancill RJ, Sheldon L. Aggression in the demented patient: a double-blind study of loxapine versus haloperidol. Int Clin Psychopharmacol 1993; 8:103–108.
75. Kane J, Honigfeld G, Singer J, Meltzer H, and the Clozaril Collaborative Study Group. Clozapine for the treatment-resistant schizophrenic: a double-blind comparison with chlorpromazine. Arch Gen Psychiatry 1988; 45:789–796.
76. Chengappa KNR, Baker RW, Kreinbrook SB, Adair D. Clozapine use in female geriatric patients with psychoses. J Geriatr Psychiatry Neurol 1995; 8:12–15.

77. Chouinard G, Jones B, Remington G, et al. A Canadian multicenter placebo-controlled study of fixed doses of risperidone and haloperidol in the treatment of chronic schizophrenic patients. J Clin Psychopharmacol 1993; 13:25–40.
78. Jeanblanc W, Davis BY. Risperidone for treating dementia-associated aggression. Am J Psychiatry (letter) 1995; 152:1239.
79. Schotte A, Janssen PFM, Megens AAH, Leyson JE. Occupancy of central neurotransmitter receptors by risperidone, clozapine, and haloperidol, measured ex vivo by quantitative autoradiography. Brain Res 1993; 631:191–202.
80. Megens AAH, Awouters FHL, Schotte A, et al. Survey on the pharmacodynamics of the new antipsychotic resperidone. Psychopharmacology 1994; 114:9–23.
81. Nyberg S, Farde L, Eriksson L, et al. 5-HT2 and D_2 dopamine receptor occupancy in the living human brain: A PET study with risperidone. Psychopharmacology 1993; 110:265–272.
82. Prado N, Kramer-Ginsberg E, Kremen N, et al. Risperidone in dementia with behavioral disturbances. American Psychiatric Association Meeting, Miami, FL, 1995 (NR6).
83. Goldberg RJ, Goldberg JS. Low-dose risperidone for dementia related disturbed behavior in nursing homes. American Psychiatric Association Meeting, Miami, FL, 1995 (NR262).
84. Van Putten T, Marder SR, Mintz J. A controlled dose comparison study of haloperidol in newly admitted schizophrenic patients. Arch Gen Psychiatry 1990; 47: 754–758.
85. Stone CK, Garver DL, Griffith J, Hirschowitz J, Bennett J. Further evidence of a dose-response threshold for haloperidol in psychosis. Am J Psychiatry 1995; 152: 1210–1212.
86. Kirven LG, Montero EF. Comparison of thioridazine and diazepam in the control of nonpsychotic symptoms associated with senility: double-blind study. J Am Geriatr Soc 1973; 21:546–551.
87. Covington JS. Alleviating agitation, apprehension, and related symptoms in geriatric patients. South Med J 1975; 58:719–724.
88. Stotsky B. Multicenter studying thioridazine with diazepam and placebo in elderly, nonpsychotic patients with emotional and behavioral disorders. Clin Ther 1984; 6:546–559.
89. Burgio LD, Reynolds CFI, Janosky JE, et al. A behavioral microanalysis of the effects of haloperidol and oxazepam in demented psychogeriatric inpatients. Int J Geriatr Psychiatry 1992; 7:253–262.
90. Schneider LS, Sobin PB. Non-neuroleptic medications in the management of agitation in Alzheimer's disease: a selective review. Int J Ger Psychiatry 1991; 6:691–708.
91. Jones DM, Lewis MJ, Spriggs TLB. The effects of low doses of diazepam on human performance in group administered tasks. Br J Clin Pharmacol 1978; 6:333–337.
92. Liljequist R, Linnoila M, Mattila MJ. Effect of diazepam and chlorpromazine on memory functions in man. Eur J Clin Pharmacol 1978; 13:339–343.
93. Ghoneim NM, Mewaldt SP, Berie JL, Hinruchs JV. Memory and performance effects of single and 3-week administration of diazepam. Psychopharmacology 1981; 73:147–151.

94. Pomara N, Deptula D, Singh R. Cognitive toxicity of benzodiazepines in the elderly. In: Anxiety in the Elderly: Treatment and Research. New York: Springer Publishing Company, 1990.
95. Lawlor BA, Radcliffe J, Molchan SE, et al. A pilot placebo-controlled study of trazodone and buspirone in Alzheimer's disease. Int Am J Geriatr Psychiatry 1994; 9:55–59.
96. Lebert F, Pasquier F, Petit H. Behavioral effects of trazodone in Alzheimer's disease. J Clin Psychiatry 1994; 55:536–538.
97. Burke WJ, Folks DG, Roccaforte WH, Wengel SP. Serotonin reuptake inhibitors for the treatment of coexisting depression and psychosis in dementia of the Alzheimer type. J Am Geriatr Psychiatry 1994; 2:352–354.
98. Geldmacher DS, Waldman AJ, Doty L, Heilman KM. Fluoxetine in dementia of the Alzheimer's type: prominent adverse effects and failure to improve cognition. J Clin Psychiatry 1994; 2:161.
99. Holton A, George K. The use of lithium carbonate in severely demented patients with behavioral disturbance. Br J Psychiatry 1985; 146:99–100.
100. Liebovici A, Tariot PN. Carbamazepine treatment of agitation associated with dementia. J Geriatr Psychiatry Neurol 1988; 1:110–112.
101. Lemke MR. Effect of carbamazepine on agitation in Alzheimer's inpatients refractory to neuroleptics. J Clin Psychiatry 1995; 56:354–357.
102. Mellow AM, Solano-Lopez C, Davis S. Sodium valproate in the treatment of behavioral disturbance in dementia. J Geriatr Psychiatry Neurology 1993; 6:205–209.
103. Weiler P, Mungas D, Bernick C. Propranolol for the control of disruptive behavior in senile dementia. J Geriatr Psychiatry Neurol 1988; 4:226–230.
104. Prien RF. Chemotherapy in chronic organic brain syndrome—a review of the literature. Psychopharmacol Bull 1973; 9:5–20.
105. Harris MJ, Panton D, Caligiuri MP, et al. High incidence of tardive dyskinesia in older outpatients on low doses of neuroleptics. Psychopharmacol Bull 1992; 28: 87–92.
106. Tepper S, Haas J. Prevalence of tardive dyskinesia. J Clin Psychiatry 1979; 40:508–516.
107. Glazer W, Morgenstern H. Predictors of occurrence, severity and course of tardive dyskinesia in an outpatient population. J Clin Psychopharmacol 1988; 8: 10S–16S.
108. Gilbert PL, Harris MJ, McAdams LA, Jeste DV. Neuroleptic withdrawal in schizophrenic patients: a review of the literature. Arch Gen Psychiatry 1995; 52:173–188.
109. McDaniel KD, Kazee AM, Eskin TA, Hamill RW. Tardive dyskinesia in Alzheimer's disease: clinical features and neuropathologic correlates. J Geriatr Psychiatry Neurol 1991; 4:79–85.
110. Blumenthal MD, Davie JW. Dizziness and falling in elderly psychiatric outpatients. Am J Psychiatry 1980; 137:203–206.
111. Davies P, Maloney AJF. Selective loss of central cholinergic neurons in Alzheimer's disease (letter). Lancet 1976; 1:1403.

112. Perry EK, Gibson PH, Blessed G, et al. Neurotransmitter enzyme abnormalities in senile dementia. J Neurol Sci 1977; 34:247–265.
113. Davis JM. Antipsychotics. In: Crook T, Cohen GD, eds. Physicians' Handbook on Psychotherapeutic Drug Use in the Aged. New Canaan, CT: Mark Powley, 1981:12–25.
114. Hicks R, Davis J. Pharmacokinetics in geriatric psychopharmacology. In: Eisdorfer C, Fann W, eds. Psychopharmacology of Aging. New York: Spectrum Publications, 1980:169–212.
115. Baldessarini RF. Clinical and epidemiologic aspects of tardive dyskinesia. J Clin Psychiatry 1985; 46:8–13.
116. Forrest FM, Forrest IS, Serra MT. Modification of chlorpromazine metabolism by some other drugs frequently administered to psychiatric patients. Biol Psychiatry 1970; 2:53–58.
117. Fann WE, Davis J, Janowsky D, Seerke H, Schmidt D. Chlorpromazine: effects of antacids on its gastrointestinal absorption. J Clin Pharmacol 1973; 13:388–390.
118. Mavroidis ML, Garver DL, Kanter DR, Hirschowitz J. Plasma haloperidol levels and clinical response: confounding variables. Psychopharmacol Bull 1985; 21:62–65.
119. Volavka J, Cooper T, Czobor P, et al. Haloperidol blood levels and clinical effects. Arch Gen Psychiatry 1992; 49:354–361.
120. Van Putten T, Marder SR, Mintz J, Poland RE. Haloperidol plasma levels and clinical response: a therapeutic window relationship. Am J Psychiatry 1992; 149: 500–505.
121. Kin NY, Klitgaard N, Nair NPV, et al. Clinical relevance of serum nortriptyline and 10-hydroxy-nortriptyline measurements in the depressed elderly: a multicenter pharmacokinetic and pharmacodynamic study. Neuropsychopharmacology 1996; 15:1–6.
122. Devanand DP, Cooper T, Sackeim HA, et al. Low dose oral haloperidol and blood levels in Alzheimer's disease: a preliminary study. Psychopharmacol Bull 1992; 28:169–173.
123. Dysken MW, Johnson SB, Holdon L, et al. Haloperidol concentrations in patients with Alzheimer's dementia. Am J Geriatr Psychiatry 1994; 2:125–133.

23
Nonneuroleptic Treatment of Complications of Dementia: Applying Clinical Research to Practice

Pierre N. Tariot
University of Rochester School of Medicine, and Monroe Community Hospital, Rochester, New York

Lon S. Schneider
University of Southern California, Los Angeles, California

I. INTRODUCTION

The purpose of this chapter is to review nonneuroleptic therapies for the behavioral manifestations of dementia. Behavioral disturbances associated with dementia are of importance to all concerned. They can cause subjective distress for the patient (1), burden caregivers, and are frequent precipitants of institutionalization (2). The health care system itself is burdened with such problems (3). Relief of behavioral disturbances could improve quality of life for the patient as well as the care providers, who play a crucial role in the fate of patients with dementia. To the untrained eye, the behavior problems associated with dementia can appear confusing, partly because they are highly variable in their presentation, frequency, severity, and duration. Studies in the last 10 years have begun to identify clusters of signs and symptoms that frequently co-occur in individuals with dementia, facilitating description and quantification of these behaviors (4–8). Examples of these clusters include delusions, hallucinations, depressive and anxious features, agitation, and apathy and withdrawal (3). Table 1 presents a summary of reported ranges of frequencies (% of patients affected in the sample) of behavioral disturbances associated with dementia, based upon reviews of the literature (3,6).

TABLE 1 Schematic Summary of Reported Frequencies of Behavioral Disturbances Associated with Dementia (% of Patients)

	Range	Median
1. Disturbed affect/mood	0–86	19
2. Disturbed ideation	10–73	33.5
3. Altered perception		
hallucinations	21–49	28
misperceptions	1–49	23
4. Agitation		
global	10–90	44
wandering	0–50	18
5. Aggression		
verbal	11–51	24
physical	0–46	14.3
resistive/uncooperative	27–65	14
6. Anxiety	0–50	31.8
7. Withdrawn/passive behavior	21–88	61
8. Vegetative behaviors		
sleep	0–47	27
diet/appetite	12.5–77	34

Reprinted from Ref. 3: based on review of approximately 50 articles found in literature search on this topic.

The median frequency reported is presented as a conservative estimate of the likelihood of encountering that type of behavioral change. Each of these constructs has individual components. For instance, depressive features may include sad affect, tearfulness, subjective reports of low mood, guilty or self-deprecatory ideation, pessimism, preoccupation with death, suicidality, and certain vegetative features. These clusters provide a useful basis on which to make decisions regarding pharmacotherapy, a point which will be expanded upon later in the chapter.

A similar approach to classifying behavioral complications of dementia was adopted by the International Psychogeriatric Association Consensus Conference on Behavioral Disturbances of Dementia (9). In essence, the Conference concluded that: (1) patients suffering diseases that cause dementia manifest clinically significant neuropsychiatric signs and symptoms; (2) these symptoms are troubling to patients and caregivers; (3) they are measurable; and (4) they are potentially treatable. These neuropsychiatric signs and symptoms include the kinds of clusters referred to above: hallucinations, delusions, misperceptions, depressive and anxious features, apathy and withdrawal, agitation, aggression, lability, and vegetative features. Such signs and symptoms do not necessarily signify syndromic concepts, but they do emerge frequently, and they can be identified, quantified, and treated.

II. BEHAVIORAL SCALES

A variety of outcome measures have been developed to assess these behavioral clusters and to assess the result of therapeutic interventions. Instrument development studies have varied widely in the manner in which patients were selected and in important clinical characteristics such as diagnosis and diagnostic ascertainment, prior psychiatric history, stage of dementia, and gender. There were also important differences in sample size, design, criteria used for characterizing behavior, reliability, type of analysis, time frame of relevance, setting, characteristics of interviewers, and source of information (3,10,11). The literature regarding measurement of behavior is therefore understandably heterogeneous. Existing instruments can also be judged by a variety of important psychometric criteria, many of which have been reviewed previously (10). Depending on the purpose for which a scale is used, one or another of these criteria may be of particular importance. In general, those with clear constructs, established reliability, demonstrated validity and sensitivity, and practical features suitable for the intended purpose will be the most relevant choices. Some key features include whether the scale is a general behavioral measure or whether it focuses on one particular behavioral domain (such as agitation); whether the instrument is based on patient interview and/or informant interview; and whether frequency and/or severity of behaviors is assessed. Given the approach adopted in this chapter, those scales which address all of the behavioral domains identified above, including the particular components of these domains, will be deemed the most adequate.

Several recent articles have surveyed the field (10–12). For purposes of this chapter, several scales are summarized in Table 2, some of which will be described in more detail below. These have a sound basis for use in dementia, and offer a spectrum of attributes from which to compare and contrast the strengths and weaknesses of each.

The Brief Psychiatric Rating Scale (BPRS) (13–15) was initially developed to provide rapid reliable assessment of psychopharmacological treatment effects in general psychiatric inpatients. Originally 16 items, it was revised to include two additional items which were to represent collectively "somewhat global, clinical familiar, symptom and behavior constructs that span much of the range of manifest psychopathology" (13). The rating constructs represent a process of abstraction and synthesis that models clinical judgment and decision making, and requires clinical experience in order to recognize mild symptoms as well as gauge the severity of more intense symptoms. The BPRS has been widely used to document treatment effects of clinical trials and also in descriptive studies of patients with dementia (11). It provides an overall indication of level of psychopathology, and change in level in psychopathology, and offers five factors that have been identified in a

TABLE 2 Behavioral Ratings Used in Clinical Trials

ADAS noncognitive subscale (101)	Assesses the following areas: tearfulness, depression, concentration, uncooperativeness, delusions, hallucinations, pacing, motor activity, tremors, appetite on a 6-point (0 to 5) severity scale. Usually rated by the cognitive tester; essentially limited for behavior during test-taking. Often combined with ADAS-Cog score for a total ADAS score.
Behavior Rating Scale for Dementia of the Consortium to Establish a Registry for AD (CERAD BRSD) (8)	A standardized, reliable semistructured interview that is administered to caregivers based on frequency of behaviors. Eight factors map onto clinically relevant domains in AD: depressive features, psychotic features, defective self-regulation, irritability/agitation, vegetative features, apathy, aggression, and affective lability.
Behavioral Pathology in AD scale (BEHAVE-AD) (101)	Assesses 25 well-defined behaviors in seven areas: paranoid and delusional ideation, hallucinations, activity disturbances, aggressiveness, diurnal rhythm disturbances, affective disturbance, anxieties and phobias. If present, behavior is rated as mild, moderate, or severe.
Brief Psychiatric Rating Scale (BPRS) (13)	Based on an interview by an experienced clinician, 18 items rated on a 7-point severity scale. Five factors are withdraw depression, agitation, cognitive dysfunction, hostile suspiciousness, and psychotic distortion.
Neuropsychiatric Inventory (NPI) (17)	Assesses 13 behaviors on the basis of frequency and severity. Structured interview of caregiver; scores range from 0 to 120.
Cohen-Mansfield Agitation Inventory (CMAI) (104)	A nurse's rating questionnaire consisting of 29 "agitated behaviors" rated on a 7-point frequency scale [1 (never) to 7 (several) times per hour]. Often used with a nurse's aide usually in nursing home. Four factors include: aggressive behavior, physically nonaggressive behavior, verbally agitated behavior, and hiding/hoarding behavior.

geropsychiatric population, including depression, agitation, cognitive dysfunction, psychotic distortion, and hostile/suspiciousness (14). To this end it can provide a profile. Because it relies on clinical experience and judgment, interpersonal and communication skills, and synthesis of information, a trained clinician is necessary to apply it reliably. It is intended as a present-state interview, and thereby ignores behaviors that occur outside the interview as well as potentially useful information available from caregivers.

The CERAD Behavior Rating Scale for Dementia (BRSD) (8) evolved from a multicenter research initiative to develop a standardized technique for reliably and comprehensively characterizing psychopathology in demented patients. It was intended to sample a range of behaviors sufficiently wide to be useful for most patients with dementia, regardless of severity, and to ensure that the scale consisted of well-anchored, homogeneously scaled items that could be administered by interviewers without extensive training. In its current revised form, the scale has 48 items. It is administered to a knowledgeable informant because of the concerns about reliability of patients as informants. Items are scaled by frequency, not intensity, because of concern that severity judgments would be difficult to anchor and hence less reliable. Only behaviors occurring within a limited period (the previous month) are rated, although provision is made for noting occurrence of behaviors prior to the last month since the illness began. Reliability has been reported as excellent, and factor analysis suggests that five to eight clinically relevant factors can be identified: depressive features, psychotic features, defective self regulation, irritability/aggression, vegetative features, apathy, aggression, and affective lability.

The Psychogeriatric Dependency Rating Scale (PGDRS) (16) is a structured, standardized, observer rating scale for the evaluation of physical function, orientation, and behavior. The behavioral subscale consists of 16 clearly anchored items that are rated according to frequency, intended to capture the time-demanding characteristics of the behaviors in question. It is self-administered by institutional staff most familiar with the subject. Reliability is excellent. It has been shown to be sensitive to change in clinical conditions in nursing home patients over time and is a result of interventions (11). The instrument is brief and has simple and clear instructions. It was developed specifically for use in the long-term care setting. The major disadvantage is that it omits several domains of interest, including depressive features, illusions, apathy, withdrawal, and vegetative features.

By way of brief summary of the topic of behavioral tools, this sampling illustrates some relative advantages and disadvantages. The CERAD BRSD is an example of a comprehensive but time-consuming instrument that is also incompletely developed from a psychometric perspective. It addresses to some extent all of the behavioral features of interest. The simplest instrument, with extensive nursing home use, is the PGDRS: its major weakness is that it is short on detail. It does not address depressive or vegetative features and illusions at all, and only partially addresses anxious and aggressive changes. The BPRS is an example of a sensitive, reliable, general measure of psychopathology used to assess changes in most realms of interest except for illusions. Since it is based on patient interview, it requires considerable training to use. It is reassuring to see that, regardless of which instrument is used, there is general convergence on the finding that the kinds of behavioral syndromes described above emerge. This is further illustrated by one of the most recent and comprehensive scales, the Neuropsychiatric Inventory, which by design addresses all of these domains in addition to euphoria, disinhibition, and lability (17). Much of the relevant clinical outcomes research entails use of instruments such as these, and some familiarity with these issues will facilitate a grasp of the clinical trials in this area.

III. POSSIBLE NEUROBIOLOGICAL BASES OF BEHAVIORAL DISTURBANCES IN DEMENTIA

Evidence is accruing that suggests, but does not establish, that functional alterations in CNS neurotransmitter systems could be identified and possibly linked to mechanism-based pharmacotherapy (18–21). Anatomical, functional, neurochemical, and pharmacological data exist to varying degrees. These will be summarized briefly, relying heavily upon these expert reviews, which can also be used to guide the critical reader to primary references in this area.

Anatomical and functional studies of brain tissues from patients with AD indicate frequent and significant deficiencies in the functional capacity of central serotonergic systems. These findings are supported by cerebrospinal fluid (CSF) studies. Other lines of evidence suggest that such deficiencies play a role in the occurrence of depressive features and of impulsive, aggressive behaviors in nondemented patients. Evidence of this nature leads to the hypothesis that serotonergic therapies might ameliorate depressive and/or agitated signs and symptoms associated with AD. As will be described later in this chapter, an increasing number of clinical trials support this hypothesis.

The data regarding the status of noradrenergic systems in AD are somewhat conflicting. Anatomical studies consistently show loss of neurons in the locus coeruleus in AD. CSF and pharmacological studies indicate increased turnover of norepinephrine in AD as well as normal and sometimes possibly episodically enhanced function of noradrenergic systems. These findings suggest the possibility that patients with AD complicated by significant depressive features might show benefit from treatment with medication enhancing central noradrenergic function. On the other hand, those with agitated or psychotic features might experience aggravation of those features with noradrenergic-enhancing medications, while they might experience reduced, agitated, or psychotic features with medications that decrease central noradrenergic function. This is supported by results from the only pharmacological challenge study in AD using yohimbine and clonidine (18). Treatment studies with noradrenergic enhancing agents in AD patients with significant depressive features are rare and inconclusive, but hint that benefit probably accrues in at least a subset of such patients (22–24). Conversely, treatment studies with agents that reduce CNS noradrenergic function (e.g., beta-blockers) in agitated patients with AD have reported benefit, but, as summarized subsequently in this chapter, have been limited by methodological shortcomings.

It is well known that anatomical and functional cholinergic deficits occur in the brain in AD, and considerable evidence supports a role for this in the cognitive dysfunction associated with the illness. Recent pharmacological studies have shown amelioration of psychotic and, in some cases, agitated behaviors in patients with AD who receive cholinomimetic therapy. This will be reviewed later in the chapter.

Dopamine nerve terminals in the neocortex appear to be spared in AD, while there is evidence of dopaminergic dysfunction in the neostriation (25, 26). This dysfunction may reflect loss of excitatory corticostriatal innervation. It is probably not reliably related to parkinsonian motor symptoms, although such signs are commonly seen in late stages of the illness. Dopaminergic dysfunction may relate to some of the slowed cognitive processing and response time seen in some patients with AD, as well as some of the affective features of the illness (26).

Finally, some evidence points toward the presence of deficits in gamma aminobutyric acid (GABA) systems in some patients with AD. GABAergic therapies are known to modulate aggressive behavior in animals, leading to the hope that the same may be true for agitated or aggressive humans with a variety of clinical syndromes, including AD. Treatment studies in AD provide some encouragement for this idea.

The neurotransmitter abnormalities described may theoretically play a role in the behavioral manifestations of AD, and suggest logical approaches to pharmacotherapy. Clinical trials, however, rarely illuminate pathophysiological mechanisms. Rather, clinical trials primarily address another question: can distress be relieved, diminished, or prevented? The remainder of the chapter will focus on a systematic approach to the evaluation of behavioral complications of dementia, and to the clinical evidence that indicates whether different classes of non-neuroleptic medications used for these features of AD have utility.

IV. A SYSTEMATIC APPROACH TO THE EVALUATION AND MANAGEMENT OF BEHAVIORAL DISTURBANCES IN DEMENTIA

In a series of previous articles, we have proposed a rational and systematic approach to the management of behavioral complications of dementia (17–30). Our current general approach to the assessment and management of these behaviors, summarized below, is generally consistent with the 1992 position statement of the American Association for Geriatric Psychiatry, American Geriatrics Society, and American Psychiatric Association (31).

1. The first step is to carefully delineate the behavioral symptoms by eliciting observations from multiple sources; clarifying aggravating and ameliorating factors as well as frequency and duration of symptoms; and yielding a simple characterization of the target symptoms. These behaviors can often be "forced" into the schematic of typical behavioral syndromes summarized in Table 1.
2. The next step is a comprehensive medical evaluation to determine whether the behavioral problem is the manifestation of a medical disorder. If this is the case, the patient is treated specifically and the target symptoms are monitored until they are resolved. Common problems include delirium, medication side effects, infection, stroke, or pain syndromes. Similarly, a standard psychiatric evaluation should be performed, and any specific psychiatric problem found should be treated until the target symptoms resolve.
3. The third step is to identify and adapt to aggravating factors. Such factors can be internal or external, and can include sensory impairment, environmental disruption, or chaotic schedules. In some cases, problem behaviors can be better understood as well-intentioned but perhaps confused or disruptive efforts to communicate or cope (32). For instance, pacing may reflect a need for stimulation, or verbally disruptive behaviors may represent efforts to obtain assistance. In each of these instances, interventions may be designed according to the patient's particular pattern of cognitive impairment.
4. Attempting to optimize psychosocial factors is an important therapeutic step. Reminiscence, encouragement, validation, maintenance of routines and religious identity, and optimization of social and physical stimulation are all means of accomplishing this end.
5. Behavior management principles are relevant in dealing with behaviors of this nature. In simplistic terms, this refers to the concept that the caregiver's demeanor has a major impact on the patient's behavior.

There are no good data to indicate the effectiveness of the general approach outlined above. It is more a matter of clinical opinion. One rough indicator is provided by unpublished data from a full-time consultation service in a long-term care facility in Rochester, New York. Roughly half of the consultations requested for management of agitation associated with dementia did not result in the administration of psychotropic medications, which at the very least, suggests that nonpharmacological approaches may be helpful.

A. Development of Psychobehavioral Metaphor

For behavioral disturbances that persist after nonpharmacological steps are taken, medications are usually considered. The choice of the optimal type and dosage of medication may involve a process of trial and error (29). In order to guide our selection of pharmacotherapeutic agents, we develop a specific list of disturbed behaviors for each patient, to identify a so-called "psychobehavioral metaphor" or cluster of the most salient signs and symptoms that are roughly analogous to a drug-responsive syndrome (27,29). The term "metaphor" refers to atypical features of classic syndromes, rather than to discrete psychiatric diagnoses.

The following provide examples of some typical "psychobehavioral metaphors," which are similar to the behavioral clusters referred to previously, and presage much of the medication review to follow.

1. *Psychotic features.* Paranoid features of hallucinations may be readily apparent, or they may be inferred from fragmented data such as poorly articulated fears, inappropriate accusations, or agitation occurring only in the presence of interpersonal interactions. This suggestion of paranoia could provide the logical basis for the choice of an antipsychotic agent first. Cholinergic agents may show benefit in some cases.
2. *Depressive features.* Patients with agitation or withdrawal may exhibit negativistic, irritable, dysphoric, or anxious symptoms in the absence of overt syndromal depression. In such cases, it might be reasonable to consider antidepressant medications first. Anticonvulsants or anxiolytics may sometimes be helpful.
3. *Manic symptoms.* Patients with hyperactivity, pressured speech, overly cheerful or irritable mood, decreased sleep, or sexual preoccupation might respond preferentially to thymoleptic agents.
4. *Anxious symptoms.* High levels of anxiety or restlessness, prominent insomnia, or the presence of a reversible situational stressor might suggest use of an anxiolytic agent. It should be emphasized, however, that it may be difficult to distinguish between anxious and depressive features in patients with dementia. Antidepressants, and possibly anticonvulsants, may play a useful role.
5. *Agitation/aggression.* This refers to disruptive physical, verbal, or vocal behaviors such as pacing, wandering, stereotypies, repetition of questions/complaints, screaming, and so on. Those that do not easily fit one of the "metaphors" may respond to virtually any class of psychotropics (see Table 3).
6. *Other behavioral clusters.* Repeated episodes of violence without other behavioral features sometimes lead to the choice of beta-blockers, anticonvulsants, or antipsychotics. Affective lability, distinct from

TABLE 3 Behavioral Clusters Matched to Potentially Relevant Medication Classes

Disturbed affect/mood	Antidepressants Anticonvulsants
Anxiety	Antidepressants Anxiolytics Anticonvulsants
Disturbed ideation/perception	Antipsychotics Cholinergic agents?
Agitation/aggression	Anticonvulsants Antidepressants Antipsychotics Anxiolytics Beta-blockers Cholinergic agents?
Apathy	Stimulants? Antidepressants? Cholinergic agents?
Vegetative features	Antidepressants Stimulants Phototherapy Anxiolytics Melatonin?

depression, may well respond to antidepressant or anticonsulsant therapy. Vegetative changes sometimes dictate the first choice of a medication.

V. THE PROCESS OF TREATMENT

Since this is a population that is medically complex and aged, and very susceptible to adverse effects of medication, the general rule is "start low and go slow." An effort is made to use the potentially appropriate medication class with the lowest risk of side effects, or an agent within the class with the most benign profile. Another aphorism is that every psychotropic trial in this population is an experiment with an *n* of 1, reflecting the confusing heterogeneity among patients resulting from variable etiology of behavioral disturbance, medical and psychiatric comorbidity, age, phenomenology, history of prior illness and treatment, vulnerability to adverse effects, and so forth. Concern about the magnitude of the danger resulting from drug therapy is well justified, although largely results from cases in which medications were used inappropriately, in large doses, or without ongoing monitoring and adjustments. The risk/benefit ratio is improved if the process for initiating treatment follows the general principles above, and if the patient is monitored on a regular basis to assess both benefit and toxicity.

Once a medication is started, both benefit and toxicity should be assessed at regular intervals. In some cases, standardized rating scales are useful for tracking change and documenting efficacy. Doses should generally be titrated upward until there is either clear benefit or early toxicity. If toxicity occurs, a "subtoxic" dose is used and maintained for some time before concluding that a trial has been ineffective. In the absence of benefit or toxicity, some medications permit measurement of plasma levels which can serve to guide treatment.

When a medication is ineffective, it is reasonable to perform the empirical trial in reverse, tapering the medication and watching for problems during withdrawal. At that juncture an alternative medication can be considered. When a treatment trial is positive, it is reasonable to continue treatment for a period of weeks to months, and at some point to taper the medication and reevaluate the symptoms, again performing a clinical trial in reverse. There is little evidence guiding decision making in this regard.

VI. EFFICACY OF DIFFERENT MEDICATIONS

With this general overview in mind, the remainder of the chapter will survey non-neuroleptic psychotropic therapies for the behavioral manifestations of dementia, organized by medication class and building on earlier publications (27,29,30,33). As with the description of prevalence of behaviors in dementia, the tremendous methodological heterogeneity in the studies summarized here will be touched on in the review but not reiterated exhaustively. Very few meet the stringent criteria applied to studies that should influence clinical practice. The purpose of this overview is to ascertain where there is at least some evidence that a form of therapy may be considered by clinicians in attempting to help their patients.

VII. ANTICONVULSANT AGENTS

A. Carbamazepine

Carbamazepine is an antiepileptic with psychotropic properties similar to lithium but with less neurotoxicity (29). The literature contains several pilot

TABLE 4 List of Possible Therapies

Anticonvulsant agents
carbamazepine
valproic acid
Anxiolytics
benzodiazepines
buspirone
Selegiline
Serotonin agents
trazodone
alaproclate
citalopram
fluvoxamine
fluoxetine
sertraline
Beta-blockers
propranolol
pindolol
Cholinergic agents
physostigmine
arecoline
nicotine
tacrine
Miscellaneous therapies
ECT
medroxyprogesterone
conjugated estrogen/diethylstilbestrol
light therapy
zolpidem

studies or case reports (34–40) suggesting that carbamazepine may be effective in relieving some agitated behaviors in patients with dementia. In these cases, plasma levels of carbamazepine ranged from 4 to 12 μg/ml.

Conflicting results have been reported from two double-blind, placebo-controlled, crossover studies evaluating the efficacy of carbamazepine for this problem. In the first study (41), 19 women with what was then termed senile dementia were treated with a maximum of 300 mg/day of carbamazepine for 4 weeks. Subjects also received thioridazine as needed in unspecified dosages. No improvement in agitated symptoms was found. While it is possible that the negative results of this study were a consequence of lack of efficacy of carbamazepine, other factors may have played a role, such as a confounding role of thioridazine, low plasma levels of carbamazepine (averaging 3.4 μg/ml), insufficient intensity of target symptoms, or too brief duration of treatment.

Markedly different results were obtained from a study of 25 patients with dementia and agitation in two nursing homes (42). In this crossover study, carbamazepine in a modal dose of 300 mg/day and placebo were administered over two 5-week periods, separated by a 2-week washout period. The drug was associated with a significant beneficial effect compared with placebo, and was well tolerated by most patients, with minimal effects on laboratory parameters. These findings suggest that carbamazepine in low doses can reduce agitated behaviors in some patients, with limited adverse effects. We have completed a follow-up study involving 51 patients in nursing homes, which was robustly positive (manuscript under review).

B. Valproic Acid

Valproic acid, along with its enteric-coated derivative, divalproex sodium, is another anticonvulsant with psychotropic effects as well as a reduced potential for side effects and drug–drug interaction compared with carbamazepine (29). Uncontrolled studies of this agent have been reported for treatment of agitation in organic mental syndromes, particularly dementia, with encouraging preliminary results. Mazure et al. (43) reported improvement in two older psychotic patients with organic mental syndromes and behavioral dyscontrol when they received valproate treatment that resulted in plasma levels ranging from 30 to 70 μg/ml. Mellow et al. (44) noted improvement in three of four cases of DAT (two of which were complicated by possible cerebrovascular disease), with doses up to 1200 mg/day and levels of approximately 50 to 90 μg/ml. Sival et al. (45) retrospectively reviewed the records of 24 patients with dementia who were treated with valproate in dosages ranging from 240 to 1200 mg/day. They found that six patients achieved a definite positive effect and six patients experienced a partial effect. Physical and verbal aggression and restlessness were the symptoms most likely to respond. Four patients with dementia and physically aggressive behavior were described who showed improvement in behavior when treated with valproate in doses ranging from 1000 to 1500 mg/day, with levels from 24.5 to 54 μg/ml (46). Some functional deterioration was described which was believed to be related to sedation and other psychotropics were used. Lott et al. (47) observed at least a 50% reduction in the frequency of agitated behavior in 8 of 10 elderly patients with dementia who were treated with valproate at dosages of 375 to 750 mg/day for 4 to 43 weeks. Horne and Lindley (48) reported improvement in screaming, uncooperativeness, and paranoia in a 96-year-old woman with Alzheimer's dementia (AD) treated with valproate, achieving a level of 62 μg/ml. Finally, some improvement in behavior was found in 11 of 13 psychogeriatric patients, of whom 12 had dementia in a recent open trial (49). As with many other strategies employed by clinicians for dementia, controlled trials will be necessary to establish whether valproate use should be considered standard clinical practice.

VIII. ANXIOLYTIC AGENTS

A. Benzodiazepines

Despite the fact that benzodiazepines are still widely used in the treatment of agitation, their role in the treatment of dementia has not been studied extensively. Reduction in agitation has been observed in some patients with short-term use (50,51). Available data suggest that agitation associated with anxiety, sleep problems, and tension may be most likely to respond (52,53). Although benzodiazepines are generally safe, they have numerous side effects including sedation, ataxia, paradoxical increase in agitation, amnesic effects, and tolerance and withdrawal when abruptly discontinued after long-term use. It is generally agreed that lorazepam and oxazepam are preferable for older patients because these agents are less likely to accumulate with repeated doses (54). Insufficient data exist at this point regarding the utility of clonazepam, although some anecdotes have been published (55).

B. Buspirone

The literature contains modest evidence that buspirone, a nonbenzodiazepine anxiolytic with partial 5HT-1A agonist effects, may be effective in the treatment of agitation associated with dementia, but well-controlled studies are needed to substantiate these findings. Two case reports describe a reduction in agitation in patients with probable AD (56,57). In an open trial of 16 patients with mixed dementias associated with agitation and aggressive features (58), buspirone in dosages of 15 to 30 mg/day was given; concomitant psychotropics were permitted. Six of the patients were judged to be significantly improved, and side effects occurred in two patients. In another open trial (59), 10 patients with DAT received buspirone in dosages of 15 to 60 mg/day for up to 8 weeks. Four patients showed significant improvement, and agitation scores for the group decreased by 22%. Buspirone appears to be associated with minimal side effects, which can include headache, nervousness, and dizziness. It is unknown whether tolerance or paradoxical effects occur with the drug (29). Low-dose (15 mg/day) buspirone was compared with 1.5 mg/day of haloperidol in a blinded trial involving 26 agitated nursing home patients with AD (60). Both groups showed improved behavior, with greater reduction of tension and anxiety occurring in the buspirone-treated patients. A multicenter trial of low and high doses of buspirone has been completed in the U.S. The results, expected by 1997, will clarify efficacy, safety, and dosing issues.

IX. SELEGILINE

Also known as L-deprenyl, selegiline relatively selectively inhibits monoamine oxidase type B (MAO-B) at lower dosages (10 mg/day) (61). It is believed to enhance dopamine and trace aminergic neurotransmission at this dose. Used primarily in the treatment of Parkinson's disease, selegiline also has been reported to have beneficial effects in some behaviorally disturbed patients with dementia. Significant improvement in anxiety/depression, tension, and excitement scores on the BPRS was observed with 10 mg/day of selegiline in a double-blind, placebo-controlled study involving 17 subjects with DAT (61). In an open pilot study of 14 AD outpatients with mild-to-moderate symptoms who were given 10 mg/day of selegiline for 4 weeks, Schneider et al. (62) found improvement in BPRS agitation factor and depression rating scores. Goad et al. (63) found both beneficial effects and a worsening of symptoms, suggesting the need to individualize the use of selegiline. In their single-blind, 8-week trial of 10 mg/day of selegiline, five of eight severely demented patients with AD who completed the study showed clinical improvement in paranoid and delusional ideation, hallucinations, activity disturbances, anxiety, and phobias. Two patients experienced a worsening of behavior, but returned to their previous improved behavioral state after a decrease of the selegiline dosage to 5 mg/day. A U.S. multicenter trial of 10 mg/day of oral selegiline has been completed by the Alzheimer's Disease Cooperative Study, the results of which, expected by 1997, may shed more light on the relevance of selegiline for treatment of agitation in dementia.

X. SEROTONERGIC AGENTS

Research provides consistent evidence that significant disturbances of 5HT metabolism are associated with Ad and vascular dementia (64). The rationale behind the use of selective serotonin reuptake inhibitors (SSRIs) and other serotonergic agents is that restoring serotonergic function will decrease some signs and symptoms of dementia. Because the evidence for SSRI efficacy in treating agitation in dementia is varied, further controlled studies are needed to guide clinical practice.

A. Trazodone

Several case reports and open studies (65–68) have reported antiagitation efficacy with trazodone, a 5HT-2 antagonist with α_2-adrenergic blocking activity. Used in daily doses typically ranging from 150 to 400 mg, trazodone has been associated with improvements in agitation and aggression in more than half of patients studied. A more recent open study of 13 patients with probable AD (69) found similar results with dosages of 75 mg/day for 10 weeks. Irritability, anxiety, restlessness, and affective disturbance were described, with no side effects observed. In another recent open trial (70), 22 patients with behavioral problems associated with dementia were treated with a mean dosage of 172 mg/day of trazodone for a mean duration of 20 days, with nine patients also receiving concurrent psychoactive medications. Decreases in irritability, aggression, restlessness, inappropriate vocalizations, sleep problems, and wandering were reported, with improvements in global measures of psychopathology. Six patients did not respond to treatment, and two patients experienced delirium. Trazodone (mean dosage, 218 mg/day) was compared with haloperidol in a double-blind, controlled study (71) involving 28 patients with dementia and agitation. Both groups had equal improvement in measures of psychopathology, with some suggestion that trazodone was more effective for repetitive behaviors, verbal aggression, negativism, and resistance to care. One-third fewer dropouts due to adverse effects were seen with trazodone compared with haloperidol. Schneider et al. (72) reported the benefit of trazodone in a case of progressive supranuclear palsy. Although these early findings are encouraging, controlled studies are needed to clarify the clinical utility of trazodone. Among the side effects that can occur with trazodone are orthostatic hypotension, sedation, and delirium (29). Data from a multicenter trial currently being conducted by the Alzheimer's Disease Cooperative Study will shed more light on the utility of trazodone treatment for agitation.

B. Alaproclate

Mixed results have been reported on the efficacy of alaproclate in treating behavioral symptoms associated with DAT. In a 2-week pilot study of alaproclate (400 mg/day) in 12 patients with DAT, Berman et al. (73) found a positive effect in five patients in whom irritability and aggressiveness were reduced. Three patients dropped out of the trial. The same dosage of alaproclate was studied in a subsequent double-blind, placebo-controlled, parallel-group study (74) involving 40 subjects with DAT or vascular dementia. In comparing subjects who received alaproclate or placebo, there were no differences in terms of efficacy or serious adverse symptoms. However, the alaproclate-treated subjects were reported to show significantly improved intellectual function.

C. Citalopram

Results from a multicenter, placebo-controlled study (64) of 98 subjects with mixed dementia suggested that citalopram may be particularly effective for behavioral symptoms associated with dementia. The investigators reported that 20 to 30 mg/day of citalopram significantly improved emotional bluntness, confusion, irritability, anxiety, fear/panic, depressed mood, and restlessness in patients with DAT, but not in patients with vascular dementia. Side effects were few and comparatively mild.

D. Fluvoxamine

Olafsson et al. (75) evaluated the use of fluvoxamine (150 mg/day) in a double-blind, placebo-controlled, parallel-group study of 46 elderly subjects with varying dementia diagnoses. They found no significant effect with fluvoxamine, although there were trends toward improvement in confusion, irritability, anxiety, fear/panic, mood level, and restlessness.

E. Fluoxetine

In an open trial (76) involving five patients with probable AD, 20 to 40 mg/day of fluoxetine was administered for 4 weeks, with no benefit observed. Three of the patients withdrew from the study. Side effects leading to discontinuation of treatment included confusion, agitation, dizziness, gastrointestinal symptoms, anorexia, weight loss, and insomnia.

F. Sertraline

Improvement was seen in 6 of 10 patients with relatively severe DAT in an open trial of sertraline (77). Beneficial effects on irritability, depression, attention, and food intake were reported, with no serious side effects. In an open series in which sertraline was administered to three patients with DAT, Burke et al. (78) found decreased depressive symptoms and psychosis. No side effects occurred.

XI. BETA-BLOCKERS

Beta-blockers have been studied in patients with mixed organic brain syndromes, but relatively little in patients with dementia. Most reports consist of open trials (79,80). One double-blind, placebo-controlled crossover study of sustained-release propranolol in doses up to 520 mg/day was performed in 10 patients with severe dementia of various etiologies (81). Aggressiveness improved in the majority of patients. In another study, six patients with dementia and agitation received propranolol in doses ranging from 80 to 560 mg/day for up to 2 months: all were described as improved (82). Two studies reported beneficial effects of pindolol in patients with organic brain syndrome and agitation, but no dementia diagnoses were given (83,84).

The literature regarding use of beta-blockers for agitation associated with dementia is limited, and a number of reports came from the same investigative group, which limits their generalizability. Most of the studies permitted use of concomitant psychoactive medications. Adverse reactions, which appear to be more likely with propranolol than pindolol, included bradycardia, hypotension, the potential for worsening of congestive heart failure or asthma, sedation, confusion, hallucinosis, depression, and increased AV block. In our experience, bradycardia is frequently the dose-limiting factor in open clinical trials. Where target symptoms are identified, impulsivity, hostility, and assultiveness have been reported to be most responsive.

In the absence of controlled investigations, and the limited available literature, it seems reasonable to suggest that this medication may have a tertiary role in the treatment of agitation associated with dementia, but only after safer and more conventional therapies fail, and even then it should be used with full awareness of the potential for toxic effects.

XII. LITHIUM

The available literature regarding lithium is limited. It was originally advocated for use in dementia by analogy to its putative antiaggression efficacy in patients with mental retardation, traumatic brain injury with manic complications, and stroke patients suffering lability (85). One patient with AD was part of an open series treated with lithium in doses up to 1200 mg/day, and no improvement in agitation was found (86). A single case report showed improvement in agitation, wandering, hostility, and sleep disturbance within 4 days of initiation of lithium therapy at a dose of 300 mg/day (87). Another case report of a patient with dementia and agitation indicated partial improvement on lithium, with a more complete response, subsequently, to carbamazepine (36). There was another report of lack of efficacy in an open trial in patients with unspecified organic brain syndromes (88).

The limited literature indicates that the majority of patients with dementia and agitation did not show improvement with lithium, although there were some exceptions. There are no controlled clinical studies. In theory, one might expect maniclike symptoms to be most responsive, such as pressured speech, motor hyperactivity, irritable or elevated mood, and so on (85). However, toxicity is common in the elderly and can include confusional states, extrapyramidal features, ataxia, and other CNS and neuromuscular toxicity (33,85). Given the state of the field, it is hard to justify using lithium in an older patient lacking a syndromal diagnosis of bipolar disorder.

XIII. CHOLINERGIC THERAPY

Several investigators have reported behavioral effects of cholinergic agents including physostigmine (89–92). Of these studies, the tacrine experience may be the most relevant. Several multicenter trials of newer cholinesterase inhibitors are planned which will clarify the role of these medications in ameliorating behavioral disturbances in dementia.

XIV. MISCELLANEOUS THERAPIES

A. Electroconvulsive Therapy

The beneficial use of electroconvulsive therapy (ECT) in screaming, demented patients was described by Carlyle et al. (93). The investigators reported on a series of three verbally agitated elderly patients whose symptoms were refractory to treatment with an antipsychotic, antidepressant, anticonvulsant, or a benzodiazepine. Early in the course of bilateral ECT, each patient showed a dramatic improvement, with a rapid resolution of the screaming behavior. Holmberg et al. (94) also presented a single case report of the efficacy of ECT for a patient with life-threatening agitation.

B. Hormonal Therapy

Estrogen and progestogen therapies have been reported to be effective in treating demented elderly men who exhibit physical aggression, including sexual aggression. Kyomen et al. (95) administered estrogen to two physically aggressive elderly men and reported a reduction in the number of incidents of physical, but not verbal, aggression or physical or verbal repetitive behaviors. Cooper et al. (96) reported success in using medroxyprogesterone acetate (MPA) to suppress disruptive sexual behavior in four elderly men with dementia. Within 2 weeks of initiating MPA therapy, the sexual acting out had stopped. Neither estrogen nor MPA therapy was associated with serious side effects.

C. Phototherapy

Interesting work has been reported examining the theory that bright-light pulses administered in the evening may ameliorate sleep–wake cycle disturbances and reduce agitation in patients with AD who have sleep disorders and severe "sundowning" (a syndrome of recurring confusion and increased agitation in late afternoon or early evening). In an open trial of 10 inpatients with AD whose symptoms included sundowning behavior and sleep disturbances,

Satlin et al. (97) evaluated the use of bright-light treatment for 2 h/day between 7:00 and 9:00 p.m. for 1 week. Clinical ratings of sleep–wakefulness on the evening nursing shift improved in 8 of the 10 patients treated.

D. Zolpidem

Zolpidem is a nonbenzodiazepine sedative hypnotic shown to have efficacy in older subjects with psychiatric disorders (98). Two patients with Alzheimer's disease and agitation were reported to show improvement in agitation in an open trial with this medication in doses from .5 to 5 mg/day, both of whom received other psychotropic therapy (99). There are no controlled data available.

XV. SUMMARY

Significant behavioral disturbances are common in patients with dementias of varying etiologies and pose a major challenge for clinicians. It is imperative to undertake a logical sequence of evaluations and interventions in such patients to establish whether nonpharmacological approaches can help. Only after they fail should pharmacotherapy be considered.

Clinical custom has resulted in the use of antipsychotics first, without necessarily paying close attention to differential efficacy for different target symptoms, and ignoring the fact that they only show moderate efficacy. We propose the classification of behavioral disturbances into clusters to provide a meaningful guide to pharmacotherapy. Using the "psychotherapeutic metaphor" approach, patients with psychoticlike symptoms would be treated first with antipsychotics. Such symptoms have been shown to improve with the administration of low doses of traditional antipsychotic agents such as haloperidol and thioridazine, with data minimally available so far regarding the efficacy of atypical antipsychotic agents clozapine and risperidone. Some evidence also suggests the cholinesterase inhibitors as well as some SSRIs may improve psychotic symptoms in patients with dementia.

Other target symptom clusters can be used to guide the initial selection of a medication for other subtypes of disruptive or agitated behaviors. Literature exists describing the use of anticonvulsants, anxiolytics, various antidepressants, beta-blockers, and serotonergic and other agents to manage disturbed behaviors in dementia. Available evidence regarding non-neuroleptic therapies ranges from minimal case reports to the occasional well-designed, double-blind, placebo-controlled, randomized, parallel group study. Each of the medications presented has at least some theoretical as well as clinical rationale. Those with more compelling evidence for efficacy, as well as evidence for safety, and most relevant for the cardinal target symptoms in an individual, should be considered first for a careful clinical trial. This of course entails close monitoring of target symptoms as well as toxicities. Drug levels are sometimes useful as a guide in the absence of efficacy or toxicity. Both clinical experience and a little published evidence about withdrawal of psychotropics suggest that it is desirable to consider judicious, empirical discontinuation trials in most, if not all, patients to learn whether the medication is still necessary.

Encouraging early findings have been reported for the antidepressants trazodone and selegiline. Varying results have been obtained using SSRI therapy, with citalopram and sertraline showing more promise than other SSRIs in treating behavioral symptoms in patients with dementia. Antidepressants as a class, particularly the serotonergic agents, may have the most benign side-effect profile, although paradoxical agitation can sometimes occur. Among anticonvulsants, carbamazepine and valproate have shown efficacy in uncontrolled studies; carbamazepine has produced conflicting results in two published controlled studies. The potential for drug–drug interactions and toxicity resulting from carbamazepine dictates caution. Such issues may be less pressing if valproate is shown to have similar efficacy. In either case, it is likely that the long-term toxicity of anticonvulsants will be shown to be less than for the antipsychotics. Most of the benzodiazepine data are old and suggest mild efficacy overall, although some individual patients do well. What we see clinically tends to be nonspecific sedation, with relatively little responsiveness that suggests a specific "antiagitation" effect. The anxiolytic buspirone was shown to be effective in reducing agitated behaviors in some case reports and open trials, relatively free of significant toxicity, but extensive data are lacking at this point.

The available data indicate that there can be alternatives to the use of neuroleptics in the treatment of behavioral disturbances associated with dementia. There are almost no comparison studies; those available suggest that efficacy of such agents is roughly equal to that of antipsychotics (e.g., trazodone, benzodiazepines). The side-effect profiles of these agents, however, are substantially different and should influence clinical decision making. It remains to be seen whether and to what extent newer agents with different side-effect profiles (e.g., nefazodone) will have on efficacy and toxicity profiles in these populations.

There will be data in the near future from controlled studies of nonneuroleptic therapies. The Alzheimer's Disease Cooperative Study (funded by the National Institute on Aging) has conducted a multicenter study of selegiline as well as a study comparing haloperidol, trazodone, or caregiver training techniques. A confirmatory follow-up study of carbamazepine will be presented shortly. Further data are pending regarding the efficacy of valproate. Multicenter studies have been or are being conducted of buspirone, sertaline, queriapine, olanzepine, risperidone, and second-generation cholinesterase inhibitors such as clonepezil and ENA 713. Such studies will provide useful guideposts for future clinical decision making.

REFERENCES

1. Doernberg M. Stolen Mind. Chapel Hill, NC: Algonquin Press, 1989.
2. Ferris SH, Steinberg G, Shulman E, et al. Institutionalization of Alzheimer's patients: reducing precipitating factors through family counseling. Arch Found Thanatol 1985; 12:7.
3. Tariot P, Blazina L. The psychopathology of dementia. In: Morris J, ed. Handbook of Dementing Illnesses. New York: Marcel Dekker, 1993:461–475.
4. Teri L, Larson E, Reifler B. Behavioral disturbance in dementia of the Alzheimer's type. J Am Geriatr Soc 1988; 36:1–6.
5. Reisberg B, Franssen E, Sclan S, Kluger A, Ferris S. Stage specific incidence of potentially remedial behavioral symptoms in aging and Alzheimer's disease: a study of 120 patients using the Behav-AD. Bull Clin Neurosci 1989; 54:95–112.
6. Wragg R, Jeste D. Overview of depression and psychosis in Alzheimer's disease. Am J Psychiatry 1989; 146:577–582.
7. Devanand DP, Brockington CD, Moody BJ, Brown RP, Mayeux R, Endicott J, Sackeim HA. Behavioral syndromes in Alzheimer's disease. Int Psychogeriatr 1992; 4:161–184.
8. Tariot PN, Mack JL, Patterson MB, Edland SD, Weiner MF, Fillenbaum G, Blazina L, Teri L, Rubin E, Mortimer JA, Stern Y, and the Behavioral Pathology Committee of the Consortium to Establish a Registry for Alzheimer's Disease. The Behavioral Rating Scale for Dementia of the Consortium to Establish a Registry for Alzheimer's Disease. Am J Psychiatry 1995; 152:1349–1357.
9. Finkel S, Costa de Silva J, Cohen G, Miller S, Sartorius N. Behavioral and psychological signs and symptoms of dementia: a consensus statement on current knowledge and implications for research and treatment. Int Psychogeriatr 1996; 8(suppl 3):497–500.
10. Teri L, Logsdon RG. Methodologic issues regarding outcome measures for clinical drug trials of psychiatric complications in dementia. J Geriatr Psychiatry Neurol 1995; 8 (suppl 1):S8–S16.
11. Tariot PN, Teri L, Porsteinsson A, Weiner M. Measurement of behavioral disturbance in chronic care populations. J Mental Health Aging, in press.
12. Weiner M, Koss E, Wild K, Folks D, Tariot P, Luszcynska H, Whitehouse P. The measures of psychiatric symptoms in Alzheimer's patients: a review. Alzheimer Dis Related Disord 1996; 10:20–30.
13. Rhoades HM, Overall JE. The semistructured BPRS interview and rating guide. Psychopharmacol Bull 1988; 24:101–104.
14. Overall JE, Beller SA. The Brief Psychiatric Rating Scale (BPRS) in geropsychiatrics research: I. Factor structure on an inpatient unit. J Gerontol 1984; 39:187–193.

15. Overall JE, Gorham DR. The Brief Psychiatric Rating Scale: recent developments in ascertainment and scaling. Psychopharmacol Bull 1988; 24:101–104.
16. Wilkinson I, Graham-White J. Psychogeriatric Dependency Rating Scale (PGDRS): a method of assessment for use by nurses. Br J Psychiatry 1980; 137:558–565.
17. Cummings JL, Mega M, Gray K, et al. The Neuropsychiatric Inventory: comprehensive assessment of psychopathology in dementia. Neurology 1994; 44:2308–2314.
18. Raskind MA, Peskind ER. Neurobiologic bases of noncognitive behavioral problems in Alzheimer's disease. Alzheimer Dis Assoc Disord 1994; 8(suppl 3):54–60.
19. Zubenko GS, Moossy J, Martinez AJ, et al. Neuropathology and neurochemical correlates of psychosis in primary dementia. Arch Neurol 1991; 48:619–624.
20. Zubenko GS, Moossy J. Major depression in primary dementia: clinical and neuropathologic correlates. Arch Neurol 1988; 45:1182–1186.
21. Palmer AM, Stratmann GC, Procter AW, Bowen DM. Possible neurotransmitter basis of behavioral changes in Alzheimer's disease. Ann Neurol 1988; 23:616–620.
22. Reifler BV, Teri L, Raskind M, Veith R, et al. Double-blind trial of imipramine in Alzheimer's disease patients with and without depression. Am J Psychiatry 1989; 146:45–49.
23. Reynolds CF III, Perel JM, Kupfer DJ, et al. Open-trial response to antidepressant treatment in elderly patients with mixed depression and cognitive impairment. Psychiatry Res 1987; 21:111–122.
24. Greenwald BS, Kramer-Ginsberg E, Marin DB, et al. Dementia with coexistent major depression. Am J Psychiatry 1989; 146:1472–1478.
25. Blennow W, Wallin A, Gottfries CG, et al. Significance of decreased lumbar CSF levels of HVA and S-HIAA in Alzheimer's disease. Neurobiol Aging 1991; 13:107–113.
26. Palmer AM, DeKosky ST. Monoamine neurons in aging and Alzheimer's disease. J Neurol Transm (Gen Sect) 1993; 91:135–159.
27. Leibovici A, Tariot PN. Agitation associated with dementia: a systematic approach to treatment. Psychopharmacol Bull 1988; 24:49–53.
28. Tariot PN. General approaches to behavioral disturbances. In: Reichman ME, Katz P, eds. Psychiatric Care in the Nursing Home. Oxford Press, 1996:10–22.
29. Tariot PN, Schneider LS, Katz IR. Anticonvulsant and other non-neuroleptic treatment of agitation in dementia. J Geriatr Psychiatry Neurol 1995; 8(suppl 1): S28–S39.
30. Tariot PN. Treatment strategies for agitation and psychosis in dementia. J Clin Psychiatry 1996; 57[suppl 14]:21–29.
31. Board of Directors of the American Association for Geriatric Psychiatry, Clinical Practice Committee of the American Geriatrics Society, and Committee On Long-Term Care and Treatment for the Elderly, American Psychiatric Association. Psychotherapeutic medications in the nursing home. J Am Geriatr Soc 1992; 40:946–949.
32. Cohen-Mansfield J, Marx MS, Werner P. Agitation in elderly persons: an integrative report of findings in a nursing home. Int Psychogeriatr 1992; 4(suppl 2): 221–240.
33. Schneider LS, Sobin PB. Non-neuroleptic treatment of behavioral symptoms and agitation in Alzheimer's disease and other dementia. Psychopharmacol Bull 1992; 28:71–79.

34. McAllister TW. Carbamazepine in mixed frontal lobe and psychiatric disorders. J Clin Psychiatry 1985; 46:393–394.
35. Anton RF, Waid LR, Fossey M, et al. Case report of carbamazepine treatment of organic brain syndrome with psychotic features. J Clin Psychopharmacol 1986; 6:232–234.
36. Essa M. Carbamazepine in dementia. J Clin Psychopharmacol 1986; 6:234–236.
37. Leibovici A, Tariot PN. Carbamazepine treatment of agitation associated with dementia. J Geriatr Psychiatry Neurol 1988; 1:110–112.
38. Patterson JF. A preliminary study of carbamazepine in the treatment of assaultive patients with dementia. J Geriatr Psychiatry Neurol 1988; 1:21–23.
39. Gleason RP, Schneider LS. Carbamazepine treatment of agitation in Alzheimer's outpatients refractory to neuroleptics. J Clin Psychiatry 1990; 51:115–118.
40. Lemke MR. Effect of carbamazepine on agitation in Alzheimer's inpatients refractory to neuroleptics. J Clin Psychiatry 1995; 56:354–357.
41. Chambers CA, Bain J, Rosbottom R, et al. Carbamazepine in senile dementia and overactivity—a placebo controlled double blind trial. IRCS Med Sci 1982; 10:505–506.
42. Tariot PN, Erb R, Leibovici A, et al. Carbamazepine treatment of agitation in nursing home patients with dementia: a preliminary study. J Am Geriatr Soc 1994; 42:1160–1166.
43. Mazure CM, Druss BG, Cellar JS. Valproate treatment of older psychotic patients with organic mental syndromes and behavioral dyscontrol. J Am Geriatr Soc 1992; 40:914–916.
44. Mellow AM, Solano-Lopez C, Davis S. Sodium valproate in the treatment of behavioral disturbance in dementia. J Geriatr Psychiatry Neurol 1993; 6:205–209.
45. Sival RC, Haffmans PMJ, van Gent PP, van Nieuwkerk JF. The effect of sodium valproate on disturbed behavior in dementia. J Am Geriatr Soc 1994; 42:906–907.
46. Sandborn WD, Bendfeldt F, Handy R. Valproic acid for physically aggressive behavior in geriatric patients. Am J Geriatr Psychiatry 1995; 3:239–242.
47. Lott AD, McElroy SL, Keys MA. Valproate in the treatment of behavioral agitation in elderly patients with dementia. J Neuropsychiatry Clin Neurosci 1995; 7:314–319.
48. Horne M, Lindley SE. Divalproex sodium in the treatment of aggressive behavior and dysphoria in patients with organic brain syndromes. J Clin Psychiatry 1995; 56:430–431.
49. Porsteinsson A, Tariot P, Erb R, Gaile S. An open trial of valproate for agitation in geriatric neuropsychiatric disorder. Am J Geriatr Psychiatry, in press.
50. Chesrow RJ, Kaplitz SE, Vetra H, et al. Blind study of oxazepam in the management of geriatric patients with behavioral problems. Clin Med 1965; 13:1001–1005.
51. DeLemos GP, Clement WR, Nickels E. Effect of diazepam suspension in geriatric patients hospitalized for psychiatric illnesses. J Am Geriatr Soc 1965;1 3:355–359.
52. Beber CR. Management of behavior in the institutionalized aged. Dis Nerve Syst 1965; 26:591–595.
53. Coccaro EF, Kramer E, Zemishlany Z, et al. Pharmacologic treatment of noncognitive behavioral disturbances in elderly demented patients. Am J Psychiatry 1990; 147:1640–1645.

54. Hyman SE, Arana GW. Handbook of Psychiatric Drug Therapy. Boston: Little Brown & Co. 1987:115–123.
55. Freinhar JP, Alvarez WA. Clonazepam treatment of organic brain syndromes in three elderly patients. J Clin Psychiatry 1986; 47:525–526.
56. Colenda CC III. Buspirone in treatment of agitation demented patients. Lancet 1988; 1:1169.
57. Tiller JWG, Dakis JA, Shaw JM. Short-term buspirone treatment in disinhibition with dementia. Lancet 1988; 2:510.
58. Herrmann N, Eryavec G. Buspirone in the management of agitation and aggression associated with dementia. Am J Geriatr Psychiatry 1993; 1:249–253.
59. Sakauye KM, Camp CJ, Ford PA, et al. Effects of buspirone on agitation associated with dementia. Am J Geriatr Psychiatry 1993; 1:82–84.
60. Cantillon M, Brunswick R, Molina D, et al. Buspirone vs haloperidol: a double-blind trial for agitation in a nursing home population with Alzheimer's disease. Am J Geriatr Psychiatry 1996; 4:263–267.
61. Tariot PN, Cohen RM, Sunderland T, et al. L-deprenyl in Alzheimer's disease: preliminary evidence for behavioral change with monoamine oxidase B inhibition. Arch Gen Psychiatry 1987; 44:427–433.
62. Schneider LS, Pollock VE, Zemansky MF, et al. A pilot study of low dose l-deprenyl in Alzheimer's disease. J Geriatr Psychiatry Neurology 1991; 4:143–148.
63. Goad DL, Davis CM, Liem P, et al. The use of selegiline in Alzheimer's patients with behavior problems. J Clin Psychiatry 1991; 52:342–345.
64. Nyth AL, Gottfries CG. The clinical efficacy of citalopram in treatment of emotional disturbances in dementia disorders: a Nordic multicentre study. Br J Psychiatry 1990; 157:894–901.
65. Simpson DM, Foster D. Improvement in organically disturbed behavior with trazodone treatment. J Clin Psychiatry 1986; 47:482.
66. Tingle D. Trazodone in dementia. J Clin Psychiatry 1986; 47:482.
67. Greenwald BS, Marin DB, Silverman SM. Serotoninergic treatment of screaming and banging in dementia. Lancet 1986; 2:1464–1465.
68. Pinner E, Rich CL. Effects of trazodone on aggressive behavior in seven patients with organic mental disorders. Am J Psychiatry 1988; 145:1295–1296.
69. Lebert F, Pasquier F, Petit H. Behavioral effects of trazodone in Alzheimer's disease. J Clin Psychiatry 1994; 55:536–538.
70. Houlihan DJ, Mulsant BH, Sweet RA, et al. A naturalistic study of trazodone in the treatment of behavioral complications of dementia. Am J Geriatr Psychiatry 1994; 2:78–85.
71. Sultzer DL, Gray KF, Gunay I, et al. A double-blind comparison of trazodone and haloperidol for treatment of agitation in patients with dementia. Am J Geriatr Psychiatry 1997; 5:60–69.
72. Schneider LS, Gleason RP, Chui HC. Progressive supranuclear palsy with agitation: response to trazodone but not to thiothixine or carbamazepine. J Geriatr Psychiatry Neurol 1989; 2:109–112.
73. Bergman I, Brane G, Gottfries CG, et al. Alaproclate: a pharmacokinetic and biochemical study in patients with dementia of Alzheimer type. Psychopharmacology 1983; 80:279–283.

74. Dehlin O, Hedenrud B, Jansson P, et al. A double-blind comparison of alaproclate and placebo in the treatment of patients with senile dementia. Acta Psychiatr Scand 1985; 71:190–196.
75. Olafsson K, Jirgensen S, Jensen HV, et al. Fluvoxamine in the treatment of demented elderly patients: a double-blind, placebo-controlled study. Acta Psychiatr Scand 1992; 85:453–456.
76. Geldmacher DS, Waldman AJ, Doty L, et al. Fluoxetine in dementia of the Alzheimer's type: prominent adverse effects and failure to improve cognition. J Clin Psychiatry 1994; 55:161.
77. Volicer L, Rheaume Y, Cyr D. Treatment of depression in advanced Alzheimer's disease using sertraline. J Geriatr Psychiatry Neurol 1994; 7:227–229.
78. Burke WJ, Folks DG, Roccaforte WH, et al. Serotonin reuptake inhibitors for the treatment of coexisting depression and psychosis in dementia of the Alzheimer type. Am J Geriatr Psychiatry 1994; 2:352–354.
79. Petrie WM, Ban TA, Berney S, et al. Loxapine in psychogeriatrics: a placebo- and standard-controlled clinical investigation. J Clin Psychopharmacol 1982; 2:122–126.
80. Greendyke RM, Schuster DB, Wooton JA. Propranolol in the treatment of assaultive patients with organic brain disease. J Clin Psychopharmacol 1984; 4:282–285.
81. Greendyke RM, Kanter DR, Schuster DB, et al. Propranolol treatment of assaultive patients with organic brain disease: a double-blind crossover, placebo-controlled study. J Nerv Ment Dis 1986; 174:290–294.
82. Weiler PG, Mungas D, Bernick C. Propranolol for the control of disruptive behavior in senile dementia. J Geriatr Psychiatry Neurol 1988; 1:226–230.
83. Greendyke RM, Kanter DR. Therapeutic effects of pindolol on behavioral disturbances associated with organic brain disease: a double blind study. J Clin Psychiatry 1986; 47:423–426.
84. Greendyke RM, Berkner JP, Webster JC, et al. Treatment of behavioral problems with pindolol. Psychosomatics 1989; 30:161–165.
85. Risse SC, Barnes R. Pharmacologic treatment of agitation associated with dementia. J Am Geriatr Soc 1986; 34:368–376.
86. Williams KH, Goldstein C. Cognitive and affective response to lithium in patients with organic brain syndrome. Am J Psychiatry 1979; 136:800–803.
87. Havens WW, Cole J. Successful treatment of dementia with lithium. J Clin Psychopharmacol 1982; 2:71–72.
88. Holton A, George K. The use of lithium in severely demented patients with behavioral disturbance. Br J Psychiatry 1985; 146:99–100.
89. Cummings JL, Gorman DG, Shapira J. Physostigmine ameliorates the delusions of Alzheimer's disease. Biol Psychiatry 1993; 33:536–541.
90. Tariot PN, Cohen RM, Wilkowitz JA, et al. Multiple dose arecoline infusions in Alzheimer's disease. Arch Gen Psychiatry 1988; 45:901–908.
91. Newhouse PA, Sunderland T, Tariot PN, et al. Intravenous nicotine in Alzheimer's disease: a pilot study. Psychopharmacology 1988; 95:171–175.
92. Kaufer DI, Cummings JL, Christine D. Effect of tacrine on behavioral symptoms in Alzheimer's disease: an open-label study. J Geriatr Psychiatry Neurol 1996; 9:1–6.

93. Carlyle W, Killick L, Ancill R. ECT: an effective treatment in the screaming demented patient. J Am Geriatr Soc 1991; 39:637–639.
94. Holmberg S, Tariot PN, Challipalli R. Efficacy of ECT for agitation in dementia: a case report. Am J Geriatr Psychiatry 1996; 4:330–334.
95. Kyomen HH, Nobel KW, Wei JY. The use of estrogen to decrease aggressive physical behavior in elderly men with dementia. J Am Geriatr Soc 1991; 39:1110–1112.
96. Cooper AJ. Medroxyprogesterone acetate (MPA) treatment of sexual acting out in men suffering from dementia. J Clin Psychiatry 1987; 48:368–370.
97. Satlin A, Volicer L, Ross V, et al. Bright light treatment of behavioral and sleep disturbances in patients with Alzheimer's disease. Am J Psychiatry 1992; 149: 1028–1032.
98. Scharf MB, Roth T, Vogel GW, Walsh JK. A multicenter, placebo-controlled study evaluating zolpidem in the treatment of chronic insomnia. J Clin Psychiatry 1994; 55:192–199.
99. Jackson CW, Pitner JK, Mintzer JE. Zolpidem for the treatment of agitation in elderly demented patients. J Clin Psychiatry 1996; 57(8):372–373.
100. Rosen WG, Mohs RC, Davis KL. A new rating scale for Alzheimer's disease. Am J Psychiatry 1984; 141:1356–1364.
101. Reisberg B, Borenstein J, Salob SP, et al. Behavioral symptoms in Alzheimer's disease: phenomenology and treatment. J Clin Psychiatry 1987; 48(suppl 5):9–15.
102. Cohen-Mansfield J, Billig N. Agitated behaviors in the elderly: I. a conceptual review. J Am Geriatr Soc 1986; 34:711–721.

Index

Acetophenazine, psychosis, 305
Acetylcholinesterase (AChE), AD, 15
Acetylcholinesterase (AChE) inhibitors:
  AD, 383–388
  APP, 388
Activities of daily living (ADLs), depression, 62–63
Adipose tissue, drug distribution, 32
Age-associated memory impairment, 3
Aging:
  brain, 3–10
  etiology, 1–2
  neurochemistry, 1–18
Agoraphobia, beta-blockers, 375
Agranulocytosis, 316, 338, 416
Akathisia, 312–313, 374
Alaproclate, behavioral complications, dementia, 442
Albumin, 34
Alcohol withdrawal, anxiety, 370
Alexithymia, 64
Alprazolam:
  CYP 3A3/4, 51
  digoxin, 53
  panic disorder, 373
  SSRIs, 51
Alzheimer's dementia, 10–16
  clozapine, 306–307
  depression, 137–138, 227, 230
  paroxetine, 138
  resperidone, 309–310
Alzheimer's disease (AD):
  CRH, 10
  neurochemical changes, pharmacological implications, 16–18
  prevalence, 381
  treatment, 234
    acetylcolinesterase inhibitors, 383–388
    cholinergic compounds, 382–388
    cognitive enhancers, 395–396
    future, 390–395
  WMLs, 6
Alzheimer's disease-associated protein (ADAP), 6
Amantadine:
  AD, 17
  DIP, 313
  PD depression, 204
Amitriptyline:
  anticholinergic effects, 53
  antihypertensive effects, 144
  clearance, 35
  DD, 105
  dementia, 235–236
  depression, 81
  postcancer depression, 193
  poststroke depression, 167
Amobarbital, 373
Amoxapine, dd, 106
Ampakines, AD, 392
Amphetamine:
  dementia, 235

[Amphetamine]
depression, 245–254
history, 245–246
mechanism, 252
methylphenidate, 249–250
mood change, 253–245
PD depression, 214
side effects, 252
Amphetamine psychosis, 246
Amyloid cascade hypothesis, 10–11
Amyloid protein precursor (APP), 5, 394
Aniracetam, AD, 391–392
Antacids:
adsorption, 44
neuroleptic interactions, 319
Antiarrhythmic drugs, interactions, 55
Anticholinergic drugs, 9
AD, 418
interactions, 53, 319
mood effects, 203–204
side effects, 311–312, 412
Anticoagulant drugs, interactions, 54–55
Anticonvulsant drugs:
behavioral complications, 437–440
bipolar disorder, 258–296
Antidepressant drugs, 375–376
2D6, 47
cardiovascular effects, 144–151
clinical trials, 229–230
sedative, 362
selection, 81–84, 121
side effects, 73–74, 169–170
studies, 71–72, 119–120
Antihistamines, anxiety, 375
Antihypertensive drugs:
depression, 234
interactions, 55–56
Anti-inflammatory drugs, AD, 390–391
Antioxidants:
AD, 393–394
tardive dyskinesia, 315
Antiparkinsonian drugs, side effects, 329–331
Antipsychotic drugs:
anxiety, 374
hepatic clearance, 29
Anwesenheit, 330
Anxiety, 367
alcohol withdrawal, 370
antihistamines, 375
antipsychotic drugs, 374
caffeine, 370
DD, 103
depression, 370–371
differential diagnosis, 368
epidemiology, 371–372
insomnia, 370
left ventricular failure, 368
PD, 204
Anxiolytic drugs, behavioral complications, dementia, 440
A1-acid glycoprotein, 34, 304
Apathy, poststroke, 178
Aphasia:
apomorphine, 235
bromocriptine, 235
Apolipoprotein E (ApoE), AD, 12–13
Apomorphine, aphasia, 235
Apoptosis, defined, 2
Aricept, AD, 386
A68, 6
Aspartate, AD, 391
Aspirin, depression, 234
Astemizole, CYP 3A3/4, 51
Astrocytes, 4–5
Atypical depression, 373

B-amyloid protein (AB), 5
AD, 10–12
Behavioral complications:
dementia
assessment, 429–432
classification, 428
guidelines, 433–436
neurobiology, 432–433
nonneuroleptic treatment, 427–448
treatment, 405–419, 433–448
evaluation, 405–406, 433–436
Benign senescent forgetfulness, 3
Benzodiazepines, 350–359, 373–374

adverse effects, 358–359, 414–415
anxiety, 377
behavioral complications, dementia, 440
biochemistry, 351–352
bipolar disorder, 267
clearance, 29, 35
dementia, 235
impulsive aggression, 287
lithium, 264–265
pharmacodynamics, 352
pharmacokinetics, 352–355
absorption, 352
drug interactions, 355
elimination, 353–355
lipophilicity, 352
metabolism, 352–353
protein binding, 352
poststroke anxiety, 177
side effects, 374
SSRIs, 51
Bereavement psychopathology, 122
Bereavement depression:
depressive syndromes, 117
diagnosis, 117–119
risk factors, 118
drug selection, 121
future studies, 122–123
philosophy, 116–117
psychotherapy, 121–122
selection, 121
studies, 119–120
Beta-blockers:
agoarphobia, 375
behavioral complications, dementia, 443–444
impulsive aggression, 287
social phobias, 375
Biologically informed psychotherapy, bereavement depression, 121–122
Biperiden, PD depression, 204
Bipolar depression, 68
Bipolar disorder:
adjunctive antidepressants, 265
adjunctive nonsomatic treatment, 267–268
anticonvulsant drugs, 258–296
assessment, 259–260
examination, 260
history, 259–260
laboratory tests, 260
behavioral intervention, 261
characteristics, 285–286
environmental control, 261
lithium, 259–268
adjunctive medication, 264–265, 267
continuation therapy, 265
dose, 266
efficacy, 261–262, 266
guidelines, 262–263, 266–267
maintenance therapy, 265
selection, 261
resperidone, 308
treatment setting, 260–261
Brain, 3–10
involution, 1–3, 9
compensatory mechanisms, 2–3
morphological changes, 4–6
neurochemical changes, 6–8
pathological, 10–18
neuroendocrine functions, 9–10
pharmacological implications, 9
weight, 4
Brain lesions, cognitive impairment, 228
Brief Psychiatric Rating Scale (BPRS), 429–430
Broca's aphasia, 163
Bromides, 372–373
Bromocriptine:
PD depression, 204
serotonergic effects, 56
Brotizolam:
elimination, 354
metabolism, 353
Bupropion:
cardiovascular effects, 149
depression, 68, 71, 81, 83
PD depression, 202, 210–212, 232
postcancer depression, 194

Buspirone, 374
Butyrophenone, side effects, 311
Buxpirone, behavioral complications, dementia, 440

Caffeine, anxiety, 370
Cancer, depression, 187–195
Capgra's syndrome, 331
Carbamazepine, 52
  behavioral complications, dementia, 437–439, 447
  bipolar disorder, 288, 294–295
  impulsive aggression, 286, 290–291
  interactions, 355
  neuroleptic interactions, 319
  poststroke mania, 176
  valproate, 294
Carbidopa, serotonergic effects, 56
Cardiac arrhythmias, lithium toxicity, 276
Cardiac conduction, TCAs, 146
Cardiac disease:
  depression, 143–156
  prognosis, depression influence, 152–154
CAST I (Cardiac Arrhythmic Suppression Trial), 148–149
CAST II (Cardiac Arrhythmic Suppression Trial), 148–149
CERAD Behavior Rating Scale for Dementia (BRSD), 431
Cerebral amyloid angiopathy (CAA), aging, 5
Chloridiazepoxide, 373
Chlorpromazine:
  behavioral complications, 411
  dopaminergic blockade, 331
  side effects, 416
Cholestyramine, absorption, 44
Choline acetyltransferase (CAT), 7
  AD, 15, 17, 382
Choreoathetosis, 275
CI-789, AD, 382–383
Cimetidine:
  metabolism, 46
  side effects, 312
  2D6, 47
Cisapride, CYP 3A3/4, 51
Citalopram:
  AD, 17
    depression, 230–231
  behavioral complications, dementia, 442–443
  emotional lability, 180
  OCD, 375–376
  panic disorder, 375–376
  poststroke depression, 168–169
  vascular dementia, depression, 230–231
Clomipramine:
  antihypertensive effects,
  OCD, 373, 375
  panic disorder, 373
  PD depression, 206
  serotonergic effects, 56
Clonazepam:
  clearance, 35
  lithium, 264–265
Clonidine, poststroke mania, 176
Clorazepate, 358
Clozapine:
  lithium, 264
  PD depression, 212, 332–333
  side effects, 413, 416
Codeine, anticholinergic effects, 53–54
Cognex, AD, 16–17
Cognition:
  antidepressants, 82
  resperidone, 309
Cognitive impairment:
  bipolar disorder, 285
    valproate, 292
  depression, 226–228
  poststroke depression, 171–172
    treatment, 172
Congophil angiopathy, aging, 5
Cortical dementia, 229
Corticotropin-releasing hormone (CRH), 10, 16
CYP 1A2, 52

CYP 2C9, 47–50
CYP 2D6, 46–47
CYP 3A3/4, 51–52
Cytochrome P450, 45–46
SSRIs, 319

Delirium, 233, 328–330
Delusional depression (DD), 99–110
assessment, 103–104
diagnosis, 100–104
differential, 101–103
natural history, 107–109
pharmacotherapy, 104–107
TCA combination therapy, 104–06
phenomenological factors, 100–104
postrecovery pharmacotherapy, 107–109
temporal factors, 100–104
treatment guidelines, 109–110
Delusional disorder:
depression, 102
resperidone, 308
treatment, 302
Delusions, defined, 330–331
Dementia, 2–3, 6
behavioral complications
nonneuroleptic treatment, 433–448
treatment, 405–419, 436–448
cognitive enhancers, 381–396
depression, 66, 223–237
assessment, 223–225
differential diagnosis, 224
PD, 329
treatment, 234–236
Deprenyl:
AD, 234
PD depression, 208–209
Depression, 61–86
Alzheimer's dementia, 137–138
anxiety, 370–371
cancer, 187–195
biological markers, 189–190
diagnosis, 187–188
differential, 188–189
somatic symptoms, 188
treatment, 190–194
bupropion, 194
MAOIs, 194
mood stabilizers, 192–193
nefazodone, 194
SSRIs, 193–194
tricyclic antidepressants, 193
venlafaxine, 194
cardiac disease, 143–156
CRH, 10
dementia, 66
diagnosis, 63–66
differential, 65–66
functioning, 62
medical illness, 62–63
Parkinson's disease, 199–216, 371
prevalence, 61
prognosis, 128
recurrence rate, 128
reversible dementia, 225–228
subtypes, 67–70
treatment, 67, 70–81, 230–233
augmentation, 84–85
drug treatment predictors, 70
efficacy, 71–72
medical illness effect, 80–81, 245–254
resistance, 78–80
selection, 81–84
sensitivity, 73–78
stimulants, 245–254
Depression–dementia, 223–227
assessment, 223–225
all-inclusive approach, 225
diagnosis, 228–230
diagnostic approach, 225
differential diagnosis, 224
rating instruments, 224
prognosis, 225–228
reversible dementia, 225–228
treatment, 230–236
Depressive syndromes, 232
Desipramine:
bereavement depression, 119–120
cardiovascular effects, 56, 144, 154
clearance, 36
dementia, 236

[Desipramine]
depression, 68, 73–75, 78, 81, 231
metabolism, 46
PD depression, 232
postcancer depression, 193
Desmethyldiazepam, 358
Dexamethasone, interactions, 355
Dexamethasone suppression tests (DST), 168, 189–190
Dextroamphetamine, 245
pharmacokinetics, 247
poststroke depression, 170
side effects, 252
therapeutic use, 247–249
Dextromethorphan, serotonergic effects, 56
Diagnostic and Statistical Manual of Mental Disorders—Fourth Edition (DSM-IV)
delusions, 330–331
GAD, 369
major depression, 118
OCD, 369
panic disorder, 369
poststroke depression, 162
Diazepam:
distribution, 348
interactions, 355
lipophilicity, 352
protein binding, 34, 352
research design, 37
sedative, 358
Digoxin:
anticholinergic effects, 54
clearance, 53
side effects, 312
Diltiazem:
2D6, 47
antiarrhythmic effects, 55
CYP 3A3/4, 51
Diphenhydramine:
2D6, 47
anxiety, 375
Diphenyl-butylpeperidine, antiarrhythmic effects, 55
Dipyridamole, anticholinergic effects, 53–54
Donepezil, AD, 395–396
Donepezil hydrochloride, AD, 386
Dopamine:
psychosis, 331–333
serotonin, 203
Dopamine agonists:
PD, 332
serotonergic effects, 56
Dopamine receptors, PD, 332–333
Dopaminergic drugs:
mood effects, 203–204
side effects, 330
Dopaminergic neurons, 8
Dopamine system, PD, 201–202
Dopamine theory of depression, 253
Doxepin:
antihypertensive effects, 144
cardiovascular effects, 144, 147
depression, 81
postcancer depression, 193
Drug-induced parkinsonism (DIP), 313
Drug interactions, 43–57
pharmacokynamic, 53–57
antiarrhythmic, 55
anticholinergic, 53–54
anticoagulant, 54–55
antihypertensive, 55–56
serotonergic, 56
pharmacokinetic, 44–53
absorption, 44–45
distribution, 45
excretion, 52–53
metabolism, 45–52
Dysmentia, 3
Dysthmia, 69
Dystonia, 313–314

E2020, AD, 386
Early-onset pure Alzheimer's disease (AD), 10
Early-onset schizophrenia (EOS), treatment, 301–302
EG6761, AD, 389–390

Elderly, medication use, 43
Electroconvulsive therapy (ECT):
anxiety, 376–377
behavioral complications, dementia, 444
DD, 109
lithium, 265
PD, 335
PD depression, 214, 230, 232
poststroke depression, 171
Emotional lability, poststroke, 178–179
Emphysema, panic disorder, 368
ENA-713, AD, 386–387
Encainide, 148
Eptastigmine, AD, 387
Ergotamine compounds, AD, 234
Erythromycin:
CYP 3A3/4, 51
interactions, 355
Estazolam, 355–356, 362
elimination, 354
Estrogen, AD, 388–389
Extrapyramidal symptoms (EPS), 304, 312, 327, 412

Family education:
bipolar disorder, 267–268
lithium toxicity, 278
Fenfluramine, PD depression, 203
Fever, lithium toxicity, 276
Flecainide, 148
Fluent aphasia, 163
Flunitrazepam:
elimination, 354
metabolism, 353
Fluoxetine:
2D6, 47
behavioral complications, dementia, 443
bereavement depression, 120
cardiovascular effects, 150
CYP 3A3/4, 51
dementia, 236
depression, 68–69, 71, 81–82, 85
interactions, 355
metabolism, 46
OCDS, 375
P450, 319
panic disorder, 375
PD depression, 208–209
postcancer depression, 193
valproate, 294
Fluphenazine, 305–306
Flurazepam:
absorption, 352
elimination, 354
lipophilicity, 352
Fluvoxamine:
2D6, 47
behavioral complications, dementia, 443
CYP 3A3/4, 51
DD, 106
depression, 72–73
distribution, 45
interactions, 355
OCD, 375
panic disorder, 375
PD depression, 208
postcancer depression, 193
warfarin, 55
Food, absorption, 44–45
Free fraction (FF), 34–35, 304
Free radical scavengers, vascular dementia, 234
Frontal lobe dementia, 229
Frontal lobe syndromes, 224

Gabapentin, bipolar disorder, 288
Galanin, AD, 16
Galanthamine, AD, 387
Gangliosides:
AD, 13
depression, 234–235
Gender:
delirium, 233
drug distribution, 32
Generalized anxiety disorder (GAD), 367–368
DSM-IV, 369
prevalence, 372
treatment, 372–378

[Generalized anxiety disorder (GAD)]
pharmacokinetics, 372
Genral Life Functioning (GLF) scale, 134–135
Gerontokinetics, 303–304
Gingko Biloba, AD, 389–390
Global aphasia, 163
Glutamate, AD, 15, 18, 391
Granulovacuolar degeneration (GVD), 6
Grapefruit juice, CYP 3A3/4, 51
Grief, 118

Haloperidol, 235, 304–306, 332
behavioral complications, dementia, 412, 416, 447
dopaminergic blockade, 331
dose, 418
pharmacokinetics, 417
rifampin, 319
Hamilton Depression (Ham-D) Rating Scale:
anxiety, 103–04
depression–dementia, 225
ND vs. DD, 100–101
Heart rate variability, 152
Hemodialysis, lithium toxicity, 280
Hepatic biotransformation, psychotropic drugs, 28–29
Hepatic blood flow, 29
Hepatic extraction ratio (ER), 30
High-fiber supplements, absorption, 44
Homovanillic acid (HVA), 8, 15
Hormonal therapy, behavioral complications, dementia, 444
Hydrophilic drugs, Vd, 32
Hydroxynortiptyline, depression, 75
Hydroxyzine, anxiety, 375
Hypothalamic–pituitary–adrenal (HPA) axis, 10
AD, 18
cancer, 190
Hypothyroidism:
depression, 65
lithium, 192–193

Idazoxan, AD, 395
Idebenone, AD, 393–394
Idiopathic dementia, 10–17
Imipramine:
AD, depression, 230
antihypertensive effects, 56, 144
bipolar depression, 265
cardiovascular effects, 56, 144, 147
clearance, 35
cognitive impairment, 227
DD, 100
depression, 68–69, 72, 74, 81
panic disorder, 373
PD depression, 232
postcancer depression, 193
Impulsive aggression:
carbamazepine, 286, 290–291
characteristics, 286–287
valproate, efficac, 189–190
Informed consent, psychosis, 318
Insomnia:
anxiety, 370
nonpharmacological therapy, 348–349
Insomnophobia, 370
Interpersonal psychotherapy (IPT), depression, 130–138
Involution, 1–, 9
compensatory mechanisms, 2–3
Isosorbide, anticholinergic effects, 53–54

Jealous delusions, 31

Ketoconazole, CYP 3A3/4, 51

Lamotrigine:
bipolar disorder
valproate, 294
Language impairment, poststroke, 162–163
Lanoxin, anticholinergic effects, 54
Late-onset depression, 69–70, 119
maintenance therapy, 127–139
clinical trials, 129–138

problems, 128–129
Late-onset schizophrenia (LOS), treatment, 302
L-deprenyl, PD depression, 206–207
Left ventricular failure, anxiety, 368
Left ventricular function, TCAs, 146
Leukocytosis, lithium toxicity, 276
Levodopa, 202
absorption, 44
AD, 17
cognitive impairment, 227
DIP, 317, 331
PD depression, 203, 206–207
poststroke mania, 176
serotonergic effects, 56
Levodopa abstinence syndrome, 205
Levodopa psychosis, PD, 332–333
Lidocaine, CYP 3A3/4, 51
Light therapy:
behavioral complications, dementia, 444–445
PD depression, 214
Limbic striatum, 253
Lipofuscin pigments, 6
Lipophilic drugs, Vd, 32
Lithium:
behavioral complications, dementia, 444
bipolar disorder, 259–268
dose, 263, 266–267
efficacy, 262, 266
pretreatment assessment, 262–263
selection, 261
clearance, 28, 53–53
cognitive impairment, 227
DD, 107, 208
depression, 84–85
ECT, 265
hypothyroidism, 192–193
impulsive aggression, 287
mania, efficacy, 261–262
PD depression, 212
postcancer depression, 192
poststroke mania, 176
serotonergic effects, 56
Lithium toxicity, 273–281
delayed recovery, 281
manifestations, 274–277
cardiovascular, 276
gastrointestinal, 276
mania, 276
nephrotoxic, 276
prevention, 278–279
risk factors, 277–278
cardiovascular, 277
treatment, 279–280
Loratidine, 51
Lorazepam:
lithium, 264–265
protein binding, 352
Lormetazepam:
elimination, 354
metabolism, 353
Low-salt diets, lithium, 53
Loxapine, behavioral complications, 411, 416
L-tryptophan:
cognitive impairment, 227
PD depression, 202
serotonergic effects, 56
L-tyrosine, 202

Maintenance therapies trial in late-life recurrent major depression (MTLLD), 130– 138
ethics, 135–136
future, 137–138
patient compliance, 133–34
patient selection, 133
preliminary data, 131–132
quality of life, 134–135
Mania, lithium toxicity, 275
Maprotiline, PD depressino, 212
Meclobamide, 375
Medazepam:
elimination, 354
metabolism, 353
Melancholia, 68–69, 151
Memantine, AD, 17
Meperidine, serotonergic effects, 56
Meprobamate, 373

Metachlorophenylpiperazine (m-CCP), 51–52
Methamphetamine, 246
Methylphenidate, 246
  amphetamine vs., 249–250
  dementia, 235
  pharmacokinetics, 247
  poststroke depression, 170
  therapeutic use, 247–249
Metocopramide, 51
Metrigonate, AD, 387–388
Mianserin:
  postcancer depression, 191–192
  poststroke depression, 168
Midazolam:
  elimination, 354
  hepatic clearance, 29–30
  interactions, 355
  metabolism, 353
  SSRIs, 51
Milacemide, AD, 391
Milameline, AD, 382–383
Mirtazepine, depression, 83
Moclobemide, PD depression, 207
Monoamine oxidase inhibitors (MAOIs):
  antihypertensive effects, 55
  anxiety, 373
  depression, 68–69
  PD depression, 206–207
  postcancer depression, 194
  serotonergic effects, 56
  social phobia, 375
  SSRIs, 83
Monoamine oxidase (MAO), AD, 15–8
Morcizine, 148–49
Multi-infarct dementia, depression, 227
Muscarinic receptor agonists, 382–383
Muscarinic receptors, 7–8
Myelin lipids, AD, 13
Myocardial infarction, depression, 65

Nefazodone:
  antihypertensive effects, 55
  CYP 3A3/4, 51–52
  depression, 82–83, 376
  hepatic clearance, 29–30
  postcancer depression, 194
Nefazone, interactions, 355
Nerve growth factor (NGF), AD, 392–393
Neurofibrillary tangles (NFTs), 5–6, 11
Neuroleptic malignant syndrome (NMS), 315–316, 374, 416
Neuroleptic drugs, 305–310
  absorption, 303
  atypical antipsychotics, 306–310
  benzodiazepines vs., 414
  distribution, 303–304
  dose, 413–414
  EPS, 304
  impulsive aggression, 287
  lithium, 264
  liver metabolism, 304
  protein binding, 304
  renal function, 304
  side effects, 310–316, 412, 415–416
  2D6, 47
  typical antipsychotics, 305–306
    clincial trials, 305–306
    low- and high-potency agents, 305
Neuropeptidergic systems, AD, 16
Neuropeptide Y, AD, 16
Neuropil, AD, 12
Neuropsychiatric Inventory, 432
Neurotransmitters, 6–9
  AD, 13–15
Nicotine, AD, 383
Nicotinic receptors, 7–8
Nifedipine:
  anticholinergic effects, 54
  side effects, 312
  Nimodipine:
  AD, 394
  depression, 234–235
Nitrazepam, elimination, 354
NMDA blockers, AD, 17
NMDA receptor, AD, 15
Nocturnal asthma, panic disorder, 368
Nomifensine, PD depression, 202
Nonbenzodiazepine hypnotics, 360–362

Nondelusional depression (ND), 99–101
Nonfluent aphasia, 163
Nonsteroidal anti-inflammatory drugs (NSAIDs), lithium, 52–53
Nootropics, AD, 390
Noradrenergic neurons, 8
Norepinephrine:
  orthostatic hypotension, 145
  poststroke depression, 166
Nortriptyline (NT):
  bereavement depression, 120
  cardiovascular effects, 144–45, 147, 150–151
  clearance, 36
  cognitive impairment, 172
  dementia, 235
  depression, 68–69, 71–72, 74–75, 81, 85, 231–232
    maintenance, 129–138, 172
  emotional lability, 179–180
  PD depression, 232
  postcancer depression, 193
  poststroke depression, 166–167
  safety, 132
Nucleus accumbens, 253

Obsessive–compulsive disorder (OCD), 368
  DSM-IV, 369–370
  prevalence, 372
  treatment, 373, 375–376
Ondansetron, psychosis, 340
Orthostatic hypotension, 55, 311, 374, 412, 416
  TCAs, 144
Oxybutynin, anticholinergic effects, 53

Paired helical filaments (PHFs), 5
  AD, 11
Panic disorder, 368
  DSM-IV, 369
  emphysema, 368
  nocturnal asthma, 368
  prevalence, 372
  treatment, 373, 375–376
Paradoxical intention, 349
Parkinson's disease (PD)
  dementia, 329
  depression, 199–216, 227, 232, 371
    biological therapies, 214–215
    clinical reserach, 200–201
    diagnosis, 200–201
    drug treatment, 204–212, 308
    medication effects, 203–204
    neurochemistry, 201–203
  psychosis, treatment, 327–341
Parkinson's plus syndromes, 200–201
Paroxetine:
  Alzheimer's dementia, 138
  cardiovascular effects, 150–151
  CYP 3A3/4, 51
  depression, 82, 85, 376
  interactions, 46
  OCD, 373, 375
  panic disorder, 373, 375
  PD depression, 208–209
  postcancer depression, 193
  valproate, 294
Pathological Laughter and Crying Scale (PLACS), 179
Patient compliance:
  lithium toxicity, 277–278
  psychosis, 320
Patient education:
  anxiety, 377
  lithium toxicity, 278
  sleep, 349
Peritoneal dialysis, lithium toxicity, 280
Peroxitine, P450, 319
Perphenazine:
  metabolism, 46
  side effects, 46–47
Pharmacokinetics, defined, 303
Phenelzine, 106–107
  depression, 83
    maintenance, 129–130
  PD depression, 206–207
Phenmetrazine, 246
Phenobarbital, 373
  side effects, 317
Phenothiazine, side effects, 311
Phenytoin:

[Phenytoin]
CYP 2C9, 47
dementia, 235
side effects, 317
Phobic disorder, 372
Phototherapy:
behavioral complications, dementia, 444
PD depression, 214
Physostigmine, AD, 384, 388
Pimozide, antiarrhythmic effects, 55
Pindolol, behavioral complications, dementia, 444
Piperidine, antiarrhythmic effects, 55
Plasma drug monitoring, 45
Postpsychotic depression (PPD), treatment, 302–303
Poststroke anxiety disorder, 176–177
treatment, 177–178
Poststroke apathy, 178
Poststroke depression, DSM-IV, 162
Poststroke depression, 161–171
cognitive impairment, 171–72
treatment, 172
diagnosis, 162
duration, 164, 232
lesions, 164–166
mechanisms, 166
phemenology, 162–163
prevalence, 164
treatment, 166–169
adverse effects, 169–170
stimulants, 170–71
Poststroke mania, 172–180
lesions, 173–174
poststroke bipolar disorder, 174–175
treatment, 176
Poststroke pathological emotions, 178–180
Prednisolone:
anticholinergic effects, 54
side effects, 312
Problem focused psychotherapy, bereavement depression, 121–122
Propranolol, behavioral complications, dementia, 443–444
Pseudomentia, 66, 188–190
Psychobehvaioral metaphor, 435–436
Psychogeriatric Dependency Rating Scale (PGDRS), 431
Psychosis:
diagnosis, 317
dopamine, 331–333
drug interactions, 319
informed consent, 318
management plan, 317–318
medical comorbidity, 317
PD
clinical features, 238
treatment, 327–342
psychiatric history, 316
psychosocial assessment, 317
symptoms, 328
treatment, 301–320
dose, 319–320
maintenance, 320
patient compliance, 320
selection, 318
Psychotherapy:
bereavement depression, 121
bipolar disorder, 267
depression, 70, 79
Psychotic depression:
treatment, 99–110
history, 99–100
Psychotropic drugs:
disposition, 35–38
research design, 37–38
studies, 35–7
pharmacokinetics, 27–38
absorption, 33
clearance, 27–1
distribution, 32–33
elimination, 33
protein binding, 34–35
Quazepam, 356
elimination, 354
lipophilicity, 352
Quinalbarbital, 373

Quinidine:
antiarrhythmic effects, 55
CYP 3A3/4, 51
metabolism, 46
2D6, 47

Racemic phenylisopropylamine, 245
Rafampin, interactions, 355
Rantidine, anticholinergic effects, 53–54
Rating of Medication Influences (ROMI), scale, 320
Relaxation techniques, 349
Renal clearance, psychotropic drugs, 28
Reserpine, depression, 67
Reversible dementia:
depression, 225–228
differential diagnosis, 226
Rifampin, neuroleptic interactions, 319
Risperidone:
excretion, 52
lithium 264
psychosis, 308–309, 339
side effects, 413
Ritalin, 246
amphetamine vs., 249–250
dementia, 235
pharmacokinetics, 247
therapeutic use, 247–249
Ritaserin, DIP, 331

SB202026, AD, 383
Schizoaffective schizophrenia, DD, 101–102
Schizophrenia:
clozapine, 306
haloperidol, 417
resperidone, 309–310
Sedative antidepressants, 362
Sedative–hypnotics, 347–363
Selective serotonin reuptake inhibitors (SSRIs), 9
Benzodiazepines, 51
cardiovascular effects, 150–151
DD, 106
depression, 68, 77–79, 81–82, 85
hepatic clearance, 29
lithium, 53
MAOIs, 83
neuroleptic interactions, 319
OCD, 373, 375, 377
panic disorder, 373, 375, 377
PD depression, 207–210
postcancer depression, 193
side effects, 82, 377
2D6, 47
Selegiline, 9
AD, 393
behavioral complications, dementia, 441, 447
serotonergic effects, 56
Senile dementia of the Alzheimer type (SDAT), 10
Senile plaques (SPs), 5–6
AD, 10
Senium, defined, 1
Separation distress, 118
Serotonergic drugs:
behavioral complications, dementia, 441–443
interactions, 56
Serotonin:
dopamine, 203
poststroke depression, 166
psychosis, 333
Serotonin metabolism, 8
AD, 17
Serotonin syndrome, 56
Sertraline:
behavioral complications, dementia, 443
CYP 3A3/4, 51
depression, 68–69, 77
food, 44–45
interactions, 355
metabolism, 46
OCD, 375–376
panic disorder, 375–376
PD depression, 208–09
P450, 319
postcancer depression, 193
warfarin, 55
Sleep disorders:

[Sleep disorders]
pharmacotherapy, 349–363
guidelines, 350
Sleep hygiene education, 349
Sleep manipulation, PD depression, 214–215
Sleep restriction, 349
Smoking, neuroleptic metabolism, 319
Social phobias, beta-blockers, 375
Somatostatin, AD, 16
Spiroperidol, 253
Steady-state plasma concentration (Css), 30–31
Stimulants:
depression, 85, 245–254
side effects, 250–252
depression–dementia, 233
PD depression, 214
Stimulus control, 349
Stress, 9
Stroke, depression, 65
Subcortical dementia, 229
Substance P, AD, 16
Sudden cardiac death, depression, 151–152
Suicide, 61
Synapse, 11
Synaptic degeneration, AD, 12
Synaptic loss, AD, 12
Synaptic vesicles, 11

Tachycardia, 312
Tacrine, AD, 384–385, 395–396
Tardive dyskinesia, 105, 208, 267, 314–315, 374
τ 64/65, 6
Temazepam, 357
elimination, 357
metabolism, 353
Terfenadine, CYP 3A3/4, 51
Tetra-aminoacridine, AD, 234
Tetrahydroaminoacridine (Cognex), AD, 16τ17
Theophylline:
anticholinergic effects, 53–54
side effects, 312
Thioridazine:
behavioral complications, 411–412, 414
psychosis, 305–306
side effects, 312, 416
Thiothixene, 305
behavioral complications, 411
Thorazine, behavioral complications, 412
Ticlopidine, depression, 234
Tocopherol, vascular dementia, 234
Tolbutamide, CYP 2C9, 47
Tranylcypromine:
depression, 68
PD depression, 206–207
Trazodone:
antihypertensive effects, 55
behavioral complications, dementia, 441–442, 447
CYP 3A3/4, 51–52
dementia, 235–236
depression, 71, 83, 231
hepatic clearance, 29
poststroke depression, 168
Tremor, bipolar disorder, valproate, 293
Triazolam, 357–358
absorption, 352
CYP 3A3/4, 51
hepatic clearance, 29–30
interactions, 355
metabolism, 353
SSRIs, 51
Tricyclic antidepressants (TCAs):
bipolar disorder, 265
cardiovascular effects, 55, 144–149, 154–55
clearance, 35
DD, 104–06
depression, 68–69, 78–82, 85
depression–dementia, 233
hepatic clearance, 29
PD Depression, 205–206
postcancer depression, 193
poststroke anxiety disorders, 177–178

Trifluoperazine, psychosis, 305
Trihexyphenidyl:
PD depression, 204
side effects, 311
Trimipramine, PD depression, 206
Trizolam, elimination, 354
2D6, 36–37

Unipolar depression, 68

Valium, poststroke depression, 167
Valproate:
behavioral complications, dementia, 439–440, 447
bipolar disorder, 285
cognitive impairment, 292
drug interactions, 293–294
efficacy, 287–288
gastrointestinal effects, 293
guidelines, 291–294
hair loss, 292
hematological effects, 292–293
hepatic function, 293
tremor, 293
impulsive aggression, 189–190, 286–287
poststroke mania, 176
Vascular dementia, 17–18
depression, citalopram, 230–231
free radical scavengers, 234
tocopherol, 234
Vasopressin, AD, 16
Venlafaxine:
antihypertensive effects, 55
clearance, 36
CYP 3A3/4, 51
depression, 68–69, 71, 81, 83, 376
distribution, 45
hepatic clearance 29
postcancer depression, 194
Ventricular arrhythmias, TCAs, 147
Ventricular fibrillation, depression, 152, 154
Ventricular irritability, 153–154
Ventricular premature depolarizations (VPDs), 148
Verapamil:
CYP 3A3/4, 51
poststroke mania, 176
Vigabatrin, bipolar disorder, 288
Visual hallucinations, 330
Vitamin E, AD, 393
Volume of distribution (Vd), 32–33

Warfarin:
absorption, 44
anticholinergic effects, 53–54
CYP 2C9, 47
SSRIs, 55
Wernicke's aphasia, 163
White matter lesions (WMLs), AD, 6

Xanomeline, 383

Zolpidem, 360–362
behavioral complications, dementia, 445
Zopiclone, 361–362

About the Editor

J. CRAIG NELSON is a Professor of Psychiatry at Yale University School of Medicine, and Director of Psychiatric Inpatient Services and Geriatric Psychiatry Programs at Yale-New Haven Hospital, New Haven, Connecticut. Dr. Nelson's research interests focus on descriptions of severe forms of depression, including melancholic and psychotic depression as well as depression in the elderly, and the psychopharmacological treatment of these disorders. A member of several professional organizations, Dr. Nelson is a founding member and on the Board of Directors of the American Society of Clinical Psychopharmacology. He received the A.B. degree (1964) from Stanford University, Stanford, California, and the M.D. degree (1968) from the University of Wisconsin—Madison. Dr. Nelson completed his internship at Herrick Memorial Hospital, Berkeley, California, and his psychiatric residency training at Yale University, where he has been a member of the psychiatry faculty since 1974.